Sexuality, Marriage, and Family

Sexuality, Marriage, and Family

READINGS IN THE CATHOLIC TRADITION

edited by
Paulinus Ikechukwu Odozor, C.S.Sp.

UNIVERSITY OF NOTRE DAME PRESS
Notre Dame, Indiana

Copyright © 2001 by
University of Notre Dame
Notre Dame, Indiana 46556
http://www.undpress.nd.edu
All Rights Reserved

Manufactured in the United States of America

Library of Congress Cataloging-in-Publication Data
　Sexuality, marriage, and family : readings in the Catholic tradition/ edited by Paulinus Ikechukwu Odozor.
　　p. cm.
Includes bibliographical references.
　ISBN 0-268-01773-5 (pbk. : alk. paper)
　1. Sex—Religious aspects—Catholic Church. 2. Marriage—Religious aspects—Catholic Church. 3. Family—Religious aspects—Catholic Church. 4. Catholic Church—Doctrines.
I. Odozor, Paulinus Ikechukwu.
　BX1795.S48 S53 2001
　241'.63'08822—dc21　　　　　　　　　　　　　2001001941

∞ *This book was printed on acid-free paper.*

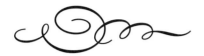

This book is dedicated to my parents,

Cordelia O. Odozor (1936–1979) and Theophilus N. Odozor,

in eternal gratitude for a nearly perfect family.

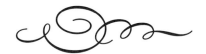

Contents

Acknowledgments	xi
List of Abbreviations	xiii
Introduction	xvii

PART 1 HUMAN SEXUALITY

1	The Witness of the New Testament *Eugene A. LaVerdiere, S.S.S.*	3
2	Sexual Salvation: Grace and the Resurrection of the Body *James B. Nelson*	14
3	Christianity and Sexuality: An Ambiguous History *Eric Fuchs*	22
4	Sexuality—God's Gift: A Pastoral Letter *Francis J. Mugavero*	76

PART 2 SCRIPTURE AND MARRIAGE

5	The New Testament Doctrine on Marriage *A. L. Descamps*	85
6	The New Testament Moral Teaching on Marriage *Edward Schillebeeckx*	131

Part 3 Marriage and Family in Christian History

7   Augustine on the Nature of Marriage 169
    Theodore Mackin

8   Sex, Marriage, and Family in Christian Tradition 183
    Lisa Sowle Cahill

9   The Family in Early Christianity: "Family Values" Revisited 216
    Carolyn Osiek, R.S.C.J.

10 The Theory and Practice of Marriage on the Eve of the Reformation 234
    H. J. Selderhuis

11 From Secular to Ecclesiastical Marriage 251
    Joseph Martos

Part 4 Marriage and Family in the Teaching of the Church

12 *Gaudium et Spes:* Promoting the Dignity of Marriage and the Family 263
    Vatican II

13 *Familiaris Consortio* (On the Family) 269
    Pope John Paul II

Part 5 Marriage in Current Theology

14 Marriage 313
    Francis Schüssler Fiorenza

15 The Sacramental Dignity of Marriage 340
    Walter Kasper

16 Marriage as a Sacrament 351
    Karl Rahner, S.J.

Part 6 Divorce and Remarriage

17 The Indissolubility of Completed Marriage: Theological, Historical, and Pastoral Reflections 369
    E. Hamel, S.J.

18 Divorce, Remarriage, and the Sacraments 385
    Richard A. McCormick, S.J.

| 19 | Pastoral Care of the Divorced and Remarried
Kenneth R. Himes, O.F.M., and James A. Coriden | 400 |

PART 7   CONTRACEPTION

20	Contraception: The Doctrine and the Context *John T. Noonan, Jr.*	423
21	*Humanae Vitae* (On the Regulation of Birth) *Pope Paul VI*	464
22	*Humanae Vitae* 25 Years Later *Richard A. McCormick, S.J.*	478
23	Some Theological Considerations on *Humanae Vitae* *Janet E. Smith*	486

Acknowledgment of Sources   509

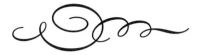

Acknowledgments

I sincerely thank Barbara J. Hanrahan, the Director of the University of Notre Dame Press, Jeffrey Gainey, the Associate Director at the Press, Wendy McMillen, Ann Bromley, Rebecca DeBoer, Anthony Barber, and all other staff of the University of Notre Dame Press who facilitated the production of this book. Many thanks to Professor Joseph Wawrykow of the Department of Theology, University of Notre Dame, and Professor Ron Mercier, S.J., Dean and Professor of Theology at Regis College in the University of Toronto, for valuable suggestions concerning the content of the book. I also thank Professor John Cavadini, chair of the Department of Theology, University of Notre Dame, Professor Fabian Udoh, Program of Liberal Studies, University of Notre Dame, and Father Daryl Rybicki, Linda Shaw, and Mrs. Dolores Ciesielski of St. Adalbert Church, South Bend, Indiana.

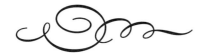

List of Abbreviations
Journals, Series, and Works

AAS	*Acta apostolicae sedis*
ACW	Ancient Christian Writers
ANF	The Ante-Nicene Fathers
ANRW	*Aufstieg und Niedergang der römischen Welt*
Antwort	Martin Bucer, *Antwort uff die zwen casus . . .* , Archive of the St. Thomas Chapter, Strasbourg, *Var. Eccl.* 2, no. 167, 64a–171
Bbl	*Biblica*
BDS	*Martin Bucer's Deutsche Schriften,* ed. R. Stuperich (Gütersloh: Mohn, 1960–)
BHT	Beiträge zur historischen Theologie
BJ	*Bible de Jérusalem*, 43 vols. (Paris, 1948–)
BJS	Brown Judaic Studies
BL	*Bibel und Leben*
BR	*Biblical Research*
BTB	*Biblical Theology Bulletin*
CBQ	*Catholic Biblical Quarterly*
CC	*Casti Connubii*, December 31, 1930
CCL	*Corpus Christianorum*
CII	*Corpus inscriptionum iudaicarum*
CSEL	*Corpus scriptorum ecclesiasticorum latinorum*
DB	H. Denzinger, *Enchiridion Symbolorum, Definitionum, et Declarationum de Rebus Fidei et Morum,* ed. C. Bannwart, S.J. (1908–13) et al. (1913–60)
DBS	*Dictionnaire de la Bible, Supplément,* ed. L. Pirot et al. (Paris, 1928–)
Dig.	*Digesta Justiniani*
DRC	Martin Bucer, *De Regno Christi Libro Duo,* ed. François Wendel (Paris: PUF, 1955)

DS	H. Denzinger, *Enchiridion Symbolorum*, ed. A. Schönmetzer, S.J., vol. 32 (Freiburg, 1963)
DTC	*Dictionnaire de théologie catholique*, ed. A. Vacant et al. (Paris, 1903–50)
EE (Selderhuis)	Martin Bucer, *Von der Ehe und Ehescheidung*, Archive of the St. Thomas Chapter, Strasbourg, *Var. Eccl.* 2, no. 167, 1a–99a
EE (Hamel)	F. Heinrich and V. Eid, eds., *Ehe und Ehescheidung* (Munich, 1972)
EKKNT	Evangelisch-katholischer Kommentar zum Neuen Testament
EKL	*Evangelisches Kirchenlexikon*
Eph. (1551)	Martin Bucer, *Praelectiones doctissimae in Epistolam D. pauli ad Ephesios*, Basel, 1562 (Bibl., no. 112)
Ev.	Martin Bucer, *Enarrationes perpetua in sacra in quatuor Evangelia*, Strasbourg, 1530 (Bibl., no. 17)
FC	Fathers of the Church
IKZ	*Internationale Katholische Zeitschrift* (1972)
ITC	International Theological Commission
ITQ	*Irish Theological Quarterly*
JB	*Jerusalem Bible*
JBL	*Journal of Biblical Literature*
JQR	*Jewish Quarterly Review*
JTS	*Journal of Theological Studies*
LG	*Lumen Gentium*, Vatican II
LThk	*Lexicon für Theologie und Kirche*
LV	*Lumière et Vie* (Bruges, Belgium, 1951–)
LXX	Septuagint
MGH	*Monumenta Germaniae Historica* (Berlin, 1826–)
MT	Masoretic Text
NKS	*Nederlandse Katholiecke Stemmen*
NovT	*Novum Testamentum*
N-PNF	Nicene and Post-Nicene Fathers
NTS	*New Testament Studies*
OTP	*The Old Testament Pseudepigrapha*, ed. J. H. Charlesworth
PG	*Patrologia graeca*, ed. J. P. Migne, 161 vols. (Paris, 1857–1866)
PL	*Patrologia latina*, ed. J. P. Migne, 217 vols. (Paris, 1878–1890)
RB	*Revue biblique*
RHPR	*Revue d'histoire et de philosophie religieuses*
RSR	*Recherches de Science religieuse*
RTL	*Revue théologique de Louvain*
RTP	*Revue de théologie et de philosophie*
SBLMS	SBL Monograph Series
SBLSBS	SBL Sources for Biblical Study
SBLSP	SBL Seminar Papers

SBLTT	SBL Text and Translations
SC (Fuchs)	Sources chrétiennes
SC (Schillebeeckx)	*Studia Catholica*
SE	*Sciences ecclésiastiques*
SJT	*Scottish Journal of Theology*
SNTSMS	Society for New Testament Studies Monograph Series
SOT	Society for Old Testament Studies
SR	*Studies in Religion/Sciences religieuses*
TE	*Theologie der Ehe*, ed. H. Greven (Augsburg, 1972)
THKNT	Theologischer Handkommentar zum Neuen Testament
TS	*Theological Studies*
TT	*Tijdschrift voor Theologie*
TV	*Theologia Viatorum*
TWNT	*Theologisches Wörterbuch zum Neuen Testament*, ed. G. Kittel and G. Friedrich
TZ	*Theologische Zeitschrift*
VC	*Verbum Caro*
VD	*Verbum Domini*
WA	Martin Luther, *Kritische Gesamtausgabe* ("Weimar" edition)
WBC	World Biblical Commentary
WUNT	Wissenschaftliche Untersuchungen zum Neuen Testament
ZNW	*Zeitschrift für neutestamentliche Wissenschaft*
ZST	*Zeitschrift für systematische Theologie*

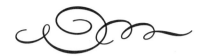

Introduction

It is a bit of an understatement to posit that human sexuality, marriage, and family have always been important issues in the Christian tradition. Peter Nichols in his book *The Pope's Divisions: The Roman Catholic Church Today* has a chapter entitled "The Failure With Sex," in which he points out the enduring preoccupation of the Christian tradition with human sexuality in general. "The question of women, the question of divorce, even the question of the priesthood, contains a powerful element of sex, and if there is one issue which it is fair to say that Christianity as a whole, and Catholicism in particular, has failed to handle successfully, it is sex."[1] If it is true, as Nichols says, that Christianity has not been quite as successful in handling the question of human sexuality as it has been in handling other issues, this failure cannot be attributed to lack of effort or clarity regarding the position of the Christian tradition on sex and sexuality. On the contrary, the tradition has had quite a bit to say on these matters, beginning from Jesus Christ himself through the early Church Fathers to our day. The present anthology bears adequate testimony to that. However, anyone who is familiar with the subject of sexuality and marriage in Christian history and tradition knows as well how complex the discussion on these issues tends to be.

The present collection seeks to highlight some of the salient elements in this rich and complex Christian tradition on sex, marriage, and family by examining the sources of this tradition in scripture, the work of ancient Christian writers, the official teachings of the Roman Catholic Church, and contemporary theological discourse. In order to achieve this purpose, we have assembled a wide array of writers from several generations as guides through the maze of the Christian tradition and in particular the Catholic tradition. These include Eugene A. LaVerdiere, James B. Nelson, Eric Fuchs, Bishop Francis Mugavero, A. L. Descamps, Edward Schillebeeckx, Theodore Mackin, Lisa Sowle Cahill, Carolyn Osiek, H. J. Selderhuis, Joseph Martos, Pope Paul VI, Pope John Paul II, Francis Schüssler Fiorenza, Walter Kasper, Karl Rahner, Eduourd Hamel, Richard A. McCormick, Kenneth R. Himes, James A. Coriden, John R. T. Noonan, and Janet E. Smith.

The choice of the articles in this anthology is determined by a number of considerations. Some articles provide a thorough historical perspective on aspects of the subject matter of this book. Others have doctrinal value as statements of the teaching magisterium of the Catholic Church. Yet others provide solid theological elaboration on some particular aspects of sexuality, marriage, and family. The choice of essays reflects a strenuous effort to avoid extremism in any form. My intention is not to provoke unnecessary debate but to present some of the finest materials available on the subjects herein treated. I am aware that there are differences of opinion on some of the issues under consideration. Where necessary, I have presented well-written materials representing the various shades of opinion on the topic. In each of these situations, I have prefaced the section with an authoritative source representing the official views of the Roman Catholic Church on the matter.

Sexuality, Marriage, and Family: Readings in the Catholic Tradition has been put together in order to make some very rich resources on Christian marriage easily available both to the professional in the field and the interested non-professional. This book is intended for use as a classroom text in colleges and universities. It is also meant for marriage instruction classes in parishes and for use by anyone who cares about the history, theology, canonical provisions, magisterial teaching, and other issues pertaining to sexuality, marriage, and family in the Catholic tradition.

Note

1. Peter Nichols, *The Pope's Divisions: The Roman Catholic Church Today* (London: Faber and Faber, 1981), 239.

Human Sexuality

1

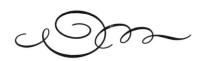

The Witness of the New Testament

Eugene A. LaVerdiere, S.S.S.

Anthony Kosnik and his co-authors [in a 1977 study entitled *Human Sexuality: New Directions of American Catholic Thought*] have raised a much needed warning against the simplistic and uncritical application of New Testament passages on sexual morality to modern situations. The basis for their *cautio* is that all such New Testament statements were occasional and historically conditioned by the various ancient contexts to which they responded. This applies to the teaching of Jesus as well as to that of St. Paul.[1]

It should be noted that the authors' contention concerning sexual ethics is not specific to this area but equally applicable to every other aspect of life, doctrinal and ethical, which is treated in the New Testament. They have thus affirmed a general principle of contemporary New Testament scholarship, which recognizes that the Scriptures must be studied historically and critically for their modern-day relevance to emerge. Only then does it become possible to discern the implications of New Testament proclamation, prophecy, and teaching for life in a vastly altered situation of Church and world.

Recourse to the New Testament in developing a contemporary sexual ethics thus includes two major investigative stages. By contemporary convention, the first, which deals with the text in its ancient context, is broadly termed exegesis. The second stage, which confronts the ancient text with our modern situation and translates it into contemporary theology, is called hermeneutics. Without the former, hermeneutics is pursued independently of any controls or limits provided by the text. Without the latter, exegesis may prove interesting to the historian of Christian origins, but the endeavor prescinds from the most important issue of the place of Scripture in the ongoing life of the Church.

In the short section of their book which formally addresses the sexual ethics of the New Testament, the authors were quite understandably unable to go much beyond their *cautio* and the affirmation of a few general principles. Their observations, however, were limited almost exclusively to the general area of exegesis. Because of this, one might be left with the impression that the New Testament is all but irrelevant in matters of sexual morality. Their effort to liberate contemporary sexual ethics from the limits imposed by past conditions which no longer obtain would thus result in an obvious injustice to the living faith of the Church which continues to draw life and inspiration from the New Testament writings.

This chapter takes up the invitation of the authors to continue and expand the discussion they have initiated. In the first section I shall explore the New Testament teaching on sexuality exegetically and historically. The second section is devoted to hermeneutics. Exploring the relationship between the Church today and the first stages of its emergence in earliest times, I shall attempt to draw out the meaning of New Testament teaching on sexual ethics for the modern situation.

I. Sexual Ethics in the New Testament: Exegesis

Within the rather ample and varied body of New Testament writings, explicit references to sexual attitudes and behavior are quite meager. In this, the New Testament stands in sharp contrast with the modern world, where sexual mores and ethics constitute a major concern. It may be that the New Testament challenges and calls into question our preoccupation with sexual ethics and the central position it has taken in a wide range of human and Christian consciousness. The relative silence of the New Testament would thus be extremely significant.

In order to explore that significance and to define its challenge, however, we cannot remain at the level of general observations. We must first differentiate the various stages in the social development of the early Church and examine the special context of the community being addressed. As we shall see, greater or lesser attention to sexual mores was closely related to the Church's evolving identity, a process in which some levels of development exhibited far greater concern with sexual ethics than others. Second, one must consider the author's stance vis-à-vis the community along with his general theological perspective and presuppositions. Sexual issues will thus be situated in the broader context of Christian life and in relation to a work's special purpose and concerns.

In this section, I shall accordingly attempt to situate sexual ethics first in the earliest stage of ecclesial development when the Church was primarily a movement characterized by a strong apostolic and evangelical outward thrust. I shall then examine those texts which pertain to the early Christian communities or churches which resulted from this creative proclamation of the gospel. At this point, our primary focus will be on the Pauline letters. Finally, I shall explore the sexual ethics of the gospel narratives, literary syntheses associated with long-established churches and with the emergence of a universal Church. Since the teaching of Jesus was integrated, interpreted, and transmitted within these post-Easter literary documents, it will be examined as part of these gospel syntheses.

I recognize that the limits of this study make a comprehensive study impossible. I have consequently selected a number of important texts and shall emphasize methodology in my analysis. I thus hope to facilitate further investigation. Like the authors of *Human Sexuality*,[2] I invite the scholarly and pastoral community to join in an ongoing exploration and discussion.

First Evangelization and the Early Churches

The earliest Christian proclamation of the gospel did not focus on the heritage of Jesus' teaching but on the absolutely fundamental event of Jesus' death-resurrection and his expected return in glory. Following the shock of Jesus' death, the apostolic community had been quickened by its experience of the risen Lord. In light of these events, previous experiences in the company of the historical Jesus and many other concerns of daily living receded temporarily into the background. Accordingly, the apostolic proclamation addressed only the most fundamental issues of human life and death.

Jesus' death-resurrection had revealed the ultimate value of life and the meaningfulness of death as life-giving. By raising Jesus from the dead, God had shown that those who gave of themselves unto death found not death but new life. Infused by the Christ-experience of God's glory, that is by the appearances of the risen Jesus, the earliest proclamation thus consisted in a communication of radical hope. In this context, which can be recovered from the early creeds, hymns, and liturgical texts cited by Paul (e.g., 1 Cor. 15:3b–5; Rom. 1:3–4; Phil. 2:6–11; 1 Cor. 11:23–25), particular ethical questions had little or no place.

First evangelization, however, was not without ethical implications. As interpreted by Luke in the various discourses of Acts, it constituted a general invitation to conversion and life's reorientation. This bond between the gospel's proclamation and a Christian's ethical stance can also be discerned in Paul's writing when he exhorts his readers to model their behavior on the attitude attributed to Christ in the Philippians' hymn (Phil. 2:3–5) or when he argues for faith attitudes and behavior consistent with the Christian credal and liturgical formulas (1 Cor. 15:12–58; 11:26–34). From a very early time, therefore, if not from the beginning, Christians were aware that the fundamental gospel proclamation had ethical implications. Only gradually, however, would the latter unfold in relation to a variety of contextual challenges. We can thus understand why the most basic evangelization included no reference to sexual issues; just as other specific issues, they were displaced by primordial concerns. Consequently, silence cannot be interpreted as implying that these were insignificant or irrelevant.

The above considerations refer to the absolute beginnings of the Church in Jerusalem as well as to its relative beginnings in the broadening geographical sphere of the Mediterranean world, as the first apostolic figures gradually reached out to people who had not yet heard the good news of salvation and new life in Christ.

Those who first heard and accepted the gospel in any given social context were bonded into communities of Christian solidarity. Together the Christians gradually worked out the implications of gospel living. Relatively little primary data is available to demonstrate this process in the earliest days. However, thanks to Paul's first letter to the Christians of Thessalonica (*circa* A.D. 51) we do have some material on developments in that community, including an important passage which refers to sexual ethics (4:1–8).[3]

In a brief introduction (4:1–2), Paul first exhorts the Christians to develop along the lines he had already presented and personally demonstrated during his brief period of evangelization at Thessalonica. The unit is thus important not only as the earliest Pauline literary statement on the subject of sexuality, but as an indication of the role played by sexual ethics in the apostolic teaching which spelled out the implications of the gospel's first proclamation. It may be that the earliest preaching at Jerusalem had not moved so quickly to particular issues. The Thessalonian mission, however, benefited from Christianity's twenty-year experience of evangelization.

Paul then summarizes his teaching as follows. Since God had given the Thessalonians the Holy Spirit, they were called to holy living (vv. 7–8), and sexual immorality was not consistent with the gift and call they had received (vv. 3–8). This gift, be it recalled, had come through Paul's word or gospel proclamation, a word which they had received, not as the word of men, but as it truly is, the word of God at work within the believers (2:13). The gospel thus constituted an internalized life principle[4] which called for certain attitudes and behavior in sexual matters. This new life or Christian nature was consequently the wellspring of right living as well as the point of departure for ethical reflection.

For sexual immorality, Paul uses the term *porneia*, a generic term whose specific meaning must be determined from the context. In vv. 4–6, he discusses two fairly specific but complex issues. First, each one must guard his body, taking a wife for himself, that is have sexual relations with his own wife, and he must do so in holiness and honor (v. 4), not in the passion and lust of the gentiles who do not know God (v. 5). Second, he must not transgress and wrong his brother in this matter (v. 6).

From the point of view of the Christians' relationship to God, sexual ethics is thus grounded in the will of God who called them to holiness (v. 3) as well as in the gospel gift of the Holy Spirit (v. 8) through which they know God (v. 5). From the point of view of the Christians' relationship to one another, sexual ethics is grounded in their specifically Christian nature, a nature which calls for honor and respect for one's marital partner, for oneself, and for one's brother and which therefore precludes adultery as a breach of Christian community solidarity. The passage thus approaches sexuality with a strong appreciation for human and Christian dignity and for interpersonal relationships within the Christian community.

While the passage is short, it does reveal that sexual ethical considerations were extremely important as a consequence of the gospel, even in a social context strongly focused on eschatological realities and the Lord's parousia (4:13–5:11). The remarkable thing is not so much that the passage is short, but that it is present at all in a brief exuberant letter which takes up none but the most pressing issues.

In the second letter to the Christians of Thessalonica (*circa* A.D. 52), which develops some of the issues taken for granted or inadequately treated in the first, Paul does not allude to sexual issues. In the letter to the Galatians (*circa* A.D. 54), however, where he argues strongly for the freedom which characterizes Christians and for the kind of behavior which springs from that freedom, he includes a number of sexual aberrations in a partial list of evils which proceed from the flesh (Gal. 5:19–21).[5] The terms which Paul uses in the list are rather general, evoking a whole range of overlapping attitudes and behavior. Concrete application to specific cases is then left open to the Christian sensitivity of the addressees.

The fruits of the internalized Spirit are listed in 5:22–23. They had already been summarized in 5:13–14, however, as Christian love of neighbor, in which each one is at the service of the others. The deeds of the flesh (5:19–21), on the other hand, had been summarized in 5:15, where Paul turned to graphic metaphors in warning against biting and devouring one another unto mutual destruction. Along with other evils, immorality (*porneia*), impurity (*akatharsia*), licentiousness (*aselgeia*), and carousing (*komoi*) are consequently to be avoided because they are inconsistent with the nature of the Christian and destructive of the new Christian self and of the community. As in 1 Thess. 4:1–8, Christian dignity and community solidarity are thus given as the norm of sexual attitudes and behavior.

Ultimately, human sexuality is governed by the biblically founded Christian law of love (5:13–14). Everything which stands contrary to genuine love of neighbor and of oneself must be considered aberrant. When sexual behavior is a concrete expression of this love it is properly Christian and one of the fruits of the Spirit. It is thus integrated in a life characterized by love, joy, peace, kindness, goodness, faithfulness, gentleness, and self-control (5:22). This does not occur, however, unless the unredeemed flesh has been crucified with Christ (5:24). In sexual matters, as in other areas of life, Paul does not allow us to escape the challenge of the crucifixion.

The first letter to the Corinthians 5–7 is the longest Pauline treatment of sexuality. Called forth by a deeply troubled situation, the letter (*circa* A.D. 56–57) confronts a general community context of factional and destructive divisiveness and lack of solidarity (1:10–17). In 5:1–13, a particular case leads Paul to deal with the question of excluding immoral persons from the community. To appreciate the unit's significance, we must carefully distinguish the Church's development at Corinth from its first evangelization. The party in question, who was having sexual relations with his father's wife, that is his stepmother (5:1–2), had already responded to Paul's gospel proclamation and was now a member of the Christian community.

As we indicated earlier, the initial proclamation had been issued to all without distinction, calling them to conversion and new life. Those who accepted the gospel, however, were distinguished from those who did not, and their membership in the community of salvation placed certain demands on them and created legitimate expectations in their regard on the part of others. When these were unfulfilled, they returned to their pre-evangelical condition and once again stood in need of evangelization. Recognizing that they no longer served the community in its internal life and missionary efforts, they were to be excluded from the community and treated as non-members. Toleration of their presence could only weaken the community and its efforts for Christ. Exclusion from the community, be it noted, was in view of the destruction or crucifixion of the flesh that once again such persons might be gifted with the Spirit and saved on the day of the Lord (5:5).

Paul's teaching is thus to be approached from the standpoint of a community which had but recently been evangelized and which retained a strong sense of its evangelical mission to the non-Christian world all about it. It did not stem from a Church with a strong sense of its universality, which was politically and socially established, and whose primary concern lay in its internal development. Had the latter been the case, Paul's teaching might have been quite different.

Matters at Corinth had fallen to such a state that Christians were even dragging one another into civil courts (6:1–8). This situation, however, was but one of many symptoms of disintegration which Paul discusses in a warning against self-deception (6:9–20).

Along with idolaters, thieves, misers, drunkards, slanderers, and robbers, Paul lists fornicators, adulterers, and sensually soft men who lie with males (6:9–10). The behavior of all such men, summarized in the term unholy (cf. 1 Thess. 4:3, 7), is deemed unworthy of those who have been sanctified in baptism and justified in the name of the Lord Jesus Christ and in the Spirit of our God (6:11).

Unlike Gal. 5:19–21, the Corinthians list does not refer to the vices themselves, but to categories of people who are characterized by the vices. Nevertheless, it clearly approaches the latter from the point of view of their relationships and behavior. Deceiving themselves, some Corinthian Christians have committed themselves to an evil course of life, and consequently they will not inherit the kingdom of God (cf. Gal. 5:21).

The modern distinction between a person's basic sexual orientation and sexual behavior itself does not enter into this picture. Paul's warning, therefore, cannot be interpreted as a condemnation of homosexuals as such, for example. In the case of all behavior, sexual or other, the question remains one of living according to one's fundamental Christian nature, which calls not for self-service, but for the service of the community. Paul does not consider homosexual behavior to be consistent with the nature of the Christian who has been freed by the gospel and whose life must unfold for the development of the community.

In 6:12–20, Paul turns to a particular case of immorality, that of sexual intercourse with a prostitute. General principles had sufficed to establish the need for moral living and for seeking what is right and good. A particular case, however, calls for further reflection and specification of these principles. Paul therefore points out that some forms of living in freedom are actually self-enslaving (v. 12). In this he responds to the Corinthians' self-deception which saw a normal link between the body and sexual expression, just as the stomach and food are made for one another (v. 13a). In a sense this was an argument from nature, not unlike Paul's own approach to such questions. The problem with it lay in the perception and appreciation of the Christian nature and in particular of the Christian body which is related to the Lord and which will join him in the resurrection (vv. 13b–14). Members of Christ, the Christians are members of one another and this excludes relationships which are incompatible with the members' Christian identity and solidarity.

Paul's point becomes extremely clear if the prostitution in question is sacred prostitution. The latter would then establish a relationship to a form of worship and religious allegiance other than Christian and would therefore work for the disintegration of the body of the Lord. Paul's mention of idolaters between fornicators and adulterers in 6:9 supports this interpretation, as also the manner he has linked relations with a prostitute (vv. 9–20) to recourse to the law courts of unbelievers (6:1–8), a link which remains otherwise enigmatic. The enslavement mentioned in v. 12 thus consists in a return to one's pre-Christian state from which the Christian had been liberated (cf. Gal. 5:13), that is cleansed, made holy, and justified (v. 11).

We must not conclude, however, that Paul tolerated other forms of prostitution. The list in 6:9–10 includes many categories which are enslaving of self and destructive of community, quite apart from incompatible relationships with the non-Christian political, juridical, and religious world of Corinth. In Pauline terms, the question thus remains whether relations with any prostitute can be considered consistent with the development unto resurrection (6:14) of one who has been redeemed at a price in view of God's glory (6:20) and whose body is sanctified by the Holy Spirit (6:19).

In chapter 7, Paul's entire teaching concerning marriage and various states of life is conditioned by the general rule that each one should remain in the state of life, married or other, in which he was at the time of the Lord's call (vv. 17, 20, 24). In v. 26 this general rule is reiterated in a statement which also discloses its basis: the Christians were living in a time of stress, a time which would be short (v. 29) and soon climax in the passing away of the world as we know it (v. 31). Given this eschatological view, it is thus better for Christians not to assume a new state of life and its responsibilities. The concerns and trials involved in changing their state would divide their attention and distract them from the affairs of the Lord (vv. 32–35). As Paul perceived it, the time in which they were living also called for detachment from all concerns, attitudes, and activities which were intrinsically associated with this passing world (vv. 29–31). In all these matters, Paul recognizes that the ideals he has presented are contingent on the experiential situation of his addressees and that their personal needs might call for another course of action (vv. 2, 9, 28, 36, 39). Although all have been gifted by God, all have not been gifted in the same way (v. 7). In all the cases discussed, save the question of divorce (vv. 10–11), Paul presents his teaching as his preference (v. 7) or opinion (v. 12) as one who by the Lord's mercy is trustworthy (v. 25). As Paul himself notes, such teaching must not be placed on the same level as those commands which are from the Lord (vv. 12, 25).

The above analysis and reflections illustrate how sexual issues arose and were treated in several of the early churches which emerged in response to the proclamation of the gospel. In each case, while local histories and contexts varied, sexual matters joined other areas of ethical concern as Christians gradually positioned themselves with regard to their world environment. In places as diverse as Thessalonica, Galatia, and Corinth, the fundamental determinant of sexual attitudes and behavior always remained the Christian nature of those who had accepted the gospel and were bonded by the Spirit in developing communities.

Toward a Universal Church

With the passing decades, the early evangelical movement and the emerging communities developed into consolidated churches with a carefully defined sense of their identity vis-à-vis the greater world and the challenge of history. The articulation of this identity can be found in each of the four gospel narratives and their presentation of the teaching of Jesus. Contextualized by Jesus' death-resurrection and his expected return in glory, the latter had been shaped and interpreted by tradition, that is by the very life of the churches which ever sought to affirm Jesus' message in its relevance to their concrete historical situation. In this process, the Gospels constituted syntheses of basic Christianity in which the various issues of life were presented in their relationship to the entire Christian challenge.

Apart from Mark (*circa* A.D. 70), these Gospels reveal a growing sense of the Church's universality. Matthew and Luke, writing in the ninth decade, and John, whose gospel was completed in the tenth decade, thus prescind from questions of purely local or immediate concern and deal with issues of universal application. Although Mark may not have possessed this same awareness, his Gospel was received by communities as varied as those of Matthew and Luke, for whom the first gospel synthesis provided an important literary source. Mark thus constituted a transitional factor in the development of ecclesial universality. Accordingly, both the formulation and the relative position of sexual ethics in the four Gospels must be taken very seriously within the context of each Gospel's articulation of Christian identity.

The most important passage in Mark's Gospel concerning Christian sexuality is 10:2–12, where Jesus' careful response to a test of the Pharisees is situated in a long unit on discipleship as the way of Jesus' cross (8:27–10:52). In that unit, Jesus affirms the value of marriage and the evil of its dissolution. Husband and wife are one (10:8) as they follow in Jesus' steps (8:34), not seeking their own importance but as servants of all (9:35). The demands of the cross thus transcend the ethic of Moses, who allowed divorce (vv. 3–5). To accept this teaching without fear, however, those who accept Jesus' call must want to see and have their blindness removed by Christ (10:46–52).

Within the second part (9:30–10:31) of the unit on discipleship, the question of marriage is associated with Jesus' teaching on attachment to riches (10:17–27). In both matters, Christians must share the simplicity of a child as they accept God's reign (10:13–16). The Gospel thus addresses various aspects of life in the world, while recognizing that in the future risen life even the marriage relationship will be transcended (12:25). In this, as in the remainder of his Gospel, Mark responds to the apocalyptic tendencies of the community, for whom earthly realities and relationships held no hope and were about to be destroyed (13:5–7). His affirmation of the marriage bond is thus a positive value judgment on life in history. Passing through difficult times, the Christians must be faithful to the end. Responding to a crisis situation, the author presents all aspects of the Christian challenge in absolute terms calling for a renewed firm decision to follow Christ. Hence his unyielding position on the indissolubility of marriage (10:9–12), whose formulation betrays a marked egalitarian attitude toward men and women.

Mark's position on marriage and divorce (10:11–12) was retained by Luke, who included it in Jesus' teaching (16:18) along the great journey to Jerusalem (9:51–24:53). In Luke, however, the question received far less emphasis. Writing for communities called to a long-term insertion in history, Luke tempers the absoluteness of the Markan challenge (Mk. 8:34; Lk. 9:23). Confronting the day to day of Christian life in the world, Luke recognizes human lapses and places great emphasis on forgiveness and reconciliation in the teaching of Jesus (7:36–50). His pastoral intention is consequently directed, not so much to bringing the community to a radical and staunch decision and fidelity, but to the continual need to extend a gesture of peace and solidarity to those who drifted away and who returned with love (17:3–4). Going beyond hospitality, the community must actively seek out and find those who had been lost (15:1–31; 24:13–35). Although the Gospel shows little concern for specific sexual issues, it does reveal a general attitude toward all who have sinned, whether sexually or otherwise.

It should be noted that, unlike Mk. 10:29 and Mt. 10:37; 19:29, Luke includes the wife among those persons whom Christians must leave for the sake of the kingdom of God (19:29–30). For Luke, however, leaving is a matter of attitude and not of physical abandonment, as we observe from the story of Levi, who left everything to become Jesus' follower (5:28) but who then gave a large reception for Jesus in his house (5:29). Leaving everything or someone is thus a state of detachment in which values are respected and properly subordinated. To leave one's wife is consequently not necessarily an option for celibacy. Christians frequently appear as couples and families in the Lukan communities (e.g., Acts 5:1; 10:1, 44, 48; 18:2–3, 18–19, 26).

Matthew's teaching on sexual matters is included first in Jesus' discourse on the mount (5:27–32), a synthesis of Christian life attitudes which focused the community's identity in relation to the synagogue from which it had been ejected. At this point two important questions are treated, the need for a chaste interior attitude (vv. 27–30) and the matter of divorce (vv. 31–32). In 19:3–13, the author presents and adapts Mark's teaching (10:2–12) and discusses the difficulty of accepting it even in its modified form.

The community must disassociate itself from the hypocrites and not perform religious acts for others to see (6:1–18). The value of such acts stems from the Christians' hidden interior attitude which the Father both sees and rewards. The same principle applies to acts such as adultery, whose evil resides not in the act alone but in the interior disposition which precedes it and which it fulfills (cf. 15:17–20).

Adjustment to an ongoing mission to the gentile world (28:18–20) and to the realities of this challenge also led Matthew to temper Mark's position on divorce and adultery. While the prohibition of divorce remains the general rule, the author recognizes situations which may call for divorce and he accepts possible exceptions in cases where unchastity has disrupted marital solidarity. The same exception is introduced in 19:9, where it modifies Mark's unconditional view. In the latter context, Matthew goes on to respond to the objection that this teaching, even in its tempered application, is too difficult and makes marriage impossible. To accept Jesus' demand concerning marriage, one must be gifted to do so (19:11). Christians are thus asked to call on their nature as Christians; so transformed they should be able to accept Jesus' teaching in their new life context just as some of their fellows are able to accept life outside of marriage (19:12). Like Paul (1 Cor. 7:7), Matthew thus recognizes a variety of gifts and corresponding lifestyles within the Christian community.

From the above presentation, it appears that the Gospels considered marriage and fidelity to be extremely important in Christianity. At the same time, we note that the matter was but one of many realities in Christian life. The synoptic Gospels reflect this relative position of sexuality and concentrate their attention on issues which are of deeper import and which give meaning to the marriage commitment. The same is even more striking in John's Gospel, where little attention is paid to sexual matters apart from the narrative of the wedding at Cana (2:1–11) and Jesus' discussion with the Samaritan woman at the well (4:16–18). The value of marriage is implied in Jesus' very presence at the feast and marital fidelity affirmed by his observation that the woman's successive husbands were not really her husbands.

John's relative silence in relation to the other Gospels is understandable in light of the fundamental problem he meant to counter. Addressing a community whose tendency was to escape the flesh, his concern was not so much with the difficulties which issued from the flesh as with the need to affirm its importance and value. For John, the glory of God was manifested in the Word become flesh (1:14), a position which has profound implications for the sexuality of all who receive that Word while living in the flesh. The Christians' association with the Word become flesh constitutes a deep interior source for ethical living and the point of departure for reflection on what is right and what is wrong in the area of sexual morality.

II. The New Testament and the Life of the Church: Hermeneutics

A hermeneutical interpretation of the New Testament's teaching on Christian sexuality must respect the nature of its various documents. Since without exception all New Testament writings were fundamentally apostolic and pastoral by intent, their primary application must consequently reside in the area of apostolic and pastoral practice. Our task is thus to discern the position of the Church today in relation to that which underlies the various letters and Gospels which we accept as challenging and normative for Christian living. In light of this relationship, the significance of New Testament ethical teaching for modern life should emerge with considerable clarity.

Some general observations are warranted at the outset. First, at no time in the development of the New Testament did sexual issues displace the central message of Christianity from its position at the heart of the Church's efforts. There were situations, such as that which obtained at Corinth, where they drew more attention than usual. Even there, however, preoccupation with sexual matters was clearly related to deeper realities such as the gospel of the cross. Given the modern world's preoccupation with sexual gratification, does it not then become part of the Church's mission to strive for balance and perspective in human sexual attitudes?

Second, in all the passages we have examined, sexual ethics is grounded in a strong sense of the Christians' new identity in Christ as well as in their community solidarity. Human dignity and respect for other persons are constants of New Testament teaching concerning sexuality. In a world which manipulates human beings by subliminal appeals to the sex drive as isolated from the full reality of personhood, must the Church not use every means to emphasize the dignity of human beings?

Third, the New Testament approaches sexual issues by appealing to the Christian nature of its addressees, men and women gifted by the Spirit and transformed by the gospel which provided an interior principle of moral living and of discernment. All was not specified. Rather, Christians were expected to be able to recognize in individual cases what was in keeping with the Christian self and what was not. Too minute a specification constitutes a return to a law extrinsic to the human person and fails to recognize the new law which is inscribed in the heart. Our fundamental questions should then concern what actually reflects the Christian self in practice and what contributes to the development of a Church community with a mission to the world.

First Evangelization and the Early Churches

As we learn from the New Testament, the Church's initial efforts at evangelization focused on the fundamental reality of the gospel and its call to conversion. Only later did the more specific ethical implications of the gospel come to the fore. At that point, appeal would be made to the Christians' internalized sense of gospel in sorting out moral options and orienting Christian life in the world. Does this not constitute a legitimate pattern for evangelization today? In recent times, the Church no longer assumes that populations which have known Christianity for a long time are actually evangelized. Ethical teaching to such populations has all too often been ineffective precisely because the basic gospel proclamation had not been heard and accepted. Without a personal experience of the Lord, the demands of the gospel in sexual matters make little or no sense.

Only after hearing the gospel and encountering Christ do Christians personally assume their Christianity. Membership in a Christian community then provides a point of insertion into the universal Church. It is there in the local community of believers that moral values develop and the challenge of living according to the gospel is first confronted. As in the case of evangelization, the Church has come to realize that the existence of a true community cannot be assumed. Without a sense of community solidarity, however, and the needed social context for developing one's Christian selfhood, the Christian sexual ethic, which is a personal and social ethic, has no experiential basis. The New Testament thus challenges the Church to build genuine communities in which sexual behavior can be recognized as disruptive or constructive of community life.

Our major difficulty in interpreting Pauline passages such as 1 Corinthians 5–7 lies not in Paul's actual teaching but in recognizing the community's level of development. The fact that Paul excludes an incestuous person from the community in order that this person might be open to salvation is especially difficult to understand. However, once we recognize that this community had no sense of the indelible character of baptism, Paul's position makes sense. For a Church which baptizes infants and maintains baptism's irrevocability, Paul does not provide a warrant for exclusion from the community. His message does imply, however, that a renewed effort at evangelization must be made.

In chapter 7, Paul's expectations with regard to the imminent passing of this world condition the entire statement concerning marriage and various states of life. In a Church which no longer has such expectations, Paul's positions consequently become highly relativized. They do remind us, however, of the ultimate realities which govern all of our life choices and introduce a note of seriousness as decisions are made in light of the passing of each one's world.

Toward a Universal Church

Recent times have seen a resurgence of the Church's sense of its universal mission to the world. This renewed attitude gives the gospel syntheses and their effort to formulate a Christian ethic of universal scope great importance for our time. Like the early churches which gave birth to the Gospels, the modern Church is no longer preoccupied with its life as set apart from the world but with life as set apart for the world.

In a world which provides few supports for faithful married life and where family relationships have become tenuous or non-existent, the strong affirmation in all four Gospels of the value of married life, sex, and fidelity is extremely important. Mark's absolute rejection of divorce counters tendencies to take the marriage bond lightly. Luke challenges the Church to extend a welcoming hand of forgiveness and peace to those who have not lived up to their commitment. Matthew emphasizes interior dispositions for a world which values performance and productivity. At the same time, he opens our eyes to possible exceptions to the indissolubility of marriage.

Through the years, every effort has been made to explain away the exception clause which he included in his statement on the indissolubility of marriage. It appears better to accept the obvious and to recognize that Church practice is at variance with the openness which Matthew felt free to affirm even in the face of Mark's absolute position. Following Matthew, the Church would hold that while the marital intention must be unconditional and maintained until death in fidelity, conditions could well arise in which this intention is unfulfilled and the marriage relationship dissolves. Semantics aside, this is quite different from affirming that the marriage never existed.

Joining John's Gospel as well as the other Gospels in affirming the Christian value of married love, the Church is thus challenged to adopt an apostolic and pastoral attitude in sexual matters which is appropriate for its universal mission to the world.

Notes

1. *Human Sexuality: New Directions in American Catholic Thought* (New York: Paulist Press, 1977), pp.17–29.
2. Ibid., pp. xiv–xv, 241.
3. The passage includes a number of interpretive difficulties. While in itself the reference to wronging one's brother *en to pragmati* (v. 6) could mean "in business," the context, which refers to sanctification (*hagiasmos,* v. 3) and opposes the latter to uncleanness or impurity (*akatharsia,* v. 7), renders this interpretation quite improbable. Wronging one's brother is thus related to matters of sexual immorality (*porneia,* v. 3). It is most unlikely, however, that the brother in question would have been a prostitute. Paul would not have referred to him as a brother without qualification. Paul could then have been referring to a Christian's forcing himself on his brother or to transgressing his marital rights. Since the text is open to both interpretations, we have no grounds for limiting it to one or the other.

In itself, the expression *to heautou skeuos ktasthai* (v. 4) could refer to control of one's own body, or member, as well as to having sexual relations with one's own wife. Given Paul's subsequent reference to wronging or cheating one's brother, the latter is very likely the primary meaning. At the same time, a secondary meaning for what might well be an intentionally general or open expression should not be excluded, especially when the two meanings are so closely related.

4. Cf. 2 Cor. 3:1–3 and Jer. 31–34.
5. The "flesh" in this context must not be interpreted as a sensual or sexual reference. Rather it refers to the whole person from the point of pre-Christian existence and is opposed to the whole person as gifted by the Spirit of God.

2

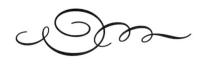

Sexual Salvation: Grace and the Resurrection of the Body

James B. Nelson

"Sin is estrangement; grace is reconciliation."[1] Salvation, in its original meaning, is healing. It is the reuniting of what has been torn apart and estranged. It is the recovery of a center and a wholeness in that which has been split asunder. It is the overcoming of alienation within the body-self, between the person and the world, between the person and God.

Salvation is sexual. This does not mean that we are saved by our sexuality. We are saved by the grace of God—God's unearned, healing, life-giving love. But "sexual salvation" does mean that we are given new life not in spite of the fact that we are sexual body-selves but precisely in and through this entire selfhood which we are.

The focus for this chapter is not on salvation generally, the incredibly broad and rich dimensions of divine grace and human healing. Rather, the focus is more particularly on the healing and augmented wholeness we experience both in and through our sexuality, those dimensions of us which have been wounded and divided by spiritualistic and sexist dualisms. Our concern is the process and meaning of the resurrection of the sexual body.

Three attitudes toward sexuality have appeared most commonly in Christian thought.[2] The Medievalists typify one of them: control by reason and will. After all, is it not our experience that we can more easily master other appetites than we can master the sexual? We can come to terms with our greed. We can repress or sublimate our aggression. But our sexual desires seem to leap up at inconvenient moments, revealing to us our animal state, taking possession of us with forces we do not understand. Instead of being our own master, at times we seem to become our own monster. Thus, we seek to control our sexuality for higher purposes through reason and will power.[3]

But self-control easily slips into bodily mortification—the death of the flesh. In reaction to this, a second attitude emerges. Over against the stringency of "the Apollonian," some would have us exalt "the Dionysian" within us. This may be the oldest attitude of all, though it is forever being rediscovered. Sexuality, it is said, has been artificially repressed. We must throw off the social masks, reclaim our inner forces and feelings, and in this way be united with a cosmic vitality. While there are many secular advocates of the Dionysian, there are articulate Christians as well. But, curiously, the members of this school do not seem to regard sexual expression and sexual love as truly personal.

Then there is a third attitude: sex is unimportant. It is simply there. This is the approach of detachment in some form or another. Sexuality is neither divine nor demonic. Jesus demythologized sex, and we can have freedom over our sexuality, too, only if we can "take it or leave it." Indeed, we must be able to laugh at sex or we shall be humiliated by it, for it is an irrational, impersonal force which threatens to turn even the best of us into caricatures of ourselves.[4] Odd and laughable, sexuality becomes almost inconsequential.

If there are hints of truth in each of these orientations, there also is something basically amiss. A common thread unites persons of each of these apparently widely-differing views. Dan Sullivan says it well: it is "the unyielding determination to locate sex somewhere—or anywhere—outside the human self, the authentic 'me,' that inner core of personhood which makes humanity distinctive. In this one crucial respect there is no difference between the Christian Fathers' conviction that sex is a 'beast in the belly,' and Norman Brown's that it is 'Christ in me.'"[5] And, if sexuality is still experienced as being outside of and apart from the authentic self, there is still alienation.

To Christian faith, however, alienation is never the last word. The Apostle speaks with power of both alienation and reconciliation. Of the former, he exclaims, "Wretched man that I am! Who will deliver me from this body of death?" (Romans 7:24.) It is not inconsistent with the Gospel to alter Paul's words at this point: "Wretched person that I am! Who will deliver me from this death of the body?" Then, with him we can continue, "Thanks be to God through Jesus Christ our Lord!" Because fear is at the root of our alienation, merely an intellectual understanding of the problem will not release us. But the Gospel does not announce salvation through correct understanding. Rather, it comes through the gracious love of God received in human openness and trust.

It is quite possible that the term "salvation" may not be particularly helpful to many contemporary Christians. In spite of its widespread traditional use in the church (and perhaps because of it), the term is fraught with numerous associations which may mislead rather than assist. We need then to be flexible and pluralistic in vocabulary, as, indeed, the Bible is. Different nuances will attach themselves to different words, and that is all to the good. A variety of polar concepts thus can be used, bearing common meanings with different shadings: sin and salvation, alienation and reconciliation, fragmentation and wholeness, death and life, law and gospel, death and resurrection.

The experience of the new life is a relational reality in which the miraculous and the everyday stuff of life are interwoven. The incarnation of God, the divine presence in and through human flesh, is always a miracle. We celebrate its decisive and normative occurrence in Jesus Christ. We also celebrate faith's conviction that God's incarnation continues to occur. The resurrecting power is beyond our own. It is the mysterious creativity and renewal of life itself, God's power in our midst. And the miracle of the body's resurrection is all the more awesome because it occurs through human gestures, human words, human touch and caress, human intimacy.

We experience new life of the body-self as a gift. A dead body cannot raise itself, nor can we lift ourselves by our own bootstraps. It is the eternal paradox of life and of the gospel that our own strenuous and strident efforts to possess renewal seem to shut us off from it more completely. This is inevitable, for the self who so strives to be changed is the very self who is organized by means of a dualism, which itself must be challenged and overthrown, not simply confirmed by effort. The latter is the trap of both sexual ascetics and libertines who, in trying to overcome the alienation of their bodies, only seem to establish it more firmly since their weapon is the dualism which has nurtured the alienation in the first place.[6]

The miraculous dimension in sexual salvation lies not in the fact that it is necessarily dramatic, which it may not be, nor that it interferes with the "natural world" (if by that we mean an external structure working according to its own laws). It is in our discovery of what we really are. As H. A. Williams declares, "The discovery is miraculous because the previous organization of our being provided no vantage point from which we could have seen what now we do see. Our new vision has come to us. It has arrived from we know not where."[7] To be sure, there is a paradox here. Significant change in the body-self does not usually occur without effort, risk-taking, courage, and pain. So Paul counsels, "work out your own salvation with fear and trembling." But the point is that the effort, risk, and will are expended within the context of a creative Power for change which is neither our invention nor possession: "for God is at work in you . . ." (Philippians 2:12–13).

The experience of reconciliation of the body-self surely is not the exclusive possession of any sect or creed, Christian or otherwise. In point of fact, because both sexist and spiritualistic dualisms have so plagued Christianity, many people have left the church to seek the wholeness of their sexual humanity elsewhere. And, for our own understanding we must draw on the experiences and insights of numerous non-Christians who have realized something genuine of that sexual salvation to which we point with Christian symbols. But those of us who find ourselves within the church, both by fate and by free choice, will use also those faith symbols which for us best express that universal and gracious Reality which the words themselves cannot possess but in which they meaningfully participate.

Within the experience of sexual salvation there seems to be a double movement. It is not simply a temporal sequence, though there are elements of that. Yet, Christian experience throughout the centuries has found articulation in two distinguishable and complementary dimensions of reconciliation. Again, these have been given different names bearing different nuances: justification and sanctification, God's power over us and God's power within us, gift and response, acceptance and growth, forgiveness and fulfillment. We can begin with the reality to which the first term in each pair points.

Grace and the Sexuality of Jesus

That we experience God's gracious justification or acceptance in and through Jesus Christ has profound sexual implications. "The Word became flesh." Jesus was a sexual being. And here is God's affirmation of our own sexuality.

Nevertheless, the most common Christological heresy is still the docetic heresy, spiritualistic dualism applied to Jesus. It is the conviction held in varying forms by countless Christians past and present that Jesus Christ could not have been fully human, that God (acting in proper taste) would not have expressed the divine Spirit through human flesh, and that in Jesus we see true God but only in the appearance of a human body. Unfortunately, the record is clear; for the most part the church has presented Jesus as sexless. Because the human body is vitally and spontaneously sexual, many Christians in their dualistic alienation have been offended by the radical implications of the incarnation. And, to deny Jesus sexuality in one way or another "for most people today is about the most effective way of saying that he was not fully human."[8] The Victorian within still winces at the thought that the incarnation might be "a tale of the flesh."

Yet, the gospel has always had elements of scandal about it, and it has never shied away from offending the tastes of the respectably righteous. On this particular issue, however, theologians have been slow. Until recently it was more often the writers and artists who wrestled openly with the question of Jesus' sexuality—D. H. Lawrence, Nikos Kazantzakis, the rock opera Jesus Christ Superstar, and the like. If their conclusions were not altogether persuasive, at least they sensed, with an urgency greater than that of most orthodox Christians, that what is at stake in this question (as in every Christological issue) is the possibility, meaning, and nature of human salvation.

In recent years, however, several theologians have voiced their positive beliefs on the matter. A considerable part of the concern is the realization that sexuality appears to be intrinsically and not accidentally related to one's capacity to love. Thus, John Erskine writes of Jesus, "His character renders it for me utterly impossible that his youth and manhood could have been unmoved by warm, human emotions.... If he really took our nature upon him and was human, then he had our equipment of sex."[9] Similarly, Tom F. Driver observes, "The absence of all comment [in the Gospels] about Jesus' sexuality cannot be taken to imply that he had no sexual feelings.... I cannot imagine a human tenderness, which the Gospels show to be characteristic of Jesus, that is not fed in some degree by the springs of passion. The human alternative to sexual tenderness is not asexual tenderness but sexual fear."[10] Likewise, psychiatrist-theologian Jack Dominian reflects upon the necessary connection in Jesus between self-acceptance and genuine openness to others: "This response was unhampered by any need to reject, deny, or condemn any part of himself, hence of others.... Although the evidence is extremely limited, it is hard to see how such total self-acceptance and availability could have been present without including full awareness of his sexuality."[11]

William Phipps has been the most vigorous in pursuing the question. He argues that while Jesus' celibacy is a possible interpretation, his marriage is much more probable. The evidences, he believes, are multiple. The Gospels do not record Jesus as having stated either that he was born of a virgin or that he himself was a virgin. Nor does the book of Acts indicate that those closest to him knew of any special virginal conditions about him. In addition, while Jesus was sharply critical of certain aspects of Judaism, he was thoroughly Jewish in most respects, and that faith-culture rejected celibacy both in theory and in practice. Since we have no information about Jesus' life between his ages of twelve and thirty (the customary time for Jewish betrothal and marriage), it is likely that he followed prevailing Jewish custom and married as a young man. Indeed, his delight in women and his understanding of them seems to contrast markedly with the style of an ascetic, as is apparent when one compares Jesus' manner and personality with that of the Essene ascetic John the Baptist. Phipps concludes that the notion of a celibate savior is not the product of the apostolic age but rather grew out of Christianity's later contact with Hellenistic dualism.[12]

The conclusion remains, I believe, highly debatable. It is possible, to be sure but the arguments from silence are not convincing enough to make it probable. In any event, Jesus' marriage is not the crux of the issue. His sexuality is, and the virtue of at least pressing the possibility of marriage is to help us take his fully human nature with greater seriousness. Even if his celibacy remains probable, the possibility of genital expression and, most likely, the temptation toward it need affirmation. If we are offended at the thought that Jesus was ever inclined toward a *fully* sexual union, such offense might simply betray the suspicion that sex is unworthy of the Savior because it is unworthy of us. But we need not project our own alienation upon him. If he at times was so inclined, we can well assume that he did not think of it as a temptation toward something intrinsically tainted and suspect, but rather as a temptation to turn aside from a growing conviction of his compelling vocation toward a unique role in God's kingdom.[13]

John A. T. Robinson quite appropriately links the issue of Jesus' sexuality with the question of the manner of his birth.[14] A non-physical interpretation of the Virgin Birth story still leaves unresolved the manner of Jesus' conception, and Robinson, together with several other biblical scholars, raises the possibility of an irregular sexual union. This question, like that of Jesus' marriage, remains debatable, but this line of inquiry should not be rejected out of hand because of its supposed impropriety. At the very least, it should prompt us to view God's incarnation in Jesus of Nazareth in a fresh and scandalous light, a perspective that is hardly out of character for a gospel which proclaims that the divine love is often a surprising affront to our assumptions of human righteousness.

In addition, we might need to take another look at the debates of Nicaea and Chalcedon.[15] On those occasions there was a persistent worry that any insistence on Jesus' full humanity would lead to a denial of his divinity. The fears of Athanasius and Cyril led them to insist that the Word *became man* but did not come into a *man*. "And they were prevented from understanding that men like Theodore and Nestorius really were arguing (as we can now see) for a genuine and deeply *personal* union of God and man in Christ—however inadequate their vocabulary. . . ."[16]

Thus, the issue of Jesus' sexuality is not simply a curious historical debate. Nor is it an inappropriate sort of "prurient interest." If the docetic heresy, though early condemned by the church, continues to linger in current Christian mentality, this suggests something about our own salvation and possibilities for wholeness. For, if we are not really sure about the full humanity of the one whom we call Truly Human, we can only be confused about what authentic humanity might mean for us. If we try to take Jesus with utter seriousness and yet uneasily retreat from thoughts of his sexuality, or even recoil with repugnance, it is also likely that we shall either deny much of our own sexuality or else find considerable difficulty integrating our Christological beliefs into the reality of our lives as body-selves.[17]

But the Word did become flesh. Logos, Cosmic Meaning, was embodied, and our own embodiment has been given definition and vindication in Jesus Christ. What is at stake—and here the Nestorians were right—is whether or not it is possible, however partially we may experience it, that there be a genuine and deeply personal union of God and our embodied selves. If we deny the radicality of God's incarnation in Jesus, we may well persist in a vain attempt to be more spiritual than God. The possibility of our own full humanity, after all, decisively hinges upon "the humanity of God" (to use Karl Barth's fine phrase). That humanity of God is an unexpected scandal, and the issue of Jesus' sexuality is an important place to test our commitment to it. In those central symbols of incarnation and resurrection Christian faith affirms that God embraces fleshly, bodily life. God invites us to do so.[18]

Justification as God's Acceptance of Our Bodily Life

Grace is "God's generosity in personal action."[19] It is not a supernatural "something" which God gives to us. Rather, it is a gracious personal relationship, the gift of the accepting personal Presence itself. Gregory Baum puts it well in saying that "the author of reality is on our side. The ground of being is not far away, hostile or indifferent to us: the deepest dimension of the total reality facing us is for us. There is no reason to be afraid of the world . . . for the ultimate root of all being protects and favors human life. Despite the suffering and evil in the world . . . we are summoned to believe that the ultimate principle of reality is love itself."[20]

God's radical, unconditional, and unearned acceptance of us is a fitting contemporary translation of justification by grace. In his powerful sermon, "You Are Accepted," Paul Tillich evocatively states, "It strikes us when our disgust for our own being, our indifference, our weakness, our hostility, and our lack of direction and composure have become intolerable to us. It strikes us when, year after year, the longed-for perfection of life does not appear, when the old compulsions reign within us as they have for decades, when despair destroys all joy and courage. Sometimes at that moment a wave of light breaks into our darkness, and it is as though a voice were saying: 'You are accepted. You are *accepted*, accepted by that which is greater than you, and the name of which you do not know. Do not ask for the name now; perhaps you will find it later. Do not try to do anything now; perhaps later you will do much. Do not seek for anything; do not perform anything; do not intend anything. *Simply accept the fact that you are accepted!*' If that happens to us, we experience grace."[21]

When we have experienced that kind of acceptance, even momentarily, we know that everything is transformed. Though recognition of this frequently has been neglected in Christian theology, God's word of acceptance is addressed to the total and sexual self, not simply to a disembodied personality. We might extend Tillich's language in this manner: You are accepted, the total you. Your body, which you often reject, is accepted by that which is greater than you. Your sexual feelings and unfulfilled yearnings are accepted. You are accepted in your ascetic attempts at self-justification or in your hedonistic alienation from the true meaning of your sexuality. You are accepted in those moments of sexual fantasy which come unbidden and which both delight and disturb you. You are accepted in your femininity and in your masculinity, for you have elements of both. You are accepted in your heterosexuality and in your homosexuality, and you have elements of both. Simply accept the fact that you are accepted as a sexual person! If that happens to you, you experience grace.

An incarnational, non-docetic understanding of acceptance takes seriously its enfleshed mediation. Such grace can be mediated by words of Scripture and tradition. It can be conveyed through the church's liturgy. Yet, in regard to sexual acceptance, tradition and liturgy at times are more alienating than gracious, and Scripture is frequently interpreted docetically. So the gracious Word often becomes flesh in ways not usually labeled religious. It is mediated through sexual communion in ecstasy and playfulness with the beloved partner. It comes as healing through "the laying on of hands"—the spontaneous hand of a friend on one's shoulder. Such grace is mediated by parents when the child receives (as in breast feeding, sensitive toilet training, physical expressions of affection, and appropriate sex education) a sense of the trustworthiness and goodness of his or her own body rather than a legacy of mistrust and shame. Grace comes through human agency in struggle and judgment as well—as when the Women's Movement gives a woman new self-respect and power born from her pain, and when in judgment on distorted masculinity it opens a man to new ranges of emotion and bodily self-acceptance.

Thus, beyond the dualistic alienations we experience the gracious resurrection of the bodyself. I really am *one* person. Body and mind are one; my body is me as my mind is me. Beyond the imprisonment of rigid sex roles I am freed to be a *person*. And in such resurrection I discover that I belong intimately to others and intimately to the world.

We live in grace, but we also continue in sin, and the experience of radical acceptance and God's resurrection of the body is never unambiguous. Reinhold Niebuhr thus declares, "The element of sin in the experience is not due to the fact that sex is in any sense sinful as such. But once sin in presupposed, that is, once the original harmony of nature is disturbed by . . . self love, the instincts of sex are particularly effective tools for both the assertion of self and the flight from self."[22] In our experience of sexuality there is often a bewildering confusion of elements. If in our estrangement we never utterly lose our original unity, so also in the gracious experience of acceptance and reunification, estrangement is not totally or permanently conquered. The glorious oneness I experienced begins to disintegrate as body and mind once more compete for the title of being me. And the glorious liberty of the children of God once more submits to old and fearful assumptions as men and women imprison themselves and each other in dominance and submission.

Thus, to speak of—and to celebrate—God's radically accepting love does not require us to engage in a romanticized idealism about human perfection under grace. Nevertheless, when we are open to the divine acceptance, in some measure everything is transformed. If the old fears and sexual dualisms do return, still we are not the same as before. "Grace aims at fulfillment," as Harold Ditmanson rightly affirms. "It is the operative power of God's personal action, moving us toward that which God intends us to be. The purpose of creaturely existence is that each of God's creatures achieves the fullest excellence of which its nature is capable. Any thwarting of fulfillment, therefore, is really a wrong against the basic purpose of creation itself."[23]

This affirmation leads us to grace's second dimension: sanctification. If that traditional word is less than intelligible to many modern ears, contemporary equivalents are appropriate: growth, fulfillment, God's empowerment toward our greater wholeness. To explore what this might mean sexually, I have selected several facets of our bodily experience: growth in self-acceptance, in sensuousness, in knowing, in freedom, and in androgyny.... Each of these is an expression of love's fulfillment....

Notes

1. Paul Tillich, *Systematic Theology*, Vol. II (Chicago: University of Chicago Press, 1957), 57. Cf. 166. See also Harold Ditmanson, *Grace in Experience and Theology* (Minneapolis: Augsburg, 1977), esp. Chaps. 4, 6.
2. See Dan Sullivan, "Introduction" to Abel Jeanniere, *The Anthropology of Sex,* trans. Julie Kernan (New York: Harper and Row, 1967), 15f.
3. See Leslie Paul, *Eros Rediscovered: Restoring Sex to Humanity* (New York: Association Press, 1970), 142f.
4. See Tom F. Driver, "Sexuality and Jesus," in Martin E. Marty and Dean G. Peerman (eds.), *New Theology* No. 3 (New York: Macmillan, 1966); also, "On Taking Sex Seriously," *Christianity and Crisis,* Vol. 23 (Oct. 14, 1963).
5. Sullivan, 17.
6. See Harry A. Williams, *True Resurrection* (London: Mitchell Beazley, 1972), 50f.
7. Ibid., 51.
8. John A. T. Robinson, *The Human Face of God* (Philadelphia: Westminster, 1973), 64.
9. John Erskine, quoted in William E. Phipps, *Was Jesus Married?* (New York: Harper and Row, 1970), 9.
10. Driver, "Sexuality and Jesus," 243, 240.
11. Jack Dominian, *The Church and the Sexual Revolution* (London: Darton, Longman and Todd, 1971), 66.
12. See Phipps, *Was Jesus Married?*, esp. Chaps. 2, 3, 4.
13. See Lewis B. Smedes, *Sex for Christians* (Grand Rapids, Mich.: Eerdmans, 1976), 78f.
14. See Robinson, *The Human Face of God,* 57ff. If we interpret the Virgin Birth as a non-literal way of attempting to affirm something about Jesus as the Christ, we are left, according to Robinson, with only three possibilities concerning Jesus' conception. One is that Joseph was his human father who impregnated Mary inside wedlock; another is that Joseph impregnated Mary outside wedlock and subsequently legitimized this action by marriage. But both of these possibilities are not strongly supported by biblical evidence. Hence, a third possibility presents itself: that the conception took place outside wedlock by a man unknown to us, and this was subsequently accepted by Joseph. In pressing this point Robinson may be stretching the available evidence, but his overall contention concerning the radical scandal of the Incarnation is clear and appropriate.
15. See ibid., 197ff.
16. Ibid., 199.
17. Both Driver, "Sexuality and Jesus," 236, and William E. Phipps, *Recovering Biblical Sensuousness* (Philadelphia: Westminster Press, 1975), 158, make this point.
18. In speaking of God's incarnation in Jesus Christ, we do well to remember why Paul Tillich was hesitant about the term. The notion that "God has become man" is nonsensical because God cannot become something else—God cannot cease to be God. There is, then a danger that the doctrine of the Incarnation will be interpreted as a mythological transmutation. Rather than speaking of the divine nature and human nature wedded in Jesus Christ, Tillich finds it more appropriate to assert that in Jesus the Christ

"the eternal unity of God and man has become historical reality" and in Christ we meet the manifestation of God "in a personal life-process as a saving participant in the human predicament." See *Systematic Theology,* Vol. II, 148, 95.

19. Ditmanson, 58.
20. Gregory Baum, as quoted in ibid., 24.
21. Paul Tillich, *The Shaking of the Foundations* (New York: Scribner's, 1948), 162.
22. Reinhold Niebuhr, *The Nature and Destiny of Man,* Vol. I (New York: Scribner's, 1941, 1943, 1949,), 237.
23. Ditmanson, 60.

3

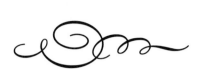

Christianity and Sexuality: An Ambiguous History

Eric Fuchs

  Any research on the Christian ethic of sexuality can not bypass the history of the difficult and ambivalent relations of Christianity to sexuality (unless it be frivolous or in bad faith). No one could ingenuously claim to go straight from the Bible to our time while ignoring, or pretending to ignore, the impact which this tradition has had on the consciousness or the unconsciousness of Christians in our day. This could only reveal presumption or childishness. Presumption, if we want to claim that we are our own beginning or to think that we ourselves are the initiators of Christianity; childishness, if we believe that shutting our eyes dispenses with reality! One cannot refute, whether we rejoice in it or denounce it, that our western morality largely flows from the past that belongs to Christian tradition. But it is equally true that more often than not we are unfamiliar with that tradition and that we rarely attempt to place it in its real intentions and in its confrontations within the theology of a time very different from our own. Because of this, my fourth chapter [of the author's *Sexual Desire and Love: Origins and History of the Christian Ethic of Sexuality and Marriage*] tries to measure the real value of the Christian moral tradition and tries to understand, with supporting texts, how and why Christianity took a particular stand on sexuality, wherein was merged, at least from our contemporary viewpoint, the best and worst of things. I shall also examine why, on certain important points, Christian tradition distanced itself from the scriptural tradition, and to discern thereby what is at stake in the ethical interpretation which the Church has made and continues to make of its sources.

  This intention summarizes my field of interest here: it is less a question of reporting the whole history of the rapport between Christianity and sexuality than of highlighting the major trends, particularly those that defined what we finally have come to call "Christian morality." The first category is composed of reflections by the Church Fathers in the second, third and fourth centuries. As members of ancient society, they sought to formulate a morality (they preferred to call it an "asceticism") whereby gnostic dualism would be repulsed and an eschatological tension be maintained. This patristic ethic will be taken up and elaborated with great precision by Augustine (too great, in fact), whose teaching clearly dominated all of medieval western morality. The Augustinian position represents a second category. The third concerns the Protestant Reformation, which in its deliberate return to scriptural sources for morality as well as for faith, develops a morality which is clearly at odds, particularly in the area of sexuality and marriage, with Catholic morality.

At the end of the sixteenth century, we can say that in its broad outlines, Christian morality in the West vis-à-vis sexuality and conjugality is constituted under two forms—Catholic and Protestant. I will define the characteristics of both in a concluding section. I have decided not to follow the evolution of these two moralities down into our modern era (from the seventeenth to the nineteenth centuries) because that development has not been influenced by any internal theological necessity but has been a reaction (positive or negative) to the general evolution of a society where the influence of the Church and of theology has been progressively diminishing. In fact, a close look reveals that the evolution altered nothing fundamental in the two moralities, but only accentuated, by emphasizing the difference, the essential characteristics of Catholic and Protestant morality. The models already set up in the course of history were not essentially affected by that evolution. Only in the twentieth century, more precisely in the mid-twentieth century, did certain Catholic moralists begin to discuss the validity of the foundations of traditional Catholic morality and did Protestant theology begin to question its links to bourgeois society with its moral ideals. This critical review has only just begun; it is certainly rich in promise, but it cannot be included in a chapter devoted to the history of the problem! Therefore, in my last chapter [of *Sexual Desire and Love*], I will try to deal with the necessity of reinterpreting scriptural and ethical tradition in a critique vis-à-vis the ideology of our contemporary culture.

1. THE EARLY CHURCH AND SEXUALITY (UP TO CA. 250)

During this time the Church insists above all on the necessity for *moral discipline*. In so doing, the Church joins the ranks of a polemic tradition existing in Judaism as well as in Hellenism, which pronounces judgment on ancient customs (particularly sexual customs) that is often quite harsh. Thus the indictment of Paul against the immorality of pagans in Romans (1:18–32)[1] takes up the terms of the traditional polemic in Judaism against the idolatry of ancient religions and its dual consequence in the area of sexual morality: sex made sacred and homosexuality.[2]

In the New Testament, the denunciation of the ancient Greek world is frequent, Here, for example, is a list of sins which provoke indignation on the part of the author of the first epistle to Timothy who is faced with the moral situation of his day: "... the law is not laid down for the just but for the lawless and disobedient, for the ungodly and sinners, for the unholy and profane, for murderers of fathers and murderers of mothers, for manslayers, immoral persons, sodomites, kidnappers, liars, perjurers...."[3]

In the midst of this kind of society, Christianity proclaimed itself the messenger of a religious morality which linked concrete practice to religious faith and sought thereby to express the cohesiveness of the Christian anthropological scheme.[4] Here are some examples from Christian texts of the end of the first and second centuries. In opposition to the popular practice of the *exposure of children*,[5] Justin writes: "Lest we molest anyone or commit sin ourselves, we have been taught that it is wicked to expose even newly-born children, first because we see that almost all those who are exposed (not only girls, but boys) are given over to prostitution. As your forefathers are said to have raised herds of oxen, or goats, or sheep, or grazing horses, you now raise children only for this same disgraceful purpose, for in every country there is a throng of females, hermaphrodites, and degenerates, ready for this evil practice. And you who should eradicate them from your land, instead accept wages, tribute, and taxes from them. Anyone who consorts with them, besides being guilty of a godless, impious and shameful action, may by some chance be guilty of intercourse with his own child, relative, or brother.... Still (another reason against this practice is) lest some of them would not be (discovered and) taken home, but die, and we would then be murderers."[6] Thus the exposing of children is denounced first of all because it encourages prostitution and immorality, and secondly because it is often equivalent to homicide. This link between respect for life and respect for the other is clearly evidenced in the *Didache:* "You shall not commit murder. You shall not commit adultery. You shall not corrupt boys. You shall not commit fornication. You shall not steal. You shall not practice magic. You shall not practice sorcery. You shall not kill an unborn child or murder a newborn infant."[7] The same teaching is found in the *Epistle of Barnabas* (19:4a, 5d). Along with a very unusual exegesis of Leviticus (chap. 11), this epistle condemns sodomy, adultery, homosexuality and the practice of *fellatio*.[8] The same condemnation is perhaps found in the list of vices in the *Epistle of Clement of Rome to the Corinthians:* Christians should be ". . . fleeing from evil speech, and abominable and impure embraces" (30:1).

The Christian ideal exalts fidelity and purity in marriage. "Tell my sisters to love the Lord and to be satisfied with their husbands in the flesh and spirit. In the same way tell my brothers in the name of Jesus Christ to love their wives as the Lord does the Church. If anyone is able to persevere in chastity to the honor of the flesh of the Lord, let him do so in all humility. If he is boastful about it, he is lost. . . ."[9] The ideal of chastity must here be understood as the quest for a moral discipline capable of checking the current immorality. Thus Hermas sees himself commanded to "guard purity. Let it not enter your heart to think of another man's wife, nor about fornication, nor any such thing. If you do, you will commit a serious sin. Keep your wife in mind always and you will never fall into sin."[10] There is as yet no exaltation of the spiritual virtues of celibacy, but only concern for safeguarding a sexual ethic by and in marriage that respects, among other things, the person of the woman. And so Tertullian affirms: "So, we who are united in mind and soul have no hesitation about sharing what we have. Everything is in common among us—except our wives. In this matter—which is the only matter in which the rest of men practice partnership—we dissolve partnership. They not only usurp the marriage rights of their friends, but they even hand over their own rights to their friends with the greatest equanimity."[11] This text is important because it brings out the fundamental justification for the moral discipline called for by the Christians; it holds to an absolute distinction made between the relationship of man to things and the relationship between a man and his wife: the latter is structural and thus cannot be lived out according to the model for the former without fundamentally altering humanity.

In their insistence on the value of moral discipline, the first Christians met the expectation of a great number of their contemporaries.[12] Stoicism, which I shall come back to later, had already raised the ethical issue but its morality of moderation was not sufficient to respond to the most pressing questions. "One must admit that the Hellenistic and Roman world lived in the greatest sexual confusion. Nor did it find itself more 'liberated' or happier as a result. Certain societies outside of Europe that have perpetuated these customs (condemned on the surface) to this day certainly do not give the impression of having blossomed! We can well understand that the moral requirements of Christianity should have appeared as true liberation for those with sensitive consciences and for the victims of that kind of anarchy."[13] As an example, among many others, of this expectation and of the quest for a more exacting morality, here is an extract of ordinances of a private shrine founded at Philadelphia in Lydia in the first century B.C., dedicated to the goddess Agdistis: "Let men and women, slave and free, as they come to this shrine swear by all the gods that they will not knowingly devise any evil guile or harmful poison against man or woman; that they will neither know nor employ baneful spells; that they will neither themselves use nor recommend to others nor be accomplices in love charms, abortives, contraceptives, robbery, murder.... No man shall have intercourse with any married woman other than his wife whether free or slave, nor with any boy, nor with any virgin, nor advise another to do so, but if he shares another's guilty secret, he shall make public such an one.... A married woman who is free must be chaste, and know the bed of no man but her husband: if she know another, she is not chaste but impure, infected with incestuous pollution and unworthy to venerate this god whose shrine is erected here.... These commandments were set up by Agdistis the most holy guardian and mistress of this shrine. May she put good intentions in men and women...."[14]

Pliny the Younger, describing Christians in one of his letters to Trajan, particularly highlighted the moral discipline they submitted to: "... (they met) regularly before dawn on a fixed day to chant verses alternately among themselves in honour of Christ as if to a god, and also to bind themselves by oath, not for any criminal purpose, but to abstain from theft, robbery and adultery, to commit no breach of trust and not to deny a deposit when called upon to restore it."[15]

Meanwhile, the same dual struggle which was outlined in our study of Paul's teaching continues on within the church and becomes intensified. On one hand, certain ascetic excesses must be restrained and on the other, certain antinomian tendencies linked to Gnosticism must be repelled. The first Christian theologians (Clement of Alexandria, Irenaeus, Tertullian) are the witnesses and the actors in this struggle which will mark Christian moral tradition for many centuries.

Clement of Alexandria,[16] with regards to marriage and sexuality, fights against encratic movements on one hand and licentious gnostic sects on the other. The whole third *Stromata*[17] is devoted to this battle.

Encraticism is more of an extreme ascetic attitude than a philosophy of a particular sect;[18] Clement sees it as defended by Marcion and his disciples, by Tatian[19] and his movement, and by Julianus Cassianus[20] and his school. It strongly influenced certain apocryphal texts like the *Apocryphal Acts*, particularly the *Acts of John*[21] (second century) and the *Gospel of Thomas* (early third century). That influence is essentially defined as a rejection of marriage. The encratic arguments, judged frm Clement's refutation, are as follows. First, marriage is sin because it is stained by the uncleanness that comes from sexual relation; it (therefore) discourages any spiritual relationship with God and only perfect chastity can signify the resurrection, and is the means whereby one can experience that reality even here on earth. Second, marriage belongs to the old order of reality, that of the Law, which has been abolished: "The Savior has transformed us and set us free of the error of the union of sexes."[22] Finally, since Christ was not married, chastity is part of the imitation of Jesus. The Encratites freely cite, as does Clement himself elsewhere, passages from the apocryphal *Gospel of the Egyptians*, a text which seems to have been authoritative in Alexandria. This text, or at least the fragments which have come down to us through Clement, link sexuality and procreation with the continuation of the reign of death. Marriage is thus in service to death[23] and the Kingdom is characterized by the abolition of sexual difference.[24] It is clear that encraticism displays a profound pessimism toward creation, a pessimism which naturally engenders disdain for the body since it is mortal and inhabited by desire and passion.

In the face of this asceticism, Clement defends the dignity of marriage. First of all, marriage is instituted by God. It is in no way the consequence of sin, and sexuality was willed by God for the propagation of the human race.[25] Moreover, marriage joins man to the creative work of God: "This is to share in God's own work of creation, and in such a work the seed ought not be wasted nor scattered thoughtlessly...."[26] Following Ephesians 5, Clement especially interprets marriage from the starting point of the bond that unites Christ to His Church. This battle for marriage is a battle for the positive affirmation of divine Creation; it becomes part of the broader debate on the meaning of Christian eschatology. The Encratites, like certain Gnostics who will be discussed later, set redemption in opposition to creation and sought to manifest the already active presence of the *eschaton* by their unworldly attitudes. This was carried to the point where they denied all value or goodness to creation and became more and more systematic (one thinks of Marcion) in their juxtaposition of creator-god to God-the-savior. Under the conditions, we can understand Clement's forceful insistence on the fact that marriage is in collaboration with the divine work of creation.[27] So now, the principal end of marriage can be nothing other than procreation. We can see how the concern to fight for the value of the order of creation led to an emphasis on the procreative function of marriage. Against those who scorned marriage for spiritual reasons, it was necessary, in line with 1 Timothy 4:3[28] and Hebrews 13:4,[29] to honor the marital institution and consider how an authentic spirituality could be lived out in it—which idea was not self-evident in the stoic and dualistic context that the Christians were living in. The problem seemed to be solved by insisting on the link of sexuality to procreation.

Clement meanwhile clashes with certain *gnostic groups* in Alexandria who have very unusual views[30] on marriage and sexual life.

First of all, there are the disciples of the Gnostic Basilides and his son Isidore, who were Alexandrians at the beginning of the second century. From what we can reconstruct of their doctrine, it seems that Basilides recommended to the disciples who could not live in total sexual abstinence—which was his ideal—that they practice free sex without scruples, as long as no domination or compulsion by amorous desire was allowed. He preaches a sort of indifference to sexuality, an indifference which can as easily end up in continence as in immorality. In a very characteristic proposition, possibly inspired by epicureanism, Basilides distinguishes between love and sexual desire: he condemns love as a sign of aspiration contrary to nature and as a revolt against the limitations that it imposes on man, and he exalts sexual desire as a sign of man's participation in the spermatic power of God. One must thus satisfy sexual instinct, which is in conformity with nature, and therefore moral, without becoming dominated by love. Sexual desire is good, but love, which disturbs *mystical agnosia*,[31] is not. Where Christianity defends the indissolubility of monogamous union and tries to promote the idea that the morality of that union is linked to the love between the partners, Gnosticism proscribes sexual promiscuity which abolishes all love and authorizes spermatic communion. Even if at the beginning Basilides may have had the lofty ideal of the total adhesion of man to nature, of man's complete immersion in a sort of primitive and innocent ignorance whence all passion would be abolished, it is readily apparent that his less scrupulous disciples would have conserved only the simplest and grossest elements of that doctrine and that the sect would have degenerated progressively into immorality, going as far perhaps as establishing a spermatic cult (cf. Irenaeus *Adv. Haer.* I, 19).

Next (in *Strom.* III, ii), Clement calls to mind the sect of Carpocrates and his son Epiphanes. They preached total communism especially with regard to women: "God made all things for man to be common property. He brought female to be with male and in the same way united all animals. He thus showed righteousness to be a universal fairness and equality. But those who have been born in this way have denied the universality which is the corollary of their birth and say, 'Let him who has taken one woman keep her,' whereas all alike can have her, just as the other animals do."[32] Thus sexual desire is an original expression of God's will, and it is the Law, promulgated by the evil god of the Jews, which has disturbed the good order of things. According to Clement, the Carpocratians gathered together for sacred meals which ended in orgies; after the meal, ". . . they have intercourse where they will and with whom they will" (III, 2, PG 8, 112).

Against all these movements (he further cites the Nicolaitans, the disciples of Prodicos, the Antitactes), Clement opposes an all-encompassing refutation which has bearing on two points: the meaning of freedom and the religious justification for morality.

As to the meaning of freedom, the debate on the gnostic position is not new;[33] the claim of absolute freedom (which is measured by significant transgressions against moral laws) is illusory; it is nothing but a theoretical justification for the concrete enslavement to instinctive drives. "We have learnt to recognize as freedom that which the Lord alone confers on us when he liberates us from lusts and desires and other passion."[34]

As to the second point, the battle is against moral indifference that the Gnostic extols (since he believes himself to be already in the perfection brought by salvation); the most effective weapon for this battle is a theology of creation which on one hand challenges any dualism between Old and New Testament (evil creator-god of the Jews vs. the good-god of Jesus), and on the other hand assures the moral and theological value of natural law. We must pause to consider this point because its historical importance was so great in the future development of Christian morality. It was for pastoral and theological reasons that the first Christian theologians (especially Irenaeus and Clement of Alexandria) had recourse to the concept of natural law, because it seemed more effective than any other argument against Gnosticism. But in so doing they accepted a problematic attitude that was more stoic than biblical.[35] The concept of *nature* has three meanings for the Fathers at the end of the second century: a) a disposition is natural when inscribed in a process which is not contaminated by sin or by human error (for example, the sexual process is "natural" to the extent that it is analogous to the sowing of seed in a field); b) whatever animals do is "natural": here again is the conviction that the universal models that are useful to man can be found where man's sin is absent, i.e., in the animal kingdom; c) finally, nature is a structure belonging to the realm of the human body: we could say that the most evident function of a particular bodily organ is "natural" (the eye is made to see).[36] This recourse to stoic values sought to anchor morality in an objectivity no longer conferred by the Old Testament and disqualified by gnostic arguments. But instantly the accent was removed from the morality of a faithful and loving covenant between man and woman and placed upon a morality of objective principles (or so-claimed!) which ratified the dualism between spiritual love (agreed as belonging to the Christian vocation) and bodily, sexual love (excluded as not natural).

We can see how, in order to fight against the aberrations of certain gnostic propositions, Christian thinking made use of stoic arguments which allowed a defense of marriage, while meanwhile excluding bodily love and sexual desire. Clement declared that Christian law intended ". . . husbands to cohabit with their wives with self-control and only for the purpose of begetting children" (*Strom*. III, xi, 71); and that "to indulge in intercourse without intending children is to outrage nature" (*Paidagōgos* II, x, 95). As Noonan correctly remarks,[37] "in Clement this view was linked to his basic position that desire as such was evil. . . . It is the purposeful, non-desirous act of intercourse which he defends." Love is certainly not excluded between the partners, but it is a spiritual love which can really be expressed only by continence. "A man who marries for the sake of begetting children must practice continence so that it is not desire he feels for his wife, whom he ought to love . . ." (*Strom*. III, vii, 58). This kind of moderate asceticism[38] which Clement preaches concerning conjugal ethics is indicative of Christian ethics at the end of the second century; it is a question of defending the necessity for moral discipline without falling into the excesses of an asceticism that disdains the body, and thus disdains divine creation. The goal is to gain some distance from a society where the disregard for others is so often manifested in sexual license (slave-concubines, easy divorce, homosexuality, sodomy. . .), while simultaneously avoiding the creation of a Christian ghetto—but also to allow for the practice of an uncompromising morality. The ethical responsibility which the Christian has a duty to assume in and for the world must be taken even more seriously, since the world was created by God for all men so that they could enjoy His material and spiritual blessings. It is thus correct to take inspiration from what is best in the moral values of philosophers and sages who also fought against moral disorder and thus to enter resolutely into the mainstream of the moralizing on sexuality and marriage which was operative at this time in Roman society.[39]

We can see already why stoic ideas had such a great influence on Christian morality. There will be more than one opportunity of confirming that as we continue.

2. The Early Church and Conjugal Rights

The moral trend on this issue is similar to the Church's attitude toward the institution of marriage. Modern historians today by and large agree on the fact that early Christianity did not evidence any originality in the realm of laws, rites or customs concerning marriage. As the author of the *Letter to Diognetus* says: "They [Christians] marry like the rest of men and beget children, but they do not abandon the babies that are born."[40] Christians readily adopted Roman law and traditional pagan custom.[41] The celebration of marriage, as practiced in the Empire by Christians as well as by pagans, "was accompanied by various ceremonies . . . the later custom of . . . *usus* as a condition of matrimonial authority . . . disappeared in Imperial Rome. Marriages were concluded at this time without any form of law, and merely by mutual consent, though in traditional circles, this was supplemented by the ancient religious customs. The two concrete elements necessary to make the marriage valid were the *consensus,* or mutual consent of both partners, and the *domum-ductio,* or leading of the wife to her husband's house. The *domum-ductio* and the community of the partners, the *individua vitae consuetudo,* together formed, at least for those who were not slaves, a . . . valid and lawful marriage. . . . In the Christian era, stated Justinian finally, the mutual consent of both partners was sufficient for a valid marriage without any further formalities: *nuptias non concubitus, sed consensus facit;* in other words, marriage was not brought about by *usus,* or actual sexual intercourse, but by the partners' mutual consent."[42]

There is no such thing during this whole period as a "religious marriage." Marriage remains essentially a familial and earthly affair, even if it is acknowledged as a gift from God. Anything to do with marital rights comes from civil legislation. The concern of the Church in the matter is neither juridical nor liturgical, but pastoral: marriage between Christians must be protected from harmful pagan influence. That is the thrust of two texts which have sometimes been interpreted (incorrectly) as an indication that the Church intervened from the very beginning in matrimonial jurisdiction. Ignatius of Antioch requests that when "men and women marry the union should be made with the consent of the bishop, so that the marriage may be according to the Lord";[43] Tertullian speaks of "that marriage which the Church arranges, the Sacrifice (of the Eucharist) strengthens, upon which the blessing sets a seal, at which angels are present as witnesses, and to which the Father gives His consent. For not even on earth do children marry properly and legally without their fathers' permission."[44] However, in both cases, the goal is to call to mind the spiritual link between the wedded couple and the community, which alone can guard that marriage in its spiritual richness and authenticity. So then, there is here a pastoral and spiritual concern which seeks to suffuse the earthly affair of marriage with a Christian spirit, but there is no juridical concern whatsoever.

Of course, certain concrete problems were quickly raised, such as divorce, the remarriage of widowers and widows, and the sensitive question of "mixed marriage" with non-Christians. Paul had already dealt with these problems and the early Church would take its inspiration chiefly from his teachings.

Here are some examples that concern *divorce*.[45] We read in Hermas's *The Shepherd*: "'Sir,' I said, 'if a man has a wife who believes in the Lord and surprises her in adultery, does he commit sin if he lives with her?'—'Before he finds out,' he said, 'he does not. But, if her husband knows the sin, and she does not repent, but persists in her fornication, he becomes guilty of her sin, so long as he lives with her, and an accomplice in her adultery.'—'Sir,' I said, 'what then is he to do, if the wife continues in this passion?'—'Let him divorce her,' he said, 'and remain single. But, if he divorces her and marries another woman, he himself commits adultery.'—'But, if, sir,' I said, 'after the divorce the wife repents and wishes to return to her husband, will he refuse to receive her?'—'No, indeed,' he said, 'If the husband does not receive her, he sins. He incurs great sin. The sinner who has repented must be received. However, not often, for there is only one repentance for the servants of God. To bring about her repentance, then, the husband should not marry. This is the course of action required for husband and wife,'"[46] We can see how the question presented itself in the middle of the second century: divorce was authorized, and even recommended so that one should not take part in error. But, as in the scriptural tradition, remarriage was not authorized, so that the door to forgiveness and reconciliation could remain open.

The same motive authorizing divorce is found in Tertullian: "You will find him (Christ) also, in whichever direction you will, taking forethought regarding marriage: while he will not have it dissolved, he forbids separation: and while he will not have it continue under stain he permits divorce."[47] Thus, once the marriage tie has been severed by the adultery of one of the partners, divorce only ratifies an existing fact, and as such is legitimate and so allows for remarriage.

These two examples are interesting in that they clearly manifest the pastoral concern of theological reflection; there was a concern to safeguard the dignity of marriage, which adultery precisely destroys, and a desire that those who experience failure in conjugal life should not be crushed by legalism.

Another problem, remarriage for widowers, is commented upon by Hermas: "'Sir,' I said, 'If a wife or husband is deceased and either one of the survivors marries again, does he or she sin by marrying?'—'There is no sin,' he said. 'But, anyone who remains single achieves greater honor for himself and great glory before the Lord. But, even in remarriage, there is no sin.'"[48] He expresses a point of view that is to become traditional: remarriage is allowed, it does not constitute sin, but the widower who can remain in that state follows a better path, that of continence and chastity.

Finally the question of *mixed marriages* is equally preoccupying. In Paul's teaching (I Corinthians 7:12–17), the Fathers see an opportunity for the Christian member of the pair to be a witness. But, probably judging from the experience of many couples, they fear the risk and the problems involved; the non-Christian partner can hinder his mate (by his demands) from living out the requirements of faith. This tension becomes more and more vigorously described by authors, as shown in the following choice example from Tertullian: "Her duties to the Lord she certainly cannot fulfill according to the demands of ecclesiastical discipline, since she has by her side a servant of Satan who will act as an agent of his master in obstructing the performance of Christian duties and devotions. Thus, for example, if a station is to be kept, her husband will make an early appointment with her to go to the baths; if a fast is to be observed, her husband will, that very day, prepare a feast; if it be necessary to go out on an errand of Christian charity, never are duties at home more urgent! Who, indeed, would permit his wife to go about the streets to the houses of strangers, calling at every hovel in town in order to visit the brethren? Who would be pleased to permit his wife to be taken from his side, when she is obliged to be present at evening devotions?"[49]

In general, the Christians aligned their juridical conception and their practice of marriage with those of the Roman world. There is one point however, where their Christian convictions led them away from adherence to common laws: the *marriage of slaves.*[50] No right protects or recognizes the marriage of slaves. The union of two slaves is neither *connubium* (fully legal marriage) nor *matrimonium* (marriage in the general sense), but rather only a *contubernium* (intimate relationship, concubinage). With no legal guarantees whatsoever, slave couples were at the mercy of their masters' discretion.[51] Very quickly, it seems, the Church afforded aid and protection to Christian slave couples and recognized the validity of these unions in her eyes. Pope Calixtus (217–222) acknowledged as licit and honorable what would be called "marriages of conscience" which were contracted without the knowledge of the civil authorities but with the bishop's approval. These marriages particularly involved the union of a free woman with a slave. The Church stood as guarantor and witness to this marriage just as a family would have in the case of a legal marriage.

To conclude: up until the middle of the third century, the ethical thinking of Christians on marriage and sexuality was essentially in defensive reaction against the quasi-obsessive and aberrant practices of certain hyper-ascetic Christians or against libertines. In a reaction against the moral eschatology of the latter group, i.e., their affirmation of an already actualized salvation which authorized transgressions of the moral laws of this condemned world (which has already been transcended), the Fathers wished to root ethics in a theology of creation (which allowed the theological justification for recourse to natural law). They indeed defended marriage, but insofar as it was ordained by natural law for procreation. As for conjugal love, it was described as a chaste respect for one's partner, which was more threatened by sexual desire than expressed by it.

On the other hand, the formal and juridical aspect of the problem was never really approached: the Christians essentially adopted the laws and customs of the Roman world.

3. The "Yes, but" of the Great Patristic Tradition in Regard to Marriage and Sexuality (Fourth and Fifth Centuries)

The most systematic thinking of the great moral theologians of the fourth and fifth centuries (Gregory of Nyssa, John Chrysostom, Ambrose, Jerome, Augustine) leads to two conclusions which will mark the Christian morality of marriage and sexuality for many centuries: 1) sexuality is completely separate from love; it is aligned with sin with which it secretly connives; 2) virginity is superior to marriage since the latter continually threatens to turn one away from God.

Let us examine these two affirmations more closely.

Ambrose writes: "For now (since the fall), although marriage is good, it includes something that makes even married people blush at themselves."[52] This quotation is typical: it affirms the goodness of marriage, but with some reservations, since marriage implies sexuality (which is felt to be shameful).

This feeling of shame which accompanies sexuality can be observed in Augustine's statement: "... in all united pairs ... there has been a permanent necessity of avoiding the sight of man in any work of this kind (sexual intercourse), and thus acknowledging what caused inevitable shame, though a good thing would certainly cause no man to be ashamed."[53] To interpret the private, secret and intimate character of human sexuality by the single category of shame reveals the inability in patristic thought of conferring positive value on sexuality (other than procreation).

The subject of shame is explained by Augustine in a very interesting way: "The undeniable truth is that a man by his very nature is ashamed of sexual lust.[54] And he is rightly ashamed because there is here involved an inward rebellion which is a standing proof of the penalty which man is paying for his original rebellion against God. For, lust is a usurper, defying the power of the will and playing the tyrant with man's sexual organs. It is here that man's punishment particularly and most properly appears, because these are the organs by which that nature is reproduced which was so changed for the worse by its first great sin."[55] What causes shame is the discovery of the irrational power of the libido, which challenges the rational and free-will ideal of the self. If all of man's dignity lies in this rational capacity, one can only fear and repel this disturbing force: "Such lust does not merely invade the whole body and outward members; it takes such complete and passionate possession of the whole man, both physically and emotionally, that what results is the keenest of all pleasures on the level of sensation; and at the crisis of excitement, it practically paralyzes all power (*acies*) of deliberate thought (*quasi-vigilia cogitationis*)."[56] It is clear that for the Fathers, this kind of loss of self in the sexual act was felt to be a humiliation and therefore was a denunciation of the secret complicity between sexuality and sin—the latter being interpreted as revolt, disorder, irrationality. From this vantage point, it is not surprising to read this sentence from the great thinker of the West: "I have decided that there is nothing I should avoid so much as marriage. I know nothing which brings the manly mind down from the height more than a woman's caresses and that joining of bodies without which one cannot have a wife."[57]

Sexuality is evidently so linked to sin that the question of how to avoid its culpability takes on more and more interest! And naturally, we find arguments, which have been defended by tradition until now, on the value of procreation. But the perspective has changed slightly: where the theologians of the third century defended procreation in order to defend the theology of creation, now the Fathers of the fourth century see procreation as the excuse for exercising sexuality. As Jerome said, "The activities of marriage itself, if they are not modest and do not take place under the eyes of God as it were, so that the only intention is children, are filth and lust."[58]

This excuse becme more and more relative, especially with the eastern theologians, who under Origen's influence, came to consider marriage and sexuality as consequences of original sin. But how can the texts in *Genesis* which state the contrary and affirm that God created man "male and female," thus as sexual beings, from the beginning be explained? Here is Theodoret's answer: "Foreseeing and foreknowing that Adam would be liable to death because of the violation of the command, He already fashioned a nature of this kind beforehand, and formed it into a male and female body. The reason, of course, was that this is the design of bodies that are mortal and need the procreation of children to conserve the race."[59] By this kind of exegetical sleight of hand, the principal notion in *Genesis* of the goodness of sexuality—the notion that it was given by God to man and to woman so that they could learn to recognize the call of God's own love—was swept aside completely.

In this patristic perspective, God desired, in creating man and woman, that they should live as angels, in virginity and chastity.[60]

If challenged, the theologians, at least the western theologians, would not say that sexuality is sin, but they would indeed emphasize its connection to sin—the signs being sexual desire, irrational instinct and pleasure. Had there been no sin, sexuality would have been pure love, free from all desire whatsoever. Sexuality would have existed—and on this point, western Augustinian theology differs from eastern theology (cf. above)—but it would have existed without libido; it would have been a sign of differentiation calling for a relationship that was purely voluntary and without concupiscence. Augustine attempted to describe it: "'Increase and multiply and fill the earth.' Although it seems that this could not happen without the intercourse of a man and woman . . . still we may say that in mortal bodies there could have been another process in which, by the mere emotion of pious charity, with no concupiscence, that sign of corruption, children would be born."[61] "Who denies that marriage would have existed even if sin had not preceded it? But it was to have existed so that the reproductive members would be moved by the will, like the other members, not aroused by lust; or (not to burden you with sorrow about lust) they would not have been aroused by lust such as now exists, but by lust obedient to the will."[62]

Such a devaluation of sexuality must necessarily be accompanied by an exaltation of virginity. And this is the second line of thought in patristic teaching. As we have seen when discussing Clement of Alexandria, this element is already quite present in the Church of the second and third centuries[63] under deviant forms that Clement had to fight against.

However, it is especially in the fourth century that Christian theology develops systematic thinking on the value and dignity of virginity. A whole series of writings comes forth on this theme,[64] which aims at eulogizing virginity.

Virginity makes one divine, or as John Chrysostom says, it makes "mortals like unto angels." In the words of Ambrose, "A virgin marries God."

To better understand the rationale for this glorification of virginity, let us take the example of Gregory of Nyssa and his *Treatise on Virginity*.[65] Written in 371 by a man who, according to his own memoirs (cf. 3:1, 5–15) was himself married (even at the time of his bishopric), this treatise is very representative of the manner in which the Fathers of the fourth century approached these questions.

Gregory proposes first that virginity is a perfection that belongs to divine and incorporeal nature: "Virginity is exceptional and peculiar to the incorporeal nature, and, through the kindness of God, it has been granted to those whose life has been allotted through flesh and blood, in order that it may set human nature upright once more after it has been cast down by its passionate disposition, and guide it . . . to a contemplation of the things on high" (II, ii, 5–10). For "purity alone is sufficient for receiving the presence and entrance of God" (II, ii, 12). On the other hand, marriage is the proper state for those who cannot renounce passion: "However, the one who is stupid looks downwards and hands his soul over to the pleasures of the body . . . being alienated from the life of God . . . considering nothing else to be good than pleasing the body" (IV, v, l ff.). The "intelligible and immaterial contemplation of the beautiful" (V, 19) is incompatible with a subjection to "the afflictions that accompany mankind" (IV, viii, 9). Certainly, marriage as such is not to be condemned, but it does become a risk for those who are in that state, i.e., the risk of forgetting the spiritual because of sensual pleasure (*hèdonè*) (IV, v, 7) and of being dragged along by nature (IV, v, 8). Moreover, marriage "was contrived as a consolation for death" (XII, iv, 23); it is thus a consequence of sin, a lesser evil which collaborates in the end with the reign of death because it constantly furnishes that kingdom with new occasions for triumph (XIV, 2).

On the other hand, virginity "is stronger than death (by promising a spiritual fruitfulness which escapes death)" (XIV, 3). He who practices virginity "reaps the choicest goods in the resurrection and in the present life. For if the life which is promised to the just by the Lord after the resurrection is similar to that of angels—and release from marriage is a peculiar characteristic of the angelic nature—he has already received some of the beauties of the promise..." (XIV, iv, 13–18).

Of course one must practice the virtue in a temperate way, nor should one believe that avoiding shameful pleasures automatically safeguards a person from the attraction of the more subtle pleasures of honor or power (XVII, i, 1). With great finesse, Gregory warns against the danger demonstrated by those "who, by reason of much fighting against pleasures, are somehow easily overcome by an opposite kind of weakness and spend their lives in grievances and irritations and malice..." (XVII, i, 9–12). And there is always the fact that "... if you are longing for God to appear to you, why do you not listen to Moses who ordered the people to abstain from (the privileges of) marriage in order to be present at the appearance of God?" (XXIII, vii, 36–39). To see God, one must be chaste and pure.

As we can see, the word "virginity" has a very broad meaning: *parthénia* means the uprightness of a body consecrated to God; absolute continence; exclusion of all moral error; virtuous life considered in its totality; the fullness of divine life communicated to man; a state of life in contrast to normal life; finally, one of God's own perfections. The warnings of Gregory against those who are excessive and who in the last analysis show themselves to be more obsessed with their bodies than freed from its needs, demonstrate clearly that, for him, virginity is altogether different from sexual abstinence alone; it's a whole way of life centered on seeking God. But, since sexuality is linked to passion, to the body, to pleasure (all negative terms), it is an obstacle to the contemplation of God. It must be renounced because it drags man downward, toward the material and the temporal. For isn't it linked to death, being "life in the flesh which death normally follows upon?" (XIII, 3). For this reason, one should choose virginity, which is love for eternal and spiritual things, which uproots passion for carnal things; it is a quest for the incorruptible, an angelic life. It is a way of anticipating even here and now heavenly divine life. It is also a way of reversing the movement of Adam's sin—Adam, who was condemned to sexuality after his disobedience.

This kind of exaltation of virginity (while disqualifying marriage and sexuality) is classic in most of the texts cited above. The only exception, it seems to me, is in the *Symposium* by Methodius[66] where virginity is presented less as a return to the lost paradisiac state than as an ultimate step in the evolution of humanity according to God's plan: "It was a most extraordinary disposition that the plant of virginity was sent down to mankind from heaven. Hence too, it was not revealed to the first generation" (I, ii, 16). "To begin with, they were to advance from brother-sister unions to marriage with wives from other families. Then they were to give up practicing, like brute beasts, multiple marriage (as though men were born merely for intercourse!). The next step was to take them from adultery; and the next to advance them to continence, and from continence to virginity...." (I, ii, 18).

This extraordinary (and very modern!) way of describing the progressive moralization of mankind does not devalue marriage since it is a step on the road to the highest morality; it is not, then, a result of the fall. And this viewpoint allows Methodius in a treatise exalting virginity, to describe the force and complexity of sexuality without seeking to disqualify it: "... this was perhaps the symbolism of that ecstatic sleep into which God put the first man, that it was to be a type of man's enchantment in love, when in his thirst for children he falls into a trance, lulled to sleep by the pleasures of procreation, in order that a new person, as I have said, might be formed in turn from the material that is drawn from his flesh and bone. For under the stimulation of intercourse, the body's harmony... is greatly disturbed, and all the marrow-like generative part of the blood, which is liquid bone, gathers from all parts of the body, curdled and worked into a foam, and then rushes through the generative organs into the living soil of the woman" (II, ii, 31 ff). And thus, one could write an apology for virginity—which is the thrust of the second discourse (cf. 7:49)—without necessarily disqualifying the material, corporeal and sexual world.

But this text, so vitally interesting because of its scientific imagination, is isolated. Gregory's position is the classic stance. We need not number the patristic texts which heavily insist on the inferiority of marriage while glorifying virginity. One main argument, which was already mentioned by Gregory, reappears constantly: marriage turns one away from God. The next four examples prove the point.

First of all, Jerome: "Do you think that it is one and the same thing to spend days and nights in prayer and fastings, and to paint the face in anticipation of the arrival of a husband, to break step, to feign flattery? . . . Add to this the prattling of infants, the noisy clamoring of the whole household, the clinging of children to her neck, the computing of expenses, the preparing of budgets. Then there is the pounding of meats by a busy band of cooks; there is the chattering of a crowd of women weavers. In the meantime, she is told that her husband has arrived with friends. Like a swallow, she flies over the entire interior of the house, to see if the couch is properly arranged, if the floors have been swept, if the drinking bowls have been set in order, if the dinner has been prepared. Tell me, I ask you, where is there an opportunity to think of God in the midst of all this?"[67]

This pessimism (or realism) about marriage is common. Augustine says: ". . . nothing seems more certain to me than that he was unwilling to reveal and explain in words that same tribulation of the flesh which he had predicted for those who chose marriage, in the suspicions of marital jealousy, in the bearing and the raising of children, in the fears and anguish of bereavement. For, what man is there who, when he has bound himself by the bonds of wedlock, is not torn and harrassed by these emotions?"[68] The same echo, the same description is found in John Chrysostom: "It is an evil thing to wed a very poor wife, or a very rich one; for the former is injurious to the husband's means, the latter to his authority and independence. It is a grievous thing to have children, still more grievous not to have any; for in the latter case marriage has been to no purpose, in the former a bitter bondage has to be undergone. If a child is sick, it is the occasion of no small fear; if he dies an untimely death there is inconsolable grief; and at every stage of growth there are various anxieties on their account, and many fears and toils. . . . Is this then life, Theodore, when one's soul is distracted in so many directions, when a man has to serve so many, to live for so many, and never for himself?"[69] One should note in passing the high esteem John Chrysostom has for the woman whose only "usefulness" is to provide a lineage for her husband; the conjugal bond, already quite arduous, has no other meaning!

Ambrose sees the cares and the trials of marriage which turn one from God already symbolized in the sleep Adam was put into by God when He took one of his ribs to fashion Eve: "What does the phrase 'deep sleep' signify? Does it not mean that when we contemplate a conjugal union we seem to be turning our eyes gradually (away from) the direction of God's kingdom? Do we not seem as we enter into a vision of this world, to partake a little of things divine, while we find our repose in the midst of what is secular and mundane?"[70] The encounter between man and woman is no longer compared to the love of Christ for His Church, as in the scriptural tradition (cf. Ephesians 5), but interpreted as the occasion of allowing oneself to be turned away from God, the one relationship which truly fulfills human destiny. Whereas the Scripture made of the male/female relationship a privileged place of experiencing otherness, and consequently, the sign of the human vocation to relationship with God, the Fathers, on the other hand, insist on the spiritual dangers in the male/female relationship, which tie man down to his material body and to temporal cares.

From this point on, what could possibly excuse, let alone justify, marriage? "Procreation and the education of the children are obviously the first excuse (and for many the only valid one).

A concern to avoid even worse sexual impurity (adultery, fornication, etc.) or the fear of disrupting the fidelity which is indispensable to the survival of the marital institution are equally valid excuses: these are the three 'goods' of marriage. More precisely, the evil that would come if these three goods were destroyed justify exercising sexuality, which is indispensable in their service; in brief, the lesser of two evils must be chosen."[71] Sexual practice is excused, although it nonetheless is an admission of spiritual weakness (if not error) because it is required for the procreation of children and for maintenance of marital fidelity. But, things become pushed to this point: "The wife will be saved if she engenders children who will remain virgins, i.e., if that which she has lost (virginity) is regained through her progeny, if the fall and corruption affixed to the root (of sex) is compensated for by the flower and the fruit."[72] This astonishing passage unabashedly avers that sexuality is so sinful that even procreation does not sufficiently excuse it and that the children who have been conceived must in some way expiate for the fault of the parents by themselves renouncing any practice of sexuality!

Such a perspective immediately risks heading into deviant forms of asceticism that lead closer to Gnosticism and Encraticism than to Christianity. But doesn't the exaltation of virginity risk leading, on the theological level, to disdain for the creation of God, and on the pastoral level, to the formation of an elite kind of Christianity that is cut off from the people? Augustine saw precisely these problems in his debate with the Manicheans.[73] If sexuality is condemned as sin, there can be no response to the attacks of the Manicheans against the theology of creation which is delineated by the Old Testament. The "be fruitful and multiply" of Genesis 1:28 must be upheld against the radical pessimism of the Manicheans. But to do that, any disdain of sexuality must necessarily cease; or, rather, it must be demonstrated that sexuality is linked, because of procreation, to the creative act of God Himself. This is a repetition of Clement's debate with the Gnostics. Like the Gnostics, the Manicheans scorned sexuality precisely because it had a procreative function; they urged those who could not altogether abstain, to at least avoid procreation, since it subjects a soul to the domination by matter: ". . . the unrighteous law of the Manicheans, in order to prevent their god, whom they bewail as confined in all seeds, from suffering still closer confinement in the womb, requires married people not on any account to have children—their great desire being to liberate their god."[74] It must be remembered that ". . . eternal law—that is, the will of God the Creator of all—for the preservation of the natural order, permits the indulgence of bodily appetite under the guidance of reason in sexual intercourse, not for the gratification of passion, but for the continuance of the race through the procreation of children."[75] Thus to preserve the theological value of sexuality, which is linked to the recognition of the value of creation, its procreative function is unilaterally emphasized, and that even more since the Gnostic and Manichean opponents devalue this function and seem to justify sexuality sometimes only by the satisfaction of desire. Everything, then, conspires to narrowly link sexuality to procreation in the discussion of Christian ethics.

Exaltation of virginity and a condescending acceptance of marriage (justified by procreation): these are the two fundamental thrusts in patristic teaching which will mark Christian practice and thought for many centuries. Eusebius of Cesarea summarizes it quite well: "Two states of life have been established in the Church of Christ, one of which is actually superior and goes beyond the normal capacity of man. . . . The other . . . permits a modest use of marriage and procreation of children."[76]

Why was the theological reflection in the early Church incapable of maintaining itself within the perspective of scriptural tradition? Why was sexuality never thought of in terms of tenderness or love? Why was marriage never described as the privileged locus of an existential experience of God's love? For, as we have seen, these very issues incorporate the sense and the meaning of the scriptural teaching on this area.

In order to answer these questions, a distinction must be made between what could be called the *external causes* of the patristic evolution—essentially, the influence of the ideology of ancient society on Christianity—and the *internal causes*—the interpretation of the gospel in theological (and particularly eschatological) categories that were insufficiently criticised.

The External Causes

The influence of ancient society on Christianity is evidenced in at least four areas. The first is that of customs. In a clear reaction against a social setting where the breakdown of traditional societies had encouraged a great relaxation of moral standards (particularly in the sexual domain) and where consequently Christian authors constantly emphasized that the weak—the "little ones," i.e. the children, slaves, women, were being sacrificed to the covetousness of the strong, the "great ones," Christianity defended the necessity of a moral discipline. The apparent "puritanism" of the early Christians is best understood as a reaction against a world where sexual practice was effectively often lived out in the mode of "murderous" violence. In this kind of atmosphere, the "test of procreative intentions seemed to many Christians, as it had to the pagan Stoics and to Jewish thinkers like Philo, the measure by which sexual promiscuity might be rationally criticized."[77] It should be repeated that this "puritan" reaction occurred not only on the part of Christians but also on the part of a whole strata of society at the turn of the second century. Christianity certainly reinforced this current of thought but it in no way created it. Having become the major religion, it allowed its extension to the whole population, uniting in one common development of morality both the aristocrats' need for respectability and the sexual conservatism of plebeian milieus.[78]

Thus, the moral context made even the possibility of thinking of sexuality in terms of affection and love quite difficult for the Christians. The *juridical* status of marriage, governed by Roman law, accentuated the difficulty; Roman law had established the procreation of children as the only goal of marriage—whence the custom at the end of a wedding for the father to read a declaration calling to mind that the engaged couple are marrying *liberorum procreandum causa* (in order to procreate children). There is no mention in the law, nor in customs, of the value of the affective bond which unites the pair, or of the reality of communion within the marital bond. On the juridical level, the marital institution leaves no room for love; it is essentially defined as a contract. As we have seen, the Christians had readily accepted this juridical situation; here again, the social influence greatly affected Christian thought and practice.

But even more central, I believe, is the influence of ancient man's *mentality*. Even if a critique of that mentality appears here and there among the theologians, as we will see further on, it is itself determined by the categories of ancient thought. This thought is marked especially in the first centuries of the Christian era, by a deep pessimism, clearly revealed in philosophical and religious thinking.[79] Thus the Stoic seeks to abolish his temporary character: "The essential part of man is the Logos, and the Logos is timeless. So the Stoic concentrates exclusively upon his Logos-being, thus rising superior to all obligations and denying himself any future. But in this repudiation of the future, he deprives the present and the past of their temporal character as well."[80] In a denial of temporality, salvation comes from making man equivalent to the divine law that is immanent in the universe. It is a negative ethic, where liberty consists in freeing oneself from whatever turns one aside from this equivalence where man saves himself by denying himself. We could certainly consider Stoicism as the most positive attempt at handling the deep pessimism of ancient man in some way, for its fruits are incontestable. But it structures itself completely into a framework where man perceives (and even feels) himself to be an exile in the world, a stranger to himself, having come from somewhere that is now forgotten, but for which he is nostalgic. The mystery religions, Gnosticism, popular astral religions, each express it in their own way; human destiny is a source of anguish, for man knows that he is the victim of strange forces, exterior and interior, that dominate him.

Even if Christianity reacted strongly against this tragic dualism by affirming the value and goodness of divine creation, it also at the same time quite "naturally" admitted that contingency and temporality could not express the divine.[81] Thus the contingency of marital existence cannot truly signify man's call to the divine, the spiritual, the eternal. As for sexuality, which is evidently a sign of our temporality in its irregularity, its instinctive force, its brutality, it is even more surely excluded from the "noble" part of man. This perspective prohibits ever discovering its humanizing value. The best people will renounce it; as for the others, let them consent to it only in order to avoid even greater disorder.

On another level, Christianity was not able to question one of the most significant points of Indo-European culture, i.e. the juxtaposition of marriage and passion-love. This subject has been admirably researched by Marcel Detienne[82] who shows that the mythic opposition of Adonis and Demeter actually evokes the opposition of amorous seduction and marriage. He shows in particular how society, by means of aromatic spices seeks to arouse passionate love at wedding time, but how, except for this brief time, society considers it antithetical to marriage. We can ask, along with J. L. Flandrin[83] whether or not this paradox constitutes a real social prohibition that aims at discouraging any spiritual and affective intimacy between the spouses which could threaten social unity and cohesion. The early Christians shared this conviction, even to the point of no longer hearing the radical biblical contestation of it.[84]

Finally we must reemphasize the considerable importance of the influence of *Stoicism* on the Christian *ethical discourse*.[85] Not only did the Christians find a very elaborate and lofty ethical system in the Stoics, they also shared with them the same criticism of current sexual customs. The theologicians, in their battle against the Gnostics, borrowed the concept of natural law from the Stoics, which allowed them to define an objective moral standard, as well as to give themselves a principle for an ethical interpretation of the theology of Creation. Furthermore, Stoicism had some reflections on the meaning and value of the couple that were already developed. It insisted on the quasi-biological unity of the man and woman,[86] all while affirming the social value of fidelity.[87] But Christianity also inherited from Stoicism its distrust of the imagination and of passion, both of which upset the equilibrium of the sage.[88] Pleasure is an enemy because it links one to ephemeral and deceptive things, and therefore one must maintain detachment even in affective relationship: "How, then, shall I become affectionate?—As a man of noble spirit, as one who is fortunate; for it is against all reason to be abject, or broken in spirit, or to depend on something other than yourself; or even to blame either God or man. I would have you become affectionate in such a way as to maintain at the same time all these rules; if, however, by virtue of this natural affection, whatever it is you call by that name, you are going to be a slave and miserable, it does not profit you to be affectionate."[89]

If tender affection can be considered weakness, how much more should one indeed guard against sexual desire! This is why one must be careful about love. "Any love for another's wife is scandalous; likewise too much love for one's spouse is adultery. The wise man should love his wife with his head (with discernment, *iudicis*), not with his heart (not with affection, *non affectu*). He should control his passions and not let himself be dragged along into intercourse. Nothing is more impure (*foedius*) than to love one's wife like a mistress. Surely those who claim to unite themselves to their wives to beget children for the good of the State or for the human race should at least imitate the animals and once their wives are pregnant, not destroy the offspring. Let them approach their wives as husbands and not as lovers." This surprising passage from Seneca has come down to us only through Jerome's respectful quoting of it. He precedes this quote with one from Sextus the Pythagorian[90] whose original text he corrects: "An adulterer is also he who is shamelessly immodest with his own wife." This quote becomes a formula that is closer to Seneca: "An adulterer is one who too passionately loves his wife."[91] This sentence will often be quoted, with complete approval, by Christian moralists up until the time of Gratian and Peter Lombard. We find an almost identical version of the saying in Augustine: "For he who is intemperate in marriage, what is he but the adulterer of his own wife."[92]

"The conclusion is inescapable. Christian moralists owe a large debt to philosophy, especially stoic philosophy . . . in the moral domain its influence (stoic philosophy) is primary and can be clearly discerned. Stoicism furnished Christianity with a series of concepts and theories; it dictated—even in the wording—its practical morality. These concepts are sometimes adapted or transposed, but Stoicism is everywhere discernable, and its overall place during the first centuries of the Church is very significant in all the questions that concern man."[93]

There is no doubt that these external causes carried significant weight in the evolution and development of Christian ethics. However, it is clear that they had that influence only because they were in fundamental agreement with Christianity itself. This point should be elaborated.

The Internal Causes

In the gospel there is a twofold manner of presenting the kingdom of God and of calling for its acceptance: on one hand, it is the presence of another world which can neither be perceived nor received without leaving one's own way of life behind; on the other hand, it is presented as the way which God, through Christ, and next through His disciples, takes to penetrate reality and "act" on it from within in order to bring about its ultimate fulfillment. These two elements—a break (or separation from the world) and the taking hold of present reality—are in the gospel. The whole issue consists in maintaining this twofold requirement and of understanding the reasons for it. The temptation is always to present only one of these aspects. Thus, if the accent is placed upon the break (with the world) the immediate consequence is that this world becomes a place of exile; if, on the contrary, the emphasis is unilaterally placed upon the responsibility of taking a firm hold of things here, the consequence is that any challenge or criticism about the way in which this responsibility is exercised is posited as proceeding from an evil intention. In the first case, the other world is posited as the real world, a someplace else; but then there is no longer any possibility of concretely signifying the reality of this world. The Kingdom becomes unutterable, inexpressible except through a dream, utopia, or wordless cry. In the second case, one leaves behind the eschatological and critical perspective of the Kingdom when applying oneself to a task or project and risks having it marked by covetousness more than by responsibility.

The question, then, revolves around the meaning of Christian eschatology. As the horizon of this world, simultaneously the goal or end of all accomplishments and the reversal of judgment, eschatology has bearing on all personal and social existence. If it calls for a separation, it is with the idea of recapturing the plan of God for man in its essence, as already attested to in the history of men.

How did the early Church understand and experience this eschatological tension? It certainly had a vivid consciousness that it was a witness to ancient society of another way of living. Although the primitive Church united concrete morality and spiritual reference, and called for moral discipline but only so that it would be a sign of submission to the requirement of love, i.e. an indication of willingness to incarnate the love of God here and now, the early Church instead progressively dissociated the two streams of morality[94] and spirituality. The battle against the gnostic movements played an important role in this. Because the Gnostics wanted to live an "already-realized-eschatology," and manifested that by transgressing common moral laws, it was necessary to insist on responsibility with regard to morality, i.e. to insist on discipline which is the refusal of disorder, and on facing concrete reality. All at once, the eschatological accent on separation was displaced onto the side of spirituality only; it is through spiritual life, as opposed to sensual or corporeal life, that the Christian can enjoy a real apprehension of the divine world, and can participate here and now in the eschatological work of beatitude.

The willingness to break (with the world) did not remain on the ethical level, but manifested itself more strongly than ever on the spiritual level. Morality, in reaction to the aberrations of certain Gnostics, became conformist and aligned itself with the highest values of the ethics of the Stoics. There was no doubt a desire in this on the part of the Church to be recognized and accepted by society, and not to appear as a destructive social factor. But all this took place as though eschatology was of no consequence whatsoever to morality, that it really was only a promise of another world, celestial and eternal, which man could only participate in down here by contemplation and prayer. Morality, then, remains entirely in the realm of this present world and is not in any way qualified by the *eschaton* of the Kingdom. Man connects with this *eschaton* by spirituality, and not by morality.[95] Morality belongs to provisional, contingent reality and is only needed to make a space for man which is sheltered from passions and wicked desires, so that man can devote himself to the only thing that's important: God. In this realm of contingent reality, everything can be regulated by reference to natural laws without ever suspecting that such laws might be cultural rather than natural, i.e. that they signify in reality a fixed social order.

This eschatological reference afforded no criticism of the type of society that existed in the Empire; on the contrary, it led the Church on many points to reinforce the dominant ideology of ancient society. In fact, by presenting itself as the voice of the other (eternal and celestial) world, Christian eschatology, as proclaimed by the Church, called for a separation indeed, but a purely spiritual separation, like the quest for the long-lost real world, which this one only shadows and reflects. The gospel, meanwhile, was speaking of another kind of separation—one which concerned the mode of relationship a man had with himself, with others, with the world, and with God. As Christ had lived it, it was accomplished by a critique of social ideology (religious in that case) and it proposed to the disciples another mode of community life, founded on other values. This critical dealing with reality was not imitated with the same enthusiasm in the following centuries. Why not? Essentially, I repeat, because of a misunderstanding of biblical eschatology. This misunderstanding was the source of a double morality in the Church, illustrated by its stand on virginity and marriage: there are those who can, through asceticism, anticipate the other world more directly and clearly and there are those who content themselves, due to a lack of spirituality, with general morality, described mostly in negative terms.

But the paradox is really only an apparent one: the groups with the strongest will to break with the "world" (for example, the anchorite movement and the first monastic communities) are in fact the very ones who reinforced the contemporary dominant ideology the most. They did so on two decisive counts: whereas Christ had proclaimed the possibility of new relationships between men and women because of the Kingdom, Christian asceticism reinforced the ancient disregard for women; whereas the Gospels and Paul had presented a new understanding to the Christians of their bodies, a new way of living, this same Christian asceticism tended to devalue, along with all ancient thinking, the corporal by juxtaposing it to the spiritual.

In a discussion of the first point, it is easy to verify the good intention of the Church when it uncritically adopted the dominant ideology of the age, even though the gospel gave it the means for a critique—I am referring to society's disdain for women.[96]

It is not necessary to recall at length the rigid subordination of woman to man in ancient society, Greek as well as Jewish. "It's a truism to say that man in Greek culture congratulated himself for being born human and not animal, man and not woman, Greek and not barbarian."[97] The same concept is found in Judaism: it is taken up by the liturgy of the synagogue and three times daily the Jew thanks God for not having made him a Gentile, a woman, or a slave.[98] Given this state of affairs, we can measure the revolutionary character of Paul's affirmation in Galatians 3:28: "There is neither Jew nor Greek, there is neither slave nor free, there is neither male nor female, for you are all one in Christ Jesus." This affirmation of the principle of equality, which did have some practical consequences in the first years of the Church's existence,[99] was never forgotten in following centuries; however, it remained for the most part an affirmation of principle, sufficiently there to oblige the Fathers to multiply explanations and interpretations which justified (sometimes in bad faith) the marginal position of woman in society; but it never brought the principle of the subordination of the woman into question.

When Augustine recalls that, according to Genesis, "human nature itself, which is complete in both sexes, has been made to the image of God, and he does not exclude the woman from being understood as the image of God,"[100] he openly affirms the dignity of woman before God, but he draws no social consequences from it that would modify woman's status. As Jean-Marie Aubert says, "we can summarize this traditional concept of woman by the words *equality* and *subordination*: equality in God's eyes and in terms of the possibility of perfection; subordination to man in terms of temporal, earthly work down here."[101] Such a separation between theological thinking and social practice is proof of the misunderstanding of eschatological meaning that was discussed above: there is no attempt to orient reality toward the eschatological kingdom, or to transform it with a view to fulfilling the sense of divine creation, but instead two separate worlds are postulated. In one, man and woman are fully equal, and in the other woman is entirely subordinated to man.

The influence of such a mentality could exercise itself without restraint since the critical function of the gospel was reserved purely for inner spirituality. Something of the gospel, of course, would cross over into Christian practice;[102] but in the end, the most influential thing for the longest time would be the theological justifications (although it would be better to call them ideological) which the Fathers multiplied in ratification of social reality, i.e. society's disdain for women. This disregard is translated into a refusal of the otherness of woman: the way in which she is different (sex, weakness, sensitivity) is exactly what is disqualified by the Fathers. And so for Augustine, only the masculine is specifically human; woman participates in being human only by having a soul. But she is definitely inferior in regard to her body—which is how the second account of creation (Genesis 2) is to be understood, where the distinction is made that man is created first and in the image of God whereas woman is created second and comes from the man.[103] With this kind of mentality, Christian theology showed itself incapable of going beyond the level of ideological justifications on this point;[104] it took up instead the most traditional interpretations, like, for example, that of the Jewish philosopher Philo: "For progress is indeed nothing else than the giving up of the female gender by changing into the male, since the female gender is material, passive, corporeal, and sense-perceptible, while the male is active, rational, incorporeal and more akin to mind and thought."[105]

Thus in spite of continual affirmations of principle, the Fathers of early Christianity did not acknowledge the otherness of the woman. The disqualification of feminine sexuality by patristic theology is indicative of this misunderstanding. Tertullian, for example, reduces the role of woman in procreation to that of a field which receives seed sown: "she brings neither sperm nor pneuma, nor substance for the embryo, but only nourishment for it, whereas the man produces pneuma and substance."[106] Man alone, then, is the source of the embryo, and he transmits the soul along with the flesh. "Finally . . . is it not a fact that in the moment of orgasm, when the generative fluid is ejected, do we not feel that we have parted with a portion of our soul? As a result, do we not feel weak and faint, along with a blurring of our sights? This, then, must be the seed of the soul which proceeds from the dripping of the soul, just as the fluid which carries the bodily seed is a species of droppings from the body."[107]

A similar theory is found in Clement of Alexandria.[108]

The man thus furnishes all that is necessary to constitute a new being; the woman only receives the seed and nourishes it. Thus even in the area of generation, the woman is still dependent on man and subordinated to his creative force. Woman creates nothing, but receives everything, her role being only to bear the fruit of what she has received from the man.[109]

Consequently, anything that indicates active sexuality on the part of the woman appears as an abnormal and dangerous phenomenon. Once the woman does not accept being reduced to submissive passivity, she becomes a threat. Her apparent weakness covers up dangerous and mysterious powers which fascinate man and cause him to lose control and reason.[110] "Hurtful are women, my children; because, since they have no power or strength over the man, they act subtly through outward guise how they may draw him to themselves; and whom they cannot overcome (they draw) by craft."[111]

The only thing that remains to be done is to convince woman to accept the disqualification of her sexual otherness, to propose consecrated virginity as the best means of being liberated from submission to the man. Ambrose of Milan will use this argument frequently, which consists of denigrating marriage to cause virginity to appear as a liberation for the woman. Of course, from a certain point of view that was not false, but it is revealing that the Fathers presented liberation to the woman by her acceptance of that which denied her womanhood, in the rejection of what really seemed like an inexplicable otherness in the eyes of the Fathers.[112]

If woman hides that which designates her otherness in the eyes of man (cf. for example the importance in the Fathers of the discourse on modesty of conduct in women and the dangers of coquetry[113]), then could she perhaps be forgiven for being a woman; by denying herself she could attain a certain kind of recognition, entirely determined by her rapport with man.

In a certain way, a call for consecrated virginity affords, through the detour of a negation of sexuality, the discovery of something in the evangelical affirmation on the equality of man and woman in the presence of the Kingdom of God. It is a sure proof that Christ's and Paul's teachings have not been forgotten, but actually it succeeds in making the most of that teaching only by accentuating the subordination of the woman to masculine models of ancient society. In order to escape rigorous submission to man, as was the case in marriage, woman must accept and interiorize a totally androcentric vision of herself!

It seems established, then, that the disdain for woman is closely linked to an incapacity to conceive of sexuality in terms of positive value. Anything that recalls sexuality is by that fact disqualified; insofar as she has sexuality woman is disqualified. But keeping in mind the gospel teaching where there is no value differentiation between men and women, a second trend appears, parallel to the first, which exalts the countervalues of the woman. Over against Eve—the tempting seductress by whom man loses himself in losing his liberty, his authority, his reason—Mary, virgin and mother, is raised up, symbol of unsexed love, of a gentle love that is wholly spiritual which no contingency threatens. The ground is now laid for the birth and development of the typical stand on woman in our western society, the stand which will be repeated throughout the Middle Ages under diverse forms: seductress or inspiration, Eve or Mary, a double image of the one same desire which bespeaks both the search for affectionate love and the impossibility of linking it to sexuality, because desire is firmly rooted in flesh.

The elements of the twofold stance, disdaining and exalting the woman, are easily seen in the Fathers of the fourth century. It is clear that this position reflects the desire of man, for only man has the right to speak about woman. In the case of the Fathers, the difficulty is increased: only men can speak about women and, what is more, celibate men (since the vast majority of them had chosen consecrated celibacy). Theology, from the third century on, and then more and more as time goes on, is the work of monks for whom women symbolize what they have renounced and who constantly threaten their special devotion to God. Without over-emphasizing this fact, it is necessary to at least recognize that it carried some amount of weight. Celibate monks whose experience with women was through sins in their youth (like Augustine and Jerome) or through maternal love (like John Chrysostom) are not particularly equipped to recognize women as the "other" whose otherness signifies the very otherness of God. For them, the otherness of woman signaled instead the otherness of the devil!

*   *   *

This ends the analysis of the patristic tradition. I have tried to draw out the major trends. It is indeed difficult to do justice to all the theologians of an era which is distant and foreign to us. Nevertheless, it may perhaps be safe to conclude that a study of patristic texts does seem to bring out the Church's difficulty in its attempt to maintain itself within the eschatological tension. In breaking with the basic assumptions of contemporary society on the spiritual level only, patristic theology failed to exercise any criticism of that society's dominant ideology. And on the contrary, its own theological presuppositions, on matters of sex and marriage, led Christian morality to reinforce some of the most debatable assumptions (judging by the Gospel norm) of ancient society: fear of sexuality, disdain for women, pessimistic dualism in anthropological matters, reinforcement of "natural" hierarchies.

In all fairness, it must also be acknowledged that the gospel was certainly not forgotten, and that even within this moral conformity it exercised a critique which during the Middle Ages ended in radically challenging the ancient model.

4. SAINT AUGUSTINE AND THE MEDIEVAL MORAL TRADITION

Although Augustine has already been quoted several times, a special section is devoted to him as the master of medieval thought; for, through him, the Middle Ages was furnished with a framework of ethical reference in the area of sexuality and conjugality. Right up to the twelfth century, theologians, moralists and jurists systematically referred to him whenever discussing these ethical issues.[114] There are two reasons for this: Augustine expressed himself quite completely on these questions,[115] and he did so with a remarkable spirit of clarity, allowing him to present a genuine synthesis of the patristic theology of his time, leaving to his successors all the elements of an elaborated doctrine.

This synthesis hinges on three points: the link between sexuality and concupiscence, a description of the triple goal of marriage, and the beginnings of a reflection on the sacramentality of marriage. Since these three elements dominate medieval thinking, they should be briefly examined.

a) Sexuality and Concupiscence

Augustine is the first Christian theologian to have systematically analyzed the link between sexuality and sin.[116] Briefly, these are the elements of his analysis. Sexual diversity comes from God, as well as sexual union in its procreative aspect: "For God made the sexes.... But how could it possibly happen, that they who were to be united together... were not to move their bodies?"[117] On the other hand, that which comes not from God but from the devil is concupiscence, manifested by passion which, outside the control of reason, subjects genital organs to its empire. Incontrollable erection of the male organ whenever desire comes upon man is the sign of the irrationality of concupiscence, and a clear indication that it is evil. It is concupiscence "over which even marriage blushes, which glories in all these before-mentioned goods. For why is the especial work of parents withdrawn and hidden even from the eyes of their children except that it is impossible for them to be occupied in laudable procreation without shameful lusts? Because of this it was that even they were ashamed who first covered their nakedness... when... they felt their members disobedient to themselves."[118]

If there had not been a fall, sexuality would have been exempt from concupiscence: "... the seed would have issued from the human being by the quiet and normal obedience of his members to his will's command."[119] "That concupiscence... had no existence in the body during its life in paradise before the entrance of sin.... Without this concupiscence it was quite possible to effect the function of the wedded pair in the procreation of children: just as many a laborious work is accomplished by the compliant operation of our other limbs, without any lascivius heat; for they are simply moved by the direction of the will, not excited by the ardour of concupiscence (*aestu libidinis*)."[120]

Clearly, Augustine does not fall into the Manichean trap of confusing sexuality with sin. He firmly holds to the original goodness of sexuality. Even if there had been no "fall," Adam and Eve would have had intercourse for procreation, but without passion, that is, without the shame, without having their bodies affected in spite of themselves by "libido." Thus concupiscence is the consequence of original sin, and it forever marks sexuality with ambiguity, making it a threat wherein man is ceaselessly separated from himself, stripped of his reason and his control. Concupiscence manifests the state of enslavement to sin in which man finds himself. Thus in opposition of Manicheanism, Augustine maintains the goodness of procreative sexuality and in opposition to the Pelagians he maintains the force of concupiscence which links sexuality with sin. In so doing, he systematized and crystallized the intuitions of previous tradition which had effectively sought to avoid rejecting sexuality by focusing only on its bad aspect and to avoid misconstruing the tragic aspect of human existence, in which sexuality so often plays a death-dealing role. But in distinguishing as he does between a good sexuality (procreative) and a bad sexuality (concupiscent, passionate), Augustine plunged Christian ethics into the old stoic impasse whose difficulties we have seen. Moreover, when he interprets the "covetousness" in Romans 7:7, that sin reveals, only in terms of sexual concupiscence, Augustine considerably diminished the theological depth of Pauline anthropology. While Paul was evoking fundamental human idolatry (covetousness toward all things that can permit man to escape God), Augustine speaks only of sexual relations. As a result, all of Christian ethics became almost fixated upon sexuality as the very symbol of the idolatrous covetousness of man. From this point on and for many centuries, sexuality could not be spoken of without simultaneously evoking the thought of sin.

b) The Goals of Marriage

"These are all goods on account of which marriage is a good: offspring, fidelity, sacrament (*proles, fides, sacramentum*)."[121] This Augustinian formula is repeated through all of the Middle Ages. It is the necessary conclusion to the preceding propositions: since God willed the "human couple" before the fall, one must meditate on the meaning that God wished to confer on this privileged relationship where sexual difference could not be reduced to the functional role of procreation. Augustine refuses this reduction, and rightly comments that if it were only a question of ensuring the continuation of the species, marriage would not have been necessary. "You are entirely mistaken if you think that marriage was instituted to compensate for the departed dead through the succession of those who are born. Marriage was instituted so that through the chastity of women sons would be acknowledged by their fathers and fathers by their sons. It was indeed possible that men be born through random or unregulated intercourse, but there could not have been a bond of kinship between fathers and sons."[122]

Marriage allows for a major social experience, summarized by the term *fides* (pact of faithfulness). It is not only a means of socializing and regulating the anarchic impulses of the libido (*quod carnalis vel iuvenilis incontinentia . . . redigitur; De bono conjug.* III, iii), but it is also a possible means of experiencing what could be called the institutionalization of love. The pact of faithfulness guarantees life by permitting the existence of a locus where fathers and sons can recognize each other.

Evidently, the problem is that in this familial institution the values of socialization are dissociated from sexuality. It is not by chance that Augustine speaks only of the bond between fathers and sons here. Women are excluded from the familial and social acknowledgment. So then the pact of fidelity between a husband and wife makes possible a family, but it gives no meaning to the sexual relationship. So, if it happens that, in order to avoid a greater evil (like adultery for instance), the spouses have sexual relations with no intention of procreation, it would be as a concession to weakness and not as a conviction. Again this reveals the whole ambiguity of the matter: on one hand, the spouses are called upon to discover a social value in their conjugal relationship which goes beyond the procreative function, but at the same time this value is divorced from the sexual relationship which ever remains a lesser evil. Augustine, although he was more sensitive than others to the social dimension of the couple, was unable to conceive of the possibility that sexuality could hold tenderness, friendship, spirituality, and this lack of insight was very influential on later tradition.

c) Marriage as Sacramentum

Augustine sought to give Christian marriage its own theological status. This status, both juridical and spiritual, is expressed in the word *sacramentum*. "It is certainly not fecundity only, the fruit of which consists of offspring, nor chastity only, whose bond is fidelity, but also a certain sacramental bond in marriage which is recommended to believers in wedlock. Accordingly it is enjoined by the Apostle: 'Husbands, love your wives, even as Christ also loved the Church.' Of this bond the substance undoubtedly is this, that the man and woman who are joined together in matrimony should remain inseparable as long as they live; and that it should be unlawful for one consort to be parted from the other except in the case of fornication. For this is the case of Christ and the Church; that, as a living one with a living one, they are forever united with no possibility of divorce or separation. And so complete is the observance of this bond in the city of our God, in His holy mountain—that is to say, in the Church of Christ—by all married believers who are undoubtedly members of Christ, that, although women marry, and men take wives, for the purpose of procreating children, it is never permitted one to put away even an unfruitful wife for the sake of having another to bear children. And whosoever does this is held to be guilty of adultery by the law of the Gospel, though not by this world's rule.... Thus between the conjugal pair, as long as they live, the nuptial bond has a permanent obligation, and can be cancelled neither by separation nor by union with another."[123]

Marriage, then, is *sacramentum* insofar as it allows a comparison of the union between man and woman with that of Christ and the Church. This third "good" is more vital than the other two (fruitfulness and faithfulness), for it establishes the indissolubility of the conjugal bond. Now the question remains as to whether or not this good is recognized and given to Christians only (because of their incorporation into the body of Christ through baptism) or if it applies to all couples. Augustine hesitates on this point. The passage just cited seems to lean to the first hypothesis, but elsewhere Augustine affirms that from the beginning, before the fall, marriage had a sacramental character as the mysterious prefiguration of the union of Christ and His Church; nevertheless, he is hesitant: "(in addition to faithfulness and offspring in marriage) a third good, which seems to me to be a sacrament (*aliquod sacramentum*) should exist in the married, above all in those who belong to the people of God, so that there be no divorce from a wife."[124]

Augustine, along with his time, seems to have hardened his position and to have considered all remarriage, even if between pagans, as adultery because of the indissolubility of marriage, its sacramental aspect.

But it remains nevertheless that the word *sacramentum* is somewhat indefinite with Augustine. It is only used to explain the rationale for the indissolubility of marriage. But marriage does not produce what it prefigures: it does not make the partners members of Christ—only baptism accomplishes that. So two themes overlap here: a juridical-ethical theme and a symbolic-religious theme. The first relies on the real meaning of the Latin *sacramentum* (commitment, oath, juridical tie) which emphasizes the ethical imperative of the indissolubility of the marital bond. The second theme calls to mind the text in Ephesians 5:32, where the Greek *mystérion* is translated as *sacramentum* in the Latin versions of the New Testament; here the word evidently refers to the symbolism of the conjugal bond as a sign of the bond between Christ and the Church. This evokes the theological depth of the ethical reality of indissolubility. Augustine wished to go beyond the tenuousness of morality in basing indissolubility instead on a broader consciousness of the meaning of the marital relationship, on the awareness that analogically, it signifies the meaning of a love relationship and faithfulness between Christ and the Church. Even if the conjugal commitment is juridical, it is much more than juridical: it has a theological signification.

By reintegrating the profound viewpoint of Ephesians 5 with theological reflections on marriage, Augustine rescued the Christian ethic of marriage from a dull theologizing that viewed marriage only in its normal function. But it must also be noted that in so doing, he opened the door to a more objectifying conception of *sacramentum,* i.e. an objectively real bond that nothing can dissolve, in the name of which a very legalistic conception of marriage would finally be established. The introduction of *sacramentum* in the thinking on marriage certainly afforded a positive broadening of consciousness as to the implications of the male-female rapport, but it also led to a solidification of the juridical character of conjugal indissolubility, now made sacred.

The Middle Ages received the heritage of Augustine with great devotion. The next part of this chapter is devoted to the twofold juridical and theological problem that scholastic theology had to resolve as a result of Augustinian concepts: the validity of marriage and its sacramentality.

But first, a few examples of how Augustinianism was taken up, and often caricatured, in later medieval reflections on sexuality.

*   *   *

Bishop Caesarius of Arles, the embodiment of the sixth century, endeavored throughout the troubled period of the great barbarian invasions, to maintain some moral standards in the Church. In his fight against concubinage, fornication and sexual disorders, he repeats (and solidifies even more) the Augustinian teaching on procreation as the single final goal of the marital sex act.[125]

Invoking Psalm 51:5 ("Behold, I was brought forth in iniquity, and in sin did my mother conceive me") and Exodus 19:15 ("Be ready by the third day [to meet God on Sinai]; do not go near a woman"), Caesarius emphasized the idea that all sexual relationship is sin.

At the end of the same century, Gregory the Great (Pope from 590–604) follows the same line, i.e. an Augustinianism that is reducd to a few major themes that constantly recur. For example, the link between sexuality and sin: "Because the first man fell from his state of innocence by sinning, he transmitted the punishment of sin to his children. For sexual appetite is the punishment of sin, and comes from the root of sin, so much so that no one is born into the world without its exercise."[126] The reduction of sin to sexuality is unreserved, and Augustine's subtle distinctions are forgotten. Married couples always sin when they have intercourse by the very fact that pleasure accompanies that act.[127] "But since even the lawful intercourse of the wedded cannot take place without the pleasure of the flesh, entrance into a sacred place should be abstained from, because the pleasure itself can by no means be without sin. For he had not been born of adultery or fornication, but of lawful wedlock who said, 'Behold I was conceived in iniquities and in my sin my mother brought me forth.'"[128]

As Noonan pointed out in his study of penitentials from the sixth to eleventh centuries, such a perspective resulted—in pastoral practice—in a condemnation of any form of sexual activity that did not specifically aim at procreation.

Peter Lombard, named bishop of Paris in 1159, expresses the traditional point of view quite well, taking up all the elements of the Augustinian elaboration which justify sexuality through the procreative intent: "original sin is transmitted by the act of generation, which act is preceded by concupiscence. The descendants of Adam are in their turn affected by concupiscence."[129] The result of this transmission of original sin and its consequences is the "law of deadly concupiscence in our members, without which no carnal union would be possible"; therefore, "coitus is reprehensible and evil unless excused by the bonds of marriage."[130]

In a similar manner, when the fourth Lateran Council (1215), against catharism, declares "Not only virgins and celibates, but also married people who please God by right faith and good conduct merit to arrive at eternal happiness,"[131] it is understood that the "good conduct" in question equals practicing sexuality with only procreative intention.

But from the twelfth century, powerful intellectual and spiritual mutations appear which are evidenced by certain movements outside the Church (for example, the courtly tradition and the catharic heresy) as well as by a new approach to a theology of the couple, love, and marriage (in particular by Abelard and Hugh of Saint Victor).

Peter Abelard (1079–1142) deserves particular mention because he knew how to transfer the elements of his century's new consciousness of love onto the theological and philosophical level; he had, through his relations with Heloise, experienced the human and spiritual values of it. Because of this he is recognized as one of the precursors of courtly love.[132] He defines a doctrine of pure love for God, of love for the perfection of God, which could go to the point of renouncing the happiness He promised to man. God should be loved precisely because He is God, and not because of what one might get from Him. Etienne Gilson has shown that this concept had been furnished to him by his love-relationship with Heloise: "The description of disinterested love that Abelard, turned theologian, proposes is that very same with which Heloise bitterly reproached him with never having understood when he pretended to love her. The Abelardian doctrine of Divine love amounts to this, that God is not to be loved as Abelard loved Heloise, but as Heloise loved Abelard."[133]

Accepting the loss of oneself by and through love is the very meaning of Heloise's obedience: "Not, however, by another, but by thee thyself, that thou who art alone in the cause of my grief may be alone in the grace of my comfort! For it is thou alone that canst make me sad, canst make me joyful or canst comfort me. And it is thou alone that owest me this great debt, and for this reason above all that I have at once performed all things that you didst order, till that when I could not offend thee in anything I had the strength to lose myself at thy behest."[134] There is a tragic aspect to love, a denial of self for the sake of the other which, beyond the framework of morality, unites and opposes human and divine love at the same time in one single cry. "But in the whole period of my life (God wot) I have ever feared to offend thee rather than God, I seek to please thee more than Him. Thy command brought me, not the love of God, to the habit of religion. See how unhappy a life I must lead, more wretched than all others, if I endure all these things here in vain having no hope of reward in the future."[135] Heloise speaks of Abelard like she does of God, while yet admitting, with the bitter lucidity that makes her letters so moving, that these two loves destroy one another.

Surely this is a singularly striking proof of the new sensibility which appears in the twelfth century, very close indeed to courtly love which exalts a love that is fully sexual (considered as the most concrete example of mutual love of man and woman!) and highly spiritual (since sexuality, when sexual activity is denied, is a call to a love that is completely sacrificial). This sensibility exalts the bond of love more highly than marriage: "... thou has not disdained to set forth sundry reasons by which I tried to dissuade them from our marriage, from an ill-starred bed; but wert silent to many, in which I preferred love to wedlock, freedom to a bond. I call God to witness, if *Augustus*, ruling over the whole world, were to deem me worthy of the honour of marriage, and to confirm the whole world to me, to be ruled by me for ever, dearer to me and of greater dignity would it seem to be called thy strumpet than his empress."[136] For marriage not only enslaves the philosopher and impedes him from freely applying himself to his intellectual tasks, but it also reduces love to a vested contract. "Nothing have I ever (God wot) required of thee save thyself, desiring thee purely, not what was thine. Not for the pledge of matrimony, nor for any dowry did I look, nor for my own passions or wishes but thine (as thou thyself knowest) was I zealous to gratify. And if the name of wife appears more sacred and more valid, sweeter to me is ever the word friend."[137] Heloise, furthermore, reproaches herself more for having consented to marry Abelard than for having been his mistress. For she thereby seemed to have contradicted her fundamental conviction of the value of simple disinterested, pure love. And so begins a critique of marriage in the name of love: "Question: Can true love exist between married people? Answer: We state and affirm, according to the tenor of those present, that love cannot extend its rights to two married people. For lovers are freely in mutual accord without constraint of necessity, whereas spouses are bound to the duty of a reciprocal submission of their wills and of not refusing anything to each other. May this judgment which we have renounced with much deliberation, according to the opinion of a great number of Ladies, be for you a sure and indisputable truth. Adjudicated in the year 1174, the third day of the Calends of May."[138]

This critique of marriage is actually at the very core of *courtly eroticism*.[139] In its traditional perspective, marriage is primarily a contract which stringently subjects the wife to the desires of her "lord and master," reducing her to being merely the procreatrix of his children; marriage, then, cannot allow for a personal relationship between man and woman, but justifies only a functional relationship.

As opposed to the marital institution, courtly love appears as a vindication for the woman, a recognition of who she is, i.e. a person. The rejection, not of pleasure, but of sexual fulfillment in the "fin' amors" stems from this; woman is vindicated in her right to be a man's friend, which implies that the man accepts a reduction of his male power, a humbling of himself. "It is necessary, in the discovery of love, that the woman, freed from the threat of masculine omnipotence, be solicitous of the desire she arouses. It is thus necessary, in order to love, to renounce oneself and be noble and strong.... Paralleling feudal service, love becomes a service. Voluntary (or converted) humiliation abolishes the misogyny that would hinder love."[140]

The "couple" can only spring from a real recognition of the two partners, of their otherness, and from their mutual right to speak: the woman can also express her preference and pleasure.[141]

But this kind of couple—marginal by necessity since it is the countermodel to the contractual and hierarchical couple, is stamped with deadly ambiguity: it exalts erotic pleasure without being able to bring it to full term; by the technique of *asag* (lit. "putting to the test"),[142] it postulates that pleasure is never so pure and so great as when it is renounced while one is in a position to have consented to it. The prohibition against orgasm that *asag* presupposes signifies that one's desire is only finally fulfilled in death, and not in life. Only death can fulfill love. Time and history must be distanced from the game of love, that is, the child that signifies these contingencies; thus the child, which is the single justification for sexuality according to orthodox Catholic morality, is here totally negated. Along with the child, the assignment of love into the risk of a creative project is also denied.

It is as though, in this twelfth century so rich in so many kinds of renewals, the discourse of sex and marriage hesitates between two paths that are equally blockaded: a traditional morality, inspired by Augustine which links the male/female relationship to a social contract aimed at ensuring descendants to the family group and stability to social order; and courtly love which exalts love by tearing it away from the temporal reality of a conjugal couple to bestow it upon the marginal couple which consists of passionate and provisional lovers.

Thus love is opposed to marriage, because true love (whether it be erotic love for the troubadours or mystical love for the theologians) can be nothing less than perfect, that is to say, eternal and non-contingent. The ideal Woman becomes the image of this Love which is elevated to the rank of essence: unreal, inaccessible woman, infinitely respectable and at the same time altogether unattainable.[143] Thus what courtly love had bestowed upon woman is cancelled out by making her vindication only an abstraction!

Wasn't it possible to think of the conjugal couple as capable of a love encounter? Wasn't it possible to go beyond the Augustinian position without falling into the "courtly" critique of marriage? Hugh of Saint Victor (1096–1141) is worthy of mention here, for he is the only one to consider marriage in terms of love.[144]

According to Hugh, the origin of marriage, or what constitutes its foundation, is the bond beween a man and a woman:[145] marriage is first of all and essentially a conjugal community. This community was not abolished by the fall but it is threatened by a concupiscence which could possibly overshadow the friendship-love which unites the partners. Marriage is not primarily destined to allow procreation nor is it a remedy for concupiscence; it is primarily a community in service to the couple and their love. This is the sense in which it is sacramental, and Hugh rediscovers here the rich symbolism of Ephesians 5.

"Hugh is clear: he does not conceive of marriage as the institution for parenthood but as the institution for the tenderness and intimacy of the couple."[146] The important point is that love unites the married couple, and whatever leads to it or affirms it, including intercourse, is good. But sexual desire constantly risks shutting the couple up into egoism or violence, and therefore continent love is a more sure and noble path. The couple who can thus live in chaste love (an obvious parallel to courtly love) really know what love is, the sign in the life of man of the perfect and inaccessible love of God. Such a love is possible *within marriage!* This is undoubtedly Hugh's originality, for up until this point, in order to partake in perfect love, one had either to make vows of religious virginity or, as a courtly lover, to try to escape the extremely contingent bonds of marriage.

Hugh was thus rediscovering essential elements of the biblical strain and his reading of the texts in Genesis is not as whimsical as Marie-Odile Métral says.[147] For the first time, perhaps, a somewhat coherent theological attempt was made to consider marriage in terms of love and to associate sexuality with affection and friendship. Agapè-love was not opposed to eros-love! It must unfortunately be admitted that this attempt had no echo in subsequent moral theology. Why not? For two reasons, in my opinion: one historical and the other ideological. The ideological reason (which I will come back to in the comparison of Catholic and Protestant moralities) is rather obvious: to reestablish the human couple as being the "original man," as Hugh did, is to radically challenge the whole social and ecclesiastical structure founded on a strict hierarchy which postulates the superiority of the man over the woman and the superiority of the ecclesiastical celibate and virgin over the married (and incontinent) man of that time. To give woman personal value is to challenge the power of clerics who are justified precisely by the essential inferiority of woman!

As for the historical reason, it is connected to the appearance of the catharic heresy at that same era. Faced with a movement which recalled many elements of the old gnostic heresy, the Catholic Church naturally had recourse to classical arguments, which reinforced its long-standing distrust of sexuality. Catharism[148] is, in fact, a resurgence of gnostic dualism, by way of a Manicheanism that was reworked and corrected by Bogumil, a Bulgarian priest at the beginning of the tenth century. It took root in the West during the eleventh century and became a dangerous concurrent to the Catholic Church in the twelfth century. In the area of sexual morality, many elements noted in ancient Gnosticism resurface. The rigorous dualism which undergirds it results in a rejection of sexuality, especially insofar as it participates in the malignance of this world by procreation. There is only one sin: submission to the world, that is, attachment to the flesh. Sexual relations and sensual pleasure signify submission to the world. Thus any sexual activity whatsoever is sin, every marriage is lewd, *jurata fornicatio*. There are no distinctions in sexual activity, for it is all equally grievous: the Catholic distinction between sex authorized by procreation and perverse sex aiming only at pleasure is abolished. And, furthermore, procreation, to some extent, is a more serious sin than pleasure. Therefore pregnant women were not admitted into the catharic church.

But the simple faithful of the sect, who were not required to submit to the rigid ascetic prescriptions reserved for the "Perfect," very quickly deduced that since all sexual activity was equally wicked, the very notion of sexual perversion could be abandoned! Thus a double morality arose: "the sage, illuminated by the Spirit, denied himself the carnal act, but the believer, who had not evolved to such a total liberation, was supposed to obey his 'natural' desire, and it mattered little if he sinned (in spite of himself and in spite of the Spirit) either in marriage or outside of marriage."[149] Once again, there is proof (for the paradox is only a surface one) that an absolute disdain for sexuality corresponds to very "permissive" morality in practice.

This explains the disregard of Cathari for marriage, which placed them in opposition to the Catholic Church. The Perfect is absolutely chaste; his nature is thereby changed and he resembles God Himself. He is free of the world, of contingency. On the other hand, no sacrament whatsoever is capable of making marriage innocent, or purifying it of the stain of physical love which condemns man to a submission to Satan. From this point on, what is required of the simple believers, who yet experience the disjunction of body and soul, is an adherence to the true doctrine; apart from that, whether they sin in or out of marriage is irrelevant. It is even probable that the Cathari were more lenient about a free union than about marriage, because marriage constituted a permanent wicked state whereas a free union could only be temporary, and therefore a lesser evil. Furthermore, marriage is fruitful in principle whereas free union could pass for a kind of sterile friendship or purification of passionate love. Love outside of marriage could partly escape evil and matter if it manifested at least the desire (if not the reality) of chastity.[150]

Without entering the complicated discussion on the rapport between catharism and *courtly love*[151] one can at least recognize the similar atmosphere in catharic heresy and the work of the troubadours. The shared insistence on continence gives rise to a new consciousness of love as purifying pain and a new consciousness of Woman—who moves from being the devil's bait to lure men into perdition to being Virgin Mother, protectress and inaccessible. For the troubadours and the best of the catharic believers, sexuality can be the locus of a spiritual experience. In any case, sexuality is no longer justified by procreation only. Whether it be through disdain for procreation and horror of submission to the evil world (as for the Cathari) or whether it be through the recognition of the value of the woman (as for the poets of courtly love), the dissociation of sexuality and procreation is important to notice. I will return to it later.

The Church, opposing the Cathari, affirmed, as it had before with the Gnostics, the goodness of divine creation. In its refusal of dualism, the Church recognizes the human and Christian values of sex within the framework of marriage. It denounces, and rightly so, the ambiguities of a dualism whose negative spirituality leaves the door wide open for moral indifference. But at the same time, by affirming the superiority of virginity, the Church supports a double morality that is equally ambivalent and which does not succeed (any more than its opponents did) in finding a correct rapport between spirituality and sexuality.

The catharic crisis, as well as the whole trend in the twelfth century which tried to reinvest value in human love by spiritualizing eroticism, would force the Catholic theology of marriage to take up and pursue its reflections on the sacramental value of the conjugal couple. And so the great scholastics of the thirteenth century would set themselves to the task of completing, nuancing, and correcting the traditional Augustinian doctrine.

Actually, the first signs of a new language were already appearing and manifesting a new consciousness whose values the Renaissance, the Reformation, and the Counter-Reformation would express. Some of these signs are:

1) Theologians discover the value of conjugal love: they are no longer satisfied to justify marriage by its social function of procreation, but discern (probably through the influence of courtly literature) that in male/female relationships something occurs which is neither in the order of (wicked) concupiscence nor in the order of procreative duty. However, this love is disquieting: it could be concurrent to that love which is owed to God alone: "Now amongst all relationships the conjugal tie does, more than any other, engross men's hearts. . . . Hence, they who are aiming at perfection must above all things avoid the bond of marriage. . . ."[152] If it can rival the love of God which leads to perfection, it must indeed be an extraordinary force! In their commentaries on Aristotle's ethics, both Albertus Magnus and Thomas Aquinas describe the beauty of special friendship which is born between a man and his wife, a friendship based on sexual pleasure, the usefulness of creating a family together, and virtuous and reciprocal attachment. Bonaventure speaks of love and is amazed by it: ". . . there is something miraculous in the fact that a man finds an attraction, an appeal in a particular woman that he finds in no one but her."[153]

2) Another sign is the growing importance that medieval thinkers attribute to the education of children. It is not enough to bring children into the world; they must be educated, i.e. nourished morally and spiritually. And thus sexual relations cannot be justified in marriage by procreation alone; the married couple must assume all the consequences of that procreation. This argument is used by Thomas against fornication,[154] but it is also a way of giving value to the family setting and to the quality of the marital relationship. Conjugal love becomes the condition of the true education of children and by the same token the importance attributed to education reinvests value in the conjugal bond.[155]

3) Within the framework of Augustinian doctrine, theologians highlight the value of "conjugal duty." Up until this point, Paul's words—"The husband should give to his wife her conjugal rights, and likewise the wife to her husband" (1 Corinthians 7:3)—had been interpreted in a restrictive sense, as the authorization of a lesser evil. Reflections on conjugal fidelity (a sufficiently important value so that it is preferable to abstinence if abstinence "pushes one of the partners to adultery) lead theologians to reflect on the purpose of the sexual act in a more subtle manner. All sexual activity cannot be justified solely by procreation because it can play an important role in conjugal fidelity.[156]

4) Along the same lines, and even more original, there is an attempt to restore value to pleasure. Under the influence of Aristotle, who defined pleasure not as an action in itself but as a subjective feeling which accompanied an action, theology, and particularly that of Thomas, ceases condemning pleasure as such. Henceforth pleasure is to be condemned only if it accompanies an indecent action. Conversely, it is recognized as good and desirable if it accompanies a good action.[157] With Augustine, as we have seen, sexual pleasure, since it is outside of reason's control, had been condemned per se, for it was the sign of concupiscence; in Paradise there was sexual activity but without "libido." This opinion is not shared by Albertus Magnus who thinks that Adam experienced pleasure in Paradise; and he adds that even if sexual relations recall original sin, it is not because they are accompanied by pleasure, but because the pleasure is not as great as it could have been: "I heartily concede that there would have been a greater and more genuine pleasure in the (sex) act at that time but it would have been under reason's control."[158]

Thomas shares the opinion of his former professor. His refusal to take on the Augustinian dualism of charity and cupidity leads him to see in all forms of love, even bodily love, something that shows forth the love of God.[159] Thus pleasure, willed by God, cannot be declared evil in itself. However it cannot be separated from the fidelity of the act that it accompanies; we cannot seek pleasure for its own sake. But if it be a licit act, as is the sexual union of the married couple desiring to procreate, it can in no way be condemned.

John T. Noonan[160] reports the arguments of an English theologian, Richard Middleton, who, in 1272, presented a defense of pleasure as a legitimate goal: pleasure, moderated by temperance, is part of the good that belongs to the sacrament of marriage. But it must be acknowledged that this point of view is isolated among medieval theologians. On the moral plane, Augustine remains the recognized authority.

5) Among the factors that contributed to a certain evolution of consciousness, as previously discussed, is the very distinct promotion of woman during the twelfth and thirteenth centuries. This phenomenon is of course reserved for the intellectual elite, but the impact of this new light on woman is striking and corresponds in the religious domain to the development of the Marian cult.[161]

In any case, women speak out[162] on sexuality, love and marriage, and express some thoughts and feelings which correspond very little to the rigid Augustinian traditions! There is an appeal for love, which by dint of customs and traditions, becomes more often than not a critique of marriage and a defense of adultery. As Evelyne Sullerot says so well: "The vigorous and constant revolt against marriage is a remarkable trait in the writings of women. Marriage imprisons them much more than men, and the disproportion in ages almost always is not in their favor. A young maiden is often handed over to an elderly man, or to an old man whom she hates...."[163]

This is a surprising kind of literature: women speak of themselves as subjects and their lovers as objects which they do away with at will! An expression like this, even if it is limited to a small elite, could not remain without influence on theological reflections, even that of celibate men! This is especially true since it did not come about by chance at that very moment of history: it exteriorized the expression of a slow but sure mutation that had been operating all along and to which Christianity, in spite of Augustinianism, was certainly not a stranger. The Christian discourse on marriage and sexuality, although in an apparently fixed state through Augustinian morality, was evolving and that evolution will be better perceived through an examination of how the questions of the validity and sacramentality of marriage were resolved in the Middle Ages.

5. The Evolution of Conjugal Rights from the Fourth Century to the End of the Middle Ages

As we saw in section two, Christians up until the third century adopted the laws and customs which regulated the conjugal and family questions in the Roman world.

Once it came out of hiding from the fourth century on, the Church was able to exercise a greater influence on laws which corresponded with its influence on morals. The collapse of the Western Empire conferred upon the Church (now the only stable juridical institution) a legal and moral importance that was considerable.

This reinforcement of the social importance of the Church is marked by the growth, from the fourth to the eleventh centuries, of a stronger emphasis on the ecclesiastical character of the celebration of marriage. The Church intervenes to recall that marriage, for Christians, has a religious and social significance. As Edward Schillebeeckx notes,[164] "increasing emphasis was placed on the church aspect of the marriage contract, without prejudice to its legal validity, by surrounding it with liturgical ceremonies." The bishop plays a more prominent role than in the first centuries and is more and more associated with marriage ceremonies.[165] The aim in these ceremonies is not to juridically validate marriage but to relegate onto a moral and religious plane any marriage contracted according to different national laws and customs. Therefore these ceremonies were not obligatory except for priests. One of the first detailed descriptions of a marriage liturgy has come down to us through the work of Paulinus of Nola (beginning of the fifth century): the ceremony is held at the church, the groom's father leads the couple to the altar where the bishop gives his blessing. The prayer is probably spontaneous, during which the couple's heads are covered by a veil that the bishop has stretched over them.[166]

It is important to note that all these rites remain absolutely optional. In the ninth century, Pope Nicholas I, in answer to a question from Bulgarian Christians, writes: "The Greeks, you say, insist that all these matrimonial rights are obligatory under pain of sin. We do not agree, especially since so many poor people cannot afford the expense. Only consent, exchanged according to law, is necessary. Conversely, if consent be the only element lacking, all the other rites and even conjugal union are without value."[167] This passage clearly shows the maintenance of the tradition which distinguishes between the validity of marriage, which is conferred according to Roman law by the mutual consent, and the religious ceremonies, which are personal testimonies, desirable, certainly, but not obligatory.

On the question of *divorce,* the Church which had now become official sought to reinforce the civil laws which prohibited it. With little success: the emperor increased the punishment meted out to adulterers, but divorce by simple mutual consent remained authorized, according to the tradition of Roman law.[168] Many Fathers loudly expressed their disapproval on this point—like Jerome who recognized with bitterness that "the laws of Caesar are different...from the laws of Christ"[169]—but the Church never tried to impose its laws on the State: the State was allowed to legislate, while the Church retained the right of calling the Christians to the imperatives of the gospel. Even within the Church, the most rigid position on divorce, defended by Jerome and Augustine, was not established in the West until the ninth century. Up until then, in the West as well as in the Eastern Churches, a more tolerant and pastoral attitude prevailed: "The right to remarry was not denied to the husband victimized by adultery or abandoned for no reason, according to Origen, Lactantius, Basil, or Chrysostom. They interpret Matthew's famous interpolation as support for this concession and liken adultery to the death of a spouse. That opinion becomes canonized in the East by the Council at Trullo in 692."[170]

In 395 Jerome wrote: "A husband may be an adulterer or a sodomite, he may be stained with every crime and may have been left by his wife because of his sins; yet he is still her husband and, so long as he lives, she may not marry another."[171] But in the middle of the eighth century Bishop Ekbert of York, a disciple of the Venerable Bede, translated the opinion received from the Church during the first millennium in this manner: "No one infringes on the Gospel of Paul with impunity; we are therefore against adultery completely. But we refuse to burden whomsoever, if it risks crushing him. We fearlessly proclaim the desires of the Lord. As for him whose weakness hinders him from fulfilling them (the Lord's desires), we prefer to leave judgment to God alone. Consequently, so that our silence be not encouragement to adulterers or that the devil who lures adulterers may not find his joy in them, we say to them, 'What God has joined together, let no man put asunder.' But we add, 'Let him who can, understand.' Often the experiences of life actually compel a violation of the law. What did David do when he was hungry (Mark 2:25–26)? We cannot accuse him of transgression. Thus, in difficult cases let us not be so definite: let us accept instead seeing our fixed notions jeopardized so that others may be saved."[172] It is regrettable that such an attitude was abandoned. Under the influence of the works of Augustine and Jerome which were enormously prestigious in the Middle Ages, the Carolingian theologians established an inflexible point of view in the Western Church, breaking with its own tradition[173] as well as with that of the Eastern Church. Here is a significant echo of that tradition: "He who cannot remain continent after the death of his first wife or who is separated from his wife for a valid reason like fornication, adultery or other cause, if he takes another wife (or if the wife takes another husband) Sacred Scripture does not condemn him nor exclude him from the Church or from life, but supports him because of his weakness. Not that he can have two wives, with the first one continuing a relationship with him, but if he truly be separated from the first wife, he may legally unite with another if the situation presents itself. For Sacred Scripture and Holy Mother Church take pity on him, especially if the man is otherwise pious and living according to the law of God."[174]

It was during the ninth century in the West that the situation evolved perceptibly. The juridical and cultural importance of the Church, since it seemed able to ensure a link with the prodigious past of the Roman Empire that the Carolingians were trying to restore, was henceforth very evident. Thus developed ecclesiastical legislation on marriage, which aimed at blocking incestuous marriages, "mixed" marriages (i.e. where one of the spouses was an "infidel" or a Jew), and forced marriages following abduction or rape. In order to avoid these cases, the publication of marriage, i.e. the celebration of marriage before the Church, became obligatory.

But it is the apocryphal writings of Pseudo-Isidore (ca. 845),[175] a collection[176] of False Capitularies (royal or conciliary decrees) and False Decretals (pontifical letters), which would modify the situation in a decisive way. Henceforth the nuptial blessing became canonically required and the civil forms of marriage were absorbed into ecclesiastical law. From that point on, the Church tended to add civil juridical forms to its jurisdiction.[177] However, one important note is that tradition was respected, i.e. the validity of marriage which throughout the Middle Ages never depended on the ecclesiastical celebration of marriage; the Church celebration was obligatory for Christians but it did not validate the marriage, which only the consent of the spouses could guarantee. It is the Council of Trent, in the sixteenth century, which finally mingled licitness and validity in one single obligation and declared civil marriage invalid.

From the eleventh century on, theological reflections concentrated on two problems, which were closely linked: the sacramentality of marriage and the validity of marriage.

"Since the church had in fact taken over complete jurisdiction in matters of marriage, from the tenth to the eleventh century, she was faced in matrimonial lawsuits with the question as to what really constituted marriage as a valid contract between husband and wife.... The church discovered that it was a highly complex issue.... First there was the Roman conception of the marriage of mutual consent—marriage by *consensus*. Then there was the Germanic, Frankish, Gothic, and Celtic *mundium* form of marriage in which the marriage contract was formally regarded as a handing over of the bride by her father to the marital control of the bridegroom. Finally, the very ancient idea that the marriage was not consummated until cohabitation and sexual intercourse had actually taken place played an important part in the minds of all peoples. The *domum-ductio*, or the solemn taking of the bride in procession to the bridegroom's house, was thus regarded both by the Greeks and the Romans and by the Western tribes as the consummation of the marriage contract. In the Middle Ages, these did not exist side by side as three distinct systems of law; they interacted upon each other."[178] From that time on, the debate concerned the rapport between the old Roman idea of mutual consent and the Germanic law which insisted on the importance of sexual union to validate the marriage. Already around 860, Hincmar, the archbishop of Reims, in response to Count Regimond's question, created a breach in the old Roman juridical tradition: "But I must tell you this: there is a valid marriage between people when the girl, who is asked for in marriage from the rightful authority—be it parents or tutors—, is properly engaged, duly equipped with a dowry, united in public nuptial ceremony in the bonds of marriage, becomes one body and one flesh with her husband, as it is written 'the two shall become one flesh'; notice, I did not say two, but one flesh."[179] Thus bodily union was recognized in the Frankish churches as necessary for the marriage to be completed; there must be cohabitation and sexual union for the mutual consent to constitute the "sacrament" of Christ and the Church.

The debate over Roman law, in full resurgence in the eleventh-century West, and the Germanic concept which linked the indissolubility of marriage to the accomplishment of the sexual act, continued on throughout the whole Middle Ages.[180] Two great schools opposed each other on this matter: the theologians of the French school (Hugh of Saint Victor, who died in 1141; Peter Lombard, who died in 1164) and the canonical writers of the school in Bologna (Gratian, who died ca. 1160). The first school continued in the old tradition: it is the consent which makes the marriage and not the promise to marry (*desponsatio*) or the consummation, i.e. sexual union. The second school distinguished between marriage "begun" (engagement, wedding, consent) and marriage "consummated" (sexual union and cohabitation). For the latter, only consummation creates the marriage because only that transforms the *sponsi* (the promised one) into *conjuges*. While the French school insisted on the sacramental representation by marriage of the *love* of Christ for His Church, the canonical writers in Bologna emphasized the representation of the *union* of Christ with His Church by the physical union of the spouses.

The results of these discussions, summarized under the form of articles of law, are to be found in the Fourth Book of the *Decretals* of Gregory IX which is entirely devoted to marriage.[181] The importance of consent is immediately reaffirmed: "marriage is contracted only by consent" (I, 1); as well as the importance of a free decision without which the marriage is invalid: "in marriage and espousal, there must be liberty, otherwise the promise is not binding" (I, 29); and "no one can make a fiancée become a spouse by intercourse" (I, 32). But at the same time it must be recognized, because of the issue of sexual impotence, that physical union constitutes the aim of marriage: "an impotence to perform intercourse is impotence to contract marriage, whether that impediment is from age or from nature" (XV, 2); and "any natural impediment to intercourse, if not reparable by the art of medicine, impedes a marriage" (XV, 3). He is concerned to avert clandestine marriages (cf. all of chapter III); to protect the spouses from the whims of parents: "a father may contract a marriage for his son if he is under age, but if he is not under age, the father can only do so with the son's consent" (II, 1, cf. also I, 11); and to affirm the church's right to control the juridical (and not only the liturgical) practice of marriage: "marriage cannot be contracted contrary to the interdict of the church or its judgment, because it alone has jurisdiction" (XVI, 1); or "a man may not dismiss his wife, without ecclesiastical permission . . ." (XIX, 3). Consider also the three important chapters on divorce (XIX, XX) and remarriage (XXI), both issues being subject to specific interdictions. In the discussion between theologians and jurists the debate on the validity of marriage could not be divorced from the issue of sacramentality, i.e. the debate on the value of the Christian tradition of marriage.

Augustine had closely connected his thoughts on *sacramentum* (the third good in marriage) to his pastoral concern for theologically establishing the indissolubility of the conjugal couple. Marriage, insofar as it is a "sacrament" or sign of the union between Christ and His Church, is indissoluble. This is precisely what the liturgical practice of the Church wished to emphasize by the benediction and the bestowal of the veil.[182] Through it, the Church called the faithful to discern in the terrestrial reality of marriage a spiritual truth which, aside from the moral requirement of indissolubility, recalled and signified the love of Christ for His Church.

From this point on, and because of the historical necessity of promoting marriage anew in opposition to the heretical movements of the twelfth century (which rejected marriage as a radical evil), scholastic theologians applied themselves to determine more precisely the nature of the mystery (Ephesians 5: *mystérion* in Greek, translated into Latin by *sacramentum*) that links Christ to the Church and which marriage signifies. The twelfth- and thirteenth-century theological reflections on the validity of marriage are divided into two camps on the question of sacramentality: some, like Anselm of Laon, believe that the sacrament is in the union of the bodies, that human sexual union symbolizes the union of Christ and the Church; others, like Hugh of Saint Victor, assert that the bond of love is the element that constitutes the marriage and the sacrament, the physical union depends on it but a marriage could be perfectly valid without sexual relations (like the marriage of Joseph and Mary!). An emphasis on union is an emphasis on love: in the end, the best theologians refused to choose, preferring instead a synthesis, and thus Thomas Aquinas defines marriage as "a certain joining together of husband and wife ordained to carnal intercourse, and a further consequent union between husband and wife. . . ."[183] What the spouses consent to is more than the sexual act; it's a whole life together, a unity of life which can exist without this act, but whose profound meaning is manifested in the conjugal sexual act. Sacramental grace, then, is not directly linked to the physical act but to the conjugal love which is actualized through it. The grace which is exercised in marriage makes of a specifically human community, a community of grace.

What such a theology highlights is the discovery that through the gospel the male/female relationship has its most profound signification revealed, its ultimate meaning: to signify the very love of Christ for His Church. This kind of theology affords an understanding of how the most human of acts can become the sign and the object of the most divine love.[184]

6. The Reformation and Protestantism

The Reformation was essentially a conflict over authority—in all areas, but primarily in the area of theology. Breaking with the oldest of traditions, Luther dared to affirm the primacy of Scripture over ecclesiastical magisterium. In the name of the Word of God, which he considered to be alive in the Bible, he questioned not only certain abuses of Roman power but even the very principle of that power. The consequences of this crisis were enormous, as we know. This was no less true in the area of morality since the challenge to Church authority was necessarily accompanied by a critique of its moral teachings and its claims to define the very details of the conduct of believers.

Certain facts, demonstrating the failure of the Church's teaching, caused that criticism to be even sharper. The more canon law tried to precisely elaborate regulations concerning marriage[185] the more it moved away from the real needs of a society that was trying to organize itself more autonomously. On two particular points the new lay spirit was in conflict with clerical authority: divorce and clandestine marriages. Sacramental theology, which had been superimposed little by little, led to almost insurmountable problems in these two areas when transposed to the level of civil law. Spouses, even though separated by the adultery of one partner, could not be divorced, because the indissolubility of the conjugal sacramental bond was absolute; the marriage bond had an objective reality that no one had the power to annul. Naturally, in practice the harshness of this kind of principle resulted in situations that were more immoral than those it was fighting against.[186] As for the second issue—how could clandestine marriages, contracted without the parents' consent and in the absence of a priest, be prohibited if the consent of the spouses is really the material cause in the conjugal sacrament? The union could not then be dissolved even if, under certain circumstances, things went as far as the excommunication of the spouses. Such were the difficulties that threatened a social order that had been founded on the quasi-absolute paternal authority, and constituted a ferment of anarchy for a society on its way to secularization, searching for new standards by which to establish its social and moral order.

There was another area that revealed the failure of the Church's teaching on sexuality: the customs of the clergy itself! The clergy at that time interpreted required celibacy as an obligation not to marry, but not as an obligation to renounce living with a woman. As we know at the end of the fifteenth century, the great majority of priests were living with concubines. And this of course could not fail to provoke questions about the validity of the official theological stand which exalted the virtues of virginity and chastity. A choice had to be made: either authorize the marriage of ecclesiastics (the choice made by the Reformation) or restore moral discipline within the ranks of the clergy (the work of the Counter-Reformation).

In this context, it is clear that the crisis effected by Luther concerning the Church was going to appear to many as a possibility for liberation from the legalism and casuistry then in effect. The reception given to the Reformation by the urban bourgeois class was related to this ethical (and therefore spiritual) liberation, which appeared to many as the prerequisite for any attempt at "remoralizing" the social practice of the time. Countless voices at the end of the Middle Ages in fact protested against the presence of a clergy who had no well-defined professional activity; they were often described as social parasites who were ill-equipped for the role of moral guidance which had been delegated to them. Thus, in the minds of many, the demoralization of society was linked to the existence and status of the clergy.

The essential points of the Protestant perspective, outlined by men as different as Erasmus, Luther, Butzer, Zwingli, Calvin, Bèze,[187] can be summarized in these following four theses:

1) The Reformers aimed at freeing consciences from the yoke that canon law and pastoral practice had placed upon the believers, clerics as well as laymen.
2) The basic theological discussion concerned the relationship of marriage to the order of God's creation and ended in refusing to consider marriage as a sacrament.
3) The Christian doctrine of marriage, thus liberated from the canonical and theological constraints of ecclesiastical legislation, could once again play an important role (even a major one) in the social and ethical order. The underlying tone of Reformation teaching on this point came forth in the praise given to the beauty, dignity, and the deep-seated morality of the conjugal bond which is the foundation of all social life.
4) This kind of teaching was easily adaptable to the perspectives of the new western society which came about during the Renaissance. It tended towards flexibility by liberalizing divorce, and it reinforced social and economic structures by justifying a super-valuation of the family, now more tightly knit under the authority of the father as family head.

Let us briefly examine these four points.

1) In 1520, Luther, in his call *To the Christian Nobility of the German Nation,* had listed, among the propositions destined to favor the reform of the Church, freedom for the clergy to marry or not.[188] "You will find many a pious priest against whom nobody has anything to say except that he is weak and has come to shame with a woman. From the bottom of their hearts both are of a mind to live together in lawful wedded love, if only they could do it with a clear conscience. But even though they both have to bear public shame, the two are certainly married in the sight of God. And I say that where they are so minded and live together, they should appeal anew to their conscience. Let the priest take and keep her as his lawful wedded wife, and live honestly with her as her husband, whether the pope likes it or not, whether it be against canon or human law. The salvation of your soul is more important than the observance of tyrannical, arbitrary, and wanton laws which are not necessary to salvation or commanded by God."[189]

"Let consciences be free" is the cry repeated a thousand times by Luther, and echoed by so many Christians (cleric and lay) who found in the rediscovered gospel the courage to break with a legalism that led to hypocrisy and guilt. "(And) Christ has granted to Christians a liberty which is above all laws of men":[190] here we have the boldness of new liberty which so strongly marked the beginnings of the Reformation, along with a call to oppressed, "miserable consciences." Of course the time would quickly come when a morality would have to be constructed, a guideline to distinguish the do's and don'ts, but Luther's thrust would be sufficient forever to impede any return by Protestantism to a strict and contemptible casuistry in the realm of conjugal and sexual practice. "I would have nothing decided here on the mere authority of the popes and the bishops; but if two learned and good men agreed in the name of Christ and published their opinion in the spirit of Christ, I should prefer their judgment even to such councils as are assembled nowadays..."[191] Rejecting clerical casuistry, Luther appeals to individual conscience, enlightened and sanctified by the gospel; in some ways this defines the whole of Protestant morality!

"Christian or evangelical freedom, then, is a freedom of conscience which liberates the conscience from works. Not that no works are done but no faith is put in them."[192] Because of this, Luther undertakes a struggle against obligatory vows of celibacy and against the absolute prohibitions against divorce which in practice end in greater social disorder and in the personal despair of so many men and women.[193]

With Calvin,[194] typically, the struggle for the freedom of conscience takes on a more social and political aspect. With regard to divorce, he distinguishes between the will of God and the constraints upon political power which necessitate choosing the lesser of two evils. In contrast to an idealist morality, which on the social plane can only lead to legalistic "tyranny" or to a loose and carefree attitude, Calvin proposes a realism which seeks to safeguard liberty: "It was the same as with the magistrate, who is constrained to bear many things which he does not approve; for we cannot so deal with mankind as to restrain all vices. It is indeed desirable, that no vice should be tolerated; but we must have a regard to what is possible (i.e. to consider what is possible in a given situation [author's note])."[195]

In virtue of the twofold principle of realism and of freedom of conscience, Calvin sanctions divorce in certain cases, as does Luther: "But if a comparison be made, Malachi says that it is a lighter crime to dismiss a wife than to marry many wives ... for the husband ... then not only deals unfaithfully with his wife to whom he is bound, but also forcibly detains her: thus his crime is doubled" (*idem*). In opposition to those who prohibit any remarriage of divorced people who are the victims of adultery, Calvin also writes: "Our impartial moderators bind them to perpetual celibacy. What if they need a wife? No help for it; they must just fret on and atone for another's crime with the destruction of their soul. Thus a Christian man will be forced either to cherish adultery and swallow the dishonor of an unchaste wife, or be cruelly subjected to perpetual disquietudes, if the gift of continence be not bestowed upon him. While they provide so ill for miserable consciences, shall we aid their inhuman tyranny by our assent?"[196] As to the ecclesiastical obligation of celibacy, he sees it as stemming from the same tyranny: "The prohibition, however, clearly shows how pestiferous all traditions are since this one has not only deprived the Church of fit and honest pastors, but has introduced a fearful sink of iniquity, and plunged many souls into the gulf of despair. Certainly, when marriage was interdicted to priests, it was done with impious tyranny, not only contrary to the word of God, but contrary to all justice. First, men had no title whatever to forbid what God had left free; secondly, it is too clear to make it necessary to give any lengthened proof that God has expressly provided in his Word that this liberty should not be infringed."[197]

Opposing the tyranny exercised on oppressed consciences, the Reformation points to an ethic of individual responsibility, which is capable of determining one's obedience to the gospel and of accepting earthly reality as a place for service to that gospel.

2) As we have seen, the whole juridical and moral construct of medieval Catholicism relied on the doctrine of the sacramentality of marriage. And to that doctrine was linked the rejection of divorce and the requirement of ecclesiastical celibacy. Actually, marriage had become gradually recognized as a sacrament partly in response to the diminished value that the religious exaltation of virginity and celibacy risked assigning to marriage in the West. This was clearly seen by the Reformers, who attacked both the ecclesiastical requirement of celibacy and the sacramentality of marriage. Erasmus,[198] in his *In Novum Testamentum Annotationes* of 1518,[199] had already inaugurated a very pointed criticism against the sacramentality of marriage. He developed three arguments which reappear in the writings of the Reformers and which form the core of the polemic against the Catholic doctrine of marriage-as-sacrament. The first argument is historical. Marriage as a sacrament is a new thing: it is unknown in patristic tradition, and when the Fathers speak of marriage they describe it as an image of the union of Christ and the Church: "The Fathers followed Paul in calling marriage a sacrament; by that, they meant that the union of man and woman, being a very close-knit friendship, represents the figure and a certain kind of image of the union of Christ with the Church, His spouse."[200] It is therefore not a sacrament in the scholastic sense of the word. The second argument concerns the precise nature of the sacrament. If a sacrament is a sign of God's grace which also confers grace, how can marriage, which scholastic tradition says is a remedy against concupiscence, be a sacrament? And if it is a

sacrament, what bearing does that have on the free consent of the spouses? Finally, the third argument, which had by far the greatest success later on, is the scriptural argument. The classical interpretation was based on the Vulgate's translation of the Greek *mystérion* in Ephesians 5 by the Latin word *sacramentum*. This translation lends itself to serious misunderstandings, as Erasmus points out: "*Mystérion* must be translated as 'mystery' and not 'sacrament'; furthermore, the mystery refers to the union of Christ and the Church and not to marriage."[201] In this excellent exegesis, Erasmus notes that the word "mystery" does not designate a sacrament in the New Testament, but rather a secret and hidden reality (for example, Romans 11:25; 16:25; I Corinthians 2:7) concerning the work of God.

This critique by Erasmus was often echoed later. In 1520 Luther in *De captivitate babylonica* also rejects the sacramentality of marriage: "Christ and the Church are, therefore, a mystery, that is, a great and secret thing which can and ought to be represented in terms of marriage as a kind of outward allegory. But marriage ought not for that reason be called a sacrament. The heavens are a type of the apostles, as Psalm 19 declares; the sun is a type of Christ; the waters, of the peoples; but that does not make those things sacraments. . . ."[202] Marriage belongs to the natural order that is willed by God for all men: "Furthermore, since marriage has existed from the beginning of the world and is still found among unbelievers, there is no reason why it should be called a sacrament of the New Law and of the Church alone."[203]

In his *Institutes*, Calvin systematizes this critique (IV, xix, 34–36). Sensitive to the tragic history of men marked by sin (as all the Reformers were), he defines marriage as an order of creation prior to the fall, "that order of creation in which the eternal and inviolable appointment of God is strikingly displayed."[204] Marriage is even more necessary and beneficial in a world that it threatened by the disorder of sin: "Still marriage was not capable of being so far vitiated by the depravity of men, that the blessing which God had once sanctioned by His word should be utterly abolished and extinguished."[205]

This distinction between the order of creation and the order of redemption opens the way for constructive criticism of marriage-as-sacrament. Freed from the tutelage of canon law, marriage could rediscover its own ethical importance, as will be seen in section 3 which follows.

In concluding this point, it should be noted that among the Reformers, only Butzer refined this critique: even though he rejects the sacramental character of marriage, he nevertheless admits that it has the value of a sacramental sign when it is lived out in the faith and love of Christ. God's goal in instituting marriage is the total union of the man and the woman. "In this verse (Genesis 2:23 ff.), God shows what marriage is and why He instituted it. The communion of man and woman is such that in all things they are one flesh, i.e. one being, and that each of them has a willingness and desire to remain with the other more than with anyone else on earth."[206] This final end of marriage is fulfilled when the spouses live out their relationship as a sign of the union of Christ with the Church. Butzer did not wish the necessary process of de-sacredizing marriage to lead to a suppression of its spiritual (as well as moral) values. In 1557 he proposed this beautiful definition of marriage: "True marriage, as instituted by God . . . is a society and conjunction of man and woman, in which they are obliged to mutually communicate all things, divine and human, throughout their whole life and to live together in giving their bodies to one another whenever required or because of warm affection and genuine friendship."[207]

3) Why did the Reformers criticize the sacramentality of marriage? Apart from the reasons already stated, this was the only way to give marriage a morality of its own. Marriage involves first of all the liberty of two human beings who share the duty of creating a new community. The demand for individual liberty and responsibility which characterizes the beginning of the sixteenth century finds fertile ground here. The conviction in this case is the same for the

Humanists as for the Reformers: the moral reformation of marriage occurs via a criticism of its juridical sacramental status. The grace *ex opere operato* of the sacrament must give way to the active and liberating grace of God, which stirs up the faith and the responsibility of the believer. Thus, another shift occurs in the understanding of the final end of marriage and because of it, of sexuality: no longer as a remedy for concupiscence, marriage becomes a means of exercising true charity and authentic spiritual chastity.

A new judgment is thus brought to bear on sexuality, as witnessed in the following quotations:

Against the anti-feminism of the medieval and patristic tradition, Luther declares: "So they concluded that woman is a necessary evil, and that no household can be without such an evil. These are the words of blind heathen, who are ignorant of the fact that man and woman are God's creation. They blaspheme his work, as if man and woman just came into being spontaneously!... In order that we may not proceed as blindly, but rather conduct ourselves in a Christian manner, hold fast first of all to this, that man and woman are the work of God. Keep a tight rein on your heart and your lips; do not criticize his work, or call that evil which he himself has called good."[208] He affirms the goodness of marriage and of sexuality, both willed by God: "God divided mankind into two classes, namely, male and female, or a he and a she. This was so pleasing to him that he himself called it a good creation. Therefore, each one of us must have the kind of body God has created for us.... Moreover, he wills to have his excellent handiwork honored as his divine creation, and not despised. The man is not to despise or scoff at the woman or her body, nor the woman the man."[209]

Although this new attitude on sexuality is prudent and discreet, it is nevertheless quite different from that of medieval theology, as proved by this passage from Calvin: "But that God should permit a bride to enjoy herself with her husband, affords no triflng proof of His indulgence. Assuredly, it cannot be but that the lust of the flesh must affect the connection of husband and wife with some amount of sin; yet God not only pardons it, but covers it with the veil of holy matrimony, lest that which was sinful in itself should be so imputed; nay, He spontaneously allows them to enjoy themselves. To this injunction corresponds Paul's statement: 'Let the husband render unto his wife due benevolence: and likewise also the wife unto the husband. Defraud ye not the other, except it be with consent'...."[210] The goodness of marriage is such that it can justify whatever could be "depraved" in sexuality. Fear of sexuality is not so easily surmounted, especially when it is reinforced by religious arguments. On this point, Calvin does not hesitate to denounce a diabolical scheme under "religious" appearance: "... he (Paul) knew how much influence a false appearance of sanctity has in beguiling devout minds, as we ourselves know from experience. For Satan dazzles us with an appearance of what is right, that we might be led to imagine that we are polluted by intercourse with our wives...."[211] The only means of fighting against the perversion of this human vocation is to recognize that sexuality is given to man so that he can experience love through it: "*But neither is the man without the woman.* This is added partly as a check upon men, that they may not insult ... women; and partly as a consolation to women, that they may not feel dissatisfied with being under subjection. The male sex (says Paul) has a distinction over the female sex, with this understanding, that they ought to be connected together by mutual benevolence, for the one cannot do without the other. If they be separated, they are like the mutilated members of a mangled body. Let them, therefore, be connected with each other by the bond of mutual duty."[212]

Giving this kind of value to marriage inverts the scale of medieval values: henceforth marriage is the order willed by God, and celibacy is an exception which is rarely acceptable: "I say these things in order that we may learn how honorable a thing it is to live in that estate which

God has ordained. In it we find God's word and good pleasure, by which all the works, conduct, and sufferings of that estate become holy, godly, and precious so that Solomon even congratulates such a man and says in Proverbs 5:18: 'Rejoice in the wife of your youth' and again in Ecclesiastes 9:9: 'Enjoy life with the wife whom you love all the days of your vain life.' . . . Conversely, we learn how wretched is the spiritual estate of monks and nuns by its very nature, for it lacks the word and pleasure of God."[213]

Calvin echoes this position: "If anyone imagines that it is to his advantage to be without a wife and so without further consideration decides to be celibate, he is very much in error. For God, who declared that it was good that the woman should be the helpmeet for man, will exact punishment for contempt of His ordinance. Men arrogate too much to themselves when they try to exempt themselves from their heavenly calling."[214]

From this point on, the Reformers continually reassert the dignity and the beauty of the marital bond: ". . . this great honor stems from the fact that God holds it in such high regard that He committed himself to it (symbolically) by the intermediary of His only-begotten Son and through Him united Himself to us."[215] Marriage, restored to the order of creation willed by God, must be defended not only against those who scorn or denigrate it, but against any attempt to make its moral values relative. For immorality is not only an offense to the love of God since He has made our bodies a temple of the Holy Spirit,[216] but also an attack against man and the right order he should establish in line with God's law: "For He has stamped His mark upon us, to indicate that we bear His resemblance, and doesn't this image lie partly in the fact that men do not let themselves go at every turn, whenever a man meets a woman, as a dog meets a female dog? But each one has his own match and finds therein companionship blessed by God and sanctioned by Him."[217]

4) Marriage, now de-sacredized (or should I say de-sacramentalized?), accrued extreme value within the order of social morality: the success of the family (and even more of society) hinged on its success. But, given this new perspective, it yet remained to structure marriage unto the legal level, and there was urgency on one point in particular: the validity of clandestine marriages contracted without the knowledge of the parents. According to canon law, which strictly adopted the Roman principle of *"consensus facit nuptias,"* these marriages were recognized as valid. The parents' consent was not a part of the essence of marriage. Such a position came into conflict with the needs of a society that was seeking a more open atmosphere (free from Church domination) and a more stable order. Giving marriage social importance meant fighting against clandestine marriages (which were valid according to canon law) because they threatened family order. Therefore the Reformers made this fight one of the favorite themes of their matrimonial doctrine.

Erasmus had already pointed out, with irony, that Christians (as opposed to Jews and pagans) could contract marriage very easily, but without being able to undo it![218] The Church had come to sanction hasty marriages, in bad conscience; it seemed to approve disorder and even anarchy, while preventing marriage from fulfilling its genuine social function. Therefore the authority of parents had to be restored, i.e. their consent required to validate their children's marriages.

Luther insisted on this point quite a bit. Marriage is a public event and should thus be ratified by witnesses. But even more crucial than witnesses is the parents' authorization. Thus a marriage is clandestine whenever it is celebrated without the parents' knowledge: this was the important point for the Reformers. The major scriptural argument used is that of obedience to parents: to go against the will of the parents is to disobey God. "There is a solemn commandment from God which says that children must honor their father and mother, and nature teaches us that children should undertake nothing that is not known to their parents so long as they are minors. Therefore no marriage can be founded in God when one scorns his parents and acts without their consent. This is the reason that Christian authorities must prohibit such unions."[219]

This point would be woven into the Genevan legislation on marriage by Calvin's *Ecclesiastical Ordinances of 1561:* "As for young people who have never been married, let none of them (be they sons or daughters) who have living fathers have the power to contract marriage without the authorization of their fathers, unless they have reached legal age, (20 for the son, 18 for the daughter); and if after reaching legal age, they obtain or ask their fathers for permission to marry, and if the fathers do nothing about it and that fact is known to the Consistory, after having called the fathers concerned and exhorted them to their duty, in such cases, it is legitimate to marry without the authority of the fathers.... If it occurs that two young people have contracted a marriage on their own through folly or levity, let them be punished and chastized; let such a marriage be rescinded (declared null) upon the request of those who have them under their charge."[220]

In principle this paternal authority is limited by law. And so at Geneva, these same ecclesiastical ordinances specify that: "no father [should] force his children into a marriage which seems good to him without their willingness and consent; let him or her who does not wish to accept the partner chosen by the father be excused, maintaining a humble and reverent attitude, without being punished by the father for such a refusal."[221]

But in reality,[222] the cases were rare, it seems, when paternal authority was discredited by the magistrate. Even if a consummation of the marriage (*copula carnalis*) had occurred, marriage could be annulled on request by the parents, according to the law as influenced by Calvin—which was not the case in the Lutheran countries. In the Germanic countries the trend would also be to reinforce parental authority, for example, by raising the "matrimonial age" which was 24 for the man and 20 for the woman (Strasbourg 1530) to 25 for both of them (Strasbourg 1565).

So, in general, the weakening of the authority of canon law in Protestant countries as influenced by the Reformation, was simultaneously accompanied by a strengthening of parental authority. As I have said, this new attitude fitted in with the needs of the new society. As proof of this, the very Catholic king of France, at the Council of Trent,[223] called for a reform of canon law condemning clandestine marriages, defined as (and the Council rejected this definition) those contracted without the consent of parents. The conjunction on this issue of political power and the Protestant position signifies an evolution of customs which posited a new and important responsibility to the family in the economic realm, as well as in the moral and educational realms.

This reinforcement of family order was undergirded by a hierarchical vision of relationships between men and women. The whole classical arsenal of arguments was taken up by the Reformers to affirm the rigid subordination of the wife to the husband in marriage. Luther very strongly affirms: "... it is necessary that the woman know and be convinced that man is higher and better than she is. For government and supremacy belong to man as head of the family and master of the household.... Consequently, in the conjugal state also, the woman must not only love her husband, but also be obedient and submissive; she must let herself be governed by him, reverence him, in brief, hold only to him and be directed by him; she must not only acknowledge the protection he affords her, but must remember, in seeing him, this example, and think of it: My husband is the image of the true and supreme head, Christ...."[224] This interpretation of Ephesians 5 emphasizes the authority of Christ in His rapport with the Church. But Luther is aware that the text also speaks even more of Christ's love. This is why there is a tension in Luther's writings, as well as in Calvin's, between, on one hand, the affirmation of the primacy of love as the foundation of the marital bond—a love which implies the recognition of the spiritual equality of man and woman before God—and, on the other hand, the need for maintaining a hierarchical order within the couple. That tension between theological perspective and social requirement clearly appears in this passage from Calvin: "Woman is like a branch that has come from man; for she was taken from his substance, as we know. It is true that God did this in order to recommend the union that we should have together, for He could easily have formed Eve from the earth, as He did Adam; but He wished to take one side from man so that man would not have anything apart from the woman, but that he should recognize that God created us as one body and that we cannot be separated unless we go against His will. God took that into consideration, but . . . He nevertheless placed man over the woman."[225] Thus, in Protestant ethics, the desire to construct society based on a hierarchy that is able to resist the eruption of anarchy, is coupled with the concern for maintaining the theological affirmation of the primacy of the couple over the individual, and the primacy of the structural unity of the man and woman over the contingent reality of the wife's submission.

*   *   *

The Reformation was experienced by its proponents as a liberation movement. However, the Reformers, aware that the Church in its faithfulness to the Gospel must accept social responsibility, very quickly opposed radical revolutionaries (like the Anabaptists) who attempted to bypass the gradual evolution of mentalities and structures (because of the length of time required). An old debate! Given the two extremes of Catholic conservatism and Anabaptist utopianism, the Reformers tried to maintain a course between patiently coping with the weight of reality and impatiently and urgently proclaiming the rediscovered Gospel of justification by grace and of salvation by faith.

And so in the realm of sexual and conjugal ethics the Reformation opened the way for a new consciousness which represented a sharp break with the dominant ideology in the Middle Ages. The change was crucial (and full of potential) on at least three points. First of all, there was the break with the ancient Christian tradition which exalted celibacy as the royal road to salvation and obedience to God: the Reformation strongly asserted the primacy of marriage and thereby gave sexuality a new and positive status (even if its boundaries were carefully drawn!). Sexuality was recognized as the locus of the fundamental human experience of conjugality. Man does not exist independent of woman but is a partner in humanity, in a bond that is both emotional and social. "Man was created by God to be a creature of companionship," according to Calvin. And so—this is a major point—sexuality was no longer considered a priori as a fearful menace to guard against.

Next, and following logically, the Reformation took a stand on women quite different from that at the end of the Middle Ages. Woman, although rigidly subordinated to the husband, is seen neither as a demonical creature created to test the chastity of true believers, i.e. monks, nor as just a reproductive being charged with ensuring descendancy to her "lord and master";[226] she has co-responsibility with her husband for conjugal and family life. Examples of these "stalwart women" are not lacking in Protestant tradition (and even in American westerns!), especially in the traditions of the persecuted churches (whether Puritan or from the Cévennes region.)

Finally, restored to the created order, marriage became a matter of moral and social responsibility. What is lost as to the aspect of sacred mystery is regained in the awareness of what is relevant on the human moral and social level. It seems certain that the countries influenced by the Reformation were the first to attempt basing a social order on the family as the primary nucleus for all social life. This attempt at the moralization of society through the intermediary of the family is a characteristic of the Reformation. Through marriage, which is no longer deemed a remedy to concupiscence but recognized as an aid to human weakness, man can build mankind. It is important, then, that marriage and the family be protected by law.

It is at this juncture that the fact of institutional reality weighed most heavily on the attempt at renovating society. Through fear of the Anabaptist anarchy, the Reformers gave the Church a juridical power that constituted canon law.[227] They had fought against the meddlesome domination of canon law, but found themselves obligated to legislate that which fundamentally only belongs to the responsibility of each couple before God. Thus the Protestant canonical writers throughout the seventeenth century gradually returned to notions that existed before the Reformation: "... there was a very clear reaction near the end of the sixteenth century, which tended to discard the lay concept of the first reformers and to accentuate the religious consequences of the fact that the institution of marriage was divine."[228] To structure a moral requirement into a social and political context is quite difficult, as the Reformation Churches came to see. Pierre Bels is undoubtedly right when he concludes his book with this affirmation: "... the sixteenth century ... is marked by an accumulation of serious difficulties which left reformed law quite vulnerable. For instance, the initial doctrines that set the tone for Protestant action and performance led to some inauspicious and harmful effects. These doctrines, as part of a systematically critical and anti-juridical viewpoint aiming at demolishing canon law and at attacking the Roman Church, sought their justification along moral lines; marriage was thus seen as a reformation of morals and not as an ensemble of juridical mechanisms. This perspective affected the technical aspect of law, which in turn presented insoluble problems."[229]

Thus, the essence of Protestant ethics in matters of sex and conjugality has a twofold character. On one hand, there is a liberation vis-à-vis an inquisition-like legalism in the sexual domain: "To the very extent that the Protestants consider the issues of conjugal ethics to be the responsibility of each couple before God, the pastors, although married themselves, do not 'penetrate the mysteries of the conjugal sanctuary' and in no way take on the role played by the Catholic celibate confessors with regard to their penitents. Likewise, in opposition to the verbosity of the theologians of the Roman Church, the Reformation theologians are extremely discreet on these matters."[230] But, along with this undeniable freedom of conscience, there is a real juridical and social rigidity concerning conjugal questions in the reformed tradition. Therefore, (for example) ecclesiastical control on the validity of marriage ends up being more important in Protestant law than in the post-tridentine canon law: "The direction of the evolution of the religious ceremony was exactly inverse in the two faiths. The Catholic priest was deprived of active intervention given to him by custom (to now become only a witness of the marriage [author's note]). With the Protestants, the evolution developed logically and resulted in marriage being created only through the religious ceremony and the preponderant action of the pastor."[231]

Freedom and responsibility were indeed restored to believers, but only within the framework of a social order authenticated by the Church and the bias of its ministers: this roughly summarizes the Protestant position. On the social level, it fit into the effort to moralize society that was undertaken by Christianity in the sixteenth century; what distinguishes it from the parallel effort by Catholics is its sharper emphasis on personal responsibility: it is henceforth the believer's conscience, more than the exterior control of the Church (through confession), which ratifies what is fitting and correct in moral attitudes on sexuality and conjugality. But that conscience, however, must be able to recognize and measure the social importance of a personal and conjugal practice of sexuality that is virtuous.

Notes

1. "Therefore God gave them up in the lusts of their hearts to impurity, to the dishonoring of their bodies among themselves, because they exchanged the truth about God for a lie and worshiped and served the creature rather than the Creator.... For this reason God gave them up to dishonorable passions. Their women exchanged natural relations for unnatural, and the men likewise gave up natural relations with women and were consummated with passion for one another, men committing shameless acts with men and receiving in their own persons the due penalty for their error" (Rom. 1:24–27).

2. Erich Klostermann, "Die adäquate Vergeltung in Röm. 1:22–29, *ZNW* (1933) has demonstrated that this genre of indictment was known in Hellenistic Judaism. Cf. also Joachim Jeremias "Zu Rom. 1:22–32," *ZNW* (1954). On Judaism at the time of the birth of Christianity: Emil Schürer, *A History of the Jewish People in the Time of Jesus Christ.* 2nd rev. (Edinburgh: T.&T. Clark 1897–98); and George F. Moore, *Judaism in the First Centuries of the Christian Era* (Cambridge: Harvard University Press, 1927–1930).

3. 1 Tim. 1:9–10. Similar lists are found in 2 Tim. 3:2–4; Titus 3:3; 1 Peter 4:3.

4. On the way in which Christianity took up certain moral requirements and radicalized ethics in a totally different way, cf. Alfred Darby Nock, *Early Gentile Christianity and Its Hellenistic Background* (New York: Harper Torchbooks, 1962), especially pp. 7–23.

5. The exposure of children in a public place shortly after birth is well known in literature of the Hellenistic period (cf. Gustave Glotz, *Etudes sociales et juridiques sur l'antiquité grecque* [Paris: Hachette et Cie, 1906], pp. 187–227) where it is attested to as the classical means of population control. "A son is reared even if the family is poor; a daughter is exposed even if the family is rich" (Poseidippos, *Hermaphroditos*, fragment 11). The majority of exposed children were taken to become slaves. The exposition of children was still widely practiced in the period of the empire (cf. Letters 65 and 66 from Pliny to Trajan). Cf. Claude Vatin, *Recherches sur le mariage et la condition de la femme mariée à l'époque hellénistique* (Paris, 1970), p. 234 ff.

6. Justin, *Apologia* I, 27–29, *FC*, Vol. VI, pp. 62–63.

7. *Didache*, II, ii, *FC*, Vol. I, p. 172. Cf. Jean Paul Audet, *La Didachè Instructions des apôtres* (Paris: J. Gabalda, 1958), p. 228 ff. and pp 286–289.

8. "Furthermore, Thou shalt not 'eat the hare either.' (Lev. 11:6). Why? You shall not become, he means, a corrupter of boys, nor shall ye become like such persons. For the hare gains a passage in the body each year, and every year it lives, it has that many passages. Nor shalt thou 'eat the hyena.' You shall not, he means, become an adulterer or fornicator, nor become like such persons. Why? Because this animal changes its nature every year and becomes now male, now female. Moreover he hates the weasel (Moses in Lev. 11:29), and rightly so. You shall not, he means, become like those men who, we are told, work iniquity with their mouth in their uncleanness nor shall you associate with impure women who work iniquity with their mouth. For this animal conceives by the mouth." *Letter of Barnabas*, X, 6–8, *FC*, Vol. I, p. 207.

9. Ignatius of Antioch, *To Polycarp* VI, 1–2, *FC*, Vol. I, p. 126.

10. Hermas, *The Shepherd*, Mand, IV, i, 1, *FC*, Vol. I, p. 263.

11. Tertullian, *Apologia*, XXXIX, 11–12, *FC*, Vol. X, pp. 99–100. This text can be compared to the following passage from Diogenes Laertius: "It is also their doctrine (the Stoics) that amongst the wise there should be a community of wives with free choice of partners, as Zeno says in his *Republic* and Chrysippus in his treatise *On Government*. Under such circumstances we shall feel paternal affection for all the children alike, and there will be an end of the jealousies arising from adultery." *Lives of Eminent Philosophers*, VII, 131, trans. by R.D. Hicks (Cambridge: Harvard University Press, 1950), Vol. II, p. 235.

12. Paul Veyne, in his article, "La famille et l'amour sous le Haut-Empire romain" (*Annales, E.S.C.* 33 [1978], 1, pp. 35–63), shows that sexual and conjugal morality is in full evolution at the turn of the second century in Rome. This very interesting article sets forth the following thesis: "Between the time of Cicero and the century of the Antonines, a major event transpired that is not well known: a metamorphosis in sexual and conjugal relationships. At the end of this metamorphosis, pagan sexual morality becomes identical to the future Christian morality of marriage. This transformation was accomplished independent of all Christian influence" (p. 35). In response, I would say, that even if there were a conjunction between the Christian contribution and the moral transformation from pagan origins (and that therefore Chris-

tianity is certainly not the only factor in this moral metamorphosis), one could not affirm without being dogmatic (and Paul Veyne's article is not exempt from dogmatism) that Christianity had no effect on the evolution of morality in the empire. It should be noted, however, that here we have a specialist in Roman History who would have us believe that Christianity had no effect on the victory at the heart of the Empire of what the whole world calls the "taboos of Judaeo-Christian morality"!

13. Gabriel Germain, *Epictète et la spiritualité stoicienne* (Paris: Editions du Seuil, 1964), p. 129.

14. Quoted in Nock, op. cit., pp. 20–21. Nock goes on to say that it would be a mistake to think these moral requirements represent an isolated example: "In reality they are a striking illustration of a widespread change of moral outlook"; p. 22.

15. Pliny, *Letters and Panegyricus*, X, xcvi, 7, trans. by Betty Radice (Cambridge: Harvard University Press, 1969), p. 289.

16. The whole field of conjugal ethics has been authoritatively studied by J. P. Broudehoux, *Mariage et famille chez Clément d'Alexandrie* (Paris: Beauchesne et ses Fils, 1970).

17. *Stromateis* III, trans. by Henry Chadwick in *Alexandrian Christianity* (Philadelphia: Westminster Press, 1954), Vol. II, pp. 40–93. Quotations will be taken from this edition.

18. As P. Batiffol has written, encratism is "a spirit spread throughout the Church itself in the second century," *Etudes d'histoire et de théologie positive* (Paris, 1968), p. 53.

19. Author of a work entitled *On Perfection According to the Saviour*, the thesis of which was that marriage was really only corruption and fornication; this is according to Clement, *Stromateis* III, xii.

20. His book *Concerning Continence and Celibacy* proposed castration as the ideal. Cf. Clement, *Stromateis* III, xiii.

21. For example, this passage from *Acts of John*, 113: "O thou who hast kept me until this hour for thyself and untouched by union with a woman: who when in my youth I desired to marry didst appear unto me and say to me: John, I have need of thee: who didst prepare for me also a sickness of the body: who when for the third time I would marry didst forthwith prevent me, and then at the third hour of the day saidst unto me on the sea: John, if thou hadst not been mine, I would have suffered thee to marry: who for two years didst blind me (or afflict mine eyes), and grant me to mourn and entreat thee: who in the third year didst open the eyes of my mind and also grant me my visible eyes: who when I saw clearly didst ordain that it should be grievous to me to look upon a woman: who didst save me from the temporal fantasy and lead me unto that which endureth always: who didst rid me of the foul madness that is in the flesh:.... Now therefore Lord, whereas I have accomplished the dispensation wherewith I was entrusted, account thou me worthy of thy rest, and grant me that end in thee which is salvation unspeakable and unutterable." In the *Apocryphal New Testament*, trans. by Montague Rhodes James (Oxford: Clarendon Press, 1924), p. 269.

22. Julius Cassianus, according to Clement, *Stromateis*, III, xiii.

23. Salome asks Jesus when man will cease to exist; Jesus answers that man will continue as long as women give birth to children; cf. *Stromateis,* III, ix, 64, p. 70.

24. "When Salome asked when she would know the answer to her questions, the Lord said, When you trample on the robe of shame, and when the two shall be one, and the male with the female, and there is neither male nor female." Quoted by Clement in *Stromateis,* III, xiii, 92, in op. cit., p. 83. The same idea is found in the *Gospel of Thomas*. "When you make the two one, and when you make the inside as the outside, and the outside as the inside, and the upper side as the lower, and when you make the male and the female into a single one, that the male be not male and the female not female; ... then you shall enter (the Kingdom)," *Gospel of Thomas*, v. 22, in *New Testament Apocrypha I*, ed. Willhem Schneemelcher, trans. by Robert McL. Wilson (Philadelphia, 1963), p. 92.

25. Clement, *Pedagogos*, II, x, 83, FC, Vol. 23, p. 164 ff.

26. Ibid., II, x, 91, p. 170.

27. Cf. Bourdehoux, op. cit., p. 85 ff.

28. "... some will depart from the faith by giving heed to deceitful spirits and doctrines of demons, through the pretensions of liars whose consciences are seared, who forbid marriage and enjoin abstinence from foods..."

29. "Let marriage be held in honor among all, and let the marriage bed be undefiled; for God will judge the immoral and adulterous."

30. On the licentious gnostic sects, cf. Hans Leisegang *Die Gnosis* (Stuttgart: A. Kröner, 1955); Robert M. Grant, *Gnosticism and Early Christianity*, rev. ed. (New York: Harper & Row, 1966); Werner Foerster, Ernest Haenchen, Martin Krause, *Die Gnosis* (Zürich: Artemis Verlag, 1969); as for Church Fathers, cf. Irenaeus *Adv. Haer I*, passim, Clement of Alexandria, *Strom.*, III, and Epiphanius, *Panarion* XXIV–XXVII, PG 41, coll. 307–378.

31. Hans Leisegang proposes quite similar parallels in certain expressions by Jakob Boehme and Meister Eckhart (op. cit., p. 164 ff.).

32. Quoted from Epiphanes, *Concerning Righteousness* in Clement, *Stromateis*, III, ii, 8, op. cit., pp. 43–44.

33. Cf. Rom. 6:15; 1 Cor. 5:1–8; Gal. 5:13; 1 Pet. 2:16, 2 Pet. 2:19.

34. Clement, *Stromateis*, III, v, 44, in op. cit., p. 60.

35. Michel Spanneut, *Le stoïcisme des Pères de l'Eglise* (Paris 1969). Patristica Sorboniensa I, pp. 252–257.

36. The reader can refer to further material on this point in John T. Noonan, Jr., *Contraception: A History of Its Treatment by the Catholic Theologians and Canonists* (New York: New American Library, 1965), p. 99 ff.

37. Ibid., pp. 101–102.

38. This is André Mehat's expression, *Etude sur les Stromates de Clément d'Alexandrie* (Paris: Editions de Seuil, 1966), p. 509 ff.

39. Cf. Paul Veyne, art. cited, *Annales*.

40. *Letter to Diognetus*, V, vi, FC, Vol. I, p. 361 (epistle at the end of the second century).

41. On this point, cf. Schillebeeckx, op. cit., Vol. II, pp. 3–18, and his helpful bibliography; cf. also Pierre Grimal, *The Civilization of Rome*, trans. by W. S. Maguiness (London: Allen & Unwin, 1963), Chapt. III, "Life and Customs."

42. Schillebeeckx, op. cit., Vol. II, pp. 13–14.

43. Ignatius of Antioch, *To Polycarp*, V, ii, FC, Vol. I, p. 126; for an interpretation of this text, cf. Korbinian Ritzer, *Le mariage dans les eglises chrétiennes du 1er au XIe siècle* (Paris: Editions du Cerf, 1970), pp. 81–84.

44. Tertullian, *Ad uxorem*, II, ix, in A.C.W., Vol. XIII, p. 35. Specialists like Ritzer and Schillebeeckx interpret this text as a reminder that the marriage of baptized people is ecclesiastic; its Christian and ecclesiastical character is reinforced by the fact that the spouses take part in liturgical celebration and pray together at home. The angels of God are the witnesses and guardians of this conjugal life. This is the kind of marriage the Heavenly Father approves of.

45. Cf. P. Nautin, "Divorce et remariage dans la tradition latine," *Rech. Sc. Rel.* 62 (1974), pp. 7–54 (a very well-informed article). It should be remembered that divorce in first century Rome was extremely easy: "... since marriage was neither a public nor a juridical action, nothing was easier than repudiating a spouse: one word was enough, and it was not even necessary to inform the spouse of the repudiation, which was not a solemn act." Veyne, art. cited, *Annales*, p. 42.

46. Hermas, *The Shepherd*, Mand. IV, i, 4–8, FC, Vol. I, p. 264.

47. Tertullian, *Adversus Marcionem*, IV, xxxiv, 7, trans. by Ernest Evans (Oxford, The Clarendon Press, 1972), Vol. II, p. 453.

48. Hermas, *The Shepherd*, Mand. IV, iv, 1b–2, FC, Vol. I, p. 267.

49. Tertullian, *Ad uxorem*, II, iv, in op. cit., p. 29.

50. Cf. R.C. Gerest, "Quand les chrétiens ne se marient pas à l'église: histoire des cinq premiers siècles," *Lumière et Vie*, 82 (1967), pp. 24–27.

51. Ibid., p. 25 (note 51): "It was still current practice in the first centuries of our era for masters to set aside young slaves for prostitution and to regard those who were not in any established union as being in a more flexible position than the others."

52. Ambrose of Milan, *Exhort. virgin*, VI, xxxvi, PL 16, 362.

53. Augustine, *De nupt. et concup.*, II, xxi, N–PNF, Vol. V, p. 297; cf. *De civit. Dei*, XIV, xviii, 41, FC, Vol. XIV, pp. 391–392.

54. Augustine's use of this concept signifies the sexual instinct as linked to sexual pleasure and desire which are not under reason's control. Cf. *De civit. Dei,* XIV, xv, 37, *FC,* Vol. XIV, p. 384 ff.

55. Augustine, *De civit. Dei,* XIV, xx, 44, *FC,* Vol. XIV, p. 395.

56. Ibid., XIV, xvi, 38, p. 388.

57. Augustine, *Soliloquia* I, x, 17, *FC,* Vol. V, p. 365. Augustine, recently converted, was 33 when he wrote this.

58. Jerome, *Comm. in ep. ad. Gal.* III, v, 21, *PL,* 26, p. 415.

59. Theodoret of Cyrus, *Quest. in Genesium,* ch. 3, qu. 37, PG 80, 135.

60. There is, however, an exception (the only one that I know of!). It comes by chance from the lay theologian Lactantius, who wrote in *The Divine Institutes,* VI, xxiii: "When God invented the plan of the two sexes, He placed in them the desire of each other and joy in union. So he put in bodies the most ardent desire of all living things, so that they might rush most avidly into these emotions and be able by this means to propagate and increase their kind. Ths desire and longing is found more vehement and more keen in man, either because He wished the number of men to be greater, or because He gave the power to man alone, so that it might be to His praise and glory in refraining from pleasures and in self-restraint. That adversary of ours knows how great is the force of this desire . . . and puts in illicit desires so that the foreign ones contaminate those which are proper, which it is all right to have without any fault. . . ."—in *FC,* Vol. XLIX, p. 457. This is a unique testimony which puts sexual pleasure and desire on the side of God and aligns sin with adultery, rather than with sexuality. Written between 304 and 313, this text has no echo in later tradition.

61. Augustine, *De Gen ad lit.,* III, xxi, 33; *Oeuvres,* Vol. XLVIII, pp. 264–265.

62. Augustine, *Contra Julianum,* IV, xi, 57, *FC,* Vol. XXXV, p. 214.

63. As is shown in this quote from Pseudo-Clement: "God . . . has declared that it (celibacy) is 'better than sons and daughters,' and that He will give to virgins a notable place in the house of God, which is something 'better than sons and daughters,' and better than the place of those who have passed a wedded life in sanctity, and whose 'bed has not been defiled.' For God will give to virgins the kingdom of heaven, as to the holy angels, by reason of this great and noble profession." *Epistola I ad Virgines,* IV, in *ANF.,* Vol. VIII, p. 56; cf. Justin (I *Apol.* XXIX), the story of the young Christian who asks the prefect for permission to make himself a eunuch.

64. These are the most important works: *The Symposium* by Methodius; *De virginitate* by Basil of Ankara; another by Gregory of Nyssa; and *De virg.,* and *Letters* (on virginity) by (or attributed to) Basil of Caeserea; *Exhort. Virg.* by Ambrose of Milan; *Contra Helvidius* by Jerome; *De sanc. virg.* by Augustine.

65. Gregory of Nyssa, *De virginitate, FC,* Vol. LVIII, pp. 3–79.

66. Methodius, *The Symposium,* trans. by Herbert Musurillo (Westminster, Maryland: The Newman Press, 1958).

67. Jerome, *De Perpetua Virginitate B. Mariae,* XX, *FC,* Vol. LIII, pp. 40–41.

68. Augustine, *De Sancta virginitate,* XVI, *FC,* Vol. 27, p. 159.

69. John Chrysostom, *Paraenesis ad Theodorum Lapsum,* II, v, *N–PNF,* Vol. IX, p. 115.

70. Ambrose, *De paradiso,* XI, *FC,* Vol. 42, p. 328.

71. Jean-Marie Pohier, preface to Kerns, *Les chrétiens, le mariage . . .* p. 13. The original edition: Joseph Kerns, *The Theology of Marriage* (New York: Sheed and Ward, 1964).

72. Jerome, *Adversus Jovinianum,* I, xxvii, *PL* 23, p. 260.

73. On Manicheanism, consult Henri Charles Puech, *Le manichéisme: son fondateur, sa doctrine* (Paris: Civilisations du Sud, 1949); François Decret, *Mani et la tradition manichéenne* (Paris, 1974). On St. Augustine and the Manicheans in regard to questions of sexual ethic, cf. Noonan, op. cit., pp. 137–175.

74. Augustine, *Contra Faustum,* XXII, xxx, *N–PNF,* Vol. IV, p. 284.

75. Ibid.

76. Eusebius, *Ad Marinum, PG* 22, 1107.

77. Noonan, op. cit., p. 101.

78. Paul Veyne's article already quoted (*Annales*) sheds important light on this question. But I prefer the more subtle analysis of Henri Irenée Marrou, *Décadence romaine ou antiquité tardive?: IIIe–VIe Siècle*

(Paris: Editions du Seuil, 1977); cf., for example, pp. 21–32 which describe the difficulties that Christianity had in significantly modifying ancient morals, especially in the area of entertainment.

79. Marrou's book listed above offers many proofs of the surprising symbiosis between Christianity and the spirit of Roman antiquity of the third and fourth centuries.

80. Rudolf Bultmann, *Primitive Christianity in Its Contemporary Setting,* trans. by Rev. R.H. Fuller (New York: Meridian Books, 1956), p. 144.

81. This was more and more readily admitted especially when the philosophical influence of Neoplatonic dualism supplanted stoic influence on theology in the middle of the third century.

82. Marcel Detienne, *The Gardens of Adonis,* trans. by Janet Lloyd, intro. by J.P. Vernant (Atlantic Highlands, N.J.: Humanities Press, 1977).

83. J.L. Flandrin, *Annales, E.S.C.,* 27 (1972), p. 1366.

84. For instance, the *Song of Solomon* which could be accepted and understood only when interpreted allegorically.

85. I am speaking of the ethical domain, for on the strictly theological level, the dominant influence in the middle of the third century was Neoplatonic, as we have seen from the example of Gregory of Nyssa.

86. Stobaeus reports that the Stoics would say that whereas "Other friendships and affections resemble mixtures by juxtaposition—vegetables or other analogous objects—the affection of the husband and wife is comparable to a total fusion, like water and wine," *Florilegium,* LXVII, 25.

87. Cf. Epictetus, *The Discourses,* II, iv, 1–11, trans. by W.A. Oldfather (Cambridge: Harvard University Press, 1946), Vol. I, pp. 233–237.

88. "—Can we properly have confidence, then, in something that is insecure?—No.—Pleasure contains no element of security, does it?—No.—Away with it, then, and throw it out of the balance, and drive it far away from the region of things good," Epictetus, II, xi, 20–21, in op. cit., p. 289; cf. II, xviii, 18, pp. 333–335.

89. Epictetus, III, xxiv, 58–59, in op. cit., Vol. II, pp. 203–205.

90. "Sextus was probably, in fact, a Christian philosopher who, between 180 and 210, had reworked an ancient set of gnomic sayings . . ." Noonan, op. cit., footnote #23, p. 106.

91. Jerome, *Adv. Jov.* I, xlix, *PL* 23, 281.

92. Augustine, *Contra Jul.* II, vii, 20, *FC,* Vol. XXXV, p. 81.

93. Spanneut, op. cit., p. 266. What this author says about the Fathers of the second and third centuries describes the situation in the fourth century in the ethical domain equally well.

94. The term itself is absent in patristic language. The Fathers speak of "asceticism."

95. To repeat, this dissociation will be accentuated in the third century and even more later, when Christian thinking becomes more directly inspired by Neoplatonism. Cf. Etienne Gilson, "Le christianisme et la tradition philosophique," *Rev. des Sc. Ph. et Rel.* 2, 1941–42, pp. 249–266.

96. Cf. Johannes Leipoldt, *Die Frau in der antiken Welt und im Urchristentum* (Leipzig: Koehler & Amelang, 1955); F. Quere-Jaulmes, *La Femme. Les grands textes des Pères de l'Eglise* (Paris, 1968); Jean-Marie Aubert, *La Femme. Anti-féminisme et christianisme* (Paris, 1975); Elisabeth S. Fiorenza, "Le rôle des femmes dan le mouvement chrétien primitif, *Concilium* 111, 1976, pp. 13–25; Klaus Thraede, *Aerger mit der Freiheit. Die Bedeutung von Frauen in Theorie und Praxis der Alten Kirche.* This is the first part of the work by Gerta Scharffenorth and Thraede, *"Freunde in Christus werden. . . ." Die Beziehungen von Mann und Frau als Frage an Theologie und Kirche,* Gelnhausen/Berlin et Stein/Mfr., 1977, pp. 31–182.

97. Elisabeth S. Fiorenza, art. cited, p. 17. It must also be shown that a more positive tradition existed, that "a feminist tradition fought against the misogynist tradition" (F. Quere), and that the defense of women by Plato (i.e. *Laws VII,* 804–806; VII, 833–839) tempered the narrow-minded sexism of Aristotle (cf. *Politics* I, 1254b, 1260a; VI, 1323).

98. Abraham Cohen, op. cit., p. 159.

99. "Women were not marginal figures at the heart of the movement; they exercised a leading role as apostles, prophets, missionaries." Fiorenza, art. cited, p. 18; cf. also U. Ruegg, "Marthe et Marie," *Bull CPE,* 22 (1970), 6–7, pp. 19–36.

100. Augustine, *De trinitate,* XII, vii, 10, *FC,* Vol. XLV, p. 352.

101. Jean-Marie Aubert, op. cit., p. 58.

102. Which is clearly shown by France Quere-Jaulmes, op. cit., pp. 18–38.

103. Cf. Kari E. Borresen, *Subordination and Equivalence: The Nature and Role of Women in Augustine and Thomas Aquinas* (Washington, D.C.: University Press of America, 1981). There is also an article by this Catholic theologian on this same topic in *Concilium* III, 1976, pp. 27–39.

104. This is even rooted in language itself: in Greek as in Latin, the word designating *virtue* comes from the same root word for man: *andreia* from *aner* and *virtus* from *vir*.

105. Philo, Supplement II, *Questions and Answers on Exodus 1:8*, trans. by Ralph Marcus (London: William Heinemann Ltd., 1943), pp. 15–16; cf. Richard Arthur Baer, *Philo's Use of the Categories of Male and Female* (Leiden: E. J. Brill, 1970).

106. Spanneut, op. cit., p. 181.

107. Tertullian, *De Anima*, XXVII, vi, *FC*, Vol. X, p. 244.

108. Clement, *Stomateis III*, xii, in op. cit., p. 76 ff.

109. This physiological theory (from Stoicism) will be taken up by Christian tradition from Augustine to Thomas, and even after them.

110. There is a very nice illustration of this in the way in which Philo recounts how Balaam counsels Balak to make the daughters of his people seduce the sons of Israel, cf. *Vita Mosis* I, 295–299. As a prisoner of the desire aroused by woman, man loses all faculty to judge or defend himself.

111. *The Testament of the Twelve Patriarchs*, Bk. I (The Testament of Reuben), trans. by Robert Sinker, in *ANF*, Vol. VIII, p. 10.

112. Jean-Marie Aubert quotes these theories from the historian H. Leclercq: "He [Ambrose] does not go as far as Tertullian and speak of the pregnant woman's nausea, dangling breasts and small screaming children (*Tertullian, De monogamia, XVI*); but it is Tertullian's spirit which breathes in him and inspires him to a kind of disgust for the laws and mysteries of [feminine] nature," op. cit., p. 194, note #80.

113. As for instance, among many others, Tertullian, *De cultu feminarum, FC*, Vol. XL; Clement of Alexandria, *Pedagogos* III; Gregory of Nazianzen, *Carmina moralia;* Cyprien, *De habitu virginum*.

114. The recent publication of a study by Huguette Taviani, "Le mariage dans l'héresie de l'An Mil," in *Annales E.S.C.* 32 (1977), pp. 1074–1089, convinced me that I should qualify this judgment. Even if Augustine is the main authority, the influence of Greek patristic thinking cannot be neglected; as we have seen, this thinking interpreted sexuality as the consequence of the fall and valued virginity as the paradisic state of perfect nature, i.e. non-sexed. "Gerard of Cambray (the bishop in charge of interrogating the heretics who denied marriage at Arras in 1025) is thus an heir of pre-augustinian and neoplatonic thought which was still present in the schools familiar with the teachings of Herik and Remy of Auxerre, themselves disciples of John Scotus.... The Carolingian theory of marriage is not a single unified theory. At the end of the 9th century John Scotus had reconnected neoplatonism and Greek Fathers, and his influence was still enormous in the 10th and beginning of the 11th centuries in Laon, Auxerre and Chartres" (p. 1082ff.). If these theologians defended marriage in the face of heretics (who, under the influence of encratic apocryphal texts, i.e. *Acts of Andrew, of Paul, Passio Sanctae Theclae*, made virginity the necessary condition for a return to God), they did not defend it by recalling, in augustinian style, that marriage was willed by God before the fall, but by invoking its necessity vis-à-vis maintaining a social hierarchical order. "The rule constituting the spiritual anthropology of *Ecclesia* is actually the discrimination of orders (*discretio ordinis*), which frames the whole discourse of Gerard of Cambray. To the hierarchy of values which places married-continent-virgin in ascending order on the road to beatitude, corresponds the distinction between a man of his century (*vir saecularis*) to whom marriage is reserved, and a man of the church (*vir ecclesiasticus*) who must abstain from marriage.... (To) impose on all laymen a continent state, which is the option pertaining to clerical or monastic status, disturbs *Ecclesia* as much as the fact of justifying marriage for clerics" (p. 1080). Marriage, a result of sin and a concession to the weakness of human nature, is thus not justified apart from procreation except by the social order which it allows and signifies.

115. These are the major texts: *De bono conjugali; De Genesi ad litteram; De bono viduitatis; De conjugiis adulterinis; De nuptiis et concupiscentia*. Equally important developments on sexual and conjugal ethics are found in *Contra Faustum Manichaeum, De civitate Dei* and *Contra Julianum haeresis pelaginae defens.*

116. Clement of Alexandria had already associated concupiscence and original sin, but that point of view had not been taken up by later eastern theologians, who do not ascribe a specifically sexual meaning to original sin; cf. Noonan, op. cit., p. 179 ff.

117. Augustine, *De nuptiis et concupiscentia*, II, xxxi, 53, in *N–PNF*, Vol. V, p. 305.

118. Ibid., II, v, 14, p. 288.

119. Ibid., II, viii, 20, p. 290.

120. Ibid., II, xiii, 26, p. 293.

121. Augustine, *De bono conjugali*, XXIV, xxxii, *FC*, Vol. XXVII, p. 48.

122. Augustine, *Op. Imperf. contra Jul.*, VI, 30, *PL* 45, 1582.

123. Augustine, *De nuptiis et concupiscentia*, I, x, 11, p. 268.

124. Augustine, *Contra Julianum*, V, xii, 46, *FC*, Vol. XXXV, p. 288.

125. Saint Caesarius of Arles, *Sermons* 42, 5; 43, 5; 44, 3–6; in *FC*, Vol. XXXI. On Caesarius, cf. Cyrille Vogel, *Césare d'Arles* (Paris, 1964).

126. Gregory the Great, *In 7 Pen. Ps.*, Ps. 4:7, *PL* 79, 586.

127. Gregory the Great, *Liber Regulae Pastorales* III, xxvii, *ACW*, Vol. XL, pp. 186–192.

128. Gregory the Great, *Epistolae*, XI, lxiv, in *N–PNF*, Vol. XIII, p. 79. Some authors consider this letter apocryphal; in any case, it has been held since the 8th century to represent Gregory's teaching and, as such, did influence the whole Middle Ages.

129. Peter Lombard, *Sentences*, II, xxx, 8, *PL* 1972, 722; cf. also II, xxx, 4; II, xxxi, 2–4, 7.

130. Ibid., IV, xxvi, 2, *PL* 192–909.

131. *De Fide Cath.*, Chapt. 1, *D.B.* 430.

132. "When we look for the source of the courtly conception of love, we must not forget to reserve an important place for Peter Abelard.... We know from his own account that he composed and sang a large number of songs in honour of Heloise." Etienne Gilson, *The Mystical Theology of Saint Bernard*, trans. by A.H.C. Downes (New York: Sheed and Ward, 1940), p. 158. Abelard explains this in Chapter VI of *The Calamities of Abelard* in *The Letters of Abelard and Heloise*, trans. by C.K. Scott Moncrieff (New York: Alfred A. Knopf, 1926), p. 11 ff.

133. Gilson, op. cit., pp. 162–163.

134. *Letter II of Heloise to Abelard* in op. cit., p. 57.

135. Ibid., Letter IV, p. 83.

136. Ibid., Letter II, p. 57.

137. Ibid.

138. Marie de Champagne, daughter of Eleanor of Aquitaine, text quoted by Evelyne Sullerot, *Histoire et mythologie de l'amour. Huit siècles d'écrits feminins* (Paris, 1974), p. 59.

139. There is an excellent presentation in the work of Marie-Odile Métral, *Le mariage. Les hésitation de l'Occident* (Paris, 1977), pp. 113–145; cf also René Nelli, *L'érotique des troubadours* (Toulouse: E. Privat, 1963).

140. Métral, op. cit., p. 129.

141. As in the example of this text by Marie de France (around 1170)

> "She wished to see her friend often,
> And her joy is to have him
> Whenever her Sire departs
> And night and day and early and late
> She has him at her beck and call.

142. An extreme erotic technique which excludes intercourse.

143. In 1140 at Lyon, the Canons established a feast to the Immaculate Conception: ideal christianized woman is obviously the Virgin Mary, who gives life without having to lower herself to conjugality.

144. I owe my awareness of this little-known attempt to Métral, op. cit., pp. 147–177.

145. Hugh of Saint Victor's works to be read: *The Sacraments* (*PL* 176, I, 8, 12, 314ff.; II, 11, 1–13, pp. 479–510) and *Letter on the Virginity of the Blessed Mary* (*PL* 176, pp. 857–876).

146. Métral, op. cit., p. 151.

147. Ibid.

148. On catharism and sexual morality, cf. Arno Borst, *Die Katharen* (Stuttgart: Hiersemann, 1953); René Nelli, *Le phénomène Cathare* (Paris: Presses universitaires de France, 1964), pp. 72–100; Denis de Rougemont, *Love in the Western World*, trans. by Montgomery Belgion, rev. and aug. ed. (New York: Pantheon, 1956), pp. 71–81 and passim. (Despite the attacks by specialists on this book, I continue to believe it to be one of the most illuminating books on the subject.) As for the rare catharic texts that have been preserved, they may be found in Ch. Thouzeillier, *Une somme anti-cathare. Le "Liber contra Manicheos" de Durand de Huesca* (Louvain, 1964); this historian also edited *Liber de duobus principiis* (Paris, 1973) (SC 198).

149. Nelli, op. cit., p. 78.

150. On the way in which sexuality and marriage could be lived out in a catharic milieu, consult the excellent book by Emmanuel Ladurie Le Roy, *Montaillou, village occitan de 1294 à 1324*, Biblioth. des histoires (Paris, 1976), esp. pp. 255–299.

151. I agree with Arno Borst; he notes that in southern France, countless Cathari hid themselves as troubadours and that the singers of love are often also the preachers of renouncement. René Nelli says that there are about twenty or so troubadours that can be proved to have been Cathari (among them, de Guilhem du Durfort, Piere Vidal, Raimon de Miravel). Borst add, however, that it is less through literary details than through the overall situation that Cathari and troubadours are linked. For one thing, many troubadours were vehement enemies of the Cathari. What the two groups have in common is a participation in the same Provençal culture where the whole mystique of chaste love (linked to the cult of the virgin and to convent reform) was developed.

152. St. Thomas Aquinas, *De perf. vitae spir.* VIII, trans. by Rev. Procter (St. Louis: B. Herder, 1903), p. 27.

153. Bonaventure, *Sent.* IV, xxxvi, 2, 2, *Opera omnia*, Vol. IV, p. 797.

154. "Hence it is that in the human race, the male has a natural solicitude for the certainty of offspring, because on him devolves the upbringing of the child; and this certainly would cease if the union of sexes were indeterminate." Thomas Aquinas, *Summa Theologica*, II–II, Q. 154, 2, edition of Fathers of the English Dominican Province (New York: Benziger Brothers, Inc., 1948), vol. II, p. 1816.

155. On affection for children during the Middle Ages in a peasant milieu, consult E. Ladurie Le Roy, op. cit., pp. 300–321.

156. Thomas Aquinas, *Summa Theologica*, Suppl. qu. 49.4, in op. cit., Vol. III, pp. 2739–2740.

157. Ibid., Suppl. qu. 49.6 in op. cit., p. 2742: "... pleasure in a good action is good, and in an evil action, evil; wherefore, as the marriage act is not evil in itself, neither will it be always a mortal sin to seek pleasure therein."

158. Albertus Magnus, *In 4 Sent.*, d 26, a 7.

159. Cf. Pierre Rousselot, *Pour l'histoire du problème de l'amour au Moyen Age* (Münster: Aschendorffsche Buchhandlung, 1908), p. 35.

160. Noonan, op. cit., p. 355.

161. According to the theory of Reto R. Bezzola, *Les origines et la formation de la littérature courtoise en Occident*, 2e partie, T. II (Paris, 1966), at the beginning of the courtly tradition, William IX of Aquitaine tried to thwart the preaching of the theologian Robert d'Abrissel who was defending the valuation of woman according to gospel standards. The courtly tradition would be an answer, via a secular mystique, to religious promotion of the woman. If Bezzola is right, it would be by means of theology that woman, from the 12th century on, would be called to rediscover her specific vocation.

162. Sullerot, op. cit., pp. 47–69.

163. Ibid., p. 52. The work of E. LeRoy Ladurie confirms this viewpoint, cf. op. cit., pp. 273–278.

164. Schillebeeckx, op. cit., Vol. II, p. 39.

165. The history of the evolution of liturgies is notably described by Korbinian Ritzer, *Le mariage dans les églises chrétiennes du Ier au XIe siècle* (Paris: Editions du cerf, 1970).

166. Ritzer, op. cit., p. 244 ff. It is interesting to note that Paulinus of Nola is describing here the marriage of Julian of Eclannum, Augustine's future pelagian adversary.

167. PL 119, 980.

168. On these questions, consult Henri Crouzel, *L'église primitive face au divorce* (Paris: Beauchesne, 1971).

169. Jerome, *Epistolae* LXXVII, iii, *N–PNF,* Vol. VI, p. 158.
170. R. C. Gerest, art. cited, pp. 20–21.
171. Jerome,*Epistolae* LV, iii, *N–PNF,* Vol. VI, p. 110.
172. *PL* 99, 1153.
173. P. Nautin has remarkably demonstrated this in an article in *R.S.C.* 62, 1974/1, pp. 7–54. "Divorce et remariage dans la tradition de l'Eglise latine." Here is his conclusion: "It was only in the second half of the 9th century that the doctrine of Augustine and Jerome triumphed. This was the result of the renewal in theological studies which marked the beginning of the Carolingian era. This change, which set aside the text of Matt 19:9, was not brought about by pastoral necessities but was the work of theologians who, I might add, thought that Augustine represented the whole Christian tradition."
174. Epiphanius of Salamis, *Panarion* LIX, 4, *PG* 41, p. 1024 ff.
175. On these texts, cf. Willibald M. Ploechl, *Geschichte des Kirchenrechts* (Wein: Herold, 1960), Vol. I, p. 447 ff. and Ritzer, op. cit., pp. 340–354.
176. "One of the biggest falsifications of history, and also one of the most successful," as A. Bride says in *Catholicisme,* art. "Isidoriens (Faux)."
177. Ritzer, op. cit., p. 347: "From then on, the conclusion of a wedding would take place before the Church tribunal, but at the same time, the juridical civil forms were to be included in the sacred domain of the liturgy. . . . However, toward the middle of the 9th century, things had not yet come to that point: the conclusion of a legal marriage was still regarded as within the jurisdiction of common legal rights."
178. Schillebeeckx, op. cit., Vol. II, pp. 74–75.
179. Hincmar, Letter XXII (around 860), "On the Marriage of Stephen to the Daughter of Count Regimond," *PL* 126, 132 ff.
180. Jean Dauvillien, *Le Mariage dans le droit canonique de l'Eglise, depuis le Décret de Gratien (1140) jusqu'a la mort de Clement V (1314)* (Paris: Recueil Sirey, 1933).
181. This collection, requested by the pope so as to put the various canon laws in order, is the work of Raymond of Pennafort who worked on it from 1227 to 1241: cf. A. Villien "Article Décrétales," *Dictionnaire de Théologie catholique,* IV, 1911, col. 206–212; Ploechl, op. cit., Vol. II, pp. 477–481.
182. The veil originally covered the couple, and later only the bride as a sign of her consecration to Christ with her husband as His representative, the "image of Christ." For a study on the evolution of this liturgical ritual, cf. Schillebeeckx, op. cit., Vol. II, pp. 96–108.
183. Thomas Aquinas, *Summa Theologicae,* Supp. qu. 48.1, in op. cit., p. 2735.
184. From this perspective, there is nothing that the reformed theological tradition can accept; cf. R. Grimm, "Indissolubilité et sacramentalité du mariage chrétien," *RTP* (1967), VI, pp. 404–418. I will return to this point in [chapter 5 of *Sexual Desire and Love*] in my presentation of the critique of Protestant theologians with regard to the marriage-sacrament.
185. There is an excellent résumé of this in François Lebrun, *La vie conjugale sous l'Ancien Régime* (Paris: A. Colin, 1975), pp. 9–13.
186. Anthony Meray's *La Vie au temps des libres prêcheurs ou les devanciers de Luther et de Rabelais; croyances, usages et moeurs intimes des XIVᵉ, XVᵉ et XVIᵉ siècles* (Paris: A. Claudin, 1878) speaks of the ways in which the severity of these principles could be sidestepped.
187. Cf. François Wendel, *Le mariage à Strasbourg à l'époque de la Réforme, 1520–1692* (Strasbourg, 1928); André Biéler, *L'homme et la femme dans la morale calviniste* (Genève: Labor et Fides, 1963); R. Stauffenegger, *Le mariage à Genève vers 1600* (Paris, 1968); Pierre Bels, *Le mariage des protestants français jusqu'en 1685* (Paris: Librairie générale de droit et de jurisprudence, 1968).
188. These are the major works by Luther on marriage:
—*Treatise on Good Works* (sixth commandment), 1520, in *LW,* Vol. XLIV. (The abbreviation *LW* will refer to the edition: *Luther's Works,* Philadelphia: Muhlenberg Press, 1962.)
—*The Babylonian Captivity of Church,* 1520, in *LW,* Vol. XXXVI.
—*Estate of Marriage,* 1522, *LW,* Vol. XLV.
—*Catechism* (sixth commandment), 1529.
—*Von Ehesachen,* 1530.
—*Sermon on Monday after Quasimodo for the Marriage of Caspar Cruciger,* 1536.

A good synthesis, among many others, of Luther's teaching in this area: O. Lähteenmäki, *Sexus und Ehe bei Luther* (Turku, 1955), Schriften des Luther-Agricola Ges. 10.

189. Luther, *To the Christian Nobility of the German Nation Concerning the Reform of the Christian Estate, LW,* Vol. XLIV, p. 177.

190. Luther, *The Babylonian Captivity of the Church, LW,* Vol. XXXVI, pp. 98–99.

191. Ibid., p. 106.

192. Luther, *Judgment of Martin Luther on Monastic Vows* (1521), *LW,* Vol. XLIV, p. 298.

193. On the problem of divorce, cf. Luther, *Estate of Marriage, LW,* Vol. XLV, pp. 3–35.

194. Calvin's major texts on mariage are found in *Institutes of the Christian Religion,* trans. by Henry Beveridge (Grand Rapids, Mich.: William B. Eerdmanns, 1966), in 2 Vols.; II, viii, 41–44 (commentary on the seventh commandment), in Eerdmann's Vol. I, pp. 348–350; IV, xii, 23–28 (against the celibacy of priests), in Vol. II, pp. 468–471; IV, xiii, 3 (on the vow of celibacy) in Vol. II, pp. 474–476; IV, xix, 34–37 (marriage and sacrament) in Vol. II, pp. 646–649. Cf. also Calvin, *Textes choisis,* edited by C. Gagnebin and K. Barth (Paris-Fribourg, 1948), pp. 196–216 for some excellent passages on the body, lewdness, marriage, and conjugal love.

195. Calvin, "Commentary on Malachi," (Mal. 2:16) in *Commentaries on the Twelve Minor Prophets* (Edinburgh: Calvin Translation Society, 1849), Vol. V, p. 559. (The abbreviation *CTS* will hereafter refer to the volumes in this series.)

196. Calvin, *The True Method of Reforming the Church,* in *Tracts, CTS,* Vol. III, pp. 301–302.

197. Calvin, *ICR,* IV, xii, 23 in op. cit., p. 468.

198. Cf. L.-E. Halkin, "Erasme et le célibat sacerodotal," *RHPR,* 57 (1977), pp. 497–511.

199. Written at a time when Erasmus was still close to the position of the reformation movement. Later, in 1526, especially in his treatise *Christiani matrimonii institutio,* he returns to strict orthodox Catholic positions.

200. Erasmus, *In Novum Testamentum Annotationes* (1 Cor. 7:39), in *Opera Omnia,* Vol. VI, p. 192.

201. Ibid., (Ephes. 5:32), p. 855.

202. Luther, *The Babylonian Captivity of the Church, LW,* Vol. XXXVI, p. 95.

203. Ibid., p. 92.

204. Calvin, "Commentary on I Timothy" (1 Tim. 2:13), *Commentaries to Timothy, Titus and Philemon, CTS,* Vol. XLIII, p. 69.

205. Calvin, (Gen. 2:18), *Commentaries on the First Book of Moses called Genesis, CTS,* Vol. I, p. 130.

206. Martin Butzer, *Von der Ehe* (1534), text prepared and translated by Wendel, op. cit., p. 46.

207. Martin Butzer, *De Regno Christi* (1550).

208. Luther, *Estate of Marriage, LW,* Vol. XLV, pp. 36–37.

209. Ibid., p. 17.

210. Calvin, (Deut. 24:5), *Commentaries on the Last Four Books of Moses, CTS,* Vol. III, p. 84.

211. Calvin, (1 Cor. 7:5), *Commentary on the Epistles of Paul the Apostle to the Corinthians, CTS,* Vol. I, p. 226.

212. Ibid., (1 Cor. 11:11), pp. 359–360.

213. Luther, *Estate of Marriage, LW,* Vol. XLV, p. 40.

214. Calvin, (Matt. 19:10), *A Harmony of the Gospels,* trans. by T.H.L. Parker (Edinburgh: Saint Andrew Press, 1972), Vol. II, p. 249.

215. Luther, *Sermon for the Marriage of Caspar Cruciger.*

216. "If we abhor immorality, it is because of the principle that our bodies are temples of the Holy Spirit,." *Fourth Sermon on the Epistle to the Corinthians* (10:8–9), *Opera Calvini,* Vol. XLIX, p. 624.

217. Ibid., p. 625.

218. Bels, op. cit., pp. 57–62.

219. Martin Butzer, *Von der Ehe* (1532).

220. Calvin, *Opera Calvini,* Vol. X, p. 105.

221. Ibid., p. 106.

222. On this point, cf. Wendel, op. cit., pp. 103–107 and Bels, op. cit., pp. 135–140 and 163–173.

223. His demands were inspired by the Edict of Henry II (1556) on the marriage of children which strongly reinforced parental authority. Cf. Isambert, *Receuil des anciennes lois françaises,* Vol. XIII, pp. 469–471. Quoted by J.L. Handrin, op. cit., p. 42 ff. (Who incorrectly dates the Edict at 1566—probably because of a printing error).

224. Luther, *Sermon for the Marriage of Caspar Cruciger.*

225. Calvin, *Twelfth Sermon on the Epistle to the Corinthians,* (1 Cor. 11:4–10), *Opera Calvini,* Vol. XLIX, p. 729.

226. "...Moses intended to note some equality (between man and woman [author's note]). And hence is refuted the error of some who think that the woman was formed only for the sake of propagation... as if she had been given to him only for the companion of his chamber, and not rather that she might be the inseparable associate of his life." Calvin, (Gen. 2:18), *Commentary on the First Book of Moses Called Genesis, CTS,* Vol. I, p. 131.

227. On this question consult Wendel, op. cit., and Bels, op. cit.

228. Wendel, op. cit., p. 59.

229. Bels, op. cit., p. 249 ff.

230. Lebrun, op. cit., p. 89.

231. Wendel, op. cit., p. 123.

4

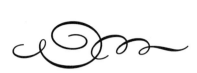

Sexuality—God's Gift: A Pastoral Letter

Francis J. Mugavero

Dearly Beloved in Christ:

Sexuality is one of God's greatest gifts to man and woman. We can say this not only because sexuality "largely conditions his or her progress towards maturity and insertion into society,"[1] but also because it is that aspect of personhood which makes us capable of entering into loving relationships with others. Theology teaches that relationship—the gift of oneself to another—is at the very heart of God. The Father and Son give themselves totally to one another and the mutuality of their total response in love is the Holy Spirit, binding them together. We honor God and become more like Him when we create in our own lives the loving, other-centered relationships which at the same time give us such human satisfaction and personal fulfillment.

Recently, the Congregation for the Doctrine of the Faith issued a "Declaration on Certain Questions concerning Sexual Ethics" to emphasize the importance of sexuality in our lives as followers of Christ.[2] Bishops are urged to share the moral wisdom of the church in a way "capable of properly enlightening the consciences of those confronted with new situations" related to the meaning and value of human sexuality.[3] It is with this hope that we share these thoughts with you, our brothers and sisters in the Lord.

Let us say clearly and without apology that chastity is a virtue which liberates the human person. Chastity means simply that sexuality and its physical, genital expressions are seen as good for man and woman—good in so far as we make them serve life and love. Any of our powers can be turned to destructive purposes due to lack of concern, weakness, or even a well-intentioned error. The excitement and adventure of human living is to take our God-given powers and talents and become someone worthwhile—lovable and loving. It should not be surprising that the power and pleasure which are part of sexuality will demand of us the intelligence, honesty and sacrifice that might test our maturity to the utmost degree. But we do not fear sexuality, we embrace it. What we fear at times is our own inability to think as highly of the gift as does the God who made us sexual beings.

Sexuality Serving Love

Sexuality is so much more than genital activity. It is an aspect of personality which lets us enter other persons' lives as friends and encourages them to enter our lives. The dimension of sexuality must be developed by all men and women not only because it is, as we have just seen, a gift making us more like God, but is also so very necessary if we are to follow Jesus' command to become "lovers."[4] It is a relational power which includes the qualities of sensitivity, understanding, warmth, openness to persons, compassion and mutual support. Who could imagine a loving person without those qualities?

Our Lord Jesus Christ was fully a man—with the sexuality of a man.[5] Some men and women choose to conform closely to His life of celibate love in service of fellow man and God's Kingdom; most people will express their love of God and neighbor through "the intimate partnership of married life and love."[6]

Does it appear unusual that as members of the same Church some can embrace married love and others celibate love as expressions of personal sexuality? It did not seem contradictory to Christ, who respected and blessed matrimony as a sacrament of His church yet chose to fulfill His own mission as an unmarried man. Far from condemning sexuality, He knew man and woman were created thus by God as "very good" and may "become as one flesh"[7] in the permanently faithful union of married love. Neither did He discourage those who would sacrifice the genital expression of their sexuality out of love for serving fellow man and God's Kingdom as priests, religious and dedicated laity.[8]

But if we are as honest with ourselves as were the Christians who have lived before us, each of us will recognize that it is not easy to integrate sexuality into our lives.[9] We all want to be loved and accepted. We want to draw close to other people, and many of us will seek fulfillment in that special closeness which married life should be. Helping our sexuality develop in a constructive way—in a way which will help us gain and give the love and affection that brings tremendous joy and peace of mind—demands that we consciously live our lives, that we don't just "let things happen." The relationships with other people which can make our lives full and enjoyable don't just "happen."

We are members of a church whose people have been part of the successes and failures of almost 2,000 years of human living. We are continually being brought out of slavery by the loving Spirit of God. One form of that slavery is the ignorance of how to love—how to use our sexuality for giving life, for truly loving, for deep and lasting relationships.

There may be no convincing way to say this to someone who does not want to listen. We know, however, that the experience of countless human beings and sound psychology support the wisdom of the church teaching regarding both the goodness of sexuality and the unfortunate ambiguity related to its genital expression. Although each of us is called to live our sexuality in the sense of the human qualities and relationships seen above, its genital expression (physical sexual contact, arousal, orgasm) needs a special context before it can serve human love and live generously and without deception.

Pre-Marital Relations

Human beings can use minerals for health and strength or turn them into bombs to kill and destroy. The pleasant smile can find its true meaning as a sign of friendship or be used to deceive. Sexuality can find its genital expression serving mutual love and new life in the total commitment of marriage, or it can easily become self-serving and stripped of its true meaning. What is meant to be the expression of the deep love of a man and woman joined forever through marriage in the service of life can be trivialized as merely a way of enjoying this person I am with.[10]

In pre-marital intercourse, the full genital expression of sexual love is robbed of its proper context of exclusive commitment, the genuine and permanent gift of oneself to one's beloved, and the possibility of the couple's love showing itself in a stable enough environment to develop new life.[11]

In truthful human communication, we must accept the meaning which is present in certain actions. A warm smile and a tender embrace are universal signs of friendship; to communicate in a human way is to be true to the meaning of a sign when I use it in my life. As much as they might like to do so, no couple can rewrite the meaning of sexual intercourse. It is tied to committed love; it is tied to life-giving. When a person engages in sexual intercourse it is a sign of giving one's very self, whether one intends to or not. To let my actions be a sign of self-gift, if my heart knows the truth to be different, is to lie.

We must pledge ourselves to be true to what is really happening. Is our love so real that it is truly permanent, exclusively centered on this one person with whom I wish to link my life forever, the kind of love which could some day bring forth children as its sign? Then we are ready not for "second best" but for the joy of marriage in Christ—not in any sense "a piece of paper from the church," but a chance to stand at the altar before God and fellow man and say: "We love one another and want our love to last forever. We ask you to respect this, to rejoice with us, to help us keep it so." This is marriage in the church.

How inadequate it would be to propose Christian marriage merely as a solution to sexual problems or needs! Those who have grown to a point where they can make that permanent, exclusive pledge of themselves one to the other in Christ are people who are alive with hope, signs of the wonderful "foolishness" of a love deep enough to face together an unknown future. They remind us that life is neither stagnant nor finished, and their total commitment to one another in Christ is broad enough to share someday with their own children. In light of this beautiful reality, don't the tentative and shallow aspects of "sleeping together" or "living together" without the maturity of a marriage commitment become painfully clear?

We know the pressures society and peers place on unmarried people. The young are made to feel "out of step" or unpopular if they avoid genital sexuality. Loneliness and searching for something or someone can lead the unmarried or unloved of any age to seek an answer to their pressing need in some passing intimacy. But this is a "solution" which is short-lived. The genital expression of sexuality is too much "myself" to let it become something commonplace or shallow, to reduce its significance to a "handshake," to lose the meaning and mystery. I am worth more than that.

Multiple Motivations

We recognize how sexual behavior is often intertwined with many other needs, often unconscious ones. Sexual behavior can be used to express nonsexual feelings and relationships such as the need to prove one's identity or self-worth, to escape from loneliness or to express strong aggressive feelings. To deny these multiple levels of motivation in the human personality would isolate the problems of sexuality from the whole reality of the person. Certain inadequacies of sexual integration must be worked on from within the person and need pastoral guidance, professional counseling and therapy. Let us not forget, however, that religious commitment has a tremendous influence on the development of our sexual perception and behavior. It is this meaning in one's life that will enable a person to discipline himself and renounce certain destructive types of activity.

We must not, therefore, presume on grace alone to heal what truly requires psychological counseling, nor feel that habit or emotional problems totally excuse one from long-proven means of asceticism and spiritual growth. Here the generosity of our response to God's love can open us to beneficial scientific and spiritual means to achieve greater personal integration.

The Practice of Masturbation

The practice of masturbation is a prime example of the complex nature of sexual behavior. It may begin in adolescence as an immature expression of "self-discovery" or enter a person's life at any time and for any number of reasons.

We wish to encourage people to go continually beyond themselves in order to achieve greater sexual maturity and urge them to find peace and strength in a full sacramental life with the Christ who loves them.

"Modern psychology provides much valid and useful information for formulating a more equitable judgement or moral responsibility and for orienting pastoral action. . . . In the pastoral ministry, in order to form an adequate judgment in concrete cases, the habitual behavior of people will be considered in its totality."[12]

Homosexual Orientation

The complexus of anthropological, psychological and theological reasoning in regard to human sexuality has contributed to the church's teaching that heterosexuality is normative. All should strive for a sexual integration which respects that norm since any other orientation respects less adequately the full spectrum of human relationships.[13]

Whatever the cause of the homosexual orientation, both to those who share that orientation and to society in general there are certain cautions we wish to put forward.

We urge homosexual men and women to avoid identifying their personhood with their sexual orientation. They are so much more as persons than this single aspect of their personality. That richness must not be lost.

Being subject to misunderstanding and at times unjust discrimination has resulted in an overreaction on the part of some persons of homosexual orientation. It is not homosexuality which should be one's claim to acceptance or human rights or to being loved by us all; it is the fact we are all brothers and sisters under the Fatherhood of God. Our community must explore ways to secure the legitimate rights of all our citizens, regardless of sexual orientation, while being sensitive to the understanding and hopes of all involved.

On a more personal level, we wish to express our concern and compassion for those men and women who experience pain and confusion due to a true homosexual orientation. We pray that through all the spiritual and pastoral means available they will recognize Christ's and the church's love for them and our hope that they will come to live in His peace.

A Call to Healing

A most important way to aid the human person achieve sexual integration and live the virtue of chastity is to provide from life's earliest years a loving and secure climate. We urge parents and teachers to examine their own attitudes toward sexuality and to set the pace for young people's pride in developing as loving and mature men or women.

We restate the Declaration's plea that responsible sex education be provided for all our people including children who should receive "information suited to their age."[14] Knowing the beauty of sexuality and the wisdom of chastity facilitates the young person's moral growth, as encouraged by the Second Vatican Council: "This Holy Synod likewise affirms that children and young people have a right to be encouraged to weigh moral values with an upright conscience, and to embrace them by personal choice and to know and love God more adequately. Hence, it earnestly entreats all who exercise government over peoples or preside over the work of education to see that youth is never deprived of this sacred right."[15]

We call on all men and women of good will to help create a more wholesome climate in society. There are still so many imprisoned either psychically or physically in the destructive activity of prostitution. The social problems of pornography must be challenged by community concern. Advertising and media too often miss vitally important opportunities to free the human spirit and instead contribute to a sex-saturated atmosphere that confuses rather than heals.

To those engaged in the ministry of healing—religious people, doctors, psychiatrists, teachers and so many others—we encourage interdisciplinary work to improve the quality of pastoral care and to help Christians in the delicate task of forming their own conscience. We hope that parish communities will cooperate in studying sexuality and chastity so these important gifts of God can enrich each of us in the way He intends.

Together

We are very conscious of the fact that all of us touch one another with our lives. What gratitude we should all have for those who have struggled with the difficulties of sexual integration and chastity in their lives and are now witnesses to us that it can indeed be done—that fidelity, commitment, self-sacrifice and compassion are realities in the lives of so many. We rejoice in you and thank you.

Yet we recognize that maturity in these areas comes only through what for many people will be a long and demanding process of growth. To our brothers and sisters of all ages who are experiencing difficulties—to those who cannot yet see that the personal and public commitment of marriage should be the context for the gift of oneself in sexual relations; to those whose homosexual orientation is causing them pain and confusion; to the widowed and to the adolescent encountering sexual needs; to those separated from their spouses by circumstances or by divorce—to all of you we pledge our willingness to help you bear your burdens, to try to find new ways to communicate the truth of Christ because we believe it will make you free. We respect you in your struggle.

Grace and peace to you from God our Father and from the Lord Jesus Christ,

Faithfully yours in Christ,
Francis J. Mugavero
Bishop of Brooklyn

Notes

1. Sacred Congregation for the Doctrine of the Faith, *Declaration on Certain Questions Concerning Sexual Ethics,* n. 1.

2. Ibid., no. 1.
3. Ibid., no. 13.
4. Mt. 22:36–40.
5. Heb. 2:14–18; 4:15.
6. Vatican II, *Pastoral Constitution on the Church in the World Today* (*Gaudium et Spes*), n. 48.
7. Gen. 1:2.
8. Mt. 19:12.
9. Evident themes in Sacred Scripture, the Fathers and the constant teaching of the living church. See also *Declaration,* op. cit., nn. 5, 12.
10. *Declaration,* op. cit., n. 7.
11. Vatican II, *Pastoral Constitution on the Church in the World Today,* op. cit., nn. 49, 50.
12. *Declaration,* op. cit., n. 9.
13. Ibid., n. 8.
14. Ibid., n. 13.
15. Vatican II, *Declaration on Christian Education,* n. 1. See also *Declaration,* op. cit., n. 13.

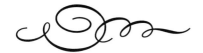

Scripture and Marriage

5

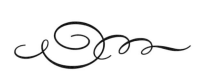

The New Testament Doctrine on Marriage

A. L. Descamps

The gospel passages on indissolubility are Mark 10:1–12; Matthew 19:3–9; Matthew 5:31–32; and Luke 16:18. To these texts must be added 1 Corinthians 7:10–11, especially since Paul there refers directly to the teaching of Jesus. Some conclusions of the exegetical and historical studies[1] of these passages are quite certain; others are controverted. However, scholarship has reached two almost unanimous decisions: (1) the apostolic Church represented in this case by Mark, Luke, and Paul taught clearly the indissolubility of marriage, and (2) this teaching goes back to Jesus himself.

The first conclusion is affected by the discussion of the two celebrated Matthean clauses "except for fornication," and the great agreement within the apostolic Church is weakened or reinforced by the interpretations given them. A few questions have arisen recently concerning the second conclusion, as we shall see below, on the basis not of definitive interpretation but of very tentative grounds. Beyond these two rather sure conclusions, a number of particular points are debated. Thus can be seen the framework in which our own conclusions are written.

This very rapid overview does not take into consideration hermeneutical analyses that today prolong exegetical and historical research. In this domain, however, we desire to take a position. We shall try to say, at the end of the chapter, how we see the scope of similar research in view of an eventual hermeneutical process.

One can surmise the essential outline of our approach. First we shall try to understand each of the texts *prout iacet*, that is, as the testimony of a redactor. From there we will go backwards, to draw out a fixed oral or written tradition. Finally, we will attempt to discover the teaching of Jesus himself. To the extent possible, this schema will appear also in the subdivisions of the article. In all this, we proceed in a manner which may appear tutioristic and almost scrupulous. Indeed, the redactional character of the passages of Matthew excepted, the wording of our texts will allow their antecedents in the teaching of Jesus to show through: from the point of view of the history of the pregospel tradition, the collection of passages on indissolubility constitutes a privileged case. Our way of proceeding is justified, however, in principle, and also because it permits us at the same time to show throughout certain characteristics of the redactional work.

In this material it is important to distinguish three things: separation *de facto*, repudiation, and remarriage. We believe, with others, that an ambiguity in the vocabulary here was the source of much confusion.

1. *Separatio de facto* refers to a simple situation with no juridical force. This is probably not involved in Mark 10:2–12. Generally speaking, separation is not taken into consideration in our texts, because Jewish law was interested only in repudiation in due form. But, in fact, the practice of separation is likely. Certainly the normal course of events was for the husband to give the decree of divorce to his spouse and then to send her away (Dt 24:1–4). But is it credible that sending her away never preceded the giving of the decree or the juridical act of repudiation? Is it even likely that there was never a *de facto* separation although the husband refused to draw up the decree? Moreover, some texts of the New Testament—rare, indeed—seem to refer to simple separation.[2]

2. Repudiation as understood by Deuteronomy 24:1 and the entire Jewish tradition concerns a dismissal which the husband alone can initiate, and it has precise juridical implications; his act—which calls for delivery of a decree of repudiation—annuls the marriage and gives both him and his spouse the right to remarry.[3]

Jewish *repudiation* then equals what we call *divorce,* on the condition that the latter term is understood as the separation by annulment of the first marriage and the right to remarry, nothing more nor less. Unfortunately, the terms *divorce* and *to divorce* are not always rigorously employed. *To divorce* is sometimes improperly used for *to separate.* And the words *divorce* and *divorced* are equally ambiguous inasmuch as they can refer either to separation with annulment of the marriage and simple right to remarry, or to separation and annulment effectively followed by a remarriage. In exegesis it would be clearer to use only the terms *repudiate* and *repudiation* and to avoid the term *divorce,* which, in any case, is not biblical. We will do this. It is better because our term *divorce* makes no important distinction between husband and wife, while *repudiation* at least among the Jews, is almost always an act of the husband.

3. Remarriage was the normal result of repudiation because the latter would give the right to remarriage and because it was without doubt motivated by the desire for a new marriage. It can nevertheless be held that remarriage, especially of the wife, would not always follow. Remarriage is called adultery by both the evangelists and by Jesus. One must ask if repudiation itself was not already tacitly considered adultery, since it gives the right to as well as the concrete occasion for remarriage, which is adultery.

I. Mark 10:2–12

1. The Redaction Of Mark[4]

a. The Controversy (Mk 10:2–9) As Understood by Mark

Mark 10:1 shows Jesus leaving Galilee for good and going to Judea on the other side of the Jordan, a stage on his way to Jerusalem; thus, this verse is one of the principal hinges of Mark's structure. Matthew 19:1–2 is an exact parallel, even stressing the departure. ("When Jesus had finished these sayings, he went away from Galilee.") Luke notes in other ways the inauguration and progress of this long journey toward Jerusalem (Lk 9:51; 13:22; 17:11; etc.).

Although it is a simple formula of transition, and not really a part of our pericope, Mark 10:1 is quite significant for the shift in perspective which was begun after the first announcement of the passion (Mk 8:31): from now on the activity of Jesus unfolds most clearly in view of his impending death. Now, if this death is necessary for the coming of the kingdom, it is without doubt normal in Mark's eyes that the progress of Jesus toward his death be accompanied by other divine requirements. In fact, in the broader context of our passage, the master makes some harsh statements (Mk 9:42–50 on scandal; Mk 10:23–27 on the difficulty of entering the kingdom);

among the actions of Jesus, he is seen cursing the fig tree and driving the money changers from the temple (Mk 11:12–25). In brief, there is here without doubt a body of statements akin to the exacting teachings of the master on indissolubility.

Mark 10:2 reads: "Pharisees came up [to Jesus], and in order to test him [in this] asked, 'Is it lawful for a man to divorce his wife?'"

As the words that we have supplied in brackets suggest, the sentence does not flow from the source, as is frequent in Mark. (Thus Jesus is no longer named after 9:39, that is, much before this.)[5] Certain manuscripts omit mention of the Pharisees and have simply *they* (that is, the crowds mentioned in 1) *asked,* a reading that is not likely to be primitive. The verb ἀπολύειν (*to dismiss*) has a precise meaning because it implies a juridical concept familiar to the Jews: it signifies repudiation with all that this means in the body of Jewish legislation and custom.[6]

Put in these terms, the question of the Pharisees is somewhat unnatural. For them, it is very evident that a man can divorce his wife, at least in certain cases. Since they are questioning Jesus to embarrass him, they would like to formulate their question in a manner that would lead him into a scandalous response through his nonconforming. For example, "Is it true that a man can never divorce his spouse?" The wording of Mark, "Is it permitted a man to divorce his wife?" would sound better coming from the lips of Jesus or from an argumentative Christian rather than from the mouths of the Pharisees. The wording is slightly awkward because Mark is not making an eyewitness report but is writing a literary composition developed at a spatial and temporal distance; this makes it difficult to preserve the nature of the original dialogue.

The redactor knows only that he is dealing with repudiation in the context of a controversy; in Mark 10:2, a somewhat Christian manner of interrogating Jesus may have seemed to Mark a valid way to begin the dialogue.

Mark 10:3: "He answered them, 'What did Moses command you?'" The way that Jesus appeals at once to Deuteronomy 24:1 is again somewhat unnatural. The master seems to call upon Moses as his best guarantee against the Pharisees when the latter held to the Mosaic text of which Jesus was to dispute the validity.[7] The verb ἐυτέλλομαι (*to command*) is also somewhat unnatural. Though Moses permitted repudiation, he did not really command it.[8]

Mark 10:4: "They said, 'Moses allowed a man to write a decree of divorce and to put her away.'" This time the verb ἐπιρέπω (*to permit*) is appropriate. The Greek text of the quotation is elliptical but conforms to Dt 24:1.

Mark 10:5–8: "Then Jesus said to them, 'For your hardness of heart he wrote you this commandment. But from the beginning of creation[9] [God] made [human beings] male and female; for this reason a man shall leave his father and mother and be joined to his wife and the two shall be one. So they are no longer two but one.'" Two subjects—God and Moses—must be supplied as well as the direct object, "human beings." In verse 8[b] the redundance is a little awkward and indicates again an unpolished redaction.

Σκληροκαρδία is not a concept borrowed from secular psychology, as would be expressed for example by the translation *intractable character*.[10] By virtue of its biblical antecedents, the term must be given a precise religious meaning: it specifically refers to the incapacity of the Israelites to submit to the divine will, their spirit of rebellion against God.[11] The Jesus of Mark thus touches an essential and constant point of salvation history, and his denunciation holds even in the present day (our hardness of heart).

Despite its brevity, this condemnation of the Pharisees by Jesus cannot be treated by the exegete as an *obiter dictum*. In the writing of Mark, it has perhaps lost its force in relation to the teaching of Jesus as it was perceived by his hearers. The evangelist was not in Palestinian territory, and criticism of Moses had been current for some time in the Church that henceforth was largely Helleno-Christian. But this was no obstacle. Mark was writing at a time when the rupture of Christianity with Judaism was far advanced but not complete. Yet the condemnation of Mosaism still has a dramatic character and the contemporary reader of Mark could not have been insensitive to it.[12] In order to perceive the audacity of this condemnation, it is necessary to place this text in its original *sitz-im-leben*, in the ministry of Jesus himself. This we will do below.[13]

Verses 6b–8a juxtapose two different quotations, Gn 1:27 and 2:24—more evidence of a developed gospel text, the work of a Christian scribe rather than the report of a witness. These quotations conform very literally to the LXX, which excludes the possibility of an Aramaic source[14] but not, however, the possibility that the texts from Genesis were used by Jesus in the context of this controversy on the indissolubility of marriage. Another revealing detail: in v. 7 the words *for this reason* (ἕνεκεν τούτου) come as the sequence of Gn 2:24 but they receive a different application. In Gn 2:24 the narrator of Genesis uses τοῦτο to refer to the words Adam spoke concerning the unity of husband and wife (Gn 2:23). Mark 10:7 has Jesus referring to Genesis 2:24, but the τοῦτο of Mark 10:7 can only refer to what he has just written (Mk 10:6), a citation of another text of Genesis (1:27). Nevertheless, this τοῦτο sounds right; for what Adam proclaimed in Genesis 2:23 about the unity of the human couple, Jesus in Mark 10:6 says in entirely equivalent terms when he announces—following Genesis 1:27—that God has made human beings male and female.

Mark 10:9: "Thus what God has joined, let no man put asunder." It is a particularly striking logion which, though presented here as a conclusion, lends itself to an autonomous use in the controversy between Christians and Jews.[15] This aphorism does not have the legal style of the following logia (Mk 10:11–12) and their parallels; thus the laws do not mention God himself directly. It is rather a matter of an exegetical conclusion phrased as a maxim in which one can hear either a sapiential tone or a prophetic accent. In any case, its scope is quite clear.

The active verb χωρίζειν means simply *to separate, to hold apart*. It would be possible to apply it to every form of physical separation.[16] One wonders whether Mark 10:9 does not condemn separation in itself; strictly speaking separation would in itself violate the union promulgated by the creator. However, this conclusion would be uncertain, for the controversy that is concluded in verse 9 pertains specifically to repudiation and so to a separation comprising annulment of the first marriage and the possibility of remarriage.[17]

On the whole, through his rather laborious redaction of verses 2–9, Mark intends to show clearly the opposition of Jesus to the divorce of a woman by her husband, in such a way that two lines of reasoning are found in the material; the teaching of Moses on divorce was a provisional concession to the Israelites' hardness of heart; this concession conflicted with the initial order of things willed by God, which the Jesus of the Gospel of Mark intends to restore.

b. The Rules of Conduct (Mk 10:11–12) As Understood by Mark

Mark 10:10: "And in the house, the disciples asked him again about the matter." This verse marks a change of scene (the house) and of questioners (the disciples). Contrary to certain real houses in Galilee, notably that of Peter (Mk 1:29; 2:1), the dwelling of 10:10—we are in Transjordania—is a literary device. The evangelist creates here a formula that reveals a different audience[18] (cf. Mk 4:10; 7:17; 9:18). In addition to the sketch of a dispute with the Jews, Mark's source material contained statements on marriage cast in legal language, namely, Mark 10:11–12. These statements could perhaps be traced back to the Q source, as claimed by some solutions of the synoptic problem which are otherwise hardly plausible.[19] It is more probable, however, that they existed alongside Q, which includes them, as we shall see. For Mark, such rules as these, proclaimed as they are within the Church, are directly meant for Christians rather than for Jews. He regards it, therefore, as more consistent to have Jesus formulate them for the benefit of his disciples rather than to have them being addressed to the Pharisees.

Mk 10:11–12: "If anyone divorces his wife and marries another woman, he commits adultery[20] against the first; and if a woman, having divorced her husband, marries another man, she commits adultery."

The form in which these verses are cast is obviously entirely different from the form of the exchange that goes before. Instead of a dispute related to the Old Testament (Mk 10:2–9), we have here assertions in typically legal style. Note the two opening formulae: "Ὅσ ἄν (*if anyone*) and καὶ ἐάν ("and if [on the contrary] a woman . . ."). More precisely, we are dealing here with one kind of phraseology proper to the legal style—the conditional style, referred to at times as *casuistic* by contradistinction to the style which is apodictic and constitutional.[21]

The content of these logia, which for the moment is to be interpreted from within Mark's own text, raises a number of problems.

The first of these is this: Does each of the verses 11–12 condemn two distinct things, or just one? Do they, first, tacitly stigmatize divorce and adultery, then go on to condemn also remarriage by branding it explicitly as adultery? Or does each of the two verses limit itself to condemning remarriage as adultery, divorce being mentioned only incidentally?

One is inclined toward the first alternative if one considers that, among the Jews, divorce includes the right to remarry, a right which Mark rejects unconditionally. The conclusion will then be that, for Mark, divorce contains the seed of adultery. Thus, we could paraphrase the text as follows: "Anyone who divorces his wife virtually already commits adultery. Should he marry another woman, adultery becomes evident." This is how many authors implicitly understand the text. Some do so explicitly. They go as far as to understand the text thus: "Anyone who divorces his wife commits adultery; anyone who marries another woman commits adultery."[22]

Dupont disagrees with this reading. "Nothing entitles us to maintain that, in the absence of a second marriage, divorce as such is being branded as adultery." Then he goes on to give his interpretation of Mark 10:11–12 as follows: "Although the charge of adultery relates grammatically to both of two distinct transactions, namely divorce and remarriage, in reality it affects only remarriage. The sin of adultery is located strictly and precisely in the second marriage, not in the divorce as such." In short, Dupont opts for the second alternative. He takes the view that verses 11–12 limit themselves to condemning as adultery, with, however, the additional stipulation that, if divorce does not fall under this condemnation, it is understood to exclude the right to remarry.

The argument on which Dupont leans most heavily is the Semitic syntax which, in his view, underlies verses 11–12. In Hebrew and Aramaic, two sentences may appear in coordination to each other, and yet the first sentence may express no more than a circumstance relative to the second. As example: "Why . . . do we fast and your disciples do not?" (Mt 9:14), or, "How many times will my brother do wrong, *and* I will forgive him?" (Mt 18:21). These two sentences mean respectively: "*since we fast,* why don't your disciples fast?" and "*Suppose that my bother should do wrong,* how many times am I to forgive him?" Dupont believes that Mark 10:11 may likewise be read as follows: "Suppose that a man divorces his wife, he commits adultery if he marries another."

There is another point to consider. If we suppose that, for Mark, divorce does not deserve to be branded specifically as adultery, is not divorce at least condemned (in 10:11–12) as being very much against the will of God which Jesus has promulgated? Here an even larger number of authors answer in the affirmative. Often they do not even bother to say so for they regard the point as self-evident. Yet Dupont dissents: "Nowhere does Jesus say: 'Divorce is forbidden'. . . . He speaks with the assumption that divorce does take place ('Anyone who divorces . . .'). The repudiation process is part of his presuppositions. . . . Jesus passes no value judgment upon the act of divorce itself; he takes a position only on its practical consequences. If the husband who has dismissed his wife, or the wife who has been dismissed, decide to remarry, they lapse into adultery."

Yet is it not true that the divorce which Mark supposedly does not condemn is in effect divorce as practiced by the Jews, that is, the kind of divorce which entitles one to remarriage and which Jesus, therefore, obviously forbids? Not so, says Dupont. Jesus retains the term *divorce* but empties it of its meaning, or gives it a whole new meaning. "The divorce of which Jesus speaks is no longer a divorce properly so called. The word is retained, but it is emptied of its substance." "Jesus may give the impression of contradicting himself, but he does not. He merely gives the verb *to divorce* a new meaning." Dupont refers here to what he regards as "one of the most characteristic traits of Jesus' teaching method." He cites several instances, especially the debate on purification (Mk 7:1–23; Mt 15:1–20), where Jesus retains the word *unclean* but only to give it the entirely new meaning of moral rather then ritual uncleanness.

All this is tantamount to saying that Jesus has in mind not Jewish divorce but what we call simple separation, a separation which does not entail the dissolution of the conjugal bond. Of course, Jesus "does not intend to issue a juridical decision as to what simple separation is as a legal concept, nor does he formally authorize such separation," yet the concept of separation "derives directly from the teaching of Jesus himself."[23]

A detailed discussion of Dupont's argument would take us too far afield. Yet the choice before us is momentous, for, as we shall see, simple separation is precisely the notion on which an entire exegetical tradition relies to resolve the difficult problem occasioned by the Matthean clauses. According to this exegesis, it is precisely simple separation (which does not include the right to remarry) that would be allowed by way of an exception (that is, in the case of fornication), and this in spite of the fact that the texts retain the phrase *to divorce* whose normal meaning is entirely different.

Which is the "good choice" as far as Mark 10:11–12 is concerned? When we earlier attempted to clarify the concepts involved here, we readily admitted that simple separation must have existed at the time of Jesus and even that it surfaces in a few New Testament texts. We may thus seem to have conceded Dupont an argument in support of his position. Yet, all things considered, we are most reluctant to go along with him, mainly for the following reason.

Even if we suppose that one could interpret the text of Mark 10:11–12 taken in isolation as Dupont interprets it, the context in Mark and in Matthew seems to call for a different reading. In Mark 10:2–9, it is obviously Jewish divorce with all its consequences that is being categorically condemned, if not as adultery, at least as a grievous fault. Since verses 11–12 follow from verses 2–9, how could they suddenly speak of divorce as if it were but a circumstantial detail? Could Mark really intend verses 11–12 to extend only to remarriage, without including the divorce that they explicitly mention? We would have a hiatus of a sort that is hardly plausible. The argument can also be turned around; if, for Mark, verses 11–12 condemn remarriage, not divorce, are we not to extend this interpretation to verses 2–9? But how can verses 2–9 be understood to refer only to a condemnation of remarriage, if remarriage is not directly at issue there? It is especially difficult to read in verse 9 in this sense because χωρίζειν, as we have shown, means *to separate* in a very broad sense, that is, to separate in any way at all.[24]

Note again that we are still reasoning here from within Mark's own text, and that we must, in consequence, pay careful attention to the context. Dupont always speaks globally of Jesus. In fact, if the logia were restored to the status of isolated units (being still regarded, however, as sayings uttered by Jesus), it would be easier to interpret them as he does. The paradox is that it is precisely Dupont who ought to be particularly sensitive to the context, since he favors Daube's view who maintains that the logia and the debate had not existed in isolation from each other but had constituted a single unit from the start.[25] We, on the contrary, see this passage as redactional and trace it back to two originally distinct situations, but both plausibly pertaining to the ministry of Jesus himself.

Be that as it may, it is by first staying rigorously within Mark's own viewpoint that we perceive a fundamental reason for dissenting from Dupont's reading of Mark 10:11–12.[26] We thus take the position that it has not been proved that Mark 10:11–12 implies the notion of a simple separation which may be looked upon as morally indifferent as long as it does not lead to remarriage.

*   *   *

A few minor problems arise if we again read Mark 10:11–12 for the purpose of discerning to whom the saying recorded there is addressed.

Verse 11 addresses the man, to whom Jewish law and custom grant the right to take the initiative in a divorce. Let us agree for the sake of convenience to call this man M1.[27] The moment M1 divorces his wife, he already transgresses the creator's will. Tentatively, we may also say that he perhaps dooms his wife (W1) to adultery. At any rate, if he takes another woman (W2) in marriage, he does commit adultery against his former wife (W1).

The last words in the preceding sentence are not verbatim in the text, which reads instead ἐπ αὐτήν (*toward her*). This is an ambiguous expression which could even more easily be read to refer to what comes directly before it, namely, to the other or second woman (W2). This is, by the way, how N. Turner interprets the expression.[28] However, the authors generally agree that the adultery spoken of here is committed against the first woman, and their consensus is good enough for us.

If, according to Jewish custom, divorce restores to a man the freedom to remarry, it restores the same freedom to the woman as well. Jesus does, of course, condemn the woman's remarriage as well, and so we are prepared for the parallel legal saying which interdicts remarriage for the woman. However, the word ἀπολύσα in this second interdiction (v. 12) creates a problem. Taken strictly, this word assumes that the wife is entitled to divorce her husband, which seems to contradict Mosaic and Jewish custom that reserves the right to divorce exclusively to the husband. In a Jewish context, we would expect something like this: The woman who has been dismissed (or repudiated, or driven out) commits adultery, if she remarries.

But here we have a prior question of textual criticism. Codex D and others speak of "the woman who has left the house of her husband."[29] J. Wellhausen adopts this reading and remarks: "This is the only wording Mark could possibly have used." Others entertain the same view, V. Taylor for example.[30] But this choice of reading conflicts head on with the well-known principle: the more difficult reading is the preferable reading (*lectio difficilior potior*). A copyist is inclined to correct texts that make for difficult reading, and so the easier reading is suspect. In textual criticism, the need to clarify always arouses suspicion. H. Zimmermann agrees with this reasoning, yet he allows for a more radical solution, which he borrows from Beyer: the entire verse 12 is unauthentic, and this for reasons internal to the text (of a linguistic kind).[31] These reasons do not, however, seem decisive; so it seems wise to retain the accustomed text, which is supported by the main uncial manuscripts, and adopted by more editors of critical editions, K. Aland included.[32]

Even so, we still need to decide what Mark intends to say as he speaks of a woman who divorces her husband. This question has been answered in several ways.

Most exegetes take the view that Mark deliberately elected to mention specifically the woman's case because of the Greco-Roman context which grants the right to divorce to a wife as much as to a husband.[33] But very few authors, who depend mainly on Josephus and the

Elephantine papyri, believe that the Jews were acquainted with the right of the wife to divorce the husband.[34] Besides, could we not suppose that the word ἀπολύσασα only exemplifies a slight misuse of language of no real consequence? The very contention that man and woman are equal before the gospel precept which enjoins indissolubility was for Mark reason enough to mention the woman's situation next to that of the man in exactly symmetrical terms. We need not suppose that Mark intended to go on record as asserting that the woman has the right to divorce her husband.

In all the possible interpretations just mentioned, it is plain that Mark has taken pains to have Jesus legislate not only with regard to the husband but also to the wife. This is a fact that deserves a mention, for in the debate just concluded (Mk 10:2–9) the husband is the sole focus of attention, which is what we would expect within the context of Jewish tradition. We will say, then, that in the present case the woman is treated symmetrically with respect to the man only in order to warn her in the same way as the man. Paradoxically, this reading discloses all the same that Jesus is determined to resist all discrimination between man and woman. His attitude is one of principle. Applied to other matters, it will afford greater protection to the woman's rights.

To bring out the content of Mark 10:11–12 we may put it this way: By divorcing W1 and marrying W2, M1 commits adultery with respect to W1. Likewise, by divorcing M1 and marrying M2, W1 commits adultery (with regard to M1). Or: no matter which spouse takes the initiative, divorce violates God's will. This initiative does not dissolve marriage, for marriage is itself proof against dissolution. In any case, any subsequent remarriage is adultery. In terms of Jewish sensitivity, and to the extent to which Mark and his readers are at home within that sensitivity, we discern in Jesus' saying a twofold revolution against accepted custom: first, the Jews permitted divorce, hence remarriage; second, the Jews would never think of equating remarriage by the man with adultery.

In sum, Mark 10:2–12 appears to be composed of two different elements: first, a remnant of a debate about scripture between Jesus and the Jews which gave him the opportunity to issue an unconditional condemnation of divorce; second, a saying which expresses this condemnation in the language of law and makes it more precise. In the scriptural debate, divorce is utterly condemned—taken in isolation, the text as word could even apply to the mere fact of separation. The saying sustains this condemnation, but moves from the statement of principle to the consideration of various cases. We thus have the conclusion that divorce—objectionable in itself—normally results in remarriage, which then earns a more precise condemnation: it is called adultery.

2. The Teaching of Jesus

To what extent can we trace back to Jesus himself the various pieces of which Mark 10:2–12 is composed?

We have already suggested a stylistic analysis that clearly distinguishes between the controversy and the teaching; this distinction will prove very useful here because our effort to explore the current of transmission will follow two different lines of reasoning.

a. Mark 10:2–9 and the Teaching of Jesus

The redactional imperfections do not hinder us from postulating the kinds of material that Mark draws upon for the controversy with the Pharisees: they were biblical quotations, memorable sayings of Jesus such as Mark 10:9, or even a fragment of dialogue which originally contained these words or into which the quotations in question were inserted. The imperfections themselves surely reveal redactional work, but it would be difficult to picture Mark as writing 10:2–9 on a blank page.

It is not foolhardy to conclude in favor of the historical reality of one of the materials suggested above: one or several confrontations on divorce between Jesus and the Jews. Whether it involved the Pharisees or another distinct group of the Jews, such controversy was a constant element in the development of the teaching of Jesus.[35] Moreover, the historicity of this particular passage can be deduced from the very audacity of the teaching.

In the time of Jesus there was no dispute over the custom or the doctrine that gave the husband the right to divorce; consequently, each spouse had the freedom to remarry. Discussion centered only on the grounds for divorce, a subject which is not treated here but will be discussed partially by Matthew, as we shall see. What Jesus challenges, then, is the steadfast conviction of the Jews on the very legitimacy of divorce. The attitude which Mark attributes to him is one of great audacity; and this, in our eyes, is one of the best guarantees of its historical authenticity.

This authenticity is confirmed by 1 Corinthians 7:10–11: "To the married I give the charge, not I but the Lord, that the wife should not separate from her husband, (but if she does, let her remain single or else be reconciled to him) and that the husband should not divorce his wife." Without going into a detailed exegesis here, it will suffice for us to note that this text, at least twenty years older than *The Gospel According to Mark,* agrees perfectly with Mark in attributing the condemnation of divorce to the historical Jesus.[36]

This attitude of Jesus is best expressed by Mark 10:9, "What God has joined let no man put asunder." And there are valid reasons for thinking that the very formulation of Mark 10:9 reflects an Aramaic substratum going back to Jesus himself.

The Greek term αυζεύγνειν, "to place under the same yoke," is practically a *hapax Novi Testamenti,* since Matthew 19:6 is little more than a copy of Mark 10:9. Indeed, it is almost absent from the LXX, where it appears only twice.[37] One may ask, therefore, whether the corresponding Aramaic term *zawwegh,* found in the *Targums,* was not in use in the time of Jesus.[38] The entire logion would seem to have been preserved, a supposition supported both by its striking conciseness, and by its vigorous antithesis between God and man: these two traits agree well with the style of Jesus and would facilitate memorization. In contrast to the rather synthetic dialogue which precedes it, here we would seem to have a logion of Jesus already present as such in the source of Mark, either as a conclusion to this dialogue (which itself would undoubtedly have been quite informal in the supposed source) or as an isolated logion that Mark himself very smoothly joined to an extant debate between Jesus and the Pharisees.

Is it possible to go even further and attribute the essential biblical argument developed in Mark 10:2–9 to Jesus? We have sufficiently indicated that this passage is not a word-for-word account of a controversy. But perhaps some evidence hidden beneath the rather unpolished redaction of Mark lets us trace back to Jesus the two arguments advanced, that the Mosaic law was only a provisional concession to the hardness of heart of the Hebrews, and that the followers of Jesus must return to the original will of God. Because these two considerations imply the nullity of the law, they are blasphemous in the eyes of the Jews. Since the historian has already traced the condemnation of divorce back to Jesus, he can seek to attribute the supporting arguments to him.

It is unlikely that the Judeo-Christian Church of Palestine or the diaspora, which would surely have been predisposed to accommodate Judaism in some ways,[39] could have invented a teaching so radical—in both thesis and argumentation—and gratuitously attributed it to Jesus in Mark's redaction. Nor would the gentile Christian Church have done so, for such a severe message would only hinder its efforts at evangelization, as 1 Corinthians 7:10–16 discreetly attests.[40] But if it is relatively easy to dispose of an anonymous milieu of the Church as *sitz-im-leben,* cannot one argue that Paul himself must be considered as a possible source here?

At first glance, one can see Paul as the true creator of an argument as anti-Mosaic as it is anti-Semitic. It suffices to recall that the Pauline system of justification (Romans and Galatians) is specifically predicated on the condemnation of the law; with its collection of weaknesses and sins, the law has been put to death on the cross, in order that grace may rule. It seems possible to explain Mark's idea of the nullity of Deuteronomy 24:1 in this approach, to focus fully on the creative genius of Paul, and to avoid the necessity of going back to Jesus. For other passages, Mark's Paulinism was and still is a theme of contemporary exegesis of the second gospel.[41] Finally, present-day exegetes of the gospels, sometimes influenced in their task by the more recent Jewish historians of Jesus, state that Jesus differed much less with his Jewish contemporaries than Christian tradition considers.[42]

But these are general considerations, and for our present purpose we must come to a precise comparison. Compare Mark's theme, that Moses watered down the original will of God on marriage to accommodate the religious indifference of his people, with the Pauline theme that Jesus Christ abrogated the Mosaic law through the reign of faith and grace. While these two themes share a common ground, namely the definitive condemnation of the teaching of Moses, the two arguments are very clearly different.

First of all, in the Gospel the nullity of the law is announced by the word of Jesus (supposed to be the very Word of God), while, for Paul, the law is conquered only by the death and resurrection of Jesus. We should not, however, insist on this difference, because it can be explained by the obvious difference in the situations (teaching of the historical Jesus, faith in the heavenly existence of Christ).

More clear is the fact that while the Jesus of Mark finds the divine will in the account of creation, Paul for his part discovers it in an event more immediately "pre-Mosaic," namely in the testament made in favor of Abraham's faith and inaugurating the rule of faith.[43]

There is another important consideration. We are fortunate enough to possess the exact teaching of Paul on indissolubility (1 Cor 7:10). Now the apostle tells us, in summary, that he conforms his teaching here to that of the historical Jesus.[44] Such a reference by Paul to Jesus contrasts with his usual development of the theme of the general nullity of the law (Romans and Galatians). To refer to rules laid down by the historical Jesus is quite another thing than to argue as a theologian the superiority of Abraham the believer to Moses the legislator. But while this argument causes Paul to exalt faith, it does not permit him to decide a question as concrete as divorce; for this question, as for others, Paul characteristically consults the exact traditions which go back to the pre-Easter Jesus (1 Cor 7). On the contrary, in his great orchestration of the antithesis law-faith (Romans and Galatians), Paul does not appeal to logia of Jesus nor to Mark's themes of the Mosaic compromise and of the necessary return to the initial order of creation.[45] We have, therefore, no reason to consider these as Pauline themes that Mark would have uncritically ascribed to Jesus.

Finally, the idea that the opposition between the law and creation (Mk 10:2–9) originates with Jesus would seem to be supported by other gospel texts. Certainly the question of the attitude Jesus took towards Moses and the law is particularly difficult, and we cannot treat it here.[46] It is probable that his attitude was complex, paradoxical, and very nuanced. It is certain in any case that Jesus distinguished the true Moses from the Moses altered by the traditions of the doctors,[47] and it may be that the master went so far as to oppose Moses to God. This is perhaps what happens, for example, when Jesus, interpreting God, proposes new rules in place of the Mosaic commandments. This is the object of the "antitheses" of the Sermon on the Mount (Mt 5:20–48), which is precisely where we find the passages condemning divorce.[48] There is possible support here for the authenticity of Mark's "reasoning" (10:2–9) on creation and the law.

In commenting on Mark 10:2–9 as understood by Mark, we have raised the question of the exact focus of the critique of the Mosiac text evoked by verses 5 and 6 on hardness of heart or, if you prefer, on the antithesis of creation-law.[49] It would be especially important to resolve this question here, that is to say, at the moment when we ask ourselves about the thought of Jesus himself. For Jesus, did Moses compromise with the hardness of heart of his people by permitting divorce? Or did he excuse Moses,[50] and reprobate the contemporaries of Moses, and even more their descendants, in this case the Pharisees? It is difficult to say. Let us say only that this second hypothesis is brilliantly defended by Dupont in a lengthy article.[51]

After having attributed to Jesus himself the use of the texts from Genesis on creation juxtaposed with the ones from Deuteronomy on divorce, can one determine their originality? It can be admitted that such conflation and precisely of marriage is attested to in a few biblical texts (Mal 2:3–16; Tob 8:6–8) and also in some Essene documents: the Documents of Damas and the Temple Scroll.[52] In one sense this observation confirms the probability of the argument *in ore Jesu*, and in another sense it does not detract from its originality: facing his surroundings and above all the Pharisees who were questioning him, Jesus employed here a nonconformist exegesis. This latter has been called "nonrabbinic" by Bundy,[53] and this is cause for reflection even if the remarks of this author are only "partially exact."[54]

b. Mark 10:11–12 in the Message of Jesus

With almost all authors we admit that these verses existed before Mark in an isolated state.

It is true that a serious attempt has been made by Daube to demonstrate that the sequence of disputed sentences, far from being redactional, is on the contrary pre-Marcan and even original.[55] This exegete appeals to the rabbinic writings, which bring two elements closely together: the teaching to the people on the outside, then in-depth explanation to the disciples. Without contesting the interest of these remarks from various points of view, we do not think that they can prevail here against an attentive examination of Mark's redaction. From the point of view of historicity, which concerns us here, the subject of this discussion is limited, inasmuch as the literary doubling Mark 10:2–9 and Mark 10:10–12 does not hinder us from recognizing for each of the two sections a *sitz-im-leben Jesu*. This solution has the advantage of suggesting that Jesus treated indissolubility on a number of separate occasions, which can only emphasize the importance that he attached to this teaching.

When attempts are made to recover the teaching of Jesus himself on marriage, present-day exegetes have a tendency to give a privileged place to the isolated logia, especially those of Mark 10:11–12. It is clear that, compared to the short sentences, the pericope on the controversy reveals very important redactional work.[56] But the verses of the genre of Mark 10:11–12 are sometimes also regarded suspiciously, especially when, as here, they take the form of legislative rules. These latter are understood better in the context of the primitive Church;[57] the historian wonders to what extent Jesus was preoccupied during his life with legislating, in the proper sense of the word, for the messianic community. But as certain writers have noted, Jesus adopted on many occasions the sapiential language of the proverb, that is to say, a style which is not far from that of rules for a way of life. Moreover and above all, in the present case evidence in favor of these logia is exceptional, since they are present (with a few differences it is true) both in Matthew and Luke, and before that in Q, Mark, and 1 Corinthians 7:10–11. This is a decisive argument in favor of their authenticity as the teaching of Jesus.

One can add that in all the forms attested to except one (Mt 19:9),[58] there are two logia; moreover, the respective subjects are different. This doubling is a sign of primitive data,[59] although the question of the identity of the two subjects remains temporarily open.

Beyond this general remark on the authenticity of the doubling, there is a body of research on the precise formulation which is equally important. In the eyes of some exegetes who have written recently, each of the gospels (Mark, Matthew, Luke) has claims to authentic value.[60] We shall examine much later the problems of the Matthean and Lukan versions. Let us content ourselves here with a few remarks on the formulation of Mark 10:11–12.

In Mark 10:11 only the words ἐπ᾽ αὐτήν ("against her") seem to be a redactional addition.[61] Without this ending, verse 11 (which is found in Mt 19:9, but with an insertion) appears to be practically identical to Luke 16:18a and even fundamentally similar to Matthew 5:32 (without the insertion). We say "fundamentally similar" because the Matthean expression "makes her an adulteress" is probably—as we shall see—a revision of the original verb: *commits adultery* (Mark and Luke).

This verb merits our attention for a moment. Although absent from 1 Corinthians 7:10–11, it has every chance of being primitive, by reason of evidence found throughout the gospels. Jesus no doubt employed it in referring directly to the decalogue (Ex 20:14). By means of this very expressive term, he will stigmatize here all remarriage during the life of the first spouse, and he will do this in a body of teaching on divorce, as the beginning of the logion indicates. It is a teaching which already condemned divorce itself, notably because it implies the possibility of remarriage and thus contains the seed of adultery. We have no reason to interpret this logion differently, as does Dupont, who holds that Jesus spoke on divorce without forbidding it as such, stating precisely throughout that it does not authorize a new marriage. In order for this exegesis to be valid, it would be necessary to suppose, that in the ministry of Jesus situations arose when the teacher considered only remarriage, and then mentioned divorce as a simple circumstance of fact; however, we have no evidence that this happened. Up to this point, in every case, the context has been a discussion of divorce: the controversy in Mark 10:2–9 and also the very formulation of Mark 10:11–12. Let us note for now that Matthew 5:31–32 also calls to mind the same context (divorce), but this time under the form of a "teaching by antitheses." We will return later to discuss the primitive context of Luke 16:18.

On the other hand, let us stress with Dupont how revolutionary[62] is the attitude of Jesus. What we have noted on this subject in the interpretation of Mark acquires its value here. It is in Jesus' own milieu rather than communities already emancipated from Judaism that the teaching of Jesus made its impact. It is in this way especially that one can speak of a true revolution in ideas. Divorce and remarriage are denounced by Jesus as contrary to the divine will. His is a unique way of going against law and custom, since the Jews admitted divorce in many cases, and thereby accepted a new marriage. Moreover, the generic idea of offense or of sin is specified by the accusation of adultery, which is applied at least to remarriage. This was a new manner of upsetting Jewish sensitivities: for a Jew, a man can never be said to be adulterous in relation to his own wife.[63]

On the whole, there can be seen behind various versions of the first logion this original form: "Every man who divorces his wife and marries another, commits adultery."

As to the second logion, let us recall the version of it given in Mark 10:12: "Every woman who, after divorcing her husband, marries another, commits adultery." The formulation alludes to Greco-Roman law (or to some particular Jewish customs), unless it is a mere carelessness of style; in any case, as it stands, the formula does not reflect the language of Jesus well.

Among the versions of Mark 10:12, that of Paul approaches that of Mark in the sense that the apostle, too, addresses himself to the man and to the woman (M1, W1), although in an order opposite to that of Mark, while Luke 16:18b and Matthew 5:32b address the new husband (M2) after having questioned the first (M1). The choice is difficult between, on the one hand, Mark-Paul and, on the other hand, Luke-Matthew (that is to say Q as well). We will leave open, then, the question of knowing if the second sentence of Jesus was addressed to the first wife (W1) or to the second husband (M2). In any case the teaching implied is the same: in each hypothesis it is a matter of denouncing remarriage as adultery as long as the spouse lives.

If our preceding analyses are correct, this last formulation summarizes the tenor of Mark 10:11–12 as these verses reflect the teaching of Jesus.

Up to this point, we have discovered nothing which confirms certain other recent hypotheses. It seems arbitrary to reduce the original passage to the single verse Mark 10:11 and to read there, either the sole prohibition of divorcing one's wife in order to espouse another (J.H.A. van Tilborg) or Jesus' exclusive preoccupation with defending the divorced woman (B.M.F. van Iersel). For this last author, Jesus would not be speaking on indissolubility but would be defending the weaker party as he did with regard to the adulterous woman, the publicans, and the sinners. What we have said about the origin of the statements of Jesus directs us toward the classical discussions among the Jews of divorce and perhaps also of the extension of the right to divorce. We have found nothing to recommend the thesis of A. Isaksson. According to this author, Jesus, in reestablishing the indissolubility of marriage, only intended to say that the Old Testament was supposed to be addressed to the members of the priestly families serving in the temple of Jerusalem. "They shall not marry a woman who has been a prostitute or who has lost her honor, nor a woman who has been divorced by her husband, for the priest is consecrated to his God" (Lev 21:7).

Even further from our conclusions about Mark 10:2–12 seem to be the ideas of B.K. Diderichsen, who simply discards Mark as a witness to the thought of Jesus, not only because he prefers Luke 16:18 but also that he may speculate, on the basis of this verse, that Jesus intends to forbid a new marriage to the one who has left or divorced his wife for the cause of the kingdom. The study of the texts of Matthew and of Luke will allow us to return to some of these hypotheses.

Only after we examine the complete collection will we attempt to state precisely the motivations and the meanings of the teaching of Jesus on indissolubility.

II. Matthew 19:3–8

The Controversy

After having commented in Part One on the texts in the oldest gospel (Mk 10:2–9 and 10–12), we present here the other elements of the record, beginning with Matthew.

We will first read Matthew 19:3–9 in comparison with Mark 10:2–12, which has already been explained.[64] Mark 10:2–12 is divided into two parts: a controversy (vv. 2–9) and rules of conduct (vv. 10–12). It is otherwise in Matthew 19:3–9. We find integrated in the account of the controversy, by virtue of the conclusion (Mt 19:9), the legislative statement which in Mark 10:10–12 was the object of a distinct pericope. However, since Matthew 19:9 requires a rather long explanation on account of the difficult exception clause inserted there, for the sake of clarity we are led to distinguish it from verse 3–8, and thus to comment on Matthew 19:3–9 in two sections, Parts 2 and 3.

We are going to comment on the Matthean form of controversy which we already met with in Mark 10:2–9 between Jesus and the Pharisees. Again, the problem of marriage is approached through divorce. This circumstance, however, cannot narrow our horizon or make us ignore the complete doctrine of marriage among the Jews.

In the time of Jesus people had an exalted notion of marriage, and there is no indication that practice varied greatly from theory. On the contrary, it is striking to note that none of the many reproaches that Jesus addressed to the Pharisees concerned marriage.[65] For the Jews of the time of Jesus, marriage was for the most part monogamous and indissoluble.[66] This is shown in two ways: the gravity of adultery is, in a sense, a subtle tribute to marriage;[67] and the regulation of the right to divorce granted the husband reveals also a care to preserve the conjugal union.

On this second point, certainly jurisprudence varied and with it the destiny of monogamous marriage. However, we have no evidence that divorce was very common. In any case, the Pharisees were rather of the rigorist school of Shammai. The gospels are silent about what in that milieu[68] would constitute noteworthy laxity in the matter. Nowhere does Jesus reproach the Pharisees or any other persons for divorcing their wives for trifling reasons.[69]

There is one more negative point for this brief summary—the very masculine approach to conjugal union. For a long time marriage has been for us a synallagmatic contract; the spouses are on an equal footing in regard to conjugal morality. Such a view was unknown to the Jews of the first century, the result of a long oriental atavism; to reproach them for it would be to commit an anachronism. For them, it was especially the woman who was guilty in cases of infidelity; moreover, only the husband[70] had the right to divorce. For them, there was no complete social equality between a man and a woman. If Jesus himself addressed the husband particularly in promulgating required conjugal morality, he doubtless did not explicitly do so in order to grant social equality to the woman. But in refusing the husband the right to divorce, he *de facto* took the defense of humiliated wives. Did Jesus express himself thus with this precise aim? The texts do not say so. We can, however, reasonably suppose that this consideration played some part in the master's thought when we bear in mind that an analogous solicitude animated him in regard to women sinners and the woman taken in adultery.[71]

In approaching Matthew's text let us limit ourselves to an understanding of the account, that is to say, the thought of Matthew himself.[72] Matthew 19:3: "Some Pharisees came up to him and said to test him, 'May a man divorce his wife for any reason whatever?'" The verse is very similar to Mark 10:2, but Matthew has placed πειράζοντες (*to test him*) in a better place. He has put the question in direct discourse (as in 12:2), perhaps to place it in higher relief. Above all, he has modified the meaning of the question in adding the words "for any reason whatever." But this addition can be understood in two different ways.

It is often interpreted as follows: the Pharisees in Matthew were interested in the various motives for divorce and not, like those in Mark, in its very possibility. More precisely, they alluded to a well-known controversy that, in the time of Jesus, divided the respective partisans of the two great Jewish doctors, Hillel and Shammai.[73] According to Shammai, divorce and remarriage were authorized only for grave reasons, most notably for the wife's lapse from fidelity and honor. On the contrary, according to Hillel, the husband could be authorized for numerous motives to divorce his wife and remarry. Hillel's position could almost be expressed in the following terms that we borrow freely from Matthew 19:3: "divorce effectively permitted *for any cause.*" Jesus would then be called upon to say whether he approved such laxity, the Pharisees being implicitly on the side of Shammai.

This exegesis offers a first difficulty, at least if we leave aside for an instant the explanation of the account in order to place ourselves in the broad context of the life of Jesus. The Pharisees could hardly be ignorant of the fact that Jesus was very far from accepting the doctrine of Hillel. In inviting him to pronounce against this doctrine, they would only draw him nearer to themselves, and would not be testing him; consequently the word πειράζοντες would be unintelligible. Nevertheless, one could object that this logic is valid in regard to oral dialogue; it is less impressive where writing is concerned. In other words, in writing on his own "for any cause whatever," Matthew could have thought of Hillel and Shammai, even if the interlocutors of Jesus could not have done so without being illogical. To this, one can retort that the writer could not have been so forgetful of historical probabilities.

The exegesis in question is open to another objection. It leads us to suppose that Matthew 19:3–9, while following Mark 10:2–12 rather closely, would have completely altered the meaning since, as we have seen, Mark 10:2–12 in no way states the motives for divorce but denies its very possibility. To conjecture that in adding "for any cause" Matthew willed to make an allusion to the laxity of Hillel is to admit that for him, Jesus is going to discuss the reasons for divorce. In fact, like Mark, Matthew is about to deny the possibility of this separation even if the exception clause justifies divorce in a unique case.[74]

We can prefer, therefore, another interpretation of the last words of Matthew 19:3, one that remains faithful to Mark in his refusal to permit divorce. Matthew prepared his readers to anticipate that there would be one exception, that of the clause (Matthew 19:9).[75] While repeating the words of Mark 10:2: "Is a man permitted to divorce his wife?" Matthew may have hesitated to stop there so as not to lead the reader to expect the absolutely negative answer that Mark gives.

Matthew 19:4–8. We refer the reader to a synopsis of the gospels or at least of the Matthean pericope. If, as we think, Matthew depends upon Mark, his essential intervention consists in reversing the latter's order of exposition. Instead of going back from Moses to the creation, the Matthean dialogue proceeds from the creation to Moses.[76] In doing this, Matthew undoubtedly thought it more natural. In reading Mark 10:3, Matthew seems to have been aware of the weakness noted above. In Mark, by alluding to Deuteronomy 24:1, Jesus appeals to Moses when the latter contradicts him.[77] The true argument of the master is found in Genesis, and that is why Jesus begins with that argument in Matthew. The Mosaic text appears in Matthew 19:7 in its true light: not as an argument in favor of Jesus, but rather as an objection to him, an objection introduced very naturally by the Pharisees in the name of scripture itself and then refuted by Jesus. Moreover, the procedure seems in conformity with rabbinical practice.[78] Let us say then with Crouzel[79] that Matthew's composition appears much better; this is a typical result when Matthew reworks Mark's text.

Having thus noted the essentials, let us add that Matthew improved Mark's account in numerous details. We will limit ourselves to a few remarks.[80] In verse 4, Matthew named a subject (God the creator ὁ κτίσας), avoiding the anacoluthon of Mark 10:6, where the subject was not named when it was apparently God, while verse 5 had Moses as the subject. Besides, in writing καὶ εἶπεν (v. 5), Matthew has at least sought to distinguish two quotations which, in Genesis, are effectively separated one from the other.[81] Moreover, Matthew 19:5 reproduces Genesis 2:24 in its entirety. Beginning with Matthew 19:7, there are other small changes, in part necessitated by the inversion in the order of exposition. The most remarkable is the addition of 8c, "from the beginning it was not so," which opposes the initial order willed by God to the Mosaic tolerance. The formula is concise and reads almost like a general principle.

On the whole, Matthew 19:3–8 is a reworking of Mark 10:2–9, and its most important change is the addition of the words "for any cause whatever" as a discreet foreshadowing of the inserted clause in verse 9.

We need not seek a way to go back from Matthew 19:3–8 to Jesus: this link can be assured only through Mark. In our understanding of the synoptic problem, Matthew gives no evidence here of any other contact with Jesus as distinct from the one we have discerned Mark.[82]

III. Matthew 19:9

The Rule of Conduct with the Exception Clause[83]

For the moment we shall limit ourselves to examining the text from the viewpoint of its composition. After 19:8, Matthew omits Mark 10:10. This perhaps is intentional, for the difficulty created in Mark by the word *house* is a real one.[84] However, in suppressing the mention of the house, the place of the disciples' questioning, Matthew was led to two small changes that in their turn raise some questions. In verse 9, Jesus directs to the Pharisees the rule that Mark 10:11 proposes to the disciples themselves. In verse 10, Matthew puts the disciples on the scene abruptly without the transition found in Mark 10:10, a transition certainly artificial in the sense that the house is "literary," but plausible in the sense that the precise laws on indissolubility are addressed to the disciples more than to the Pharisees.

Matthew 19:9 reproduces Mark 10:11 and introduces there the famous clause. Before tackling this, let us notice two minor points. After 19:9, Matthew omits Mark 10:12, perhaps because he is aware of the singularity of this verse that, by alluding to the divorce of a husband by a wife, sounds strange to all readers who know the Jewish milieu.[85] In relation to Mark 10:11, Matthew 19:9 shows, besides the insertion of the exception clause, the omission of the last two words ἐπ' αὐτήν (*against her*). The simplest explanation is that Matthew judged them superfluous, and by the single word μοιχᾶται (*he commits adultery*), he means to stigmatize divorce followed by remarriage as the adultery of the husband *vis-à-vis* the divorced wife, which we have judged to be the probable intent of Mark.[86]

Seeing the importance of Matthew 19:9, on account of the exception clause,[87] we think it advisable to consult first of all the specialists in textual criticism.

1. Lectio Genuina of Matthew 19:9

Let us begin with the form of 19:9, which is quite long if we take into account all the principal manuscripts; and for the sake of clarity, subdivide it into 9a: "I now say to you, whoever divorces his wife (lewd conduct is a separate case) and marries another commits adultery"; and 9b: "and the man who marries a divorced woman commits adultery."

At the end of a recent and thorough study, Duplacy, approved by Dupont, formulated his conclusion as follows: verse 9a is to be retained just as it is habitually presented by the editors and just as we have translated it a moment ago. The clause ought to be read μὴ ἐπὶ πορνεία. The manuscripts having παρεκτὸς λόγου πορνείας, a reading equivalent in meaning, could not prevail here, the less so as they are suspected of harmonization with Matthew 5:32. The two exception clauses, those of Matthew 19:9 and 5:32, have the same significance, and the testimony is firm in the manuscript tradition of the two passages. Only the absence of the exception clause in the patristic quotation could have led Crouzel to decide in favor of the omission; but it would be very difficult to follow the eminent patrologist on this point. For the rest of 9a, the variant ποιει αὐτὴν μοιχευθῆναι, which is rejected in the critical apparatus of the editions, is also rejected by Duplacy; it is also suspected of harmonization with Matthew 5:32.

9b or a variant is found in B, C, W, O, P, among others, but is generally not retained by the classical editors, including the most recent, K. Aland. Duplacy is not categorical, but does not exclude its authenticity. He bases his verdict on internal evidence, and he is supported by Dupont. We can only ratify this judgment, and add a remark to it. If 9b is authentic, it presents this peculiarity: it applies the condemnation of divorce to the partner M2. We do not find this in Mark, but we do find it in Matthew 5:32b and Luke 16:18b.

Having thus admitted the textual authenticity of the clause, we must now try to understand it as Matthew understood it.

2. The Clause in Itself

a. The Negation μὴ ἐπὶ

In translating Matthew 19:9 as we have done above with the majority of translators ("*except for lewd conduct*"), we have supposed that μὴ ἐπὶ very clearly marks an exception. A rather large number of authors reject this meaning of *except*. Some speak of a "preteritive" meaning and read "the case of lewd conduct not being considered," a case which would then be reserved, subject to a special solution that the evangelist does not indicate elsewhere.[88] Others defend an inclusive interpretation (the one who divorces his wife, a thing forbidden *even* in the case of lewd conduct, ...).[89]

What should we think of these two explanations? They are suspect, first from the fact that they are somewhat subtle, second because they eliminate as if by magic a difficulty that has been prominent for a long time. This leads us to think that they have been invented just in order to escape this difficulty. In favor of the idea of a true exception, we could thus apply an analogue of the principle of textual criticism, *lectio difficilior potior*.

But the decisive argument lies in the grammatical analysis of the entire verse 9. The most penetrating analysis is that of Dupont; and we conclude with him that it is necessary to read: "Whoever divorces his wife, *unless* for lewd conduct, and marries another commits adultery."[90]

In order to strengthen this interpretation, let us observe that it is already suggested, so to speak, by the expression in Matthew 19:3: "for any reason whatever." This formula would be difficult to understand if in the mind of the author there did not exist good and bad reasons for divorce. It already requires, so to speak, an answer of this kind: "No, one cannot divorce for any reason whatever, but for such or such exceptional reason."

b. The word πορνεία

In profane Greek, the normal meaning of the word, likewise attested to in the New Testament, is lewd conduct, fornication, carnal relations outside of marriage. In itself, the word πορνεία like the English equivalent just mentioned, has a generic meaning, for it is applied to all relations outside of marriage.[91] Here, however, the verse as a whole shows that the matter under discussion is the lewd conduct of the wife, hence an adultery, one kind of fornication, or something of the sort.[92]

However, some exegetes understand the word πορνεία in Matthew 19:9 quite otherwise; that is, in the sense of a marriage forbidden by the Jewish law, yet contracted *de facto*, such as, for example, marriage between close relatives. As a result, the verse would be understood thus: "if someone divorces his wife, unless it was a question of an invalid marriage ..." The exception then would not apply to true marriages, and the absolute indissolubility of the latter would be saved.

Bonsirven, an authority on Judaism, stated this hypothesis some thirty years ago;[93] it gained a rather wide acceptance, perhaps because the exegetes were happy to resolve the difficulty the clause presents by eliminating it.[94] Bonsirven bases his theory on the fact that in the New Testament πορνεία often shows its Semitic substratum to be the word *zenuth* that in post-Biblical Hebrew designates a false marriage, a union forbidden by the Law.[95] More recently, certain Essenic texts have given to *zenuth*, in the sense of a marriage between close relatives, testimony contemporary to the New Testament, and therefore more ancient than the citations referred to by Bonsirven.[96]

What must we think of this exegesis? Let us remark at once that an evangelical word does not necessarily have the same meaning as its Semitic substratum, supposing that the latter has been correctly identified. Even then one would still have to prove that the evangelist understood the Greek term in conformity with the Hebrew term and with a meaning contrary to the Greek lexicon itself. The process is delicate. What we are trying to interpret at the moment is the text such as it came from the pen of an author who was writing in Greek.

The major difficulty with Bonsirven's hypothesis is the following. If it is probable that in Acts 15:20, 29; 21:25 the word πορνεία effectively covers the word *zenuth*, we must, above all, note that these texts have a different bearing in regard to Deuteronomy 24:1 and to the problem of divorce treated in Matthew 19:9 as an echo of Deuteronomy 24:1. The apostolic decree (Acts 15) is a warning; and it is, therefore, logical that the future spouses be exhorted beforehand to avoid what could be a forbidden union. In the problematic connection with Deuteronomy, on the contrary, it is a question of a defect after marriage. As Dupont notes very justly, regarding the expression of Deuteronomy, "'if he (the husband) has found some indecency in her' (his wife), it can hardly be a question of 'discovery' of an invalid marriage or one forbidden by the Law. In short, Bonsirven's explanation also risks being only a 'loophole.'"[97]

In order to resume the reading of the clause in itself, we can translate it thus: "lewd conduct (of the wife) being a separate case."

3. The Clause in the Sentence

The real difficulty lies in the way the clause is linked to the sentence as a whole. Even if the clause is correctly translated, it remains true that the verse, read in its entirety, is not so transparent as it appears at first sight. Let us reread Matthew 19:9: "If any one divorces his wife (lewd conduct is a separate case) and marries another, he commits adultery." The thorny question is this: is the exception allowed for the act of divorce only, the prohibition of remarriage remaining the same, or is the exception allowed for both the divorce and remarriage? It is only after settling this point that we can grasp the significance of the clause.

In the first case, the verse must be paraphrased thus: if someone divorces his wife—(something forbidden) unless for lewd conduct—and marries another, he commits adultery (this in all cases, whether the divorce was legitimate or not). In the second case, the judgment comes to this, which is entirely different: if anyone divorces his wife and marries another, he commits adultery, unless it was a question of lewd conduct (on the part of the wife). In this last case, divorce and remarriage are permitted.

The problem thus caused is really difficult and its resolution is perhaps impossible. The difficulty has divided interpreters from the most ancient times. The two paraphrases above reflect the two principal types of interpretation, and we shall examine them in turn.

To begin with, let us observe with Dupont that the Council of Trent, in affirming the Chruch's right to reject *every* dissolution of the matrimonial bond, voluntarily abstained from condemning Catholic authors, among them illustrious Fathers of the Church, who admitted this dissolution in the case of adultery, either justifying this by the incidental clause or, more often perhaps, by other gospel texts.[98] From an exegetical point of view, therefore, the question remains open.[99]

a. In the Case of Lewd Conduct (on the Part of the Wife); Separation Is Permitted, Remarriage Forbidden

The reader has probably already recognized the familiar concept of *separatio tori et mensae*, a separation permitted in certain cases, the conjugal bond remaining firm and remarriage being excluded. Saint Jerome, who was no innovator in this matter, understood the text in this way and his interpretation has prevailed for a long time among Catholics, where it was classic and, moreover, has remained so in large measure. This exegesis has been brilliantly defended by Dupont.[100]

Grammatically this reading is altogether possible, as the first of the two paraphrases just given suggests. Such an interpretation has in its favor the fact that the clause immediately follows the mention of divorce and precedes that of remarriage, which could imply that the latter does not benefit from the exception, which would then be admitted only for a "simple" separation. On the other hand, the interpretation has something labored about it, for it supplies two words just before the clause: "(something forbidden) unless it be for lewd conduct . . .", which is plausible but nothing more. Dupont has explained at length the support that the grammatical order can give to this reading.[101] A detailed discussion of the subject is not necessary here, since the other interpretation is also grammatically possible; Dupont himself, as we shall see, expressly recognizes this. We cannot settle the dispute on the basis of grammar alone. Let us see then the other arguments that plead in favor of the separation of body and goods.

A major argument is that this exegesis allows Matthew's text to be harmonized with those of Mark and Luke, who without exception have condemned remarriage. This remains true for Matthew even if he is interpreted as we have just seen, since simple separation never gave the right to remarriage. Granted that Matthew thus interpreted differs from Mark and Luke in specifying that divorce not followed by a remarriage is permitted in case of lewd conduct. This had not been said by Mark 10:10–12 and, as we shall see, it will not be said by Luke. But this double silence does not contradict Matthew in any way, and a sufficient harmony is found assured among the three evangelists.

But this argument has value only insofar as it goes back to Jesus. As an echo of the master's word, the totally negative response suggested by Mark and Luke seems to prevail over the testimony of Matthew, who imputes this exception to Jesus. But this is not our point of view at the moment. We are trying here to reconstitute the Matthean writer's thought, and this person, who did not know Luke, could have added something of his own to Mark.

Another argument is that, as Jerome interpreted Matthew's text, it harmonizes well with 1 Corinthians 7:10–16; Paul, we shall see, alludes there to several forms of simple separation. In response to authors such as A. Vaccari, who object to Jerome's theory by saying that simple separation was unknown to the Jews, Dupont calls attention to the fact that it was sufficient to have simple separation known to the Christians, and this was the case in 1 Corinthians 7:10–16.[102] In relation to Matthew, the Pauline text is clearly older by about some twenty years; the practice of simple separation, tolerated by Paul, could have existed at the time of the evangelist. To admit this point it would suffice to suppose that Matthew 19:9 reflects an environment more Helleno-Christian than Judeo-Christian, which is far from being impossible. In such a milieu one can imagine for the first time separation in fact, while noting that this separation does not give the right to remarriage. The case would be strange for a Jew, but for Christians it is called to mind in 1 Corinthians 7:10–16. This is the solution preached by *The Shepherd* of Hermas.[103]

b. In the Case of Lewd Conduct (of the Wife) Divorce *and* Remarriage Permitted

This interpretation "is very generally admitted by Protestant exegetes; it is found also, with slight differences, among some Catholics;"[104] we ourselves have adhered to it *per transennam*.[105] Since Dupont's statement on the literature of the subject (1959), this exegesis has received new adherents.[106]

Let us repeat: the first exegesis, that made the text refer to simple separation, is grammatically possible. From the same grammatical point of view, the present opinion can be defended even better. Let us reread Matthew 19:9: "If anyone divorces his wife (lewd conduct is a separate case), and marries another, he commits adultery." Instead of supplying the words "a thing forbidden," we can change slightly the place of the inserted clause and read the verse this way: "If anyone divorces his wife and marries another, he commits adultery, unless the reason for the divorce is lewd conduct." Dupont himself recognized that "from the point of view of Greek grammar there is no decisive objection against this interpretation."[107] We would add that the latter is even more obvious than the other and it would have the votes of uninformed readers.[108] But it remains true that we cannot decide here between the exegetes only on the basis of grammar. Let us, therefore, see the other arguments of those who hold this second opinion.

There is, first of all, the apparently adventitious character of the clause.[109] Deprived of it, the verse Matthew 19:9 would read more smoothly; this is confirmed by its parallels, Mark 10:11–12; Luke 16:18; 1 Cor. 7:10–11. This clause appears stylistically as a parenthesis that one can easily represent as an addition. Nothing is easier for an editor than to insert some words in a sentence. It is a step made attractive by its very simplicity; it does not oblige the writer to recast his sentence entirely. A rather striking fact is that in both cases (Mt 19:9 and 5:32) the clause appears to be the result of an insertion, a kind of interruption in the sentence. Besides, we know that throughout his whole Gospel, Matthew worked into Mark's text or his other sources additions of various kinds—details, commentaries, etc. In short, this kind of editing is known in rabbinical literature; and R. Le Deaut has spoken on the subject of insertion of the halakist type.

The reasoning could be pursued in this way; if the clause is secondary, that is to say, specifically Matthean, let us try to understand it as a function of the care of the editor or of his ecclesial milieu.

What was this milieu? This is the historical aspect of the problem, already considered by the partisans of the first opinion when they supposed that certain Helleno-Christians had admitted, even created, the concept of simple separation in case of adultery. But another hypothesis is presented: the existence of Judeo-Christian communities pushing tolerance as far as to admit, in case of adultery, separation and remarriage. We perceive at least the possibility of such a *sitz-im-leben*, where the converts from Judaism did not give up the right to remarriage inscribed in the Mosaic law. Certainly, strict Judeo-Christianity must have been active before the time of Matthew's Greek. But paradoxical as this appears, it happens more than once that this Judeo-Hellenistic Gospel had echoes in more ancient communities whose tendencies were not those of Matthew as a whole. In these cases, the evangelist did not try to alter the conservative texts in order to reconcile them with a new interpretation; he preferred to leave them as they were, content to place the innovating sentences beside them.

To this recourse to Judeo-Christianity, one can object, it is true, the explanation is simply a hypothesis.[110] However, the hypothesis does not seem to us gratuitous. Before the year 70 A.D., the date of the fall of Jerusalem, conservative Judeo-Christianity was an unquestionable reality; let us think of St. Paul's combats. Again the first gospel, while not a narrowly Judeo-Christian work, contains at least some material reflecting such a tendency. It is sufficient to turn to texts such as Matthew 5:17–19 or 10:6–23; 15:24–26, and in a more general way, Matthew's presentation of Christ as the new Moses.

One will object that if Jesus condemned divorce and remarriage without reserve, it is not easy for a historian to imagine that some Christians still envisaged real exceptions. To this we can answer, at the risk of appearing subtle, that the condemnation of Jesus could have been interpreted as a general rule which left room for exceptions. Moreover, it is a unique exception; if the πορνεία is limited to the adultery mentioned, this makes the clause at least as restrictive as the judgment of Shammai, the most severe of the Jewish doctors in this matter. Such a limited mitigation of the words of Jesus doubtless did not appear to the Jewish converts as a betrayal of his message or as a return to the hardness of heart stigmatized by the master (Mt 19:8).

The matter can be explained in still another way. For strict Judeo-Christians, Jesus, in spite of his radicalism, could not have questioned what to them was obvious, namely, that an adulteress was like one dead and consequently her marriage was dissolved. We cannot forget that in Judaism, an adulteress was normally condemned to be stoned. Certainly there is every reason to think that this practice, perhaps already attenuated in the Jewish milieu surrounding Jesus, did not persist in the Judeo-Christian communities; the memory that Jesus preached mercy above all else (Jn 8:3–11, etc.) would have turned them away from a rule that was perhaps out-of-date. But even though spared, that is, not stoned, such a woman would remain the victim of an insurmountable taboo; no one could have anything to do with her, she was legally "dead." The husband who divorced her and remarried had not injured the conjugal bond that such a "death" had dissolved; in short, his remarriage was not perceived as a true exception to the rule of indissolubility.[111] In still other terms: we would have here the remnant of a Judeo-Christian practice on the margin of the Great Church; we cannot state precisely to what degree Matthew would ratify. Perhaps he merely tolerated its coexistence in a particular group with the more general and more severe standard, namely, the unconditional prohibition of remarriage.[112]

On the whole, each of the two opinions offers us a serious probability. For an exegete, the choice is presented concisely under this rubric: does Matthew's text reflect a Helleno-Christian community or, on the contrary, a Judeo-Christian milieu? Both hypotheses are plausible. Inasmuch as it was written in Greek during the eighties, the first gospel normally reflects relatively late usages, ones that are therefore Helleno-Christian, among which could be placed the simple separation evoked in 1 Corinthians 7. If the Judeo-Christian sources or customs are involved, on the contrary, Matthew may not have been familiar with simple separation, which was at best imperfectly known to the Jews, and he may therefore have retained a Mosaic tolerance regarding a standard which he otherwise interpreted strictly, holding that the adultery of the wife permitted her husband to separate from her and to remarry. Without denying that Jerome's exegesis has serious probability, we continue to incline toward this second interpretation.

IV. Matthew 19:10–12

The Word about the Eunuchs

To be complete, our commentary on Matthew 19:1–9 cannot ignore Matthew 19:10–12. Matthew 19:1–9 continues thus: "His disciples said to him: 'If that is the case between man and wife, it is better not to marry.' He said, 'Not everyone can accept this teaching, only those to whom it is given to do so. Some men are incapable of sexual activity from birth; some have been deliberately made so; and some there are who have freely renounced sex for the sake of God's reign. Let him accept this teaching who can.'"

We do not wish to explain this passage in itself, but only in the extent that it throws light on Matthew 19:1–9. Indeed, the link between the two pericopes is undoubtedly on the editorial level.

There is certainly a hiatus between verses 9 and 10. In verses 4–9, Jesus was addressing the Pharisees, while in verse 10 it is the disciples who are speaking and then receiving the explanations reserved for them.[113] This is obvious since it is a question of celibacy. Matthew, no doubt like Jesus before him, would not favor a dialogue with the Pharisees that consider indissolubility and celibacy at the same time, the more so since all husbands—the Pharisees included—are obliged to respect indissolubility. The disciples are invited to understand celibacy "if they can"; therefore, they are to be free in their choice. But in spite of this difference in audience and subject Matthew brings together marriage and celibacy; this only reveals better his intention of illuminating one by the other.

Verse 10 does not present any difficulty; "the case of a man" is that of the husbands, which Jesus has just defined with severity. Verse 10 thus confirms that the teaching of Matthew 19:4–9 clashes with the convictions and usages of the time, both in the first and the second of the two interpretations of the exception clause.

In regard to verse 11, the exegetes differ greatly on the meaning of "this teaching." For Matthew, does it refer to the sentence in verse 12 concerning the eunuchs, or to the word the disciples had just spoken in verse 10, or to the rule pronounced by Jesus himself in verse 9? Each option has its partisans. Even those who identify the "teaching" of verse 11 with the sentences on the eunuchs (v. 12) cannot deny the bond between them and verse 9 or 10, and it is this link that is important for Matthew.

Like Kittel,[114] we link verse 11 with verse 9. It seems to us that Matthew understood verse 11 this way: the prohibition to divorce and remarry can be accepted only by those to whom it has been given.

According to this interpretation, verse 12 appears as the reason for what Jesus said in verse 11, not as the content of the teaching contained in verse 11; we give full value to the initial γὰρ. For the rest, verse 12 offers no particular difficulty. The major reason that throws light on verse 11, and by that on verse 9, is that there is a third class of eunuchs, namely, those who have made themselves so for the sake of the kingdom of heaven. *In recto,* it refers to those who, in view of the kingdom, have renounced marriage. But if, as we think, Matthew links verse 11 to verse 9 in some way, he brings these voluntary eunuchs close to the married men who decided in advance to observe the strict precept of Jesus on indissolubility, and perhaps even to those husbands who have already experienced this hard observance, either in renouncing remarriage in spite of the infidelity of their wives or in not consenting to remarry in a single case of grave infidelity.

These statements are important. Apparently Matthew here tries to interpret the precept of indissolubility as if it were an ideal proposed only to the members of the kingdom. We shall come back to this clear difference from what seemed to us as a return on the part of Jesus to the absolute will of the creator above the law.

The conclusion is forced upon us that Matthew seems to be committed to such an endeavor, not only because of the choice we have made in linking verse 11 to verse 9, but in any exegesis of the expression λόγος τοῦτος. In no case, we have said, can we escape the link between the teaching of Jesus on those eunuchs and his words on marriage; it is understood, however, that we limit ourselves for the moment to understanding Matthew himself. Now voluntary eunuchs are clearly said to have made themselves so for the kingdom. Husbands who accept an indissoluble marriage are, if we dare say so, drawn along the same path: they can understand and respect indissolubility only in the perspective of the kingdom. A question remains. Does this link between indissoluble marriage and the charter of the kingdom come only from the evangelist (and his community) or has he only reproduced a preredactional chain leading back to the very discourse of Jesus?

All that we have just said of the necessary connection between Matthew 19:10–12 and Matthew 19:4–9, that is, between celibacy and marriage, is of worth for the evangelist. Let us now add that it has worth *only* for him, that is, that the joining of the words on eunuchs to the dialogue on marriage is purely redactional. Indeed, if we suppose that Matthew read Mark, he found there, immediately after the pericope on indissolubility, those presenting the little children, then the rich young man (Mk 10:13–31). We see that Matthew has used the same pericopes in 19:13–30, just after the logion on eunuchs (Mt. 19:12). This is to say that Matthew 19:10–12 is clearly a redactional insertion.[115]

In order to show that Matthew 19:10–12 is truly in place—that is, already connected thus in a former writing, even in a discourse of Jesus—those who refuse to admit the dependence of Matthew on Mark must suppose the existence of an ancient and historically privileged form of the first gospel that would have influenced Mark, since in any case we must account for the parallelism in the two gospels. We end then with a different aporia: why would Mark depend either on a proto-Matthean form of Matthew 19, presenting all the pericopes of our Matthew 19 except one (namely, vv. 10–12), or on a Matthean chapter identical with our chapter 19 but from which Mark would decide to take all the pericopes except a single one?

In short, Matthew 19:10–12 appears to be an insertion; it follows that it is the evangelist who illuminated the statement on marriage by a reference to celibacy and placed it in the perspective of the kingdom. We can even glimpse the reason why Matthew brought together marriage and celibacy. We have seen that the inserted clause probably reflected a desire to tone down the radicalism of the principal tradition. In bringing together marriage, indissoluble with a single exception, and voluntary celibacy, Matthew lessened the radicalism in another way; in a sense, marriage is indissoluble—rather, almost indissoluble—only for Christians.

V. Matthew 5:31–32

Another Rule on Indissolubility with an Exception Clause

"It was also said, 'Whenever a man divorces his wife, he must give her a decree of divorce.' What I say to you is: 'Whoever divorces his wife—lewd conduct is a separate case—forces her to commit adultery. The man who marries a divorced woman likewise commits adultery.'" (v. 32)

In textual criticism, it is doubtless necessary to read (v. 32) πας ὁ ἀπολύων as we have translated it, rather than ὅσ ἂν ἀπολύσῃ (a variant perhaps inspired by Mt 19:9 or Mk 10:11). The meaning is identical, but on the purely formal plane there is another stereotype beginning ("every man who does this or that"). This variety shows that in legislating, the community returned to traditional biblical formulas, to which perhaps Jesus at times conformed his oral style. The Greek text raises no other difficulty worthy of mention. Verse 32, which is the most delicate, is read in the same way by Nestle, Merk, Huck, and Aland.

1. The Context Of Matthew 5:31–32

Just as it is, the sermon on the mount (Mt 5:1–7:29) is evidently a redactional composition. Our two verses form part of a rather homogenous section (5:21–48), made up in its present state of six antitheses provided with a kind of introduction (5:17–20). In this section, as in the rest of the sermon, the writer's work was undoubtedly complex, since he had at his disposal various written sources that he abridged here, lengthened there—for example, by inserting parts that had already been written. Besides, the writer intervenes in a more personal way, either by constructing links or by inserting here and there a specific word or commentary on his own.

The last three of these operations will be considered here cumulatively. In introducing verses 31–32, Matthew lengthened a former series of antitheses;[116] to do this, he had to compose a formula of liaison (v. 31); finally, he inserted in the middle of a traditional logion (v. 32) the clause already examined in regard to Matthew 19:9: "lewd conduct is a separate case."

The antitheses are all formed on this pattern: "You have been given such a commandment, but I give you another." Moses is not named, but he is clearly the one aimed at. Thus we find here something of the opposition encountered above in Mark 10 and Matthew 19 between Jesus and Moses, the supreme authority for the Jews. But the grounds brought forth in Mark 10 and Matthew 19 do not appear. In Matthew 5, Jesus does not say that he means to return to the origins, beyond the laws that Moses had simply conceded to human weakness; he is rather the one who affirms with power an authority by far superior to that of the law. But the result is similar. Here, as in Matthew 19, Jesus promulgates in place of a temporary disposition or of an imperfect commandment a more exacting commandment. This is the case not only in regard to indissolubility but also in all the antitheses.

2. The Meaning of Matthew 5:31–32 for the Evangelist

Let us first read Matthew 5:31: "It was also said, 'Whenever a man divorces his wife, he must give her a decree of divorce.'" This is an allusion to Deuteronomy 24, a text already we have seen, in Mark 10:4 and Matthew 19:7.

It is important to insist on this; for the first time the question of divorce is at the center of the debate. The crux is neither the problem of adultery nor that of remarriage; the latter is considered only because it results from the divorce and makes its malice more clearly seen. The divorce by itself causes scandal. In Mark 10 and Matthew 19, we saw that a controversy concerning only divorce preceded the judgment on remarriage. But Matthew 5:31 is concerned only with divorce, not remarriage. As to the adultery mentioned in verse 32, it is the explicit object of another antithesis, that in Matthew 5:27–28.

Let us consider Matthew 5:32a, removing the inserted clause: "What I say to you is: everyone who divorced his wife . . . forces her to commit adultery." In relation to Matthew 19:9, the difference is notable. While Matthew 19:9 refers to the remarriage of the husband in addition to divorce, Matthew 5 does not mention remarriage, but affirms the husband's responsibility towards the wife he divorces: "he forces her to commit adultery"; more exactly, "he makes her commit adultery."[117] This expression is explained by the customs of the time, which scarcely had a place for the celibacy of a woman (or, for that matter, of a man). In these conditions, a divorced woman would be led to accept another marriage by which she would become adulterous, that is to say, in a state of having broken the conjugal bond that united her to her first husband. But it is the first husband who is declared responsible for this adultery. In short according to Matthew 19:9, M1, in divorcing W1 and marrying W2, committed adultery toward W1; according to Matthew 5:32, M1 in divorcing W1 led her to become adulterous toward M1, because inevitably she would marry M2.

The disastrous results of divorce differ then in the two texts. In Matthew 19:9, the consequence evoked is the remarriage of the husband who divorces, a remarriage that constitutes adultery or confirms the adultery contained in germ in the divorce. In Matthew 5:32a, the consequence to be feared is the remarriage of the wife, and it is the first husband who is responsible for it. The fundamental teaching is always identical, but its expression lends itself to variations, according as one considers a particular one of the persons concerned, of whom there are at least four.

From the Jewish point of view, Matthew 5:32a is as revolutionary as Matthew 19:9, but in a different way. In 19:9, the challenge consists in declaring a man an adulterer toward his own wife, which is contradictory. In 5:32a, the paradox consists in saying that a woman can become adulterous towards her first husband in remarrying, which is equally without precedent. One can even wonder whether in divorcing W1, M1 does not lead her to commit, in spite of herself, both adultery in regard to him and injustice in regard to him, the two aspects being linked in the eyes of the Jews. The paradox would then be at its height.

Let us go to Matthew 5:32b: "the man who marries a divorced woman likewise commits adultery." Exactly the same assertion appears in Matthew 19:9b, but we saw that the text is critically dubious there; here it is received by all editors. The assertion comes to this: if M2 marries W1, he commits adultery. This is an additional consequence of the repudiation, which is not envisaged either in Mark 10:11–12 or in Matthew 19:9a. For the first time the case of a man marrying a divorced woman is brought up; in so doing he commits adultery, that is to say, he violates the conjugal bond which joined W1 to M1, and which is supposed to remain firm.[118] We see that if the evangelist presents a new personage, it is always to teach the same message on indissolubility; one could speak of the moralist's reflex, applying the doctrine to various cases.

3. The Exception Clause in Matthew 5:32

a. The clause in itself

The particle παρεκτός, usually translated *except*, suggests to some the same problem as the words μὴ ἐπὶ of Matthew 19:9; it too would then be susceptible of receiving the preteritive or inclusive meaning of which we spoke above. It is clear that for ἐκτός and (by analogy) for παρεκτός, better than for μὴ ἐπὶ, one can quote texts which at first sight suggest the inclusive or additive sense.[119] All things considered, however, for παρεκτός as for μὴ ἐπὶ one must stay with the idea of exception. As for the sense of πορνεία we refer to the conclusions given above.[120]

One more remark: the fact that the clause is presented in Matthew 19:9 and Matthew 5:32 (its only two attestations in the whole New Testament) under two different lexicographical forms, but with an identical meaning, proves the importance of the idea of exception conveyed by the two incidental clauses. If Matthew was simply dependent on a ready-made formula, one could treat this one as an *obiter dictum;* the fact that he wrote two different formulas tends to prove that the will to posit an exception was sufficiently strong to give place to various expressions.

b. The clause in the verse

Having admitted that the incidental clause must indeed be translated "lewd conduct in a separate case" we again encounter the problem of Matthew 19:9: how to articulate the clause in the statement which contains it. On this painful point, the two principal opinions already set forth with regard to Matthew 19:9 are also the important ones here.

1) The exegesis of St. Jerome

The defenders of this explanation, already discussed in connection with Matthew 19:9, understand Matthew 5:32a as follows.

The man who divorces an innocent spouse is responsible for the adultery she will commit in remarrying; it must be implied that he cannot remarry. In the case of lewd conduct of the wife, the husband can leave her and he is not responsible for the adultery that she will commit in remarrying; but here again, it must be inferred that he cannot remarry.

2) The exegesis of numerous modern scholars

The partisans of this second exegesis, likewise presented above with regard to Matthew 19:9, understand Matthew 5:32a in the following manner.[121]

He who divorces his wife when she is innocent is responsible for the adultery she will commit in remarrying. Here also these exegetes infer that the aforesaid husband may not remarry. In the case of lewd conduct of his wife, the husband may leave her, and he is not responsible for the adultery she will commit by remarrying.[122] Moreover, the aforesaid husband may remarry.

Comparing these two paraphrases with each other, we notice again that both are probable. As in Matthew 19:9, we lean towards the second, chiefly because, in the ideas of the time, a legitimate divorce necessarily brought the right of the husband to remarry.

c. Does the Clause Apply to Matthew 5:32b?

The incidental clause of Matthew 5:32a does not reappear in 32b, and it would therefore be better not to conjecture whether it is implied there. But 32b is so complementary to 32a that the hypothesis is inevitable.

The clause of 32a, about the wife who is unfaithful to her husband, speaks of divorce under two headings: the exceptional case of the woman of lewd conduct and the ordinary case of the faithful wife. In spite of the use of the singular (his wife, W1), there are implied in 32a two categories of spouses. When one notices this, one must wonder whether, in spite of the singular ("a divorced woman"), verse 32b does not tacitly refer us back in turn to two types of the divorced woman, the innocent and the guilty.

On the whole, various indications make one think that the clause must not be 32b. First of all, a slight grammatical indication: without the article in 32b before ἀπολελυμένην, it is translated *a divorced woman* rather than *the divorced woman*, that is to say, the one just mentioned in 32a. In other words 32b seems to refer to any woman, without the evangelist's thinking of the woman of 32a, or rather, the two types of women referred to implicitly in 32a. Although complementary with regard to 32a, 32b seems to be a new sentence relatively independent of the other.

Another indication is that 32b is practically identical with Luke 16:18b and that in the Lucan text the clause could not be implied since it is ignored in Luke 16:18a and indeed appears nowhere in Luke. The presumption then is that Matthew 5:32b and Luke 16:18b come from Q, the source of words common to Matthew and Luke. Q, furthermore, is also the source of Matthew 5:32a and Luke 16:18a. It is understood, however, that Matthew 5:32a contains two important Matthean alterations, the clause and the formula proper to Matthew: "render adulterous".[123]

VI. Luke 16:18

Rules on Indissolubility

"Everyone who divorces his wife and marries another commits adultery. The man who marries a woman divorced from her husband likewise commits adultery" (Lk 16:18).

This logion is preceded immediately by two others which are summarized thus: not a minute part of a letter of the law will pass away (v. 17); and, the law and the prophets were in force until John (v. 16). Not only are the three logia rather dissimilar from each other, but they form an eccentric little block in the midst of a vast context on the use of terrestrial goods: Luke 16:1–15 (the parable of the shrewd manager, with corollaries which fit together well) and Luke 16:19–31 (the parable of the rich man and Lazarus, on an analogous theme).

Placed as a clear interruption of a homogeneous text, the three logia reveal the redactor's hand. Why such an insertion? Were an answer available, it would not enlighten us on the meaning of Luke 16:18. Let us suppose only that the three sentences were already joined in Luke's source—which could be Judeo-Christian. Indeed, if we must find at all costs an element common to the three logia, it is the problem of the value of the law in the Christian economy. Perhaps the source is quite simply Q, the classic collection of sayings of the Lord reconstructed from

Matthew and Luke, since we have already encountered the approximate equivalent of Luke 16:18 in Matthew 19:9.[124]

The content of Luke 16:18 amount to two schemata already encountered: if M1 divorces W1, he commits adultery; if M2 marries W1, he commits adultery.[125]

Apart from minor details of vocabulary and syntax which do not affect its content, the first of these two sentences appeared in Mark 10:11 and Matthew 19:9, although an exception clause complicates the version in Matthew 19:9. Even in Matthew 5:32a, the protasis is partially the same. In Mark 10:11, Matthew 19:9, and Luke 16:18, the protasis formulates the case: a husband divorces his wife and marries another. This is the most common referent of the term *divorce*.

Now that we have finished examining the various evangelical logia on indissolubility, the time has come to ask whether they are authentic *in ore Iesu*, and to choose which of them most closely approach *ipsa vox Iesu*.[126]

Together with Matthew 19:9, Luke 16:18a confirms the presence of such a saying in an earlier source, probably Q. The sentence is found elsewhere in Mark 10:11. If we admit with most exegetes[127] that Mark does not depend directly on Q, we can then posit that for this point they all depend on a small collection of logia older than Q. Moreover, the sentence is in harmony with the controversy whose intrinsic probability we have shown above; it is not far-fetched to suppose that Jesus and the Pharisees discussed indissolubility. If we add 1 Corinthians 7:10–11, we are justified in pleading for the historicity *in vita Jesu* of the message on indissolubility as formulated in Luke 16:18a, that is, its concrete phrasing in a precise and very well formulated principle and not merely in a more general sentence like Matthew 19:6a ("They are no longer two, but one flesh") or 6b ("Let no man separate what God has joined.") To specify the chances of Luke 16:18a being *ipsissimum verbum Iesu*, we must compare it more closely to its parallels. Compared with Matthew 19:9, Luke 16:18a is superior because it does not include the exception clause, which, as we have sufficiently shown, is redactional. For the rest, the two sentences agree perfectly. Mark 10:11 is identical to these two versions except for the additional two words ("against her") which only make the sense of the logion more explicit. Finally, compared to these three texts, Matthew 5:32a only partially agrees in its protasis, and has two secondary elements: the clause, which is equivalent in sense to Matthew 19:9, and the unique expression, "[by divorcing W1, M1] makes her adulterous."

It is difficult to claim literal historicity for this last unique expression; rather, it appears to be the result of Christian reflection on the responsibility incurred by the one who divorces. Such a reflection, moreover, develops what Jesus had said about divorce. In short, with its two redactional elements, clause and apodosis, Mt 5:32a is probably a revision of a logion of this type: if M1 divorces W1 (and remarries) he commits adultery. On the other hand, let us repeat, Luke 16:18a has the advantage of being both fundamentally identical with all the other witnesses, and free from the various expansions which the Matthean form chiefly exemplifies. It has the better chances of being authentic. One can attribute to Jesus an original statement like the following: the husband who divorces his wife and remarries commits adultery (towards her).

Let us proceed to Luke 16:18b: if M2 marries W1, he commits adultery. This sentence differs completely from the second rule of Mark (Mk 10:12), but it is found in Matthew 5:32b and perhaps, we have said, it lies behind Matthew 19:9b. On the basis of these statements, one may say that the assertion existed in a pre-Matthean document. Two other considerations favor its antiquity—even its presence in the discourse of Jesus.

a) In the four gospel versions, the sentences on indissolubility have a binary form. The only—dubious—exception is Matthew 19:9b, whose authenticity is barely plausible according to textual criticism. Certainly, in Mark 10:12, the second of the two elements has a strange form: if

W1 divorces M1, she commits adultery. This anomaly can be explained in various ways, all of which consider it a redactional insertion.[128] Nevertheless, this insertion in its own way is informative; Mark involuntarily attests by his imperfect editing that he has his eyes on two sayings rather than one, and that the second one, which he discarded, has all the marks of having been of the kind solidly attested elsewhere: If M2 marries W1, he commits adultery.

b) The exegetes of the Old Testament often speak of the parallelism of structure which characterizes the psalms and proverbs. One will admit without difficulty that this binary rhythm may still have marked the spoken language of the Jewish teachers in the time of Jesus, when they formulated maxims with some solemnity. The presumption would be true for Jesus also. One may specify that the present case is an example of a parallelism of complementarity, a well known type of binary construction in the psalms and proverbs. Likewise, on the level of content, a statement of the type of Luke 16:18b is truly a natural complement of the preceding one.

Granting to Luke 16:18b the greatest fidelity, after having granted it to 18a, let us say that one may ascribe to Jesus these twin statements: "if a man divorces his wife and marries another, he commits adultery, and the one who marries the divorced woman commits adultery." Of our four parallel pericopes, Luke 16:18a and b best approach the *ipsa vox Jesu*.[129]

Jesus thus takes a view contrary to even the most severe Jewish doctrine, which only rarely granted the right to divorce and then to remarry. That Jesus absolutely condemned remarriage is the almost unanimous conviction of commentators. These agree also in general in thinking that Jesus at the same time condemned divorce itself.[130]

VII: 1 Corinthians 7:10–11

Rules on Indissolubility

In 1 Corinthians, after having treated on his own authority several subjects, especially current divisive factions in Corinth, Paul comes to the questions which were put to him by his correspondents (1 Cor 7:1). The first had reference to sexual morality. After various instructions (1 Cor 7:1–9) of which the last (vv. 8–9) are addressed to celibates and widows, the apostle continues thus: "To those now married, however, I give this command (though it is not mine, it is the Lord's), a wife must not separate from her husband. If she does separate, she must either remain single or become reconciled to him again. Similarly, a husband must not divorce his wife" (1 Cor 7:10–11).

The spouses thus addressed are both Christians, since mixed marriages are treated separately immediately after (vv. 12–16). What the apostle prescribes to Christian spouses is done in the name of the Lord, that is, in conformity with the teaching of Jesus on earth, a teaching that Paul received in the Church as coming from Jesus (1 Cor 11:23).[131]

The apostle distinguishes clearly both the rules that he himself establishes (1 Cor 7:12–16) and the simple counsels that he gives (1 Cor 7:25–40) from the precepts coming from the Lord.

In 1 Cor 7:10, Paul addresses the woman first. To the extent—difficult to estimate—that this priority in attention is really intended, it breaks the tradition which took shape in the Gospels: the prescriptions there are addressed to men, not only primarily, but almost exclusively. The only exception is Mark 10:12; it forbids the woman to divorce her husband—but only after it first addressed a similar prohibition to the man. It is possible that the order Paul chooses is inspired by the same motive that, according to some, moves Mark to address the woman explicitly (after having called upon the husband): the apostle perhaps remembers that in the

Greco-Roman world, contrary to Jewish usage, it is not rare that the woman takes the initiative in the rupture.

In *commanding* (this is indeed the strong meaning of the Greek verb παραγγέλλειν) that the woman not leave her husband, the apostle surely intends to condemn the simple fact of separating, which confirms our exegesis of Mark 10:2–12 where, according to us, Jesus had already condemned the act of divorce and not only remarriage.[132]

However, the Apostle offers a hypothesis: let us suppose that a woman has, even so, left her husband (v. 11). We do not have to understand this to mean that Paul is thus attenuating the prohibition made to the wife about leaving her husband;[133] he is merely stating that she has broken the precept, no doubt because she remains under the influence of Greco-Roman customs. He sees in that, at least, a problem. We do not know whether he was the first to attempt to solve it, but the present verses are the first Christian text *ad rem*.

Pursuing our reading, let us note the importance of another precept: "if she left, she must not remarry." Although the verb is in the subjunctive, there is doubtless room here to read a prohibition pure and simple,[134] because the prohibition of remarriage was absolute in the message of Jesus: it is a point on which almost all the exegetes agree, even if some hesitate on the subject of simple separation. Certainly, with its two verbs in the subjunctive, the parenthesis which 1 Corinthians 7:11a constitutes no longer depends clearly on the expression "the Lord commands"; but one cannot suppose that Paul thinks differently from Jesus on the important question of remarriage. We must, however, recognize that for the apostle, the wife has no absolute obligation to rejoin her husband; in fact, by requiring "that she remain not married," Paul lets it be understood that in certain cases she may remain separated. So this time we are faced with what Catholic tradition will call the *separatio tori et mensae*.[135]

Moreover, Paul does ask the wife to become reconciled. But he leaves her the choice: the wife must either be reconciled or abstain from remarriage while remaining separated. The reconciliation is no doubt the ideal: and in proposing it, Paul expresses in a new way something of the message of Jesus, centered on the indissoluble union of the spouses.

To end his instruction to Christian spouses, Paul orders the husband not to divorce his wife (1 Cor 7:11b). Grammatically, these words are again governed by παραγγέλλω, like the parentheses containing the two subjunctives. They clearly convey an imperative precept of the Lord. Effectively, 1 Corinthians 7:11b partially restates an essential formula of the gospels, which we have noted goes back to Jesus: "the husband who divorces his wife and marries another, commits adultery". We say "partially" because Paul speaks of divorce without speaking of remarriage (as also does Mt 5:32a).[136] Paul uses here the mode of expression ("send away") which corresponds to the language of the Jews, without forgetting Greco-Roman manners, which also recognized, *ad sensum*, the case of the man sending away his spouse.[137]

To sum up, the two precepts formulated as coming from Jesus are: the wife must not leave her husband, the husband must not divorce his wife. These essential formulas are conformable to those of Jesus and recall once more the specific framework in which the master had spoken of the custom of divorce. Somewhat similarly, Paul addresses the woman first, which would be unexpected in the Jewish milieu. For the rest, the apostle approaches a case necessarily new at the time of Jesus: that of a wife who had left her husband, the two being supposedly Christian. The sole fact of having left the partner is contrary to the teaching of Jesus (1 Cor 7:10) but the apostle does not brandish thunderbolts; the main thing, it seems, is that the wife who has deserted the home not remarry; one would say that, on this point, the words of Jesus seem too clear to admit of violation. Besides, Paul also recommends reconciliation, which, in his eyes, would best safeguard the marriage as desired by Jesus.

Conclusions

In our analyses of the gospel texts, we have proceeded backwards, as today's method of exegesis recommends. We started from the texts as they present themselves, that is, as words of authors reflecting at the same time Church situations, and from there we went to the historical Jesus. The Pauline text made its contribution to clarity as much on Jesus as on the apostolic Church. For the sake of clarity, it is now expedient to present the conclusions in reverse order, that is, chronologically.

1. Marriage in the Message of Jesus

a. Teaching of Jesus Himself

1) Jesus understood marriage as a monogamous and indissoluble union. He therefore condemned unconditionally all remarriage in the lifetime of the partner.[138] On this subject, the consensus among the exegetes is almost unanimous.[139]

2) It is very probable that Jesus also condemned in the same manner the simple separation in itself. However, one cannot totally exclude the possibility of a tolerance by Jesus on this precise point, this notably by reason of the authority of the exegetes who are of this opinion.[140] But it remains understood, as these very exegetes agree, that separation gives no right to remarriage.

3) It is probable, in spite of the small number of texts, that Jesus spoke several times on the subject of marriage and notably on the occasion of the controversies with the Pharisees.[141]

4) The center of Jesus' argument was probably the recourse to the text of Genesis against that of Deuteronomy, that is, the appeal to the perfect will of the creator against the weaknesses of Moses; or again, the appeal to the Lord of the universe against the legislator of a particular people, even the people of the covenant.[142]

5) It is probable that Jesus concluded his responses to the Pharisees by an aphorism: "that man not separate what God has united," and that he was also led to formulate the teaching he directed to his disciples into certain practical rules. On this subject we have retained as probable *ipsissima verba* a double rule obviously addressed to the disciples, a kind of *mashal* which may have been a "canonical" rule before it was put down: "whoever divorces his wife and marries another, commits adultery; and he who marries the divorced woman commits adultery."

b. The Importance of the Teaching of Jesus in His Own Eyes

To state the essential assertions of Jesus is one thing; to establish the importance in his own eyes is another, more delicate, task. However, this brings up again the question of the competence of the historian;[143] and in addition, it sheds more direct light on hermeneutics.

1) On the basis of the text—a controversy and some statements—one cannot assume that the words of Jesus on marriage occupy an absolutely central place in the totality of his message. In any case, as always in the Gospel controversies, Jesus does not initiate the dispute; this contrasts with the proclamation *motu proprio* of the coming of the kingdom and its "constitutional laws." At the extreme, one might imagine that the result of the controversy is the simple dodging[144] in conjunction with the referral of the Pharisees by Jesus to a text of Genesis which embarrasses them.

However, if the Pharisees wish to put Jesus to the test, it is no doubt because they know that the Master has greatly criticized elsewhere and *motu proprio* the Jewish practice of divorce. One can then understand that Jesus was not content to leave the Pharisees nonplussed, but rather pronounced clearly the principle of non-remarriage and even of non-separation and made the application of it in several statements directed to the disciples.

2) The Jewish milieu, which Jesus shared, had a high regard for monogamous marriage;[145] practice largely conformed to this ideal, and it contrasts, in the eyes of today's historian, with the laxity of Greco-Roman customs. By expressing himself as he did on marriage, Jesus was not led (at least there is no indication of it) by a desire to extirpate grave abuses. Thus, one cannot invoke these as circumstantial explanations of his message. In short, nothing tells us that Jesus would have been constrained to severity in order to dam up flagrant excesses. On the contrary, the master seems to be inspired only by a concern for perfection. The Pharisees whom Jesus opposes here were, among the Jews and in comparison with other religious groups, rather severe in the matter of conjugal morality. The fact that Jesus openly confronted them is a quite striking confirmation of his radicalism.

3) It is possible that Jesus was moved to oppose divorce in part by his solicitude to defend the divorced woman. What permits us to suppose this is that Jesus often came to the defense of humiliated women.

4) To clarify this radicalism, in spite of the scantiness of our texts, we have at our disposal a vast gospel context whose historicity is not in doubt; it is clear that Jesus required of his disciples, in all domains of the moral life, a new rigor and a will for "perfection." It is in this framework of a uniformly demanding ethic that we must situate our texts.[146]

5) However, there is quite a problem here. Taking the gospels as a whole, the ethic of Jesus is polarized by two different goals, each of which would suffice to establish the ethic. On the one hand, the disciple must be capable of all renunciations because the kingdom which is to come has no price. On the other hand, if they place themselves in God's view, the disciples—and even, one would say, all men—can perceive the loftiness of the divine will, even the existence in God of a "perfection" which requires imitation. The motivation is more eschatological on one side, more theological on the other.[147]

A clear example of renunciation for the cause of the kingdom is voluntary celibacy (Mt 19:12). One would say, as we noted, that Matthew has drawn the exacting word of Jesus on marriage into the same path. But for Jesus himself, indissoluble marriage responds to the perfect will of God, promulgated from the very beginning, prior to what is properly called the economy of salvation; thus the will of God is directed to the disciples and to all men. In other words, the demand in the matter of marriage is not of the same nature as the call to voluntary celibacy or to selling one's goods; on the one hand, there is voluntary choice and an attitude of exception for the sake of kingdom; on the other, there is pure and simple submission to the absolute will of God.

Another way of expressing the same thing is to say that here Jesus presents himself as a moralist rather than as founder of the kingdom. The distinction certainly is somewhat subtle. But it seems that for Jesus, the perfect will of the creator is imposed on every upright man and not only on those who, in addition, await the coming of the kingdom and are ready to sacrifice all for it.

The "timeless" God is here the norm of morality. To walk in righteousness is to understand the height of the divine will or to live under the glance of God. The analysis, we see, is of a theological and moral type; it is centered on the sense of God and the idea of interiority. it is a question only *in obliquo* of the charter of the kingdom of God.

2. Hermeneutic Scope of the Teachings of Jesus

Let us define hermeneutics summarily as the actualization of the Word of God, the totally final manner of understanding and applying it; it is the last proceeding of the theologian and the believer.

Until recently, the assured result of exegesis, such as it is, was accepted as the norm of faith and of conduct. Thus people thought that if indissolubility is taught by Jesus it is willed by God. Even while appealing to the Jesus of history, theologians and believers knew, however, that on other issues the teaching of Jesus was sometimes only a point of departure; it remained for them to make it more precise through tradition, a tradition already attested to in the New Testament.[148]

In its evaluation of the gospel as norm, present day hermeneutics seems pulled in opposite directions.

a) On the one hand, it seems drawn by "the purity of origins" and from there is disposed to make a great case of the teaching of Jesus reconstituted with all the historical rigor desirable. Consequently, this hermeneutic sometimes treats development after Jesus as a super-structure to be criticized; it takes pleasure also in opposing Jesus to the Church.

On this subject, may we not judge that the return to the historical Jesus[149] could not give us an iron rule? The relationship between the Church and Jesus is complex. For example, from apostolic times the Church's stance has differed when it faces those teachings of Jesus which demand a hearing through their power and clarity, and when it reflects on those *dicta Jesu* which have a prophetic or apocalyptic tone. In these cases, it must be remembered that "the period of the creation of a religion can only be considered as finished when it possesses a tradition by which it is expressed and justified and when it is endowed with the necessary organs for the exercise of the functions by which its life and stability can be assured."[150]

However, the words of Jesus on marriage are dependent on cases of the first type: they were imposed on the apostolic Church as a normative fact because they appeared clear and "historically" established. Hence, a hermeneutic operating in the logic of a "return to Jesus" seems to be able to welcome the exegetical conclusions exposed above in part 1.

b) Another tendency of present day hermeneutics literally takes a point of departure from what the Jesus of history thought and willed. We allude to some markedly different types of reading—structuralist, psychoanalytical, materialistic, and so forth—which yet share a desire to make the texts speak rather than the person, or, if you prefer, to distill from the four gospels a fifth gospel,[151] which is shaped by the existential needs of modern man (in fact, of one of the many types of modern man: linguist, psychologist, economist, and so forth). This fifth gospel then functions as criteria. If it is in harmony with the rigorous exegesis of the four gospels, no problem arises; otherwise, the hermeneutic will consider that even the historically established teaching of Jesus was culture-bound and therefore is no longer valid.

Paradoxically, these attempts are an involuntary homage to the idea of tradition. The intuition of all times was also that the gospel is not a relic but a living text; however, the "fifth Gospel" is then the Church.

In the case occupying us, what was taken to be the will of the earthly Jesus was ratified for nineteen centuries by a dominant tradition, already existing and attested to in the New Testament. Can it still be so for the man of today, confronted with new situations, in some ways without precedent? Such is the question posed by some. We would say that on the plane of principles, we cannot contest the legitimacy of research; it is right indeed to be sensitive to the signs of the times, even if they reflect quite new ways of thinking and of expression. The apostle said in a somewhat analogous manner: "Do not stifle the Spirit; do not despise prophecies." (1 Thes 5:19–20) However, he added immediately: "Test everything; retain what is good" (1 Thes 5:21). It belongs to the Church to decide in the last instance.[152]

3) Marriage in the eyes of the apostolic Church

The gospels, we know, witness *also* to the ecclesial theology of the first century; and even more so does St. Paul.

a. Paul

The apostle is the most ancient witness of the memory that the Christians keep of the teaching of Jesus of Nazareth (1 Cor 7:10–11). In the present case, as in others, he has faithfully preserved the tenor of the message of Jesus: Christian spouses may not separate and in no case remarry, even if there has been a separation *de facto*. This last hypothesis appears clearly through Paul whereas we would not dare to say it with certitude for Jesus.

In the time of Paul, it evidently happened that in the pagan (or Jewish) home, one of the partners was converted.[153] In this case, if the other wished to co-inhabit peacefully, that is, without preventing the convert from practicing his (her) faith, things could remain as before (1 Cor 7:12–16); the apostle tacitly supposes that marriage between pagans (or Jews) is a true marriage. This presupposition is enlightening in that it confirms that marriage is, first of all and in itself, a natural institution; in this sense, the idea of Paul is in line with the teaching of Jesus on marriage as an element of the charter of the created world, anterior to any idea of a chosen people.

If the unconverted spouse prevents the Christian partner from practicing his (her) faith, or takes the initiative of departure, the converted party may separate (1 Cor 7:12–16). May he (she) also remarry? In exegesis, two opposite answers are possible. If one answers No, one quite confirms the remark formulated just now: the marriage which had been concluded between pagans (or Jews) is already so sacred that it is absolutely indissoluble.[154] If one answers yes,[155] one does not for all that ascribe to the apostle a vague idea of a natural (or Jewish) marriage, but rather admits that Paul, without renouncing the principle of the validity of such marriages, here creates a true exception, making allowance for the interests of faith which are sovereign. One will then speak very exactly of a *privilege* granted by Paul to the Christian party, and it is thus that the Church understands 1 Corinthians 7:15, at least since the Middle Ages.

After this almost letter-by-letter analysis, we must investigate the scope of these declarations in the eyes of Paul himself; and this is properly an exegetical question. That question is posed in the following terms: did the apostle simply adjudicate a few particular cases, or did he intend to really legislate? We need not raise the question for 1 Corinthians 7:10–11, where Paul recalls a precept of the Lord, a precept which in his eyes is assuredly imposed without reservation, but for 1 Corinthians 7:12–17, where the Apostle speaks in his own name.

The response can be found by examining the context. It would certainly be an anachronism to represent Paul as having full consciousness of promulgating a law for the universal Church and especially a law valid "forever and ever."[156] But one would fall into the opposite excess by believing that Paul aimed only at such and such a particular case. It is clear that in this chapter 7, the apostle is still thinking of *categories* of Christians, differently from chapters 5 and 6, where he treats of two problems, each time after having learned the fault of a definite individual.[157] Besides, the matrimonial morality is very important for the apostle.[158] One may then conclude that for him even *his own* instructions on this subject are imposed on all Christians concerned. This does not deny that the Pauline privilege has acquired its full force only by its ulterior ratification in the Church, as we will repeat when we speak of hermeneutics.

b. Mark and Luke

The analysis of Mark and Luke has shown that the redactional elements are not really important. There is then no need for us to stop here on what would be a very new apostolic interpretation. For what is controversial (Mk 10:2–9), we have insisted on its chances of authenticity rather than on its character of being specifically of Mark.[159] As for the statement of Mark 10:10–12, its most redactional element is the unusual Mark 10:12, addressed to a woman who is divorcing; but only the statement of the case is new, not the doctrine expressed. 1 Corinthians 7 has already made us notice this tendency to consider various possible cases: one understands from this how rules diffused with variants, which however have no effect on the content of the message of Jesus. It is probable that the Church of the first century had still other formulations, but which circumstances did not preserve for us.

Luke, let us recall, did not report the controversy, perhaps because it seemed too anchored in a Pharisaic framework which was no longer current in his day. As for his version of the statements (Lk 16:18), it is as traditional as possible, and so it reveals no intention of personal interpretation.

c. Matthew

Matthew's case is different. We are not going to recall all his redactional interventions but only the two most important ones, those which allow one to speak of an eventual "apostolic" interpretation of the teaching of Jesus.

There is first of all the exception clause, which already affects the presentation of the controversy (Mt 9:3) and still more the very formulation of the traditional rule (Mt 19:9; 5:32). If, as we have judged most probable, the exception clause permits remarriage in case of adultery, the moment has come to question ourselves on the scope of this innovation in the eyes of the Matthean editor.

Unfortunately, a certain answer is impossible. First of all the very form of the moot text—a brief parenthesis—prevents it from taking on a "coefficient of importance." Did Matthew presume that Jesus, while condemning divorce and remarriage, had to consent, in the face of his contemporaries, to grant them an exception (*Historisierung*), when for the evangelist himself, the Church had opted legitimately against all exception, thus remaining faithful to the basic teaching of Jesus? Did Matthew, on the contrary, make himself the interpreter of past or contemporary Judeo-Christian groups, admitting the aforesaid exception without, however, contesting the more strict discipline of the great Church? Such questions will remain forever without a firm answer.

In addition to the exception clause, there is another properly Matthean intervention: the linking of the teaching of Jesus on marriage with his call to voluntary celibacy. By so doing, Matthew seems to suggest that if the master has shown himself so strict concerning marriage, it is because he has made of it a law of exception, an ideal proposed "to those who can understand." For, let us repeat, even furnished with an exception, the sentence of Jesus on marriage remains severe in the eyes of Matthew.

Again, it is practically impossible for us to determine the exact scope of the link between celibacy and marriage in the eyes of the writer himself. Did he truly wish to bring the "matrimonial right" into this ethic of exception which is also expressed in texts such as 1 Cor 7:29–31: "time is short; let those who have a wife live as if they did not ...; because the figure of this world passes"? In our analysis, we have been led to speak of suggestion or insinuation: these terms mark the limits of our certitudes. The stage will have to be taken here again by hermeneutics and, first of all, by Christian tradition.

3. Hermeneutic Scope of the Apostolic Teachings

Where Paul and the evangelists merely reproduce the teachings of Jesus, their texts call for the same hermeneutic as these teachings.[160] But there is also a hermeneutic of those teachings that are properly apostolic. If the New Testament *preserves* the gospel which Jesus had preached, it also comments on it with a certain liberty. The question then arises to what extent is the specific contribution of the witnesses to Jesus normative for the theologian and the believer today?

The ancient response remains truly valid: the teaching given in their own name by the authors of the New Testament is covered by an authority analogous to that of the words of Jesus. This authority is defined by the double quality of word of God and inspired Scripture, which the Christians of today still recognize in the New Testament.[161]

Another criterion of hermeneutics applies with greater clarity to the assertions properly apostolic than to the major declarations of Jesus himself: it is the manner in which these assertions have been received in the post-apostolic Church until our day. Thus, if the Pauline privilege has indeed survived, it is because the Church has recognized in it, at least since the Middle Ages, a principle which appeared to it apt for regulating the case of mixed marriage. On the other hand, the two Mattheisms spoken of above have not benefited by such a clear reception.

The first is the exception to the rule of indissolubility in favor of the deceived spouse, at least according to the exegesis that we have considered most probable. Compared with the texts of Paul, Mark, and Luke, the Matthean interpretation has remained isolated in the New Testament and so in the Church of the first generations. Even if there were hesitations in the course of the following centuries, the Council of Trent set aside this interpretation. But in so doing, it did not wish to define the literal sense of the Gospel texts; it limited itself to claiming that the Church had the right to take a position on the points which were not absolutely clear. The prudent formulas of the council contain, then, a quite nuanced hermeneutic: total respect for the texts of the New Testament, fleshed out with the right of the Church to its own reading. What comes out of this, on the whole, is the nonconfirmation of the exception clause understood as the right to remarriage.

For its part, the insinuation of Matthew regarding indissoluble marriage, inasmuch as a voluntary choice has remained a pure Matthewism: nothing indicates that the tradition, even ancient, took this path.[162] The suggestion of Matthew cannot prevail against the manner in which Jesus, in accordance with the will of the creator promulgated in Genesis, understood the eternal attributes of marriage. In the West, a whole theological current seems to have retained this intuition of Jesus, in thinking that marriage can be regarded in itself or, if you will, in the sight of God: all marriage, and not only that of Christians, is of itself indissoluble.[163] To people tempted to prefer the interpretation suggested by Matthew, according to which indissoluble marriage is almost as specific of Christianity as celibacy for the kingdom, those who hold to a universal morality of indissolubility could answer exactly as did A. Loisy to the Greeks and Protestants concerning the exception clause. Their interpretation of the clause, said A. Loisy, "is indeed the natural meaning of the passage"—that is, its meaning for Matthew—"but it also has every chance of *not* being that of Jesus...." "The Catholic Church, by refusing to admit any case for divorce, has maintained the principle established by Jesus, and it matters little that it could only do so by sacrificing the historical sense of the passages where Matthew treats the question."[164] Applying to our subject what Loisy thus wrote of the clause, we would say that to renounce the natural indissolubility of marriage would probably be to choose Matthew against Jesus.[165]

Finally, the last criterion of hermeneutics for the teachings of the apostles as for those of Jesus is awareness of the present situation of Christian marriage. Three points pose a question: the Pauline privilege, the exception clause of Matthew, and the apparently Matthean attenuation of indissolubility (even accompanied by an exception) as an attribute of every marriage. On this triple subject, modern commentaries must, at the very least, take into account the nuanced conclusions of critical historical exegesis and the weight placed on these three problems by ecclesiastical tradition. This being said, it is also legitimate to take into account the present situation, notably the manner in which failures occur today in many families, even though the victims sincerely want to live according to the gospel and in agreement with the Church.[166] However firm the framework of the principles may be, it does not seem that accommodation should be excluded *a priori;* but the decisions, strictly speaking, belong to the Church of today and tomorrow.[167]

Let us recall in two sentences the scope of our conclusions. First we sought to establish the teaching of Jesus on indissolubility by distinguishing its tenor and scope. We then applied a hermeneutic similar to that used in the New Testament itself and in tradition, and indeed is used even today. We covered the specifically apostolic teaching in two similar stages.

Notes

1. The general bibliography on the subject includes the commentaries and annotated translations of the synoptic gospels and 1 Cor as well as the theologies of the New Testament.

The monographs are legion. For the period before 1959, we can depend on the literature used by J. Dupont all through his excellent book, *Mariage et divorce dans l'évangile* (Desclée de Brouwer, 1959). For this period, we may limit ourselves to recalling some French titles; F. J. Leenhardt, *L'enseignement de Jésus sur le divorce,* Les cahiers bibliques de foi et vie, no. 5 (Paris, 1938) 49–67; J. Bonsirven, *Le divorce dans le Nouveau Testament* (Paris and Tournai, 1948); J. Thomas, "Droit naturel et droit chrétien en matière d'indissolubilité du mariage," in *Collectanea moralia in honorem . . . A. Janssen;* "Bibliotheca Ephemeridum Theologicarum Lovaniensium, no. 23 (Louvain and Gembloux, 1948), 2 621–39; M.-F. Berrouard, "L'indissolubilité du mariage dans le Nouveau Testament," LV 4 (1952) 21–40; H. Cazelles, "Mariage," DBS 5 (1957), esp. col. 926–35. For the period 1948–59, see a very rich bibliography in J. Dupont, *Mariage,* 93–95.

For the period after 1959, let us quote first two of the bibliographical listings in existence: R. Metz and J. Schlick, *Mariage et divorce: International Bibliography Indexed by Computer* (Strasbourg, 1973); and A. Myre, "Dix ans d'exégèse sur le divorce dans le Nouveau Testament," in *Le divorce* (Montreal, 1973), 139–63 (covers the period 1963–72). We mention next some studies which have been helpful to us: B. K. Diderichsen, *Den markianiske skilsmisseperikope. Dens genesis og historiske placering* (Doctoral dissertation, Copenhagen, 1961; Glydendal, 1962); A. Isaksson, *Marriage and Ministry in the New Temple* (Lund and Copenhagen, 1965); H. Baltensweiler, *Die Ehe im Neuen Testament* (Zürich and Stuttgart, 1967); R. Pesch, "Die neutestamentliche Weisung für die Ehe," BL 9 (1968) 208–221; H. Greeven, J. Razinger, et al., *Theologie der Ehe* (Augsburg and Göttingen, 1969) with exegetical studies by H. Greeven, R. Schnackenburg, and others; U. Nembach, "Ehescheidung nach alttestamentlichem und jüdischem Recht," TZ 26 (1970) 251–77; B. Schaller, "Die Sprüche über Ehescheidung und Wiederheirat in der synoptischen Überlieferung," in E. Lohse (ed.), *Der Ruf Jesu und die Antwort der Gemeinde* (Göttingen, 1970), 226–46; E. Bammel, "Markus 10:11 f. und das jüdische Eherecht," ZNW 61 (1970) 263–74; T. A. G. van Eupen (ed.), *(On)ontbindbaarheit van het huwelijk* (Hilversum, 1970), with exegetical studies by B. F. M. van Iersel and J. H. A. van Tilborg; F. Neirynck, "De Jezuswoorden over echtscheiding," in V. Heylen (ed.), *Misklukt huwelijk en echtscheiding* (Louvain, 1972) 127–41 (into which Neirynck incorporates two of his previous articles); P. Benoit, *L'évangile selon saint Matthieu* BJ (Paris, 1972); A. Tosato, *Il matrimonio nel guidaismo antico e nel Nuovo Testamento* (Rome, 1976); J. A. Fitzmyer, "The Matthean Divorce Texts and Some New Palestinian Evidence," TS 37 (1976) 197–226; A. Stock, "The Matthean Divorce Text," *Biblical Theology Bulletin* 8 (1978) 24–33; R. Pesch, *Das Markusevangelium* (Herder, 1977) 126–27; H. Schürmann, "Neutestamentliche Marginalien zur Frage nach der Institutionalität, Unauflösbarkeit und Sakramentalität der Ehe," in *Kirche und Bibel* (Paderborn, 1979) 409–10; P. Delhaye (ed.), *Problémes doctrinaux du Chrétien* (Coll. *Lex spiritus vitae,* 4) (Louvain-la-Neuve, 1979). This latter work, a product of the ITC, has helpful references at the end of each chapter.

2. 1 Cor 7:10–11. Cf. Lk 16:18, but only in the hypothesis of B. K. Diderichsen mentioned below, n. 6; cf. Lk 18:29b (the word *woman* does not occur in the parallel texts); compare Lk 14:26, where *woman* occurs only in Luke.

3. In Judaism, Dt 24:1–4 became the legal text par excellence relative to divorce; but see also Dt 22:13–19; 28–29. Note, however, that Dt 24:1–4 does not deal with divorce as such. It touches on divorce only in order to stipulate that a former husband is not entitled to take back the wife he has previously divorced. The pas-

sage begins: "Supposing a man has taken a wife and consummated the marriage; but she has not pleased him and he has found some impropriety of which to accuse her; so he has made out a writ of divorce..." (JB).

4. The textual criticism of Mk 10:2–12 raises only minor problems, which are methodically examined by H. Zimmerman, *Neutestamentliche Methodenlehre* (Stuttgart, 1966) 107–8. The situation is different for Mk 10:12; see pp. 86–87.

5. On the syntax of Mark's Gospel, see B. Rigaux, *Témoignage de l'évangile de Marc* (Desclée de Brouwer, 1965) 96–100.

6. Ἀπολύειν is not, however, the verb used in the Greek version of the Old Testament. In Dt 4:1– is ἐξαποστέλλειν, which is very frequent in the whole LXX, whereas ἀπολύειν is rare.

In the New Testament, ἀπολύειν often occurs in the weak sense, as equivalent of *letting go* or *dismissing* (the crowds, for example). This is why it has been sometimes interpreted, at least in Lk 16:18, as meaning merely *to leave one's wife* (without divorcing her), for the sake of the kingdom, for example. Thus, B. K. Diderichsen, *Den skilsmisserperikope*, 20–47; 347. But, as J. A. Fitzmyer has recently shown, in the New Testament text on divorce (Mt 1:19 included) ἀπολύειν certainly means *to divorce* in the precise legal sense we have recalled above; see "Divorce Text," 212–13. Fitzmyer refers to hellenistic texts, and also to a text from Cave 2 of Wadi Murabba'at.

7. Similar observations in R. Bultmann, *Geschichte der synoptischen Tradition* (3rd. ed.; Göttingen, 1957) 25, ET: *The History of the Synoptic Tradition* (Oxford: Blackwell, 1963) 25–26.

We cannot agree with the suggestion of A. Loisy who maintains that, in Mk 10:3, Jesus refers to what Moses, the author of Genesis, ordains in Gn 1:27 and 2:24. See *Les évangiles synoptiques* (Ceffonds, 1908), 2, 196–97.

8. Strictly speaking, the word *prescribing* could be understood as the echo of a recommendation (suggested, perhaps, by abuses): "Do not neglect to deliver the writ of divorce before dismissing the wife, else she would risk remaining just a woman separated from her husband, and would not be entitled to remarry." See also Mt 5:31, where the text is cast in the language of obligation: "Anyone who divorces his wife must give her a writ of dismissal" (JB).

9. Κτίσις means *creation* in the sense of *created universe* that is, κοσμος, not in the sense of *act of creating*. Compare καταβολὴ κόσμου (Mt 25:34, etc.) and ἀρχὴ κόσμου (Mt 24:21; Mk 18:19).

10. Thus BJ (*hardness of heart*). This translation is not perfect, but it has the advantage of being enfranchised into religious language.

11. Ἐκληροκαρδία occurs only three times in the LXX. However, the LXX offers many expressions with similar meaning, such as σκληροτράχηλος (Vg. *durae cervicis*), σκληρότης του λαου, etc. Fr. Delitzsch's reverse translation is *geshi lebab, duritia cordis*. In the whole New Testament, σκληροκαρδία occurs only in this passage (and in the parallel text, Mt 19:8) and in Mk 16:14, but again we find in the New Testament many expressions that convey a similar meaning. See the excellent detailed presentation of all this in Dupont, *Mariage* 19–20, with the notes.

12. The precise extent of this condemnation as understood by Mark and his readers is disputed. Did they believe that Moses had been ordered by God to mitigate the original will of the creator? If so, Moses would not be at fault, whereas pre-Christian Israel would still be stigmatized as a stubborn people. Or was Moses himself guilty of this stubbornness? In this case, he would fall under the same severe condemnation as his people. The fact that Jesus appears in the New Testament as "the new Moses" does not decide the issue, for such typology is compatible with diversities and even with contrasts. As we shall see, the dilemma becomes even more acute when it comes to deciding what Jesus himself thought in the matter.

13. See the following section "2. The Teaching of Jesus."

14. H. Zimmermann, *Methodenlehre*, 110. Note that, although the interpretation of the Genesis texts in Mk 10:6–9 is not a rigorous exegesis, it nevertheless correctly captures the tenor of the these passages. See on this some remarks in J. Thomas, "Droit naturel," 625–27.

15. A slight indication of a possible autonomy is the neuter singular ὁ ("that which"; Mk 10:9), which comes after many cases where the plural occurs. Cf. G. F. Fisher, "Mariage et divorce," VC 10 (1956) 105–20.

16. Thus R. H. Charles, *The Teaching of the New Testament on Divorce* (London, 1921), 43–61.

17. Thus J. A. Fitzmyer, "Divorce Texts," 211, refers to both classical and hellenistic Greek texts, while adverting to the silence of the LXX. On 211 he speaks of "tortuous attempts" with reference to the efforts of R. H. Charles mentioned above, n. 16.

18. This is the opinion of many authors: R. Bultmann, *Geschichte*, 25; ET: *History*, 26; F. Neirynck, *Jezuswoorden*, 140, n. 22, etc.

19. On this topic see M. Devisch, "La relation entre l'évangile de Marc et le document Q," in M. Sabre (ed.), *L'évangile selon Marc* (Louvain and Gembloux, 1974), 59–91. P. G. Delling has tried to reduce Mt 5:31–32 to Mk 10:11 "Das Logion Mark. X 11 im Neuen Testament," *Novum Testamentum* (1956–57) 263–74. An opposing (and better) view is in Fitzmyer, "Divorce Texts," 202–03.

20. Both μοιχᾶσθαι and μοιχεύειν occur with the same sense (*adulterare*, to commit adultery, *Ehebruch treiben*). The two Greek verbs occur each a dozen times in the LXX; the second occurs especially in the Decalogue (Ex 20:13; Dt 5:18, οὐ μοιχεύσεις). In the New Testament, the first of the two verbs occurs only here (Mk 10:11–12), as well as in Mt 19:9 (which is a parallel), and in Mk 5:32; the second verb occurs a dozen times.

The meaning is adultery precisely as distinct from fornication, πορνεία; see J. A. Fitzmyer, "Divorce Texts," 209, n. 49.

21. On the meaning of this distinction, which derives from the Old Testament, see J. Coppens, *Histoire critique des livres de l'Ancien Testament* (3rd ed.; Desclée de Brouwer, 1942) 127–30; Dupont, *Mariage*, 53, and the authors quoted there, n. 2, including those who discuss this style in the gospels; H. W. Gilmer, *The if-you Form in Israelite Law* (Missoula, Montana, 1975). The apomictic form occurs in Mt 5:32 and Lk 16:18 (πᾶσ ὁ . . .).

This difference is regarded as important by the exegetes of the Old Testament in view of the fact that these two modes of legislation are linked to the two contexts where they originated, and these differ widely from each other. In our texts this difference has lost some of its sharpness. It is difficult to perceive a large difference between these two formulae: "if a man . . ." and "any man who . . ." (or, "anyone who . . ."). Thus in Mk 10:11 and Mt 5:32 the expressions, which differ in the original Greek texts, are rendered the same in the BJ (*Quiconque . . .*).

22. Thus J. Staudinger, *Die Bergpredigt* (Vienna, 1957) 286, n. 1; F. Neirynck, *Jezuswoorden*, passim.

23. Our quotations are taken from J. Dupont, *Mariage*, 52 (bottom); 65; 144; 69; 144; 68; 147.

24. This is also remarked by B. Schaller, *Die Sprüche*, 244, and by F. Neirynck, *Jezuswoorden*, 135.

Very briefly, here are some other considerations: 1. The instances of Semitic syntax adduced by J. Dupont seem valid in themselves, but there are reasons to wonder whether they are as parallel to our texts as it is claimed. 2. The same observation applies to instances of words which Jesus retains but gives an entirely new meaning. 3. With regard to the concept of divorce, the hypothesis of a double meaning of that concept creates a special difficulty; it supposes that Mk 10:11 suddenly fashions a new concept, which the reader can hardly understand. This difficulty is illustrated by J. Dupont himself. After completing his inquiry on the Matthean clauses, he says in conclusion that divorce is allowed in case of misbehavior. How is the reader supposed to discern that remarriage is not allowed? The author does indeed exclude remarriage because he understands divorce to be, in this case, a simple separation, but the reader is all confused. 4. Although, taken by itself, the expression, "If anyone divorces his wife . . ." in Mk 10:11 lends itself to being read, "Suppose that . . ." does this apply in the same degree to the expression, "Anyone who divorces his wife . . ."?

25. D. Daube, *The New Testament and Rabbinic Judaism* (London, 1956) 141–50.

26. One could go even further and wonder whether in Mk 10:11–12 remarriage is not condemned chiefly in order to bring out all the perversity of divorce itself. In that case, the connection established by Mark between vv. 2–9 and 11–12 would be as follows: Mark wishes to utilize, through the redactional link of v. 10, the two types of material—debate and sayings—which are at his disposal, and believes, in addition, that vv. 11–12 add to the preceding verses a welcome explicitness. They make it clear that, if divorce is already to be disavowed because, among other things, it entitles one to remarriage, a divorce "consummated" by this remarriage is to be disavowed all the more. This is a remarriage which even more explicitly may be labeled adultery. But this adultery is already seminally contained in divorce, which is what Mt 5:32 states: ". . . everyone who divorces his wife . . . forces her to commit adultery."

27. In order to perceive the redactional differences among the various logia relative to divorce, both these and those to be examined below, the following abbreviations may be helpful: M1, the man who divorces his wife; W1, the woman who is being dismissed by M1; M2, the man with whom W1 remarries; W2, the woman with whom M1 remarries.

28. N. Turner, "The Translation of μοιχαται ἐπ' αὐτήν in Mk 10:11," *The Bible Translator* 7 (1965) 151–52.
29. Ἐὰν γυνὴ 'εξηλθη απο (του) αηδρς . . .
30. V. Taylor, *The Gospel according to St. Mark* (London, 1953) 420–21.
31. H. Zimmermann, *Methodenlehre*, 108.
32. Many authors explicitly justify the current reading, for example, J. Dupont, *Mariage*, 61–63; J. A. Fitzmyer, "Divorce Texts," 205, and the authors quoted there, n. 28.
33. J. Alonso Díaz, *Proceso de dignificación de la mujer a través de la Biblia* (Madrid, 1975) 13–14.
34. J. A. Fitzmyer, "Divorce Texts," 205, and the authors quoted, n. 29; also E. Bammel, "Markus 10:11 f.," 263–74.
35. See R. Bultmann, *Geschichte*, 39–56; ET: *History*, 39–54 ("Controversy dialogues"); note, however, Bultmann's severe criticism of the literal accuracy of the debates as recorded in the synoptics.
36. The context shows that Paul addresses himself to Christian spouses. On the importance of Paul's reference to Jesus, see a long discussion in J. Dupont, *Mariage*, 57, n. 1. See also J. K. Elliott, "Paul's Teaching on Marriage in I Corinthians," NTS 19 (1973), 219–25.
37. Ez 1:11; 23.
38. In this case, the Greek has been translated into Aramaic; see R. Le Déaut, in *Biblical Theology Buletin* 4 (1974), 249–51; D. Daube, *New Testament*, 74; 368.
39. We shall see, at least by way of an hypothesis, that this is the case with regard to the Matthean clauses.
40. This clearly appears in what is known as the Pauline Privilege. Paul allows the converted spouse to leave the other, if he or she refuses cohabitation; cf. 1 Cor 7:11; 15–16.
41. See J. Weiss, A. Loisy, B. W. Bacon, C. G. Montefiore, B. H. Branscomb, W. Marxen, J. Schreiber in their discussion of the matter as noted by E. Trocmé, *La formation de l'évangile selon Marc* (Paris, 1963) 115, n. 23. With regard to Mk 10:12, A. Loisy mistakenly believes that it can depend on 1 Cor, see *Les évangiles synoptiques*, 2, 199, n. 1.
42. See among others E. Schillebeeckx, *Jezus* (Bloemendaal, 1974), passim; P. M. Beaude, *Jesus oublié* (Paris, 1977), esp. 49–75; G. Vermès, *Jesus le Juif* (Desclée, 1978).
43. L. Cerfaux, *La théologie de l'Eglise suivant saint Paul* (Paris, 1965), 71–80.
44. See L. Cerfaux, "La tradition selon saint Paul," in *Recueil L. Cerfaux*, 2, 253–63.
45. Note however that the term κτίσις occurs often enough in Paul; he uses the new-creation theme to illustrate the condition of the Christian; see 2 Cor 5:17; Gal 6:15; etc.
46. Here we touch upon a major concern of the ministry of Jesus himself and the very heart of the gospel. First, the relationship of Jesus to Judaism is a sore point for the historian who searches for the Jesus of history. The way in which historians understand that relationship is a watershed between two opposite historiographies. The first and more traditional view presents a Jesus who engaged in direct confrontation with most sacred convictions of the Jews. The second maintains that this confrontation is a misinterpretation fostered by Paul, and transmitted by the evangelists and Christian tradition. The historical Jesus, we are told, was but one of many Jewish reformers. Obviously, we cannot discuss so large an issue here, but we believe that some exegetes go too far when they describe Jesus as "not different" and attribute the break with Judaism and the foundation of Christianity to Paul. From a doctrinal point of view, the stakes are high; if Jesus is not truly responsible for the origin of Christianity, its credentials are no longer very solid. Only a kind of Judeo-Christianity would accord with what Jesus of Nazareth intended.
47. See especially Mk 7:14–23 on the rules of purity, and G. Vermès, *Jésus le Juif*, 35–36.
48. Mt 5:31–32.
49. See above, n. 12.
50. This is precisely the position of Irenaeus, who speaks of the Lord "who exonerates . . . Moses as his faithful servant." See the long quotation in J. Dupont, *Mariage*, 21, n.
51. J. Dupont, *Mariage*, 18–22; See also A. Loisy, *Les évangiles synoptiques*, 2:198 (Jesus "appeals from Moses to Moses").
52. J. Dupont, *Mariage*, 24–27; J. A. Fitzmyer, "Divorce Texts," 216–21.
53. W. E. Bundy, *Jesus and the First Three Gospels: An Introduction to the Synoptic Tradition* (Cambridge, Mass., 1955) 396.

54. J. Dupont, *Mariage*, 23, n. 2.

55. For a presentation of this view, see J. Dupont, *Mariage*, 38–45, and also A. Stock, "Matthean Texts," 29–33.

56. Hence the effort at recovering Jesus' original saying on the part of B. K. Diderichsen, B. M. F. van Iersel, J. H. A. van Tilborg, H. Greeven, all quoted by F. Neirynck, *Jezuswoorden*, 130–36, and of Neirynck himself.

57. This is already evidenced by the expression "church rules" (*Gemeinderegeln*) used in this connection; see R. Bultmann, *Geschichte*, 138–61; ET: *History*, 130–50.

58. The one exception is Mt 19:9. However, we should not forget that v. 9b does exist in an important manuscript tradition, the authenticity of which may well be only slightly probable, yet not entirely impossible; see Dupont, *Mariage*, 51, n. 3. But even if we admit that only Mt 19:9a is authentic, the difficulty thus created against a doubled saying is easily resolved. Often enough, Matthew improves Mark by abridging it. This is even one of the characteristics of his redactional technique. Cf. A. L. Descamps, "Redaction et christologie dans le récit matthéen de la Passion," in M. Didier (ed.), *L'évangile selon Matthieu* (Gembloux, 1972), esp. 363–66.

59. Neirynck, *Jezuswoorden*, 132–33.

60. B. K. Diderichsen favors Lk 16:18, and so does Neirynck. But Diderichsen conjectures that we are dealing here with something entirely different: "A man who, in order to imitate the Christ, has left or dismissed his wife, may not marry another woman." Mark, he maintains, changes this saying by linking it to the debate (Mk 10:2–9). B. M. F. van Iersel favors Mk 10:11 (he regards v. 12 as secondary). But Jesus limited himself to defending the dismissed wife. J. H. A. van Tilborg likewise opts for Mk 10:11, but reconstructs the original form of the saying and has it mean that Jesus forbade a man to dismiss his wife in order to marry another woman. Finally, H. Greeven favors Mt 5:32 (without the clause).

The efforts of Diderichsen, van Iersel, and van Tilborg seem motivated by the desire to solve problems of our time even at the expense of exegesis itself.

61. Neirynck, *Jezuswoorden*, 132; Fitzmyer, "Divorce Texts," 204–05.

62. Dupont, *Mariage*, 66–69.

63. Dupont, *Mariage*, 66–67, and the authors quoted there, especially 67, n. This is due especially to polygamy, which was allowed in Palestinian law; see the citation of Josephus in Dupont, *Mariage*, 67. On polygamy, see the authors quoted in Dupont, *Mariage*, 67, n.3, and also Greeven, et al., TE, 37–39. He concludes that only the milder wording of Mt 5:32 is authentic: "... the man who divorces his wife *dooms her* to commit adultery." This is tantamount to forgetting the very point of the proclamation of Jesus who perhaps pushed his nonconformism as far as calling divorce adultery.

64. By many authors, among them: Fitzmyer, "Divorce Texts," 206, n. 31; Neirynck, *Jezuswoorden*, 129–41; H. Zimmermann, *Methodenlehre*, 105ff., 231f; our option is for the literary dependence of Matthew on Mark; see Bultmann, *Geschichte*, 26, n. 1. On Matthew's process of composition, see Dupont, *Mariage*, 38, n. 2; Descamps, *Rédaction*, 359–415.

65. Thus the silence is rather striking in Matthew 23.

66. This was the dominant tradition for a long time in Israel: R. de Vaux, *Les Institutions de l'Ancien Testament*, 3rd ed. (Paris, 1976) 1, 45–48. See J. Jeremias, *Jérusalem au temps de Jésus* (Paris, 1976) 471–92.

67. In Israel, the lewd conduct of a married woman was severely punished. It is another thing to know whether, in the time of Jesus, the rule of stoning was consistently applied. Jn 8:5 is not sufficient to prove it, even if the pericope be retained by textual criticism (see Crouzel, *L'Eglise primitive face au divorce* (Paris, 1971) 22. The husband's infidelity was punished only if he sinned with a married woman, because he was then considered to have encroached on the right of another. See R. de Vaux, *Institutions*, 1, 62–63.

Among the prophets (Hos 1, etc.) the covenant between Yahweh and his people was sometimes symbolized by marriage; in this context, to sin with a prostitute—who represented idols—also merited the name of adultery. (Jer 5:7; LXX, ἐμοιχόντο). But it does not follow that this view had penetrated the customs or feelings of the common people.

68. It is admitted today that the evangelists reinforced the impression that Jesus ceaselessly moved in the Pharisaic milieu and often in an atmosphere of hostility; they did this to explain better the break of the Church of their day with Judaism. But their emphasis was not a complete distortion of history.

69. Although its evidential value is light, let us note that when Jesus treats the fictitious case of the woman with several husbands, he is talking about a widow, not a divorced woman (Mk 12:18–27 and parallels). Quite different is the case of the woman at the well (Jn 4:17–18), but this is situated in Samaria.

70. In any case, such was the Palestinian custom attested to by Josephus, for example (Crouzel, *Divorce*, 20). On the other hand, it is well known that the Jews of Elephantine (fifth century B.C.) allowed a woman to take the initiative in divorce. See above, n. 33, and P. Grelot, *Documents araméens d'Egypte* (Paris, 1972) 195, 214, 236.

71. See especially Luke, passim (7:37, etc.); Jn 8:3–11. This supposition has force if we consider how constantly Jesus welcomed persons considered of little worth; lepers, insane who were possessed, children, sinners, the poor, Samaritans, women, pagans, and the like. See C. Focant, *La mort de Jésus à la lumière de sa vie et de sa résurrection,* in *La foi et le temps* (1979) 137, etc.

72. On the conclusions concerning its historicity, see p. 96.

73. See Lohmeyer, *Das Evangelium des Matthäus* (Göttingen, 1956) 281, n. 1; Crouzel, *Divorce*, 28.

74. In other words, if Jesus in Matthew is preparing to side with Shammai, whose rigorous doctrine was probably shared by the Pharisees, we cannot understand why there was a controversy between them and Jesus. In fact, the exception mentioned by Matthew in v. 9—whatever its precise meaning—remains so limited that it is practically a total refusal of divorce on Jesus' part. Verse 10 confirms our exegesis; for if Jesus limited himself to the position of Shammai, we would have to suppose his disciples, who answered him by saying that it would be better then not to marry, followed Hillel, which is improbable.

75. Thus Loisy, *Synoptiques*, 2:200: "[Matthew] adds the words 'any cause whatever' with the evident intention of anticipating the addition made to the answer of Jesus 'the case of lewd conduct'. . . ." See Bultmann, *Geschichte*, 159; Neirynck, *Het evangelisch echtscheidingsverbod*, in *Collationes brugenses et gandavenses*, 4 (1958) 44–45.

76. The inversion curiously resembles Mt 15:1–9, compared to Mk 7:1–13. (Loisy, *Synoptiques*, 2:201, n. 3).

77. Let us note here that the substance of Dt 24:1 is found in Jer 3:1.

78. Lohmeyer, *Matthäus*, 282, n. 1.

79. The texts of some authors mentioned here without reference to their publications were duplicated for a colloquium held in Albano in 1977.

80. Others will be found in Loisy, *Synoptiques*, 2:200–201, and in Lohmeyer, *Matthäus*, 280–82. Curiously enough, after the author said (280) that Matthew is "literarily independent" of Mark he constantly interprets him (281–82) as if Matthew had Mark under his eyes and "was correcting" him. In our opinion, this is a good hypothesis.

81. "[Matthew] expressly presents as quotations passages from Genesis, and he gives the second entirely as the word of God, because the passage is in scripture," Loisy, *Synoptiques*, 2:201.

On the interpretation of Gen 1:27, and 2:24 in Judaism, see Pesch, *Markus*, 2:123–24.

82. See the entire section "I. Mark 10:2–12," and n. 3 and n. 11. Recently D. R. Catchpole (quoted in Pesch, *Markus*, 2:124, n. 11a) likewise has decided in favor of the authenticity of this controversy *in vita Jesu*.

83. Mt 5:32 and 19:9 are closely parallel. Although Matthew doubtless thought of 5:32 when writing 19:9, we comment first on 19:9 because this verse concludes a pericope which we obviously should examine after its Marcan parallel. Moreover, the redactor inserted a logion which comes from Mark 10 or Matthew 19 into 5:32.

84. See p. 86.

85. See pp. 89–90.

86. Understood thus, the assertion clashes with the ideas of the Jews, for even when they considered divorce reprehensible, they never considered it as adultery against the divorced wife. Neither would divorce be an adultery against the new wife, but only against her former husband if he had not divorced her. But the precise point of the present words of Jesus is to thus overturn the ideas of the Jews.

On ’ἐπ’ αὐτήν of Mark 10, there is a recent discussion (with N. Turner, P. Katz, B. Schaller) in R. Pesch, *Markus*, 2:125–26.

87. For the bibliography on the exception clause, see Dupont, *Mariage* (numerous indications up to 1959); P. Hoffman, *Parole de Jesus à propose du divorce*, in *Concilium*, n. 55 (1970): 49–62 (with a bibliographic list); L. Ramaroson, *Une nouvelle interprétation de la clausule de Mt 19:9*, in SE 23 (1971) 247–51;

H. Crouzel, *Divorce*, 11–18 (list); L. Sabourin, "The Divorce Clauses," (Mt 5:32; 19:9) BTB 2 (1972) 80–86; BTB 4 (1974) 346–48.

88. BJ, 1956 ed., 1314, n. h. Dupont, *Mariage*, 96–98 cites the following in favor of the preteritive sense for Mt 19:9: Th. Zahn, P. Dausch, W. Lauck, P. J. Arendzen, P. Benoit, E. Lohmeyer, P. Vawter.

89. See Dupont, *Mariage*, 98–99; he quotes numerous exegetes on Mt 19:9.

90. "The exception clause . . . is grammatically attached to the first subjunctive, 'if he divorces,' which it qualifies parenthetically. But the parenthesis is elliptical, it has no verb; . . . it is necessary to supply the verb 'divorce'. . . . By supplying all the terms implied, we have: 'If anyone divorces his wife, [if] this is not for lewd conduct [that he divorces her] . . .'" Dupont, *Mariage*, 102.

The correct translation of the Vulgate *"nisi ob fornicationem,"* preserved in the Neo-Vulgate, undoubtedly reflects a keen sensitivity to the Greek which is particularly striking because, for the author of the ancient Vulgate, it could only create or heighten a problem in ecclesiastical discipline, in view of its divergence from the absolute assertions of Mark, Luke and Paul.

91. According to some (see B. J. Malina, "Does πορνεία Mean *Fornication?* NT 14 (1972) 10–17, the Greek term could even have as wide a meaning as immodesty. In the present context one would expect μοιχεία.

92. Let us recall that in the Jewish milieu a husband cannot be called adulterous against his own wife. (Pesch, *Markus*, 2:125).

93. Bonsirven, *Divorce*, especially 7–24.

94. See the numerous authors cited by Dupont, *Mariage*, 107, n. More recently, J. Alonso Diaz, *Proceso*, 14.

95. Thus in Acts 15:20, 29; 21:25 (Dupont, *Mariage*, 111).

96. Fitzmyer, *Divorce Texts*, 213–21.

97. Dupont, *Mariage*, 114. It must be noted, however, that as competent an author as R. LeDéaut has recently suggested that the research ought to be continued on the pertinence of recourse to *zenuth*.

98. It is well known that some Greek tests, such as Mk 10:11 and parallels, often used καί to express purpose (semitism): "he who divorces his wife in order to marry another [the former only] commits adultery." In the ancient Church, "separation was forbidden because it led to adultery" (A. Houssiau, "Le lien conjugal dans l'Eglise ancienne," AC 17 (1973) 571. See Crouzel, *Divorce*, passim.

99. Dupont, *Mariage*, 115–22.

100. Dupont, *Mariage*, 136–57. For the ancient Greek fathers who considered that "Matthew's exception applied only to separation and never to remarriage," see Houssiau, "Le lien conjugal," 570.

101. Dupont, *Mariage*, 147–50.

102. Dupont, *Mariage*, 141–56. One can even suggest that although simple separation was juridically inconsistent for the Jews, it was perhaps less so in reality, for a husband who divorced his wife need not *de facto* remarry, although he had the right to do so; see p. 89.

103. *Mand.* IV, 1, 6–8; explanations in Dupont, *Mariage*, 153; commentary in Crouzel, *Divorce*, 44–53. As a matter of fact, the ancients and the moderns who favor simple separation generally attribute both the concept and the exception clause itself to Jesus. They do not speak of a redactor nor of a Helleno-Christian milieu as affecting the clause. To suppose that Jesus had admitted simple separation in the case of the lewd conduct of the wife is not impossible in itself. But such a conjecture depends upon a casuistry foreign to Jesus. And casuistry there would be with double force since the hypothesis appeals not only to particular cases but also to a concept, that of simple separation, that is, to say the least, rather foreign to a Jewish milieu. Besides, the conjecture neglects literary analysis, that is, the evidence of the adventitious character of the inserted clause, such as we are going to show *sub* b. Moreover, one can no longer uphold the probability of a Proto-Matthew or Aramaic Matthew very close to the time of the discourse of Jesus in the face of such literary analysis.

104. Dupont, *Mariage*, 125, which has reference to numerous authors. The ancient Protestants and also in general the Greeks attributed the exception to Jesus himself. Again, to suppose that Jesus had permitted the deceived husband to remarry is not absolutely impossible in itself. But it would scarcely be in the style of the Master. The latter has emphasized the radicalism of his requirements, and these are little compatible with the precise exceptions in regard to principles. And then there is the evidence of literary analy-

sis that we are going to show. Thus contemporary authors who have abandoned Jerome's exegesis refuse (with rare exceptions—see the quotation made by Dupont, *Mariage*, 129, n. 1.) to attribute to Jesus the clause understood as permission to remarry in case of the lewd conduct of his wife.

On the whole, the presence of the inserted clause *in ore Jesu* appears then to be excluded and in any case, unprovable.

105. Descamps, "Essai d'interprétation de Mt 5:17–48" (Berlin, 1959), 165–66.
106. See the majority of the authors cited in n. 26.
107. Dupont, *Mariage*, 147.
108. "Taken in themselves and without prejudice, Matthew's texts seem to permit complete divorce in case of adultery" (J. Thomas, *Droit naturel*, 635). The author does not accept Jerome's interpretation; such was also the opinion of G. Pouget, cited in Dupont, *Mariage*, 126, n. 2.
109. Loisy, *Synoptiques*, 1:580. W. D. Davies, *The Setting of the Sermon on the Mount* (Cambridge, 1966), 387, considers the exception clause as a sort of Christian gemara (an explanation or application) common in Matthew. Let us also observe that if Jesus had delivered the clause, its absence from Mark and Paul would be very difficult to explain.
110. R. Schnackenburg, *Die sittliche Botschaft des Neuen Testaments* (Munich, 1954), 91.
111. See Neirynck, *Echtscheidingsverbod*, 44–46. What was said above on the grammatical analysis of the exception clause evidently remains valid.
112. One could also conjecture that Matthew attributed to Jesus, whom he deliberately placed in a unique moment of history (*unwiederholbar*), an accommodation to Jewish customs which he considered outdated in the Church. Such an explanation is purely redactional and leaves out any ecclesial *sitz-im-leben*. On the general idea of such a *historisierung* in Matthew, see G. Strecker, *Der Weg der Gerechtigkeit, Untersuchung zur Theologies des Matthäus*, 3rd ed. (Göttingen, 1971); R. Walker, *Die Heilsgeschichte in ersten Evangelium* (Göttinger, 1967). In a contrary sense, (*enthistorisierung*), see H. Frankemölle, *Jahwebund und Kirche Christi, Studien zur Form und Traditionsgeschichte des Evangeliums nach Matthäus* (Münster, 1974).
113. The hiatus is confirmed by the fact that after Matthew used αἰτία in 19:3, with the meaning of *motive*, he used it with the entirely different meaning of *state of things* or *condition* in 19:10.
114. Article λέγω in TWNT 4:108. Other authors sharing this opinion are listed by Dupont who himself favors this solution in *Mariage*, 170–74.
115. It does not at all follow that, in itself, Mt 19:10–12 is not pre-Matthean and indeed an exact citation of a saying of Jesus from a different occasion. This idea of a "lost context" (T. W. Manson and others: discussed in Dupont, *Mariage*, 164–66) seems valid to us. It is reinforced by the fact that Mt 19:10–12 has no parallel in either Mark or Luke. The word *eunuch*, characteristic of v. 12, is nowhere else found in the gospels, nor in the New Testament except for Acts 8:27–39, where it designates a function.
116. Dupont, *Mariage*, 45–46. Our various observations on the redactional activity have not injured the substantial authenticity of the antitheses *in ore Jesus*. Indeed, they seem to echo the oral style of Jesus. It is not difficult to imagine the master saying with the tone of the prophets: "It has been said to you . . . but I, on the contrary, tell you. . . ." The problem is that the exception clause in Mt 5:32 breaks the oratorical thrust of the prophet with the qualification of a casuist. That is why strict authenticity can scarcely be extended to the clause, any more than it can to Mt 19:9. But in Mt 5:31–32, Matthew inserts a substantially authentic logion which he uses elsewhere; see Mk 10 and Mt 19.
117. Adultery is not yet committed at the time of the divorce (Dupont, *Mariage*, 74, n.). It does not seem that the fact of separation constitutes her adulterous.
118. This time the expression implied (M2 is adulterous toward W1) is not in itself contradictory in the eyes of a Jew for whom, on the contrary, such an eventuality would be normal if there had been no divorce; but as this is presupposed by the evangelist, his teaching on adultery thus becomes provocative.
119. Dupont, *Mariage*, 103–04.
120. What should be added here is that the λογος πορνείας is perhaps a close imitation (through the intermediary of Judaism: Moore) of the Hebrew expression *ervat dabor* of Dt 24:1; it is possible, although the LXX was translated ἀσχήμον πραγμα. We will not settle it, but this eventuality changes nothing of the meaning of Mt 5:32 with reference to Mt 19:9. Nevertheless, if the hypothesis is correct, it confirms the contact with Dt 24:1 and therefore the importance of divorce as the precise theme of our texts. (See Dupont,

Mariage, 87, n.1; Crouzel, *Divorce,* 23–29, n. 49.) On the whole, one may then read with the Vulgate and the Neovulgate: *excepta fornicationis causa.*

121. See Loisy, *Synoptiques,* 1:577–80.

122. The repeated mentioning of an adultery not followed by a stoning raises a number of problems; see Dupont, *Mariage,* 105.

123. In 19:9 Matthew thought he had to safeguard the right of the husband to divorce and probably also to remarry, in the case of lewd conduct of the woman; in the same case he has, in 5:32a, allowed divorce and freed the husband from all responsibility towards the new adultery which his wife will commit. But in speaking of another man marrying a divorced woman (5:32b), he does not seem to have distinguished between innocent and guilty women.

124. Dupont, *Mariage,* 46–48.

125. After μοιχεύει "M1 commits adultery" it is necessary to supply in 18a "against W1," which is quite contrary to Jewish thought.

126. Until now, we had touched the question of historicity only with respect to the clause.

127. M. Devisch, *La relation entre Marc et Q,* 59–91.

128. See p. 89. See also Neiryunk, *Doubets in Mark* (Louvain, 1972) passim.

129. Thus also Loisy, *Synoptiques,* 2:199; Neirynck, *Jezuswoorden,* 136; B. K. Diderichsen, *Den skilsmisseperikope,* 31–50; however, this last author understands the word quite otherwise (see above, n. 2 and n. 6). For his part, Greeven retains Mt 5:32 (without the clause) as the original form (see Neirynck, *Jezuswoorden,* 131).

130. The consensus on this second point is smaller if we take into account, for example, the opinion of Dupont, discussed above, according to which Jesus does not condemn divorce but only remarriage.

131. Cf. 1 Cor 9:14; 1 Thes 4:15, and *ad rem:* H. von Campenhausen, *Die Begründung kirchlicher Entscheidungen beim Apostel Paulus* (Heidelberg, 1957), 21–22. For Paul, the precepts of Jesus remain those of the glorified Christ. Thus also F. Hahn, *Christologische Hoheitstitel* (Göttingen, 1974), 93. In this sense, the precepts of Jesus are then supra-historical: H. Conzelmann, *Der erste Brief an die Korinther* (Göttingen, 1969), 44.

Another possibility to consider: not only does Paul *think* that the word of 1 Cor 7:10 comes from the terrestrial Jesus, but he was right; this is, for example, the conviction of F. Hahn, *Hoheitstitel,* 92.

132. On χωρίσθεναι, see Dupont, *Mariage,* 142, n; Conzelmann, *Korinther,* 143, n. 5.

133. This is also the view of Conzelmann, *Korinther,* 144.

134. This is also the view of Conzelmann, *Korinther,* 142 (*sie soll unverheiratet bleiben*); J. Héring, *La première epître de saint Paul aux Corinthiens* (Neuchâtel, 1959), 52: "I enjoin her to live without remarrying, or to become reconciled to her husband."

135. Let us repeat that there are grounds, although not conclusive, for reading even the clause of Matthew in terms of this simple separation, as St. Jerome and others do. Moreover, does not 1 Cor 7:11 give us reason to admit that, even in Mark 10:2–12, Jesus condemned not the act of divorce, but only remarriage? We think not. Mark may have remembered that the horizon of Jesus was Jewish, whereas Paul is thinking principally of converts from paganism.

136. When Paul writes "the man may not divorce his wife," does he mean that dismissal is forbidden in itself, or does he imply that divorce is forbidden because normally it ends in remarriage, which is certainly a sin? The first interpretation seems to be the obvious one.

137. On 1 Cor 7:12–16 (mixed marriages), see. "Conclusions," 3a. For now let us limit ourselves to speaking of the words of Paul which comment on the teaching of Jesus, since the master's horizon did not include the case of mixed marriages.

138. "Jesus pronounces an unconditional and absolute condemnation of divorce" (J. Dupont, *Mariage,* 75). According to the author it is a question of remarriage, that is, of "complete divorce." Let us recall that recourse to this last expression (cf. for example, J. Thomas, *Droit naturel,* 635) itself shows the ambiguity of the word *divorce,* which we have therefore completely avoided in this essay.

139. We must except B. M. F. van Iersel and J. H. A. van Tilborg, in T. A. G. van Eupen (ed.), *On ontbindbaarheid,* 19, and 26–28. See Neirynck, *Jezuswoorden,* 130–32.

140. "Nowhere does Jesus say: 'Divorce is forbidden.' Jesus does make a value judgment of the act itself...." (Dupont, *Mariage*, 144). However, "it is clear that Jesus does not wish to define the juridical status of bodily separation nor to formally authorize it." (68, n. 2)

141. Although the distinction is not really relevant to this context, it is useful to recall that the real life of Jesus was "much more varied and richer in content" than what is known from history; "the historical Jesus (that is, accessible to the historian) remains poorer than . . . the terrestrial Jesus." (A. Schilson–W. Kasper, *Théologiens du Christ aujourd'hui* [Desclée, 1978] 31).

142. It hardly need be said that our philosophical anthropology does not correspond exactly to the order of creation to which Jesus refers.

143. Delimiting the scope of the historian's competence belongs in the commentary above. In some passages we did treat it, but for clarity we will summarize our remarks here.

144. Some clear examples are Mt 21:27 and parallels.

145. Besides, we often read "that in Israel, as in Mesopotamia, marriage is a purely civil act and is not sanctioned by any religious act" (de Vaux, *Institutions*, 1, 58). These statements can be understood by comparison with Christian marriage, but taken literally, they are misleading. In a sense, nothing is purely civil in the milieu in which Jesus lived. Moreover, some texts, such as Tb 6:18, 7:11 show that marriage can be perceived as a divine blessing, calling for a feeling of thanksgiving and a prayer of petition. Although only the Vulgate version of Tb 7:15 reads "*Deus Abraham . . . conjungat vos*" (the source of the introit of the nuptial mass), it remains true that Tb develops a notion of marriage which is "Christian before its time" (BJ, 494).

146. One might say that, in the question of indissolubility, Jesus is concerned—as he is so often—about intentions, interiority, the duty of each one to assume responsibility for his acts (Mt 5:32; see also above, n. 37), and to practice a loyalty that the institution cannot always respond to. In this sense, the point of view of Jesus is that of the moralist rather than the founder of a "social order." See B. Rigaux, *Le radicalisme du Règne*, in J. Dupont (ed.), *La pauvreté évangélique* (Paris, 1971), 135–73.

147. Bultmann treats the question of how Jesus unified his eschatological preaching and his moral message at the core of his being (*Theologie des Neuen Testaments*, 2nd ed. [Tübingen, 1954], 18–21). But it is immense; to resolve it clearly is to understand the historical Jesus perfectly.

148. In a sense, tradition and the magisterium have always sought to make revelation relevant, which is a fundamental concern of contemporary hermeneutics. But this raises new problems by placing the accent more on the present than on the past, and by emphasizing the fact that all established language, even sacred, is culturally conditioned and therefore relative.

149. See above, n. 80.

150. M. Goguel, *Les premiers temps de l'Eglise* (Neuchatel-Paris, 1949), 18–19. "It was in a hellenistic milieu that Christianity had its principal development; the only one which ended in something durable." (Ibid., 39) Coming from a Protestant exegete, such remarks have a particular resonance.

Could one not apply these considerations to the oath about which one may justly raise questions in the light of Mt 5:32? If Jesus was opposed to every form of oath (Mt 5:33–37), the Church has acted otherwise and, in doing so, she surely did not feel unfaithful to her Lord. See also p. 93, n. 51, on *historisierung*.

151. The expression is not ours, but that of E. Schillebeeckx, *Gerechtigheid en liefde* (Bruges, 1977), 6.

152. *To decide* could never mean *that the Church define de fide* a particular interpretation of the Matthean incidental clause, since the exegetes remain hopelessly divided in their field.

153. The case of mixed marriage, absent from the horizon of Jesus, emerges, as we said, in the apostolic Church.

154. Does Paul believe that the Christian party who leaves a pagan or Jewish partner may remarry? Ambrosiaster thinks he can, but Augustine denies it and his opinion could perhaps be founded on 1 Cor 7:17–24 (each would do well to remain in his condition), 1 Cor 7:29–31 (time is short), 1 Cor 7:39–40 (death puts an end to marriage; however, the Christian widow can remarry but only with a Christian, but she will be happier, in my opinion, if she remains as she is.)

155. A number of exegetes think that here Paul permits a new marriage; for example, Conzelmann, *Korinther*, 149; Héring, *Corinthiens*, 54; Baltensweiler, *Die Ehe*, 192–93.

156. Paul has a clear concept of the universal Church, but lacks the perspective of duration.

157. The opening words of 7:1, "I come now to what you have written to me," show that Paul turns to another series of questions. This series takes up an entire chapter (7:1–40). It begins with a careful catalogue of various kinds of situations probably set forth more completely than in the query of the Corinthians, and it reveals concern of a pastor to distinguish different types of cases. Let us add that 1 Cor. 7:12–17 is "relatively" long and lively and that the end speaks for itself: "such is my teaching in all the Churches."

158. Let us recall the famous passage Eph. 5:22–23 which is even for those who do not admit the full authenticity of the epistle at least indirectly Pauline. Cf. 1 Tm 3:2–7.

159. See p. 90.

160. See "Conclusions," 2.

161. It follows that this teaching is normative, although it is not uniformly expressed. An intelligent hermeneutic of both the apostles and Jesus must be governed by the historically established tenor of their teachings, and also by the importance which these have in the very thought of the apostles and Jesus. This second insight is also grounded on exegesis, as we have already said.

162. The ancient Church regarded this teaching not as "an exceptional ideal" but as "the order of creation" relevant to all men. However, "this radicalism goes hand in hand with a great understanding of existing situations." (Houssiau, *Le lien conjugal*, 577). The problem involved is whether the gospel is to be viewed as a new law or as an ideal (*zielgebot*); this question has been treated especially by Protestants, often with reference to the Sermon on the Mount. See F. Montagnini, *Aspetti indicativi e aspetti precettivi della legge evangelica*, in *Paolo VI, predicatore del Concilio* (Brescia, 1967), 349–58 for an overview of different theories, borrowed from J. Jeremias.

163. For this reason, the Church, according to present discipline, does not claim that it has the right to touch the marriage of the nonbaptized.

164. Loisy, *Synoptiques*, 1:579–80.

165. We write, "for Matthew" without forgetting that the thought of Matthew on the link between marriage and celibacy is not considered in the same light by all exegetes. On the Anglican hermeneutics of marriage, see V. Taylor, *Mark*, 421.

166. "Confrontation of the sources of the faith and the experience of Christian spouses," in V. Boulanger et al., *Mariage: rêve-réalité. Essai théologique,* Montréal, 1975; "Survey of theologians on matrimonial procedures and pastoral care," in P. Hayoit, "Les procédures matrimoniales et la théologie du mariage," RTL 9 (1978): 33–58.

167. In closing let us touch on two questions which come more from hermeneutics than exegesis.

1) The moment of the completion of marriage. The texts of the New Testament are silent on this subject. The exegete can refer to the Jewish usage. The idea of a contract—if not always a written document—was a part of the betrothal rite (when the dowry was given and the penalty agreed upon in case the contract were voided). The idea of contract, in another sense, also regulated the act of divorce, and *a fortiori* the marriage ceremony. The marriage was celebrated by festivities which lasted several days and it was consummated on the first night of this festive time. These observations, which one could surely illustrate by parallels in other cultures, involve some kind of multiplicity—at least a duality—of moments (cf. *sunoikeo* in Dt 24:1) which no doubt survives in the canonical distinction *ratum—consummatum*.

2) The distinction between indissolubility intrinsic (the conjugal bond unbreakable by the couple) and extrinsic (the bond unbreakable by competent social authority). Again, our texts are silent, but the exegete can recall that for the Jews, divorce broke the conjugal bond on the initiative of the husband alone, with no intervention from any authority. In forbidding divorce, and in any case, remarriage, Jesus then wishes explicitly to oppose all divorce and all remarriage on the part of the husband and implicitly on the part of the wife. By claiming the right to dissolve certain marriages, the Church faced new problems on which Jesus left no teaching and which it had no wish to ignore. But Paul had given the example of such dissolution. That is, perhaps he gave it, in the eyes of the exegetes who believe—in opposition to others—that Paul permits the Christian party who is persecuted by the pagan party to remarry. We must rely on this faculty of dissolution, we think, to justify Paul and the Church, and not on texts concerning the power of the keys. In these texts, *to bind and to loose* do not apply to power over the conjugal bond save perhaps virtually or remotely.

6

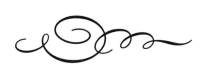

The New Testament Moral Teaching on Marriage

Edward Schillebeeckx

The Absolute Indissolubility of Marriage

The difference between the patristic view of the indissolubility of marriage and the view which came into prominence in the church in the twelfth and thirteenth centuries may be briefly summarised as follows. According to the church Fathers, marriage as a *sacramentum* in the older sense of a "life commitment" or an "oath of fidelity" was something that *might not* be dissolved, since it involved a personal commission to live married life in such a way that the bond of marriage was not broken. The indissolubility of marriage was a task which had to be realized personally. According to the later, scholastic concept of the *sacramentum,* on the other hand—a concept developed in the twelfth and thirteenth centuries especially from the idea of ontological participation in the covenant between Christ and his church—marriage was seen as something that *could not* be dissolved. There was in marriage an objective bond which—once made—was exempt from any action or interference on the part of man. These two visions—the patristic view of marriage as a moral obligation and the scholastic view of marriage as an ontological bond—are not mutually exclusive, but rather mutually implicit. Both the patristic and the scholastic doctrines are firmly based on Scripture. Since the Catholic Church at present both defends and practises these two complementary views of marriage, it is important to ascertain precisely what this biblical point of view is. It is even more important when we remember that Catholic recognition of the sacramental aspect of marriage is intimately related to Catholic affirmation of the indissolubility of marriage.

Jesus' Statement

Christ's statement on the indissolubility of monogamous marriage was absolute in an unprecedented way:

And Pharisees came up to him and tested him by asking, "Is it lawful to divorce one's wife for any cause?" He answered, "Have you not read that he [the Creator] who made them from the beginning made them male and female, and [the Creator] said, 'For this reason a man shall leave his father and mother and be joined to his wife, and the two shall become one'? So they are no longer two but one. What therefore God has joined together, let no man put asunder."

They said to him, "Why then did Moses command one to give a certificate of divorce and to put her away?" He said to them, "For your hardness of heart Moses allowed you to divorce your wives, but from the beginning it was not so." [Mt xix. 1–8.]¹

Therefore: "Whoever divorces his wife and marries another, commits adultery against her" (Mk x. 11–12)²; and "he who marries a woman divorced from her husband commits adultery" (Lk xvi. 18). In none of these texts is there any mention of an exception. Christ—and, following his teaching, the early apostolic church—allowed no scope whatever for divorce. This was in complete contrast to the teaching of the Old Testament and in express opposition to the Law of Moses. (Deut xxiv. 1–4; see Mt v. 31; xix. 7.) It also ran directly against the practice of the whole ancient world. We have already seen that in Jesus' time there was both a strict and a more lenient interpretation of the deuteronomic law, and both allowed a man to put his wife away if he had discovered "some indecency" in her. The school of Rabbi Shammai regarded adultery and moral misconduct as the only acceptable grounds for divorce; but the school of Rabbi Hillel held that all kinds of reasons, even quite trivial ones, were sufficient grounds for legal divorce, and it was this second interpretation of the law which was in fact practised. The Pharisees wanted to force Christ to choose between these two schools so that on the basis of his answer they could accuse him either of laxity or of shortsighted and narrow rigorism, and thus inflame the people against him, the leading question being: "Is it lawful to divorce one's wife *for any cause?* (Mt xix. 3). But Christ overrode the views of both schools by referring to the great marriage charter of Genesis. Marriage was indissoluble and there was no legal ground for divorce whatever; in view of the fact that marriage had been brought about by God himself, it could not be dissolved by any secular authority. "In the beginning it was not so," that is, in the beginning divorce was not permitted—Jesus was referring here to the initial phase of man's history or at least to the time before the Mosaic law. In any case, the essential meaning of this phrase is that God did not have this as his original intention when he established the institution of marriage by his creation of mankind as man and woman.

Certainly Christ's aim was not to make some kind of social statement concerning the question as to whether divorce was known or unknown in the history of man before the Mosaic period. In any case, what he asserted was that the essential indissolubility of marriage was far from being something totally new, arising only from the eschatological redemption, but on the contrary had its roots in the human essence of marriage itself as called into existence by the Creator who from the very beginning had been the God of salvation. Jesus asserted the will of the Creator as against the law of Moses.

One conclusion and one only can be drawn from these four quoted passages in Scripture: the bond of marriage cannot be dissolved by divorce. There are, however, two texts, both to be found only in Matthew's gospel, which would appear, at least at first sight, to constitute an exception to this. The first is: "And I say to you: whoever divorces his wife, *except for unchastity,* and marries another, commits adultery" (xix. 9); and the second is: "But I say to you that every one who divorces his wife, *except on the ground of unchastity,* makes her an adulteress; and whoever marries a divorced woman commits adultery" (v. 32). It would be almost impossible to estimate how much has been written about these verses in Matthew from the time of the Fathers until the present day. Does Matthew in fact claim that full divorce is permissible for Christians after one of the partners in marriage has committed adultery?

One of the points of difference between the Catholic and the Reformed Churches is the divergent interpretation of this text. Although it is not possible to speak of a clear consensus among the Reformed Churches, in general Protestant exegetes do tend to regard these two texts as saving clauses. In the non-Uniate Eastern Churches, too, remarriage after adultery committed by the other party is permitted. This does not mean, however, that adultery is regarded by any Christians as sufficient grounds for divorce. In any case of upset or disharmony in Christian marriage the Reformed Churches also maintain that "the only solution which is legitimate within the kingdom of God is a mutual return to God's order."[3] Divorce is therefore never recommended. But there are, for the Reformed Churches, some situations in which divorce with permission to remarry is the only practical solution: "There are no grounds for divorce for Christians, only situations in which divorce is inevitable."[4]

As we shall see, the Council of Trent firmly opposed any such interpretation, although its condemnation was—for historical reasons—expressed indirectly. The Catholic Church refuses to accept any grounds whatsoever for divorce in the case of sacramental and consummated marriage. All that the Council of Trent did was to confirm a long tradition in the church—that Matthew was speaking only of judicial separation "from bed and board," without any possibility of remarriage.[5]

In the middle of the second century Hermas referred to a practice in the church characteristic of the whole period before the first Council of Nicea: the husband had to repudiate his wife if she committed adultery and persisted in it, but he was not permitted to remarry; moreover, he was guilty of sinful conduct if he refused to take his wife back again on her repentance.[6] Hermas also added to this that the same was applicable both to the wife and to the husband, although if adultery was committed by the husband the wife was not obliged to send him away.[7] Apart from the obligation to send the guilty party away, it would appear that, according to the practice of the subapostolic and the ancient church, a straightforward breach between the partners in marriage did not give the innocent party the right to remarriage, even if the other party was guilty of grave misconduct. This practice was in accordance with what Paul himself, appealing to Christ's *logion,* advocated as a duty for the Christians of Corinth: "To the married I give charge, not I but the Lord, that the wife should not separate from her husband (*but if she does,* let her remain single or else be reconciled to her husband)—and that the husband should not divorce his wife" (1 Cor vii. 10–11). Remarriage was not permitted in the apostolic church, no matter what reasons were given for the separation. The *Decretum pro Armeniis* of the Ecumenical Council of Florence was later to call this a separation "from bed and board" (from the *torus*).[8] No other line has in fact ever been followed in ecclesiastical legal practice. There have been very few dissentient opinions.[9]

This apostolic and subapostolic practice gives us clear evidence that the two texts in Matthew were not understood as constituting an exception to the indissolubility of marriage. It is therefore clear that, despite the difficulty presented by these texts, the apostolic church concluded from Christ's *logion* that marriage was absolutely indissoluble, and this made it difficult to interpret the Matthaean texts as a saving clause. This extrinsic reasoning is moreover reinforced by an analysis of the texts themselves.

In the first place, there is some evidence to indicate that the two texts, which are peculiar to Matthew, are secondary. This does not mean that they are later interpolations, as some exegetes have claimed,[10] but rather that Matthew brought Christ's original *logion*—as reproduced in Mark and Luke—up to date in view of a definite problem existing in the Jewish Christian communities. The clause in Mt v. 32 is completely absent from the text of Lk xvi. 18, which gives Christ's *logion* in a more original form, and the interpolation in Mt xix. 9 is also lacking in the earlier text of Mk x. 11.[11] We are, then, fully justified in assuming that the clause does not go back to Christ himself; but this does not mean that Matthew introduced into the church an exception to something concerning which Christ himself had made an unqualified pronouncement.

Some modern exegetes have looked for a solution in the real meaning of the word *porneia* (unchastity). *Porneia,* as a translation of the Hebrew word *zenûth,* may mean not only adultery on the part of the wife,[12] or unnatural sexual intercourse, or even the marriage of an Israelite and a pagan, but also marriage which conflicted with the conditions laid down by Leviticus (Lev xviii. 1–20), or even with the rabbinical definitions of the law. All these were called "unchastity." On a basis of the various possible meanings of *porneia*, J. Bonsirven[13] reached the following solution. If the Matthaean texts are considered in connection with Acts xv. 20, 29 and xxi. 25, in which Christians are required by the apostolic synod to refrain from all "unchastity," then the *porneia* in Matthew ought to mean marriage in conflict with the Jewish definitions of the law—for example, a marriage within one of the degrees of consanguinity recognised by the Jews. Matthew wrote his gospel principally for Christians who had been converted from Judaism in Palestine and Syria, and not for converts from the Gentile world. The Jews who became Christians continued to follow the Jewish laws of marriage, while the Gentiles who were converted to Christianity kept the Greco-Roman laws of marriage. This inevitably led to a conflict, which the first council of the apostolic church solved by means of a compromise—Christians from the Gentile world were not bound by the Jewish laws, but they were subject, for the sake of peace, to the Jewish laws relating to *porneia*.

Porneia, then, was a marriage that was null and void according to the Jewish law, and thus also according to the canon law of the primitive church following the apostolic decision of Acts xv. 20–29. Consequently Matthew did not envisage any exception to the absolute ban on divorce, but only said (in parenthesis, as it were) that a marriage which was validly contracted in accordance with the Greco-Roman laws, but which was in conflict with the prevailing Jewish impediments to marriage, was henceforth to be regarded as concubinage as far as Christians as well as Jews were concerned. In such a case a Christian was bound to repudiate his wife, since she was not really his wife at all. There was absolutely no question of divorce on grounds of adultery. This, he holds, is confirmed by 1 Cor v. 1, which clearly refers to a transgression of the marriage law as stated in Lev xviii. 8, the very law which was enforced by "canon law" in the apostolic decree (Acts xv. 28).[14] *Porneia*, then, included all the various associations listed in Lev xviii.

This interpretation of the word *porneia* would appear to be generally accepted by exegetes. It does not, however, necessarily follow that the word was used in this wide sense in Mt xix. 9 and v. 32, since, if this were the case, the passages would be virtually meaningless. In any case J. Dupont has clearly demonstrated that the interpolation "except on the ground of unchastity" did not in the context relate to *de facto* invalid or illegal marriage, but was clearly connected with the saving clause in Deut xxiv. 1. This connection is apparent from the strikingly Semitic phrase in Mt v. 32, *parektos logou porneias*, which was obviously intended to be a literal translation of the technical term used in Deut xxiv. 1, namely, *'erewēth dābhār*. It is also clear that the entire context of Mt xix. 9 was dominated by the heated controversy that was raging in Jesus' time between the school of Rabbi Hillel and that of Rabbi Shammai.[15] And so the conclusion which emerges is that *porneia* referred to those cases of fornication or unchastity for which divorce was permitted according to the school of Shammai (i.e., adultery or moral misconduct on the part of the wife).

Several other interpretations have been suggested in recent years. Dupont has continued in the direction of Jerome, but has presented this view in a new way. According to Dupont, *porneia*, on grounds of which the husband was permitted to repudiate his wife, does not mean the "unchastity" that the husband might commit by contracting an illegal marriage (as Bonsirven claims), but the unchastity of which his wife had made herself guilty. In such a case the wife was repudiated according to Jewish custom, but the separated husband continued to live in continence for the sake of the kingdom of God.[16]

Another interpretation has been advanced by Hulsbosch.[17] Like Dupont, he accepts the traditional view that *porneia* refers here to adultery. Jesus, however, did not intend in this case to make a pronouncement as to whether divorce was permitted or not. He wanted rather to show who was in fact the guilty party in this case of putting asunder what God had joined together. His aim was to point out that a *de facto* separation did not change in any way the divine plan of marriage. What violated the unity of marriage was not divorce, but intercourse with a third party—in other words, adultery. According to Hulsbosch, therefore, the meaning of the two texts is this: "Whoever repudiates his wife, except in the case of misconduct, and marries another with whom he has intercourse, disrupts the unity with his first wife that was decreed by God. The addition: 'except in the case of misconduct,' is important, because in such a case of misconduct this unity has already been destroyed and the statement is not applicable to this particular case."[18]

This is certainly in accordance with Mt v. 32, which says that "whoever repudiates his wife, except in the case of misconduct, is the *cause* of her committing adultery." In the case of repudiation because of adultery, it is clear that the wife is herself the cause of the breach in the marriage. From the context it was clearly Jesus' aim to find out who was really the guilty party in an unsuccessful marriage—if the wife had not committed adultery, and her husband nonetheless repudiated her, then he was really guilty of his wife's subsequent sin with a third party. Jesus' intention, then, was to teach men the essential meaning of adultery, and in the case of misconduct this statement no longer has any meaning, since it is clear that the marriage is already violated. This view provides an adequate interpretation of Mt v. 32, since this text makes no mention of the husband's remarrying or not remarrying after repudiating his wife. It does, however, run into difficulties with Mt xix. 9, as this text refers clearly not only to the moral and religious breach of marriage, but also to the legal consequences—whether such a person was or was not permitted to marry again. This was a question that was immediately raised by the Jewish notion of "repudiation," and it is clear from the whole context that it was included in the problem.

Other modern exegetes have shown that the Greek words translated—in the RSV and in the AV/Douai respectively—as "except on the ground of" or "saving [excepting] for the cause of" (Mt v. 32) and "except for" or "except it be for" (xix. 9) do not, in this context, have any limiting meaning. In other words, the passage in Mt xix. 9 means: "Whoever repudiates his wife—this is not permissible even because of adultery or unchastity—and marries another . . ." In Mt v. 32 the word *parektos,* though normally used in an exclusive sense, has an inclusive sense, so that the text means: "Even in the case of a husband repudiating his wife because of adultery, she is driven even further into sin."[19] According to this view, Matthew must have wished to impress even more upon his Jewish readers that adultery was no reason for divorce. This interpretation is in no sense normal, though it is to some extent plausible from the philological point of view. It may not be possible to accept it on its own, but it is in any case clear enough from the preceding passage in Mt xix. 1–8 that in this respect Christ completely did away with the law of Moses.

Let us bring together all the elements which the various interpretations have established beyond dispute. First, exegetically the clause is of secondary importance. The interpolation has its original setting in a particular society, and—in view of the fact that it occurs only, and twice, in Matthew—this setting is to be found within the Matthew tradition, i.e., in Jewish Christian circles. The Greek words of the clause as it appears in Mt v. 32, *parektos logou porneias,* would seem to be a literal allusion to Deut xxiv. 1, which refers to divorce on grounds of "some indecency." In view of all this, and especially of the fact that Matthew was writing for Jewish Christians, it seems clear that he was not thinking of the Greco-Roman custom (according to which the wife could also take the initiative) but of the Jewish custom (according to which only husbands could send their wives away because of unchastity). The interpolation, then, is concerned only with unchastity on the part of the wife (contrary to Bonsirven, because contracts of marriage which were null and void also involved the husband). Consequently it should be clear that, if this secondary interpolation is interpreted as a saving clause, this not only impairs the absolute value which Mark, Luke, and Paul all placed on Christ's *logion,* but also does a certain violence to the whole context of Mt xix. 9. The deuteronomic saving clause of Mt xix. 9 would, in this case, be in flagrant contradiction to what was said in the preceding verse, xix. 8, about the abolition of this Mosaic law relating to the "putting away" of one's wife. Jesus simply refused to accept this sending away—even in the case of *porneia,* when it was permitted under the old law—and, in contrast to the Old Testament saving clause, asserted the will of the Creator.

The whole passage would have become quite meaningless if the evangelist had included this exception in the verse that followed. What is more, if Mt xix. 9 is taken to mean that Jesus was siding with the followers of the school of Shammai, who permitted divorce on grounds of adultery, then the astonishment expressed in the apostles' answer would be incomprehensible— "then it is not expedient to marry" (xix. 10). Their astonishment is only explicable if Christ in fact rejected all possibility of the dissolution of marriage. His rejection is reinforced by the statement: "Not all men can receive this precept, but only those to whom it is given" (xix. 11). It is clear too that Matthew regarded total abstinence as a possibility within marriage as well, since he linked the passage referring to those who were "unmarriageable for the sake of the kingdom of god" (xix. 12) directly to that relating to the indissolubility of marriage. The interpolated clause, which is peculiar to Matthew, is clearly connected with this merging together of the two originally distinct passages—something else that occurs only in Matthew. From a consideration of the context in Matthew itself (and so not only because of Mark, Luke, and Paul), we are bound to conclude (and whatever the interpolation may mean in the positive sense, we can and must, for purely exegetical reasons, only conclude negatively) that the inserted clause cannot be interpreted as forming an exception to the absolute indissolubility of marriage.

It is, however, more difficult in this case to establish the positive meaning of the interpolation because of its secondary character—as a later addition to an existing *logion.* In the primitive church it did happen that wives were sent away or abandoned, but remarriage was impossible. Paul based this ban on remarriage on Christ's *logion* (1 Cor vii. 10–11). It is therefore clear that the Jewish concept of "repudiation," which essentially incorporated the "possibility of remarriage," was in Christian circles divided by Christ's radical ban, so that repudiation on the ground of *porneia* was still permissible, but without the possibility of remarriage. This was further confirmed by Paul (in 1 Cor vii. 10–11) and by Hermas. The whole of the subapostolic practice of the church—repudiation without remarriage—and the closely related case of 1 Cor vii. 10–11 in the apostolic church argue strongly in favour of Dupont's view, despite the fact that this author has probably over-systematized the matter. The interpolation in Matthew is a saving clause which refers only to the "sending away" of wives, and not to "remarriage." As far as its content is concerned, the implication in Mt xix. 9 is the same as that of the less problematical interpolation in Mt v. 32. The meaning of Mt xix. 9 is, however, far less obvious, in view of the fact that the content of Mt v. 32 is closely bound up in xix. 9 with an affirmation of remarriage. Nonetheless, the idea is clearly expressed that repudiation on grounds of adultery can be understood, even if remarriage is out of the question.

Christ not only expressly condemned divorce (showing, in other words, that the indissolubility of marriage is a moral imperative); he also said that any divorce which might possibly take place had no effect whatever on the bond of marriage itself (pointing out, in other words, that the indissolubility of marriage is an objective bond). The church Fathers were to emphasize the first aspect of indissolubility, the scholastics the second. Both aspects are biblical and will have to be accorded their rightful place in our synthetic examination of the subject later on. Paul summarised Jesus' view of the indissoluble bond of marriage in these words: "A woman is bound to her husband as long as he lives. If the husband dies, she is free to be married" (1 Cor vii. 39; see also Rom vii. 2–4).

Christ went even further than this and made conjugal fidelity a matter of inward moral significance:

> You have heard that it was said, "You shall not commit adultery." But I say to you that every one who looks as a woman lustfully has already committed adultery with her in his heart. [Mt v. 27.]

Jesus' view of marriage bears undeniable witness to a radical attitude towards the principle of the holiness of marriage. On the other hand, we cannot fail to be struck by the gentleness and mercy which Jesus showed in his attitude towards sexual weakness, in contrast to the severity which he showed towards the piety of the Pharisees. (Mt xxi. 31–2; Lk vii. 36–50; Jn viii. 3–9 and viii. 11.) This redeeming mercy was also applied to married life and human sexuality.

The Becoming One of Man and Wife and the Community of Faith

On the other hand, Paul provides us with what is evidently an exception to the indissolubility of marriage. Moreover, it is clear from this exception that the absolute indissolubility of marriage is applicable only to Christian marriage.

> To the rest I say, not the Lord, that if any *brother* has a wife who is an unbeliever, and she consents to live with him, he should not divorce her. If any woman has a husband who is an unbeliever, and he consents to live with her, she should not divorce him. For the unbelieving husband is consecrated through his wife, and the unbelieving wife is consecrated through her husband. Otherwise your children would be unclean, but as it is they are holy. But if the unbelieving partner desires to separate, let it be so; in such a case the brother or sister is not bound. For God has called us to peace. Wife, how do you know whether you will save your husband? Husband, how do you know whether you will sve your wife? [1 Cor vii. 12–16.]

"Let it be so!" The question is: Should this "separation" be understood in the Jewish sense of the dissolution of marriage, or in the new Christian sense of separation without remarriage? In the first place, we should be concerned with the so-called "Pauline privilege" which conferred preferential legal treatment upon the believing party; in the second, it is probable that Paul was generalising from his own case. What is in any event clear is that Paul certainly did say that, in the case of marriage between two Christians (1 Cor vii. 10–11), those who were in fact separated were not permitted to remarry. This assertion was based on Christ's own dictum. In the case of a mixed marriage, to which he was referring in the passage under consideration (vii. 12–16), he was speaking on his own—but nonetheless apostolic—authority, and permitted separation. The contrast between the two texts shows that in the second case "separation" implies the dissolution of the marriage: "the brother or sister is not bound in such a case" (vii. 15). Although Paul does not say explicitly that the baptized party is permitted to remarry after separation, this is certainly implied in the text.

However, it must be admitted in this connection that Paul's manner of expression is to some extent forced: "he [or she] is no longer enslaved," implying that cohabitation with such a person is slavery for the believing partner. Since Christ has called the believer to peace, he may therefore withdraw from slavery in such a case. There is no clear statement to the effect that the believing party is free in the sense of being permitted to remarry.[20] This is, however, the unanimous interpretation of the exegetes—the believing party was perfectly free to remarry after separation. Paul saw this as an exception not only in respect of vii. 12–13, but also in respect of vii. 10–11. If a Christian took the initiative in the separation, either with regard to a fellow Christian (vii. 10–11) or with regard to a non-Christian (vii. 12–13), then this separation could have no legal consequences—that is to say, the marriage remained indissoluble and remarriage was not permitted. The exception here is only that if the initiative in separation was taken by a non-believer—and Paul was thinking here especially of non-Christian Gentiles—then the marriage really was dissolved. In basis the moral obligation applied to the Christian, with the result that the bond of marriage remained unimpaired even when there was a breach in his marriage with a non-Christian partner.

Paul continued to use the Jewish technical term "sending away" if the husband took the initiative; and, according to Jewish law, the husband was the only party who was permitted to take the initiative. If it concerned a wife, who could not herself write a bill of divorce, he continued to make use of the technical term "abandonment of," or "departure from," the other party. In other words, even when the separation was accompanied, according to Jewish custom, by a "bill of divorce," this legal action had no effect whatever on the bond of marriage if the initiative had been taken by the believing party—whether by the Christian husband's giving a bill of divorce, or by the Christian wife's leaving her husband and thus forcing him to issue a bill of divorce. All this indicates incidentally that separation without any possibility of remarriage was recognised as a reality in the apostolic church. The "Mosaic practice" of the bill of divorce seems to have continued among the Jewish converts to Christianity, but it took on a new meaning.

At first sight, however, this interpretation does present one difficulty. Although he was acting within his apostolic authority, Paul does appear to regard the absolute statement, proclaimed by Jesus as the will of the Creator, as applicable only to the marriages of baptized persons. It does look as if this is a rather Christian concept of the Creator. But in fact Paul, who always regarded a genuinely historical dictum made by Christ as an inviolate norm that was never contradicted by the heavenly Christ,[21] did not even here restrict the meaning of Christ's *logion*. Indeed, it is possible to say that Paul made Christ's *logion* more radical in meaning. The synoptic *logion* embraces the idea of "one flesh," the single living communion which was the God of creation's intention in marriage.

For a Christian believer this communion *in faith* is an essential element in marriage. Paul had in mind those people who were already married before they became converted to Christianity. Even then an existing marriage remained in force—unless the non-Christian partner did not wish it to continue or else made the marriage too difficult for the believing partner; but in an exceptional situation of this kind the marriage was dissolved on the very grounds of this principle of marriage itself, the biblical "one flesh," the living communion which was peace. Faith is of such essential importance in marriage, and forms such an indispensable element in its constitution, that there must have been a kind of *error substantialis* (fundamental mistake) in the conclusion of the contract if a non-Christian no longer desired to live with a believer in marriage. Paul did not say that this marriage was dissolved by subsequent remarriage, as the canonists maintain in connection with the "Pauline privilege," but that this marriage dissolved itself because of the factual situation—it was terminated as a marriage by the fact that the non-Christian partner no longer wished to live with the believing partner. We are confronted here with the self-dissolution of marriage in the interests of the baptized partner's life of faith.

It is a biblical datum that the marriage of a baptized person—a "brother" or a "sister" is a member of a community of faith, and thus a person baptized in faith—has a deeper and more radical meaning that the marriage of an unbaptized person, although the latter is certainly a real marriage. For, whereas marriage is formally indissoluble as far as a baptized person is concerned, it is dissoluble as far as an unbaptized person is concerned. (Even the marriage of a baptized person is thus indirectly dissoluble, via the unbaptized party.) The basis of absolute indissolubility is therefore to be found in Christian baptism. And so "the will of the Creator" to which Christ referred means that marriage, as a human reality, is a reality that includes a religious relationship with God—the saving relationship that was concretely provided in Christ—and thus formally falls to the share of man by faith and baptism.

Marriage is a covenant reality.[22] Eph v. 25–32 was therefore able to say that the communion to which Genesis and Jesus' *logion* about the indissolubility of marriage referred had a more profound meaning, and pointed to the indissoluble unity between Christ and his church. Jesus' *logion* about the "one flesh," on which the indissolubility of marriage is based, is essentially connected with the communion of Christ and his church. This does not mean that Paul established this connection explicitly when he confirmed separation in marriage with an unbaptized person; but this vision is certainly implied in the sheer dynamism of these texts. That is why I believe that the strongest biblical basis for the sacramental aspect of marriage is to be found in 1 Cor vii. 15—the self-dissolution of a marriage with an unbaptized person when this person refuses to live with the believing partner.

The marriage of the unbaptized person is in no way reduced in status by this view—on the contrary, Paul forbade separation if the unbaptized partner wished to continue with the marriage with the Christian partner. This view simply indicates that marriage has a special character for a baptized person. It is quite different from the situation in which a marriage "dissolves itself" on moral and religious grounds because of persistence in adultery; for in that case not only is violence done to the moral obligation, but the objective bond of marriage remains, in this biblical vision, unimpaired. This can only mean that baptism is the real and concrete bond in Christian marriage—baptism continuing to have an effect in the establishment of the marriage, and, resulting from this, the moral obligation to be "one flesh." The real bond, exempt from human intervention, is present in marriage by virtue of Christian baptism. This real bond is still present in the marriage of an unbaptized person, or in marriage with an unbaptized person, insofar as the mystery of Christ is not denied. Such a marriage can therefore be called an implicitly Christian marriage—an implicit reality which automatically disappears if there is an explicit denial of the mystery of Christ. And so if the unbaptized partner wishes to continue to live with the Christian husband or wife, this marriage remains—according to Paul—undissolved.

If, on the other hand, the unbaptized partner is explicitly confronted with the historical reality of Christianity—in this case the wife (or husband) who has been converted to Christianity—and yet refuses to continue in this living communion with her, it is evident that he is denying the implicit relationship to Christ of the marriage, and consequently also denying the real and indissoluble bond which this relationship confers upon the marriage.

It will be better to analyse the dogmatic implications of Paul's view before I proceed, in my synthesis, to discuss the power of jurisdiction which hierarchical authority has over marriage. This is to ensure that the relative indissolubility of marriage is not interpreted in a "positivist" or a purely juridical sense, by means of a simple appeal to the church's "power of the keys." The power of the keys is in any case not an authority existing independently from the authority of Christ. The two are intimately linked.

Paul did not base his reasoning on his apostolic authority, but on the objective saving reality of marriage which he, as Christ's apostle, clarified and interpreted. As a result of this, the marriage contract of unbaptized persons undoubtedly has an inner tendency towards absolute indissolubility because of this implicit relationship with Christ; but, on the other hand, it can give way to a marriage that acquires an explicit relationship, with the mystery of Christ and his church on a basis of baptism. The distinct character of the marriage of a baptized Christian also emerges even more clearly from 1 Cor vii. 14, 16, in which Paul says that the unbaptized partner in marriage is "consecrated" by the holy state of the baptized partner, and that the children of such a marriage are also "holy."

What does this signify? In the first place it is an established fact that the Jewish idea of the "uncleanness" or impurity of the Gentiles[23] was taken over by the Christians of the apostolic church and associated with the idea of the purifying effects of washing by the water of baptism. In other words, non-Christians were "unclean."[24] However, there was no need for the baptized partner to be concerned lest he should be "defiled" by an "unclean" partner's impurity, Paul reasoned. In Paul's view the very opposite was the case, for the baptized partner purified the unbaptized partner. His proof of this was that the children who were born of such marriages were "holy"; Paul clearly did not expect the Corinthians to contradict this, but rather assumed that it would be accepted in the community. There was, then, an assumption on Paul's part that the children of such mixed marriages would be "holy." Reasoning, by means of an analogy, from the fact that the children of a mixed marriage were sanctified, he went on to show that there *could* also be a consequent sanctifying effect (see vii. 16) upon the unbaptized partner.

The core of Paul's train of thought is therefore quite clear: a Christian member sanctifies the entire family. at the same time it is also apparent that in this passage the children—and not merely either the husband or the wife—are assumed not to have been baptized, otherwise the whole power of Paul's argument to prove his point is lacking.[25] This means that the "holiness" of the children is fundamentally attributable to their being members of a family with a Christian father or mother; so there is a "holiness" which is not due to personal baptism, although this holiness does in the end go back to someone who is baptized.

I do not propose at this point to provide a historical survey of the patristic and scholastic attempts to overcome this difficulty. What is, however, immediately apparent is that the terminology of 1 Cor vii. 14 is derived from the ritual terminology of the later Jews. This means that the text as such did not envisage a personal, moral-religious holiness—this, according to the New Testament view, was the result of faith and baptism, and was in actual fact associated only with adult Christians—but rather an "objective holiness" independent of personal faith.[26] Later Jewish thought also made—in connection with the baptism of proselytes—a distinction between those children who were "sanctified" and those who were "not sanctified." The children who were "not sanctified" were those born to the parents before they were converted to the Jewish faith. Such children required the baptism of proselytes. The children who were "sanctified" were those born after their parents had gone over to the Jewish faith. These children were not baptized, since they were regarded as forming an integral part of the whole Jewish family, and thus as belonging to the people of God.

This historical evidence makes it clear that, despite the fundamentally different dogmatic content of Christian baptism, the early Jewish converts to Christianity continued—as far as terminology and ritual practice were concerned, at least—to be closely associated with the practices of the Jewish baptism of proselytes. We may assume with a high degree of probability that the phrase "he was baptized with all his family" implied that the children were also baptized. Jeremias has established this on a basis of sound reasoning, but it is not relevant to the passage under consideration at present. What is of importance, however, is the fact that the primitive church continued for some time not to baptize the children born to parents who were already baptized. This practice was based on the analogy of the Jewish baptism of proselytes. The fact that there were some children who were baptized (if they were born before their parents' baptism) makes no difference to our certainty that in this passage Paul assumed that the children were not baptized. Otherwise, all his reasoning is pointless.

And yet he called these children "sanctified" and assumed that everyone would accept this. (The phrase "but as it is they are holy" in vii. 14 may be understood in the sense of "you know, they really are holy!") According to the passage as a whole, this is so even if only one of the parents was baptized. This view is closely connected with the Jewish and the Jewish-Christian idea of family solidarity and with the idea of "corporate personality" which was so fundamental to Jewish thought, and which meant that for God too the family was a single entity. For this reason, when the father of a family was converted to Christianity it generally happened that "he was baptized with all his house."[27] On the other hand, if the family was already Christian the birth of a child was regarded as an "incorporation into the Christian family." For a short period during apostolic times baptism was not administred in a case such as that, either at birth or when the child had reached adulthood. This is a fact, and it requires a theological explanation.

At this state in the historical development of the teaching on baptism, birth into a Christian family—to two Christian parents—was experienced as the sacramental equivalent of baptism. The theological explanation for this is that the essential core of the "external sign" of baptism is incorporation into the visible community of the church, made concrete by immersion in water; but that initially even this concrete sign appeared to be "plastic." Birth into a Christian family—that is to say, being accepted into a Christian sphere of life—fulfilled as such the fundamental idea of baptism as an incorporation into the visible community of the church. This situation did not dispense with the necessity of baptism, but was experienced as "baptism." The children were, so to speak, baptized in the baptism of their parents, who formed the Christian environment into which the children were accepted and incorporated.

That is why the "sanctification of the children" in 1 Cor vii. 14 does not have a purely ritual significance, despite the presence (in the background at least) of later Jewish ideas. On the other hand, the text undoubtedly lays emphasis on a state of having been sanctified (*hēgiastai,* in the perfect tense). It seems to me that there is no justification for interpreting this in the sense of "external purity"—an interpretation which is in fact based on a fear of coming into conflict with the dogma of the necessity of baptism for salvation. The objective condition of holiness is peculiar to the saving effect of baptism, and in particular to incorporation into the new people of God—the saving community which constitutes the sphere in which Christ's redemptive grace is effective in a highly concentrated form, as a powerful influence felt, so to speak, "in one's own home." This condition, then, gave members of the Christian community both the power and the duty to enter intimately into the faith and the love of this community to confess their membership of it. It was a condition of having been saved that was factually present in the Christian community of the family for those children who were not born before their parents' baptism, but who were born and brought up after their parents had been baptized.

This, in any event, appears to have been the experience of Christians at the time of Paul's first epistle to the Corinthians (i.e., in the year A.D. 54). There is no *a priori* reason for attributing to the church in apostolic times as well-developed a dogmatic awareness as we now possess with the texts of the church's councils in our hands.[28] In any case the background of the Jewish idea of sanctification, which continued to have a powerful effect among the Jewish converts to Christianity, makes the Christian view of that period quite clear. As Paul says, in a different context, but drawing on the same background thought: "If the dough offered as first-fruits is holy, so is the whole lump; and if the root is holy, so are the branches" (Rom xi. 16). Instead of forcing these texts to fit the required interpretation, the study of dogma has in fact far more to gain from trying to understand more fully the significance of the necessity of baptism as an incorporation into the community of the church during this very tentative initial period of the church. In this way it should be possible to learn how to assess theologically those "frontier" situations which are often capable of revealing in a distinctive and "flexible" way the real significance of a requirement posed by dogma.

Paul assumed that it was known that the children born to baptized parents, or to a baptized father or mother, were really sanctified, even if they did not receive baptism with immersion. From this, he went on to discuss the different situation of the unbaptized partner in marriage. In that instance, the fact that the unbaptized partner was an adult formed an essential element in the constitution of his personal response to faith, and the mere fact of his being incorporated into a Christian family did not of itself mean that he personally became converted to Christianity. This was expressed by Paul in the question: "Wife, how do you know whether you will save your husband? [= whether you will bring him to the Christian faith]. Husband, how do you know whether you will save [= convert] your wife?" (vii. 16). In such a case, a personal conversion, or repentance (*metanoia*), was necessary. This would be completed in baptism, through which salvation was accepted in faith. In the practice of the ancient church a difference was in fact experienced between the "sanctification of the children," which was objectively accomplished by the baptism of water or by the baptism of incorporation into a Christian family, the "local" community of faith, and the "sanctification of the unbelieving partner in marriage." This was so even though there was, in the latter case, an objective condition of holiness—the state of being sanctified, indicated by the use in 1 Cor vii. 14 of *hēgiasti* in the perfect tense—based on the possibility of the eventual personal sanctification of the unbelieving partner. Life in a Christian community of faith was, in other words, an objective offer of grace for the non-Christian partner in marriage.

For an adult, entry into a Christian circle could only be the result of a call to "conversion," which culminated in faith and in baptism by water. It was precisely to this end that the baptized partner had to direct his "zeal" as a believer.[29] Peter also speaks of marriage between a Christian wife and an unbaptized husband. Here, the wife's "zeal" for the faith is regarded as forming part of the total Christian experience of the domestic relationship between the husband and the believing wife: "You wives be submissive to your husbands so that some, though they do not obey the Word, may be won without a word, by the behaviour of their wives, when they see your reverent and chaste bahaviour (1 Pet iii. 1–2).

We may therefore conclude that 1 Cor vii. 12–16 not only closely follows the thought of Jesus' synoptic *logion* concerning the indissolubility of marriage, but makes if far more radical by revealing its full depths. It does this by throwing light on the idea of "peace" within the "one flesh" of marriage, and showing how Christian baptism causes the contract of marriage to become an indissoluble, objective bond. Moreover, it is clear from the text that marriage is essentially a commission—a task of apostolic sanctification proceeding from the partners in marriage to each other, and to the children and the family as a whole. Marriage does not simply enter salvation; by so doing it also becomes an instrument of salvation effective within the personal relationship of marriage. When we come to consider the increasing value placed upon the interpersonal relationship aspect of marriage—as is the case in modern marriage especially—it will no longer be possible to look to this Pauline text for the full effects of the vision of marriage it presupposes, even though it will still be necessary to be guided by Paul throughout the attempted synthesis. In my opinion 1 Cor vii. 12–16 offers the most compact "theology of marriage" in the whole of the New Testament.

Jesus' statement concerning the indissolubility of marriage, made on a basis of the Old Testament view of creation that marriage was "one flesh"—a single, living communion—is shown by 1 Cor vii. 12–16 in its full saving significance. There is an intimate connection between this indissolubility and baptism; as a result of this close interconnection the marriage of unbaptized persons has—in a sense—a lesser value (though it is in no way inferior), and lacks the special and distinct significance which characterizes the marriage of baptized partners. In its orientation towards salvation, what is usually known as "natural" marriage undoubtedly has a similar significance, but in this case an implicit one. However, if this orientation towards salvation is denied by the unbaptized partner, the marriage may be dissolved in favour of the "peace" into which salvation has incorporated the baptized partner. From this it is once again apparent that salvation in Christ, the communion with Christ, transcends married life. The moral consequences of this are very great indeed, as I shall try to show at a later stage. On the other hand, it also means that this priority is made interior in married life itself—that married life is transformed from within by the communion with Christ, who is the saving omnipotence of the living God in history. The dogmatic consequences of this will also be made clear in my consideration of marriage in the history of the church.

* * *

What is striking is that, according to Paul's view, the possibility of dissolution is *naturally* present in the case of a marriage between a baptized and an unbaptized person, but that the baptized partner may not take the initiative in the matter of dissolution. This is, of course, in tune with the apostle's view of the objective bond which baptism brings about—via the marriage contract—in marriage. It was only in the course of history that it later emerged that, if only one partner was baptized, this "onesidedness" in marriage was bound to have repercussions on the effects of baptism within the marriage bond. At a later stage, too, another problem came to be considered: Does such a case constitute an authentic sacrament of marriage? The solution of this problem will inevitably depend on whether the so-called "Pauline privilege" is only one manifestation of a definite reality which, according to circumstances, embraces other possibilities and variations that were not envisaged as such by Paul.

This brings us face to face with the fact that the Roman Catholic Church dissolves marriage between baptized and unbaptized persons, even if the unbaptized party wishes to continue the marriage. As we shall see later on, the ecclesiastical administration of the law in fact considers every marriage in which an unbaptized party is involved to be ultimately dissoluble in the interest of the baptized party's faith, even if such a marriage was concluded with the Church's permission and after a dispensation from the impediment to marriage—the *disparitas cultus*—which made this marriage invalid according to canon law. We shall also be confronted later on with the even more difficult situation in which the Church follows the legal practice of dissolving, in certain cases, a marriage concluded between two baptized parties—in other words, a sacramental marriage—if this is not sexually consummated. Undoubtedly what is in evidence here is that ecclesiastical legal practice is in this case based on the view that the biblical idea of "one flesh" ("what God has joined together" according to Christ's synoptic *logion*) gains its full significance in the explicit connection between Christ and his church, and insofar as this marital "becoming one" also gains its full form (full, that is, in the anthropological and physical sense of the word).

Paul's view of marriage has already shown that these problems cannot be solved simply by having recourse to a purely "positivist" appeal to the church's jurisdiction or "power of the keys," as the jurists and canonists are in the habit of doing, however right this may be for them. Ecclesiastical law itself must be based on dogmatic insight, and the idea of "one flesh" promulgated in the Old Testament, deepened by Jesus, and clarified by Paul, must always be the guiding canonical principle, the full scope and meaning of which can certainly be interpreted by the church, but never changed. The church's power of the keys is in no sense a high-handed authority, but a power bound to the word of the historical and risen Christ. In this way the Bible remains a critical authority from which the jurisdiction of the church is unable to emancipate itself.

In the course of history, however, the real scope and full implications of this "one flesh" as the basis of the indissolubility of marriage have been revealed through new problems in changing situations. There is also little doubt that in the future fresh problems will arise which will bring out new aspects of this idea, and which the church, guided by the vision of the Bible in the light of the tradition of faith, will be able to interpret authoritatively. Moreover, in cases such as these, particularly if they are concerned with the *dogmatic* dissolubility of a marriage which the unbaptized partner does not deny, it will be necessary to take justice into account—the humane and moral obligations that may well be present in fact—despite the fact that the marriage may be open to dissolution. In these cases, a purely dogmatic insight that there is a possibility of dissolution cannot provide the final answer to the concrete problem. But this discussion has already drawn us far from the sphere of biblical theology and into the territory to be explored in a later volume of this work.

Paul's Opposition to Mixed Marriage

In the preceding sections we have considered Paul's views on the marriages of Gentiles who were already married before one of the two partners became converted to Christianity. "Mixed marriages" of this kind were, of course, inevitable in the earliest Christian period, and Paul had only good to say of them. His reaction to "mixed marriages" contracted by those who were already baptized with non-Christians was quite different.

> Do not be mismated with unbelievers. For what partnership have righteousness and iniquity? Or what fellowship has light with darkness? What accord has Christ with Belial? . . . What agreement has the temple of God with idols? For we are the temple of the living God. [2 Cor vi. 14–16.]

Today we may well be astonished by this black-and-white picture, and by the note of triumph at the end: We are on the side of right. It is of course true that Christians of the first century had little feeling for the good in other people and their religions, whereas the spirit of the present age impels us today to acknowledge the good in others, and even to see only our own shortcomings. Paul, however, saw things in a totally different light. For him the central fact of existence was that the mystery of Christ had appeared—that redemption had come in Jesus. The "saints" were those who had turned to Christ in faith and baptism. Everything else faded into insignificance beside the explicit acknowledgement of this central fact of salvation. Christianity really appeared to the Gentile world of that time as a sun in the darkness—a phenomenon that "set the world on its head," as the Gentiles themselves put it: *hoi tēn oikoumenēn anastatōsantes* (Acts xvii. 6), surely a remarkable definition of Christians as the people who "set the world in an uproar." Both Gentiles and Christians themselves felt that Christianity was something quite unique. And indeed, it is unique, even today. What Paul said then is still applicable today. The Catholic Church still regards a marriage with an unbaptized person as invalid in principle. It is not a marriage unless the impediment to marriage has been removed by an ecclesiastical dispensation, and even then it is still dissoluble.

The New Testament of course says nothing directly about "mixed marriages" in the modern sense of the phrase (that is, marriages between Catholic and non-Catholic Christians). This particular problem will be dealt with in a later volume.

Patterns Of Behaviour

"The husband is the head of the wife": Biblical Assertion, or Simply Social Pattern?

We have already touched on the basic principle of the ethos of marriage in the New Testament in connection with the problem of "marriage in the Lord" in the context of 1 Cor vii. 39. The apostolic and the ancient church accepted man's ethical awareness as it was in Jewish and Greco-Roman society during the first century. But this ethical consciousness was incorporated into the Christian spirituality of "being in and with Christ," and thus of faith and love, and was inwardly transformed and corrected. Christians were, in everything, "in the Lord" (Col iii. 18).

This is particularly clear from the "household codes" of the New Testament.[30] These rules were modelled on the secular household codes of the Hellenistic, and especially of the Judaeo-Hellenistic, world. A form-critical analysis of these lists, which provide ethical standards for all kinds of social relationships—relationships between husbands and wives, parents and children, masters and slaves, rulers and subjects—shows that they go back to the household codes common in the popular ethics of the Hellenistic world.[31] These codes summarized the civil duties of man as a "political being," that is, as a citizen, or member of a human society. They included man's relationship towards God (since the worship of God was regarded as a political duty or civic virtue) and his relationship towards his native country (that is, towards the authority of the state) as well as relationships between husband and wife, parent and child, brother and mother, and relationships with relatives, friends, strangers, and slaves. If these civic virtues originally had a religious basis, in conjunction with the religion of the family, they were eventually "secularised"—that is, they became ethically based on "human nature" and on the human conscience.

Even before Christianity these secular household rules had made their influence felt in the Jewish world (e.g., Tobit iv. 2–23; Sir vii. 20–39), where they became intermingled with Jewish elements.[32] The New Testament took over these household codes in broad outline, but always left out the first civic duty, that of the worship of God, in view of the fact that man's relationship with God transcended his other duties and was based on revelation and faith. In this way, "religion" and "ethics" were formally distinguished, however much each was implied in the other. For the rest, "natural," secular ethics were taken over, based on God, and gradually Christianised.

This secular character is most in evidence in Paul's first use of household codes (Col iii. 18–iv. 1). All that is said here is that these ethics must be experienced "in the Lord." In Eph v. 22–33 the relationship between man and wife, following closely on the principles of these domestic rules, is interpreted in the religious sense (that is, "as Christ and his church"). 1 Pet ii. 13–iii. 7 contains many traces of Christian influence,[33] without of course Paul's theological superstructure. The planning of domestic life is the planning of a house that is the temple of God (1 Pet ii. 1–10). These household codes give the clearest possible indication of the transformation of ethical elements already present in secular society and taken over by Christianity. For they show that these ethical rules of conduct—which the New Testament raised to the level of "commandments"—were not simply experienced "in the Lord," as in Col iii. 18–iv. 1, chronologically the earliest of the New Testament household codes; the motivation of these rules became more and more explicitly Christian. Christians were exhorted to love each other "as Christ loved his Church," and to be subject to each other "as the Church is subject to Christ." The slave's submission to his master—the ethic and practice of the period—was raised to the level of a following of Christ (1 Pet ii. 19 and 21–5). And so the motivation of the current code of behaviour became formally Christian.

In other words, the "natural" code of the period was not simply viewed according to its divine basis, nor was it merely experienced as such "in the Lord." According to the New Testament, it was more than this—it acquired from Christ a formally Christian motivation. The New Testament household codes are therefore theologically the best proof that we have of the fact that a Christian moral theology was already in process of growth in the New Testament—on a basis of an ethical appreciation already existing in society, and in connection with the planning and regulation of social life, both in the smaller community of the then prevalent extended family and in the greater community of the state.

This immediately poses a delicate problem. Are we confronted here with a Christian confirmation of existing ethical forms which are thus presented in the New Testament as an unchangeable norm? Or is this just a call to experience "in the Lord" and from Christian motives the ethical values and social structures already present in society? And, if this latter is the case, is it not also the case that the New Testament, by not rejecting the contemporary situation but simply giving it a Christian motivation, has in effect put it forward as a principle that the actual, existing social structures of this world should be preserved? This question becomes particularly significant when it is considered in the context of the New Testament assertion that the husband is the "head of the wife," and of the wife's subordinate position and factually inferior social status in the ancient world which resulted from this assertion.

Before I attempt to throw light on this problem in the New Testament, a preliminary theological observation will not be out of place—especially since this observation will also prove to be in itself a conclusion from an examination of the New Testament, thus providing further substantiation of the claim that theology is regulated by the Bible.

Both in the tradition of the Old and New Testaments and in the subsequent tradition of the church, it is evident that a "human" tradition also existed alongside the divine tradition. This human tradition not only went back a long way; it is also true to say that the faithful community was, initially at least, not necessarily always explicitly aware *per se* of the distinction between the "human" and the "divine" traditions in its assertions. In the assumptions on which the community of the faithful lived and on which it based much of its thought and action, there was not only a whole area of convictions that went back to the revelation of God's word, but also a not inconsiderable group of convictions derived from the universally received ideas of a definite period of time. These convictions formed the communal property of human awareness at a given period and were only replaced when new situations and fresh discoveries showed them to be outdated.

It is only when a social or economic change takes place in human values that the believing community feels impelled to examine whether—first—the convictions that it has inherited really go back to an inner demand made by revelation or by a basic human and ethical awareness; whether their source is in fact purely human; or whether—finally—they originated in an essentially religious truth expressed thematically, either in conceptual terms borrowed from an out-of-date view of man and the world, or in outdated social structures which have in the meantime been replaced by newer ones.

Something of this kind faces us today in the matter of the married woman, in view of the changed outlook on woman in the modern world and the completely new social position which she occupies both in public life and in the circle of her own family. And so the question has arisen: Are the affirmations which the Bible makes about woman and marriage really "biblical" (that is, are they really divine declarations with the force of commandments), or are they merely structures set in an ancient historical and social framework, which Christians of that period experienced "in the Lord"?

A comparison of the structure of domestic life in the New Testament with domestic life in the secular world of the period shows that the New Testament structure contains data which are social and historical. This, however, provides no solution to the problem—at least, not to the problem of whether it is a "biblical" assertion that the husband is the "head of the wife," certainly the most important in this connection. In any case, it cannot be denied that the wife's position in the New Testament was broadly speaking very similar to the low social position of the married woman in the whole of the ancient world.[34] This is clear from minor details. A man, for example, "married," whereas a woman was "given in marriage" (e.g., Lk xvii. 27; xx. 35). A husband was to love his wife, but neither Paul nor Peter says in his epistles that a wife is bound to love her husband. She was to be "subject" to him (Col iii. 18; Eph v. 21–2; 1 Pet iii. 1, 5; Tit ii. 5).[35] This, however, still proves very little. It may well mean that the assertion "the husband is the head of the wife" was experienced by Christians in terms of contemporary social patterns, but this still does not prove that the assertion itself is anything more than an experience "in the Lord" of already present, changeable social relationships.

In a nutshell, the problem is this: Is the statement, "the husband is the head of the wife," an authentically biblical assertion, based on revelation, which was of course bound to be experienced in accordance with and within existing social structures? Or is it not a biblical assertion at all, but merely something taken over from the ancient idea of the *pater familias* and expressed in Christian terms? It is by no means easy to answer this question. First it will be necessary to examine the New Testament facts themselves, and then we shall have to go into Paul, the first epistle of Peter, and the Pastoral Epistles, since this theme is not present in the Synoptic tradition or in John (a fact which is in itself important).

In the *Corpus Paulinum* there is a double series of texts referring to this question: "the husband is the head of the wife" (1 Cor xi. 3; Eph v. 23) and "wives, be subject to your husbands" (Col iii. 18; 1 Cor xiv. 34; Eph v. 21–2; see also 1 Pet iii. 1; Tit ii. 5). This latter, this *hupotaxis* (subjection or submission) of the wife to the husband, is also to be found in the secular Greco-Roman and in the Judaeo-Hellenistic household codes. It expressed the idea. universally current in those days, of the wife's status in the *oikos*, that is to say, in marriage and in the family. It was, therefore, not an expression of the general subordination of woman in society. In 1 Pet iii. 1, Eph v. 22 and Tit ii. 5—all "household code" texts—there is explicit reference to the wife's subjection to her own husband, and consequently no direct mention of woman's subordinate position in contemporary society. What was at issue here was the wife's real place in the *taxis* (plan) of domestic life.

This was also the context in Eph v. 22–32. Eph v. 21 ("Be subject to one another out of reverence for Christ") forms an introduction to the exposition of the household codes which follows, and does not invalidate the idea of the wife's submission to the husband, as may at first sight appear. It would be completely alien to Paul's thought to suggest that he meant that the husband should also be subject to the wife. He required a mutual subjection on the part of the following groups of categories of person—husbands and wives, parents and children, masters and slaves. Even when the husband is called the "head of the wife" in Eph v. 22–3, it is quite clear that this was meant in the *domestic* sense. According to the whole context of Eph v. 22–33, the husband is the "head of his *own wife*."

In 1 Cor xi Paul appears to take quite a different point of view, both with regard to the subjection of the wife to the husband and with regard to the husband as the head of the wife. In xi. 3 the man is quite simply called the head of the woman, and the entire context refers to the subordinate position of woman in society and in the church. "But I would have you know that the head of every man is Christ; the head of the woman is the man;[36] and the head of Christ is

God" (xi. 3). The same thought is resumed in xi. 7, though now from the perspective of the concept of the "image and glory of God": "The man is the image and glory of God; but the woman is the glory of the man." It is true that Paul expresses this idea in general terms, but he certainly sees this general assertion in the light of conjugal relationships. Even in xi. 3 he states that Christ is the head of *every* man, but not that the man is the head of *every* woman. The absence of the word "every" in the second phrase can scarcely be without significance. What is more, "the man," with the Greek article, cannot mean men in general, but a concrete and particular case—"the man of the woman" is therefore "the husband of the wife," and so "the head of the wife is her husband." All the same, this text is completely divorced from any context of marriage. It cannot be denied that the text does to some extent generalise, even though it does so via marital relationships. It will therefore be necessary to examine this text before going on to discuss Eph v. 22 ff., in which the man is called the head of the family.

We have to assume that—allowing for certain gradations—woman was illiterate and had no part to play in social life, both in the Jewish and in the Greco-Roman world. She was supposed to remain silent, and her place was in the home, by the cradle and at the loom. The household codes accepted—as an ethical rule of conduct in all families which were properly regulated according to the spirit of good citizenship—that wives were obliged to be subject to their husbands. The Judaeo-Hellenistic codes even added "in everything." We may set Josephus' text, "The wife, says the Law, is subject to the husband in all things,"[37] beside that of Paul, "As the Church is subject to Christ, so let wives also be subject in everything to their husbands (Eph v. 24). What Paul aimed to do in 1 Cor xi, in connection with the proper regulation of the practice of religion, in which women had to be silent and to veil their heads, was to provide a theological basis for woman's social status and for the accepted code of behaviour which this status demanded. The pains to which he went to establish this theological basis are a clear indication of the fact that he had to go against certain strong tendencies.

It is undisputed that human values and social relationships were beginning to change in the secular world, both before and during the first century A.D., despite the existence and widespread use of the household codes in the secular sphere. A new orientation was taking place in the way that (in particular) the Greeks felt towards their fellow-men and the things that surrounded them. They were becoming aware, no doubt partly because of the contacts which Alexander's conquests had established between Greece and the known world, of the differences between themselves and other men. They were also beginning to look at the everyday things that had long been familiar to them with new eyes. Politics were becoming less and less the activity of the ordinary man and citizen and more and more the concern of "world rulers," and for this reason ordinary Greek citizens began to focus their attention on the people and the things that immediately surrounded them in their own environment.

Everyday sufferings and joys were observed with increasing interest. Epictetus, for example, comments on the growing popularity in his time of the custom of addressing girls as "madam" or "my lady" from the age of fourteen onwards.[38] A certain courtly respect for women, which up to this time had been less conspicuous, was making itself felt throughout the entire Greek world. Lovers called each other "lord" and "lady" precisely in order to testify to their mutual subjection and to their loyalty to each other. The husband remained the *pater-familias,* but a change was taking place in the sphere of human feelings, and husband and wife were gradually coming to treat each other more as equals. The ancient social structures were not swept aside as yet, but they were filled with a new spirit—a spirit of increasing equality. It is possible to detect expressions of what we should now call "female emancipation" in the world of Greek women of this time. In literature, for example, we see the beginnings of the theme of marriages of love.

The citizens of the international port of Corinth were, in Paul's time, in many ways ahead of people elsewhere. The progressive women's "movement" developed in Corinth into an unrestrained non-conformity. The women who were converted to Christianity assumed airs even in the Christian community which scandalised their fellow-Christians. Their greater freedom expressed itself, for example, in their appearing unveiled at public religious meetings, and in their rising to speak at these meetings together with the men.[39] To the Jewish converts to Christianity especially this was something quite new and unknown, and it aroused their suspicians. Paul's epistle to the Corinthians is therefore a reaction against the kind of behaviour that was threatening the normal domestic order and harmony. Was he defending an outdated social order and family pattern against the threat of a new and freer way of life? Or was he trying to show that there was much more in the older pattern of life and behaviour than simply outdated forms? This is the problem with which we must deal.

As I have already said, Paul was looking for convincing and conclusive arguments. For this reason, he points to the structure of creation. "For man was not made from woman, but woman from man. Neither was man created for woman, but woman for man" (1 Cor xi. 8–9). In 1 Tim ii. 13, too, he refers to Genesis: "For Adam was formed first, then Eve." He bases his argument not only on the creation, but also on the fall of man: "Adam was not deceived, but the woman was deceived and became a transgressor" (1 Tim ii. 14). He also uses the Old Testament, and in particular the Law of Moses, in his argument against the loose morals of the Corinthians: "As in all the churches of the saints, the women should keep silence in the churches [= in your meetings]. for they are not permitted to speak, but should be subordinate, as even the Law says. If there is anything they desire to know, let them ask their husbands at home" (1 Cor xiv. 33–5). This argument based on the Bible is clearly used to confirm Paul's main line of argument, that of ecclesiastical custom, since he stresses "as in all the churches of the saints" (see also 1 Cor xi. 16). Here he is no doubt referring to the Christian communities of Palestinian Jews in which the older social structures were more firmly rooted.

In a similar context, he also refers to the "traditions even as I have delivered them to you" (1 Cor xi. 2). It is clear from the context that the Corinthians kept these traditions, with the exception of that of the subordination of women in the community, since he makes an immediate appeal to Christology, in the text which follows: "The head of every man is Christ; the head of the woman is the man; and the head of Christ is God" (1 Cor xi. 3), which should be compared with "Wives, be subject to your husbands, as to the Lord" (Eph v. 22) and "Wives, be subject to your husbands, as is fitting in the Lord" (Col iii. 18). In Eph v. 22 ff. Paul insists that women should be subject to their husbands "for the husband is the head of the wife as Christ is the head of the church. . . . Therefore, as the church is subject to Christ, so let wives also be subject in everything to their husbands."

The whole of this argument has an unaccustomed ring, giving the impression that Paul is defending a thesis that he feels he cannot fully substantiate and must consequently reinforce with numerous supporting pieces of evidence. It is obvious that he wholeheartedly accepts the custom of women veiling their heads, but he defends this practice as a sign of the subordinate position of woman in society by a mass of arguments which seem laborious and forced. The original significance of this veiling of the head is not easy to trace.[40] The custom was in fact regarded in contemporary society as an expression of the fact that the woman was the possession and property of the man who had veiled her. Originally, however, it would seem as if the veil was used as a kind of protection to ward off the evil spirits from which the "weaker sex" especially needed to be guarded. It would also seem as if Paul had heard of this, since he comments that women must wear a veil on their heads "because of the angels" (1 Cor xi. 10).[41] But it cannot be denied that the necessity for women to be veiled is Paul's conclusion from the premise that "man was not created for woman, but woman for man" (xi. 9). This is why women must wear a veil. The argument may well be called a "biblical" argument, since the *exousia* or "power" (xi. 10) which the wife has on her head—the veil as a sign of marital power—would appear to be a translation of the Hebrew *memĕsālāh,* and thus an allusion to Gen. ii. 16 in which the woman is placed, after the fall, "under the husband's power."

A new element, this time a philosophical argument derived from the Stoics, adds weight to this reasoning: "If a woman will not veil herself, then she should cut off her hair; but if it is disgraceful for a woman to be shorn, or shaven, let her wear a veil" (xi 6). The conclusive force of this argument eludes us, but for Paul it was clearly something like an appeal to the "natural law." According to the Stoics a woman "naturally" had long hair; consequently she ought not to go against nature and allow her hair to be cut off. The Corinthian women were conscious of the shame of having their heads shaven, but they did not regard it as ridiculous not to wear a veil. For Paul, however, both were "unnatural." The impression is inescapable—Paul attached as much importance to this custom as to something very sacred indeed: "Does not nature itself teach you that for a man to wear long hair is degrading to him, but if a woman has long hair, it is her pride?" (xi. 14–15).

This was the argument of the Stoics. But Paul went further: "For a man ought not to cover his head [when he prays], since he is the image and glory of God; but woman is the glory of man ... woman [was created] for man. That is why a woman ought to have a veil on her head, because of the angels" (xi. 7–10). The biblical argument of the woman's subjection to the man was based on a divine punishment after the fall. In this text, however, Paul goes back beyond the original sin of man to the situation in paradise when the man was created as "God's image" and the woman was created indirectly, being "taken out of the man."

This final rabbinical and biblical argument marks the end of Paul's reasoning. Strangely enough, however, he does not look back over the series of weighty arguments that he has put forward convinced that he has proved his point beyond all doubt. On the contrary, he feels impelled—with a feeling of slight irritation—to conclude his case with a sentence which is highly charged with meaning and which in fact sums up the whole of his plea: "But, if any one is disposed to be contentious, *we* recognise no other practice, nor do the churches of God" (xi. 16). This is really the only argument which is fully to the point. The practice of wearing a veil was, in other words, a venerable custom both among the Jews and among the Jewish converts to Christianity. Paul attached great importance to it because, in his own time especially, it had a profound religious and symbolic value. It stressed the modesty of women before God, and was above all a social symbol of woman's subordination to man (this latter was, of course, a basic conviction of Paul's). His zeal for the veiling of women was the result of his zeal for the idea that the man is the head of the woman.

In itself, the veil is simply a fact of secular or of religious society; it possesses no constant value. Even in our own time, men remove their hats on entering church. This is a purely social and religious symbol, important to us today as an expression of respect. In one particular society and at a given period of time, the custom of wearing a veil may be extremely significant; at a later age, and in a later society, this significance may have been lost. But there is always the difficulty of transition between the two cultures. In a transitional period of this kind, a custom may be renounced for good reasons, but it may also be repudiated for less good reasons—a desire to pursue the latest fashion, a refusal to conform to established ideas, a lack of sensitivity for the condition of man, or an attitude which sets greater store by external change than by basic and intrinsic values.

Paul was in fact fighting for something which was—from the point of view of culture and society—a lost cause, but it would be wrong to accuse him of being a reactionary on that account. He had abundant reasons for suspecting that what lay behind this attitude toward the veiling of women in Corinth was a basic lack of seriousness towards religious and moral values. This accounts for his heated partisanship and his rabbinical search for arguments which probably made little impression on the Greek mind.

The pastoral epistles show clearly how this lack of modesty was to be revealed in quite a different way in an already "settled" religious community. What we have here is a case of secular fashions in head-dress among women "in church":

> [I desire that women, when they pray, should] adorn themselves modestly in seemly apparel, not with braided hair or gold or pearls or costly attire but by good deeds, as befits women who profess religion. (1 Tim ii. 9–10; see also 1 Pet iii. 3–4.)

In order to stress the relative value of the social and historical elements in this epistle, we might go so far as to say—though this is merely a debating point—that its author reaped the results of Paul's zeal for women's head-dress! On the other hand, it must be admitted that Paul was under Christ's sway and the rest was only of relative interest to him. He does not provide a "theology" of cultural and social change, or even any basic principles that underlie the changes which take place in human life and ordinary secular structures. What he does offer is that basic eschatological vision which every "theology" of society must take into account if it aims to be a Christian theology. What concerned Paul above all was man's "being in Christ," what animated and inspired the Christian. As far as the rest was concerned, the *taxis* or social order, he desired only that "all things be done for edification" (1 Cor xiv. 26). His view is confirmed by the comment with which he concludes his plea that women should be silent in the Christian community: "all things should be done decently and in order" (1 Cor xiv. 40). This order (*taxis*) does not directly imply orderliness or discipline; it is only the consequence of Paul's more profound view of "order" as "hierarchical structure." Structures of this kind were very dear to Paul:

> For just as the body is one and has many members, and all the members of the body, though many, are one body, so it is with Christ. For by one Spirit we were all baptized into one body—Jews or Greeks, slaves or free—and all were made to drink of one Spirit [= as we have all been saturated by the one Spirit]. For the body does not consist of one member, but of many. If the foot should say, . . .
> And if the ear should say . . . But as it is, God arranged the organs in the body, each one of them, as he chose . . . [1 Cor xii. 12–18.]

This passage, which continues by discussing the functions of the members of Christ's body (xii. 12–31), is a good example of one of Paul's favourite themes. It is a fruitful source, but it can easily be misused if it is taken to explain actual historical structures in terms of theology.

What we have learnt so far is that Paul's view of woman certainly contains elements which were without question determined by existing social conditions, and that to some extent the apostle was undoubtedly aware of these himself. The conclusion to his argument about the need for women to veil their heads—"be this as it may, I want women to be veiled because of their subordinate position with regard to men"—is echoed in Eph v. 25–33, in which Paul is not directly concerned to interpret marriage as an image of the covenant between Christ and his church, but concerned rather to demonstrate that the wife is subject to the husband in marriage.

What he gives us here is the exact counterpart to his argument in favour of the veil. The difference, however, is that the biblical argument—that the woman is taken from the man and thus forms one flesh with him in subjection to him—is here developed according to its relation with Christ and with the church: just as Christ and his church form one flesh, but Christ is nonetheless the head of the church (an idea which Paul had been developing throughout his epistle to the Ephesians), so also is the husband the head of the wife.

These are really the same ideas as those in 1 Cor xi. 3–16, but they have been thought over again in the light of the new idea of Christ as the head of the church. It is noticeable that Paul ends his theological argument here in Eph v. 25–33 too with a certain doubt—"that at least is my view," which is the implication of the sentence "But I take it to mean [= but I for my part relate it to] Christ and the church" (v. 32), and "However [= be that as it may] let each one of you love his wife as himself, and let the wife see that she respects her husband" (v. 33). Moreover, it is clear that, just as in 1 Cor xi. 3–16, the argument of Eph v. 25–32 (which, incidentally, occurs within the framework of a moral exhortation similar to that of the "household codes") was intended as a defence, based on formal theological lines, of the domestic relationship between man and wife that was generally accepted within the various Christian communities—a relationship which was, it should be remembered, threatened by the prevailing spirit of the age, especially in the case of the Greek Christians.

These formal theological themes are advanced with great sincerity by Paul, but he does somehow give the impression of feeling that they are not entirely convincing as a theological basis for these social relationships. (This is why, in my discussion of this passage in the section dealing with the New Testament teaching on marriage, I passed over the ultimate purpose of this text, since it to some extent distorts the legitimate image of marriage in order to defend the position of the husband as the "head of the wife.") We may therefore conclude that the New Testament ethos of marriage does contain changeable social elements, but that the relative value of these elements is recognised, even though this recognition sometimes takes a veiled form.

If scriptural statements of this and of a similar kind are to be properly understood, it is important not to forget that as a rule women received no education during the first century. I am referring to statements such as "I permit no woman to teach" (1 Tim ii. 12) because she is susceptible to heresies (1 Tim iv. 7; 2 Tim iii. 6). These are in no sense *a priori* statements, but they occur in the pastoral epistles, and these could assume that the already well-organized communities to which the epistles were addressed had gained a great deal of experience. The same kind of statement is also to be found in the secular writings of the Greeks of this period—the man's place was in the gymnasium, instructing and being instructed in physical and intellectual pursuits, whereas the woman's place was in the home, at the cradle and the distaff. The pastoral epistle, 1 Timothy, says very much the same thing:

> [During instruction] let a woman learn in silence, with all submissiveness. I permit no woman to teach, or to have authjority over men; she is to keep silent. For Adam was formed first, then Eve. And Adam was not deceived, but the woman . . . Yet woman will be saved through bearing children, if she continues in faith and love and holiness, with modesty. [Tim i. 11–15.]

This, then, is the same conduct which is expected of women by the secular Greek writers but, in the case of Christian women, experienced "in the Lord." To construct a theology of marriage on a basis of such texts—to refer to the "primary significance" of the married woman and to conclude from this that Christianity cannot, for example, accept the idea of married women working away from home—would be to violate the first principles of sound biblical exegesis.

Nonetheless, though it should by now be clear that the wearing of the veil, the insistence that women should keep silent in the community, and the similar rules of conduct which were put forward by Paul on a theological basis were really determined by existing social and historical conditions, the basic assertion of Paul—that the man is the head of the wife who is subject to her husband—is in no sense disproved by this. This, then, is the essential problem facing us: Is this doctrine, advanced not only by Paul but also by Peter (1 Pet iii. 1–7), a biblical *datum?* Or is it only a biblical *mode of thought and expression,* and as such merely a variable social and historical quantity? Contemporary thought makes this problem extremely important. Article 16 of the *Declaration of Human Rights* states that husband and wife have equal rights, before, during, and after marriage. Since the Second World War, the clause "the husband is the head of the matrimonial union" has been struck out of the legislation of most European countries. This has happened in Belgium, for example, but Holland, in contrast to the general tendency, has upheld the principle.[42] Does this modern tendency do violence to a biblical datum, and should Christians, taking their stand on the Bible, oppose it?

In the first place, it is of importance to note that Paul does not employ the term "head of the family" or *pater familias.* He refers to the husband as the "head of the woman," although it is evident that the husband exercises authority over the children.[43] This does, however, indicate that it is not simply a formal question of man as head of the family, but a more fundamental question of man as head of the woman, even though what is in the end implied is that the man is the "head of his wife." The generalisation, the "head of the woman," is derived from the Genesis account, and the fact that Paul refers his proposition to the account of the creation—this emerges from his argument in connection with the veiling of women—provides us with one element for the solution of this problem. His general proposition and his particular proposition (the place of the woman in marriage and the family) are fundamentally one, despite a certain distinction.

This is clearly so, because he advances the same biblical arguments for both: the woman must be veiled during religious meetings because "the head of a woman is her husband" (1 Cor xi. 3), and the woman must be subject to the man in marriage because "the husband is the head of the wife" (Eph v. 22–3). This position, the "head of the woman," has a biblical basis: "the woman was taken out of man." This is one element—the first—in the solution of the problem, since it is clear that Paul regards the actual social status of woman as something ordained by creation. His evidence for this is the account provided in Genesis; but it is characteristic that he blends data from the older Yahwist account of the creation with the more recent Priestly tradition.

The Yahwist account in Genesis offers an "androcentric" view of creation. First man was created, then woman. This account was, in its very formulation, dependent upon the actual social status of woman which was prevalent at the time when the tradition gained its form. First the 'ādhām was created; later, a second being was taken out of this 'ādhām, and these two beings were, in their relationship to each other, 'iš (man), and 'iššāh (woman). The 'ādhām was later identified with the 'iš, the man, and the woman was at this period regarded as a kind of "second edition" of the man.[44] The view revealed by this account of the creation without doubt relies on the actual, historically conditioned status of woman at the time. It is a biblical view, but the assertion itself is not biblical, in the sense that it is revelatory, but rather a framework within which divine revelation could come to men.

The Priestly account in Genesis is quite different. In this account, the 'ādhām existed from the very beginning as two persons in a complementary sexual relationship with each other,[45] and there is no mention of the man being the first being and the woman being the second, "taken out of the man." The Priestly account also says that this "mankind" (that is, man-and-woman) is the "image of God."

It is remarkable that Paul should follow the androcentric conception of the Yahwist account and the idea of the "image of God" of the Priestly account, but interpret this "image of God" in the light of the Yahwist tradition: "The man is the image and glory of God, but woman is the glory of man. For man was not made from [= was not taken out of] woman, but woman from man. Neither was man created for woman, but woman for man" (1 Cor xi. 7–9). That the man is the image of God and the woman the image (or glory) of the man is therefore a rabbinical and Pauline confusion of two distinct and unequal categories of data: a social and historical datum which conditioned the Old Testament view, resulting in the androcentric idea that woman was "taken out of the man," was interpreted in the light of a theological datum, namely that of mankind as the image of God, with the result that the social and historical datum itself became theology.

It is now clear what Paul means when he says that the man is "the head of the woman." *Kephalē* (head) can be the translation both of *rô'š* (head) and of *rešîth* (beginning or principle). It is true that *kephalē* was not used by the secular Greek writers to mean *arkhē* (beginning or cause). On the other hand, however, the hebrew *rô'š* (head) was translated only once by *arkhē* (beginning or principle) in the Greek Septuagint, and normally by *kephalē*, whereas *arkhē* was used to translate *rešîth* (beginning of first principle).[46] This confusion did not escape Paul. *Kephalē* (head) is used by Paul, in the context of the relationship between man and woman, to mean none other than what he was aiming to demonstrate in 1 Cor ix, namely, "first the man, then the woman," since the woman was taken out of the man. This becomes even clearer in 1 Tim ii. 13: "Adam was formed first (*prōtos*), then (*eita*) Eve." Thus *kephalē* here has not so much the meaning of "head" as of *arkhē*—the first, both chronologically and hierarchically.

I do not wish in any way to deny that *kephalē* has the maning of "head" in Paul, but simply to point to the fact that the meaning of "first" and "priority" is very prominent here, just as it is in the Latin *caput* and the French *chef* as well as the English "head" itself. "Head" therefore does not simply point to an organic unity between the "head," the man, and the "body," the woman, in Eph v. 22–32. It indicates above all a hierarchy in this organism—the first and leading function of the man, and the second and subordinate function of the woman.

To this contemporary social pattern, in which the man had priority over the woman, Paul gave a theological substructure by means of an appeal to the Yahwist account of the creation, in which the woman's position and function are a reflection of her position and function in the social system of that time—something which was to be completely overcome in the later account of the creation. In other words, although Paul had recourse to Genesis, the actual source of his assertion was still an actual social situation in which woman occupied a subordinate position. This is apparent from his argument in 1 Cor xi. 8–9, which is based on the second and older Genesis account, in which the woman was fashioned from the man's rib.[47]

Summarising the results of our investigation so far, we can say that Paul gave a theological superstructure to a factual situation which was reflected in the household codes and was accepted as a human ethos—the situation of the wife's subjection to her husband—and to the generally inferior and secondary position of woman in society, and that he did this by referring to the second and older Genesis account of the creation, in which the assertion of the woman's subordinate position was itself a reflection of an actual social situation.

This, however, still does not settle the matter finally, since Paul says in Eph v. 23: "the husband is the head of the wife as Christ is the head of the church." Many scholars have concluded from this that the ultimate establishment of the husband as the head of the family is a New Testament datum, by virtue of this analogous relationship between Christ and the church. This is, I feel, rather too hasty a conclusion. In 1 Cor xi. 3, Paul had already called the man the "head of the woman." I have already discussed in detail what Paul means by this, in my analysis of his defence of the actually subordinate, "veiled" position of woman in society. It is obvious that the epistle to the Ephesians, which continually stresses the point that Christ is the head of the church, makes use of this analogy when the "household codes" are introduced at the end of the epistle, and thus the woman's subjection to the man as the "first," and her "head."

Paul does, of course, emphasize that this situation should be experienced "in the Lord," as he does in the parallel text of Col iii. 18, in the phrase "as is fitting in the Lord." How better could he express this fact in the epistle to the Ephesians, with its repeated references to Christ as the head of the church, than by the analogy "as Christ is the head of the church"? The chief function of the man is not somehow *inferred* from the mystery of Christ as a kind of conclusion here; what Paul does is to associate the *already existing and generally accepted* position of the man as head with Christ—and there is all the difference in the world between the two. Moreover, it is already clear in 1 Cor xi that this function of the man was not a theological fact, but a situation that was already present in society to which Paul gave a theological superstructure.

We are obviously bound to conclude, therefore, that Paul is saying no more than that Christians should experience the existing social structure of marriage and the family "in the Lord"— that, in other words, the married man should "follow Christ" in marriage and family life, and the married woman should "follow the church." The biblical and dogmatic fact of the unity existing between Christ and his church and the dogmatic influence of this unity on the unity— the "one flesh"—of man and woman in marriage on the one hand, and, on the other, Paul's attempt to provide a purely social datum—the man as "head" and the woman as "subject," occupying a subordinate position—with a theological basis, cut across each other in this passage in the epistle to the Ephesians.

It is of course true that it is only now, when we are confronted with the problem of marriage in its present form, that we are in a position to make this scriptural distinction clear and to deal with it thematically. It is also true that Paul was not conscious of it, or at least not fully conscious—at a later stage I shall attempt to show that he was to some extent aware of this distinction. But the constant rereading of Scripture at different periods of man's development, and in the light of the particular situation in which a reader is placed, does not of itself result in "enegesis" rather than exegesis. The modern situation is only a stimulus which confronts us with this particular problem.

In the first place, we must always bear in mind that marriage is a secular reality which has entered salvation. As a *human* reality, this datum is based on the essence of man as an essence that only is itself, only becomes itself, within history. As a community of parents and children, marriage has essentially a social aspect—it is a community which of its very nature calls for a unifying or leading principle. In an androcentric society, a "man's world," this principle is automatically ascribed to the man. I do not mean to claim that today the woman is the unifying principle, but philosophical and other studies more and more emphasize both the husband and the wife, in their marital unity of one flesh, as the main principle of marriage and the family.[48]

It will be necessary to go into this question in the synthesis which follows, since it certainly does not come within the scope of the purely biblical examination of the subject. Whether the man or the woman should occupy the position of authority in marriage and in the family is a matter of human and historical significance. It is in any case not an arbitrary question, but arises from the essence of marriage itself. In this sense a "natural law" is involved, the inviolable norm which exists in the human values of married life; but the content of this particular norm is a question of a growing historical insight. There are societies in which the woman is the head of the family, though these are exceptional. But is this fact less "natural" than the fact of the man as the head?

This brings us to the problem of the meaning of "natural" and its evolution, which is a question that can only be answered in the synthesis. For the present I can do no more than say that the revelation of salvation does not change the essentially human and historical significance of these values. Revelation can only confirm man's consciousness of the "natural law" in this—in his search for what is objectively and essentially human in varying circumstances. But of course the whole question turns on the precise meaning of the "natural law" in this particular case, namely that of marital relationships. Moreover, it will be obvious that, before Paul, or the teaching authority of the church, can be said to *confirm* a "natural law," this natural law must first show itself as such.

How can a natural law be actually confirmed by salvation or revelation so long as the precise demands of this natural law are not apparent to the community? Revelation, it is true, does in actual fact confirm the "natural law," but for us (*quoad nos*) it cannot confirm anything that does not appear to be natural law at the time. Reflecting as a theologian on the assertions made by the exegetes, one can but say that Paul only confirms the assertion that the husband is the "head of the wife" as a natural law in the light of salvation, if it is clear that we are actually—in this instance—dealing with a natural law. So long as this is not apparent or evident—indeed, so long as it is not fully substantiated—we can only conclude that there is nothing to prove that Paul can demonstrate any more in Eph v. 22–4 and 1 Cor xi than that the Christian is bound to experience actual contemporary family relationships "in the Lord."

In Paul's own time the man, as husband and father, was the head of the wife and of the whole family. For this reason Paul was able, in his revelation of the relationship between Christ and his church, in which Christ was in fact the head, not only to disclose the very profound meaning of Christian marriage as "one flesh," but to use this reality as a suitable image for the ethos generally accepted at the time of the wife's complete subjection to her husband. In other words, it is a delicate operation which must be carried out here in connection with the dogmatic datum: the relationship between Christ and his church was made present in a special way in Christian marriage, but the idea of "head" and "subjection," which is real in the case of the relationship between Christ and the church, was in marriage only a fact determined by social and historical conditions. Paul was able to combine the two aspects of the one image, but from the exegetical and the theological point of view it is by no means evident that the man was established as head of the family *by revealed truth,* or that revealed truth confirmed natural law to the effect that the "husband is head of the wife."

At this stage of our examination of the subject it is hardly possible to reach any definite conclusions at all. The foregoing does not in itself refute the idea of the man as head of the family. All it does is to say that Paul can be regarded as having sanctioned a natural law in the light of salvation only if it is clear that there is a question of such natural law being involved in the human and historical significance of the family. Whether this is so or not will have to be made clear in our phenomenological and philosophical analysis of the relationship between husband and wife in marriage and the family. Even in the case of church pronouncements in which the man is called head of the family we are no nearer to a solution of the dogmatic part of the problem, unless such statements are borne out by an appeal to Paul. The defence of this principle can have the same significance as Paul's defence of the veil—that is, it may be meaningful but at the same time determined by social and historical factors, at least so long as it is not clearly evident that we are faced with an ethical norm of "natural law," or so long as it does not provide an intrinsically comprehensible justification which compels us to follow the particular value judgments concerned.

We may therefore conclude that what is involved in Paul's assertion, "the husband is the head of the wife," is an experience "in the Lord" of an existing pattern of society and of family life, in which an absolute—though historically conditioned—datum of "natural law" may be implied. Moreover, Paul's tendency to provide these hierarchical structures which were already present in society with a "theological" basis, and thus to give them an independent value, is clearly expressed in this assertion, with the result that we get the impression that we are dealing here with a constant and unchangeable structure bestowed on marriage by God himself. In the New Testament there is as yet no explicit recognition that revelation does not exclude the growth of human awareness, or the development of the historical significance of the values in this and similar spheres of life which have, in the first instance, a secular and existential significance.

That Paul does tend to provide existing situations with a theological superstructure is confirmed by the fact that it is apparent from the texts themselves that he is himself conscious of the relative value of his own assertions. Paul, who obviously insisted on his assertion, "the husband is the head of the wife," being accepted without question and put into practical effect by his Christians, nonetheless realised that it was necessary for him to bring out the various shades of meaning present in it. Although, as we have already seen, he was generally content to allow ordinary secular structures to take their own course, and merely to impress upon Christians the need to experience them as Christians, he clearly felt impelled, in the light of his own experience of the mystery of Christ, to place his universal vision in perspective. His general statement in the epistle to the Galatians is evidence of this: "Now [that is, in Christ] there is neither Jew nor Greek; there is neither slave nor free; there is neither male nor female [= neither man nor woman]." (Gal iii. 26–8; see also 2 Cor v. 17 and Mt xii. 25.) In the particular case of the conjugal duties of the husband and the wife, he also stated the principle of the equality of the two persons (1 Cor vii. 3–4, 12), thus breaking completely with the double morality that conceded more to the husband than to the wife. In addition to this he also modified his thesis that the husband was the head of the wife—"for man was not made from [= taken out of] woman, but woman from man" and "man was not created for woman, but woman for man" (1 Cor xi. 8–9)—in its immediate context by saying: "*Nevertheless,* in the Lord, woman is not independent of man nor man of woman; for as the woman was made from man, *so man is now born of woman.* And all things are from God" (1 Cor xi. 11–12). The inferior position of the woman, assumed in the Old Testament, though certainly not substantiated by the biblical theology of the Genesis account, is interpreted in the light of Christian experience—"in the Lord"—as a complementary interrelationship—"man is *born of* woman." From Christianity Paul came to a more anthropological view of human relationships. We have already seen how, in the light of Christianity and of Christian love, which makes use of the human interrelationships of ordinary secular structures, Paul inwardly transformed this human fellowship, and saw the woman, though subject to the man, as his "sister" in Christ. Paul was not aiming to reduce all social relationships to the same level, but rather to permeate them with the leaven of a Christian and transcendent vision. This was evident in what he had to say concerning the relationship between masters and their slaves. He was no Spartacus—not even a Christian Spartacus—but an eschatological Christian. Christian experience "in the Lord" of the actually present, existing, human and social relationships of subordination changes the real and basic meaning of this subordination for Paul. (He also attributes to Christ subordination to the Father; "subordination" is for him a matter of "hierarchical order" and has in itself no unfavourable connotation.) "Love your wives as Christ loved the Church" (Eph v. 25)—this task which husbands had with regard to their wives inwardly transformed the male position of authority and gave it a primacy of love.[49] At the same time it is important not to lose sight of the fact that Paul is here referring to *agapē*—to Christian love as a gift of God in the Spirit. The New Testament ethic is not distinguished by new norms for marriage and sexuality, but by a Christian view of man as having been received into Christ's redeeming grace. The Petrine text, "Likewise you husbands, live considerately [in marriage] with your wives, bestowing honour on the woman as the weaker sex, since you are joint heirs of the grace of life" (1 Pet iii. 7), is a typical expression of this vision. The epistle of Peter, from which this text is taken, combines a secular and a Christian datum. "Give honour to the woman as the weaker sex" is a characteristic example of the new sensitivity which was emerging in the Hellenistic world even before the coming of Christianity, but the epistle bases this courteous treatment of women on the conferment of grace equally on both men and women in Christ. There is no equality of nature between man and woman in society, but an all-embracing equality in dignity of the sexes "in the Lord."

One of the results of this Christian leavening of the "natural" social relationships is that women obtained a place in the very early apostolic church which must have caused something of a sensation in contemporary society. In the first place, Christ himself, acting in complete contradiction to contemporary custom, had talked with women in the street. The apostles were astonished by this behaviour on Christ's part, but they dared not draw his attention to it. (Jn iv. 7–11, 27; see also Mt viii. 14 ff.; Lk xiii. 10–17; viii. 1–3.) Initially, women were also permitted to speak in the community of believers. (Acts ii. 17–18; even 1 Cor xi. 5, in contrast with 1 Cor xi. 34.) They too were charismatically inspired (Acts xxi. 9). Women also took part in the election of Matthias to the ranks of the apostles (Acts i. 14, 26). There were many women in the service of the gospel (Col iv. 15; 1 Cor i. 11; Rom xvi. 1, 6, 12, 15; Phil iv. 2), and widows occupied a prominent place in the community (1 Tim v. 9).[50] Indeed, they even gave instruction in the faith (Acts xviii. 26). This was, of course, entirely alien to the Jewish spirit, and, although it was to some extent intellgible to the Hellenistic world, it nonetheless represented a distinct break with the established views of the time on the position of woman in society. It was only as a result of certain less happy experiences that the pastoral epistles show evidence of a reaction against it.

It is quite clear, then, that the Pauline (and, for that matter, the Petrine) assertions concerning the subjection of the woman to the man are not dogmatic reactions on Paul's part, but a question of ecclesiastical and hierarchical pastoral guidance within a definite historical setting—a policy in pastoral matters which required arguments to substantiate it and to make it meaningful. The theological lesson to be drawn from this is that having established that this is basically a question of a variable social and historical factor does not in fact clear the matter up once and for all—there still remain the question of the church's conduct in pastoral affairs, and the question of personal decision on grounds of individual conscience. Whether or not the attitude which Paul adopted in this matter is—from the Christian point of view—the only possible one, is quite a different question. In the history of the church there are many cases of the hierarchy taking a "Pauline" attitude, and in such cases the doctrinal background is mingled with an appreciation of the factual situation as a function of the church's pastoral guidance. The policy actually followed by the church in these cases is not the only one that she could have followed, but it deserves respect as a corporate decision on grounds of conscience on the part of the authoritative body. And so, both in the case of Paul and in the case of papal documents dealing with problems relating to this world, it is important always to distinguish betgween the "ethical norm" and the concrete "moral obligations" which are at once conditioned by the prevailing situation at the time and also present themselves as the ethical "rules of behaviour" in a given period.[51]

The Condemnation of *Porneia*

Christianity of the New Testament period accepted the "household codes" as rules of conduct in domestic life, but, as we have seen, they were deepened in the light of man's community with Christ and, where necessary, brought into line with Christian thought. The New Testament also shows a sharp reaction against both the sexual excesses of the Hellenistic world and the Manichean heretical views of marriage according to which women especially were regarded as corrupt. This is particularly noticeable in the pastoral epistles. In the first epistle to Timothy, for example, we read that these people—i.e., those who held heretical views of this kind—rejected marriage and the use of certain foods, although "God created [these] to be received with thanksgiving by those who believe and know the truth. For everything created by God is good, and nothing is to be rejected if it is received with thanksgiving; for then it is consecrated by the word of God and prayer" (1 Tim iv. 3–5; see also 1 Thess iv. 3–6). The epistle to the Hebrews has this to say about marriage: "Let marriage be held in honour among all, and let the marriage bed [= married life] be undefiled; for God will judge the immoral and adulterous (Heb xiii. 4). In the first epistle to the Thessalonians, Paul says: "Each one of you [should] know how to take a wife for himself in holiness and honour, not in the passion of lust, like heathen who do not know God" (1 Thess iv. 4–5). Chaste living within marriage as well—which here certainly does not mean abstinence, but chastity in marital relationships—is therefore a question of man's practical experience of God: "Whoever disregards this [that is, these admonitions concerning the Christian experience of married life], disregards not man but God, who gives his Holy Spirit to you" (1 Thess iv. 8).

Nowhere in the New Testament is there any explicit commandment that marriage should be monogamous or any explicit commandment forbidding polygamy. This presented no concrete problem: monogamous marriage was accepted as a point of departure. Sexual intercourse outside marriage (Jn viii. 41; 1 Cor vi. 12 ff.), sodomy, and homosexual relationships were condemned as sinful (Jude 7; Rom i. 24–7). So were prostitution (1 Cor vi. 12 ff.), which at that time was still practised in the temple, and pederasty (1 Cor vi. 9). The sexual aberrations—*porneia* in all its forms—so common in the cities of the Greco-Roman world were briefly but decisively repudiated by the New Testament.

In connection with the rejection of prostitution in the New Testament, there is a passage in Paul which shows clearly how the author had an anthropological view of marital relationships—the "becoming one" of marriage—and at the same time provided a Christological background for this:

> The body is not meant for immorality, but for the Lord, and the Lord for the body. And God raised the Lord and will also raise us up by his power. Do you not know that your bodies are members of Christ? Shall I therefore take the members of Christ and make them the members of a prostitute? Never! Do you not know that he who joins himself to a prostitute becomes one body with her? For it is written, "the two shall become one." But he who is united to the Lord becomes one spirit with him . . . Do you not know that your body is a temple of the Holy Spirit within you, which you have from God? You are not your own; you were bought with a price. So glorify God in your body. [1 Cor vi. 12–20.]

This passage ought to be an inspiration to us in our dogmatic consideration of the whole question of marriage in Paul. The apostle recognised that the Christian is closely bound to the glorified Christ even in his physical being. To emphasize this, Paul refers to the resurrection in which our bodies will reflect the glory of Christ's "spiritual" body, and this destiny is already in a sense present for our bodies by virtue of baptism. Belonging to the "body of the Lord," the Christian's own body is, so to speak, the body of Christ, so that he no longer has control of it, to use it against the will of Christ. Intercourse in marriage is a "becoming one flesh." Association with a harlot is an offence against the "one spirit" which the Christian has become with

Christ. The "one flesh" which the Christian forms with Christ in belonging to his body, the church, is here seen to be "one spirit," not in the later, "ghostly" sense of "spiritual," but in the original New Testament sense—the baptized Christian forms a *living community* with Christ. Paul is not seeking to establish a connection here between the "one flesh" which baptized partners in marriage form and the "one spirit" of the marriage covenant of the believer with Christ. All that he does is to contrast fornication with the living community with Christ. These are mutually exclusive, and Paul expresses this fact by contrasting "one flesh" and "one spirit." There is, as Eph v. 22–32 so clearly shows, no contrast between the "one flesh" of married Christians and the "one spirit" which the believer forms with Christ. This idea is a very rewarding one from the dogmatic point of view; and, from the anthropological point of view, the text implies that the sex act is not a superficial one, in which the person remains outside—on the contrary, the person is deeply involved. That is why intercourse with a prostitute is not—as the Corinthians, with their false conception of freedom, thought it to be—a "liberation" (1 Cor vi. 12–16), but rather an enslavement, of the person. True liberation consists in subjection to Christ. Paul was thinking here of the temple of Aphrodite at Corinth, in which those who gave themselves to a prostitute believed that they were dedicating themselves to the deity. This "personal" character of religious prostitution in the temple was prominent in Paul's mind throughout this argument. The idea of the body as the "temple of God" was, moreover, already well-known in Hellenistic philosophy, and had become a current term among the fashionable thinkers of those times. But this "theistic" view was given a deeper meaning by Paul: Christ had bought our bodies by his redemption, so that they belonged legally to him. In other words, they were no longer *sui iuris*, having the rights of a freeman, but *iuris Christi*—they belonged legally to Christ. (The terminology is reminiscent of that used in connection with the ransoming of slaves, vi. 20, who were regarded as bodies—*sōmata*—or things.) This vision was to have a deep influence on marriage teaching.

It should also be noted that the problem of the relationship between married love and the foundation of the family or "procreation" is not dealt with in the New Testament. It was assumed that there would be love between both the partners and the children in Christian family life. The problem of not wanting children is not discussed at all in the New Testament. Paul in fact only deals with love (especially in Eph v. 22–33) and with the need to experience sexuality in a Christian way (especially in 1 Cor vii) in his basic expositions on the subject of marriage. The problem of "children" in marriage appears not to have existed in the apostolic church, in contrast with the patristic period, when attempts were made to find a solution to such problems by abandoning unwanted children as foundlings or even by abortive means which may or may not have been effective.

The pastoral epistles show how the New Testament idea of Christian celibacy for the sake of the kingdom of God began to acquire its first concrete institutional form, and it is worth remarking that it occurred precisely in connection with those who held office in the church—*episkopoi, presbuteroi,* and *diakonoi*. True celibacy was not imposed as a condition of acceptance to office in the church, but office-bearers were forbidden to contract a second marriage on the later death of their wives, or on separation on grounds of conversion to Christianity.[52] What is more, widows who were assigned to a function within the church were not permitted to remarry (1 Tim v. 9), whereas young widows who had no function within the church were advised to remarry (1 Tim v. 14). It is clear, therfore, that the celibate ideal, which had been advanced by Paul especially, tended to be associated above all with those who held office in the church, for not remarrying was seen, in 1 Cor vii, as we have already noted, to be in accordance with the universal eschatological call to complete abstinence.

Conclusion

It would be quite impossible for me to summarize in a few words the whole New Testament conception of marriage with its dogmatically comprehensive and ethically oriented content. All that I can usefully do here is to draw attention briefly to a few points which spring to mind, since these may help to point the way in the exploration of the experience of marriage in the course of the church's history which follows.

Marriage is a secular reality with a distinctively human significance which must be experienced "in the Lord." It is not simply a fact of creation, but something which has entered salvation. Baptism has conferred a special and separate meaning on marriage. On the other hand, it is not possible to define Christian marriage without at the same time referring to the eschatological call to abstinence. A remarkable tension is disclosed in the New Testament: on the one hand there is a decisive assertion of the goodness of a morally directed sexual life within marriage, an assertion which even stresses the mutual loving sexual obligations of marriage which may not be neglected for ascetic reasons; but, on the other hand, there is a reference to the *Eskhaton* which is present in marriage itself, and because of which Christian marriage is deprived of the absolute value that it possessed in the Old Testament.

What is also especially striking in connection with the New Testament view of marriage is the definitive aspect of marriage as a commitment. It is a venture for life, a bond which is not only a call personally to forge marriage into an existential union of marital interrelationship and personally to grow together in loving fidelity into an indissoluble unity, but also—on a basis of the structure of creation made even firmer by baptism—an objective union transcending free self-dissolution and existential disruption. This fact is a unique aspect of the Christian revelation of salvation—a unique fact which, in its absolute and unconditional quality, has no natural foundation apart from the saving fact of baptism, and which can only be approached and understood as a datum or revelation. This biblical view seems the clearest basis for the sacramentalism of marriage—the phenomenon which occurs only in the sacraments of the church, whereby a secular reality, with its distinctive historical significance, is inwardly transformed into a religious reality. This definitive surrender to another person, without any foreknowledge of what may happen in the future, is the human manifestation of man's definitive surrender to the other being, God. According to Jesus' Synoptic *logion*, marriage means a consecration for life to a fellow human being—in this case, to one's chosen partner in life. Paul in his turn interpreted this as a consecration in the same sense as Christ devoted his life to the church. In utter devotion man consecrates himself, by virtue of the baptism which he has received, to God in Christ. The indissolubility of Christian marriage is connected in the most intimate way with the definitive Christian character of the community of grace with God. For this reason the New Testament ideal of marriage may be seen to reflect the unconditional and absolute quality which by definition is peculiar to the reception of grace as man's making a gift of himself to the living God. But an equally clear conclusion is that this demand can be accepted in marriage only from within the community of grace with God; outside the explicit confession of Christ it must, inevitably, have a relative value. This is apparent from the so-called "Pauline privilege," which really does no more than to say that it is only Christian marriage which possesses this distinctive, separate, and absolute value—a value which is present only as a tendency in the marriages of unbaptized persons.

The church has given form to this biblical vision of marriage throughout the course of history. It has done this in historically developing forms, some of which have been more fortunate and more successful than others. In Volume II [of the author's *Marriage: Human Reality and Saving Mystery*] I shall try to trace this historical growth, at least in its clearest and most crucial aspects, in the life of the church, before going on to provide a systematic exposition of marriage.

Notes

1. See also Mk x. 1–12; Lk xvi. 18. Paul, referring to Christ's *logion*, affirms this in 1 Cor vii. 10–11.

2. Unlike the other synoptists, who had only the Jewish legal practice of the male right to repudiation in mind, Mark interpolates a parallel text referring to the wife's repudiation of her husband. This practice was accepted in the Greco-Roman world, and the influence of Greco-Roman civilisation in this particular case was moreover already being felt in Palestine. See also 1 Cor vii. 10–11.

3. J. Rinzema, *Huwelijk en echtscheiding in Bijbel en moderne samenleving*, Aalten (1961), p. 140.

4. This is the statement of a representative of the Reformed Churches, J. Rinzema, *Huwelijk en echtscheiding*, p. 146. In fact the Reformed Churches in general accept two possible grounds for divorce— adultery and wilful desertion—although there is much more doubt concerning the second. See, among other works, the pastoral letter of the General Synod of the Dutch Reformed Church concerning marriage (*Herderlijk schrijven van de Generale, Synode der Nederlandse Hervormde Kerk over het huwelijk*, The Hague [1952]).

5. The interpretation of "separation from the body" goes back to Jerome, *In Matt.* 19. 9 (*PL*, 26. 135).

6. Hermas, *Pastor* (*Mand.* 4. 1. 5–8). The practice that the unfaithful party had to be repudiated was fairly general in the first three centuries. From the fourth century onwards, however, this obligation began to lapse. Repudiation of the guilty party was still permitted, but remarriage was still not allowed, as in the ante-Nicene period. Nonetheless, the rules of excommunication which previously applied to remarriage were abolished. See J. Arendzen, "Ante-Nicene Interpretations of the Sayings on Divorce," *JTS*, 20 (1919), pp. 230–41. For the question of excommunication on remarriage after separation because of adultery, see, among other works, the *Canones Apostolorum* which are included in the *Constitutiones Apostolicae*, viii, 47, can. 48. See also Funk, *Didaskalia et Constitutiones Apostolicae*, Paderborn (1905), pt. 1, p. 579.

7. See, for example, Tertullian, *De monogamia*, 10 (*PL*, 2. 942–3); Justin, *Apol.* 2. 2 (*PG*, 6. 443–7).

8. "Quamvis autem ex causa fornicationis liceat tori separationem facere, non tamen aliud matrimonium contrahere fas est, cum matrimonii vinculum legitime contracti perpetuum est" (DS 1327 [DB 702]).

9. Ambrosiaster, *Comm. in 1 Cor.* 7. 10 (*PL*, 17. 218). Lactantius, who was not a theologian, says more or less the same in his *Epitome* 66 (*PL*, 6. 1080).

10. See J. Dupont, *Mariage et divorce dans l'Evangile*, Bruges (1959), pp. 83–4; especially *n.* 2, in which the author refutes the hypothesis of a post-apostolic interpolation.

11. See, for example, H. Braun, *Spätjüdisch-häretischer und frühchristlicher Radikalismus*, BHT, pt. 2 (1957), p. 89, *n.* 3; p. 109, *n.* 1; p. 1210, *n.* 4. This author, however, concludes that Matthew impairs the authentic tradition of Jesus. The priority of Mark is moreover denied by J. Bonsirven, *Le divorce dans le Nouveau Testament*, Paris and Douai (1948), p. 27.

12. See, for example, Num v. 11–33.

13. *Le divorce dans le Nouveau Testament*; see also "'Nisi fornicationis causa.' Comment résoudre cette 'crux interpretum'?", *RSR*, 35 (1948), pp. 422–64. Many exegetes follow Bonsirven's interpretation, including H. Cazelles, "Mariage," *DBS*, 5 (1957), p. 934; M. Berrouard, "L'indissolubilité du mariage dans le Nouveau Testament," *LV*, 4 (1952), p. 26. See also J. Kahmann, "Evangelie en echtscheiding," *NKS*, 49 (1949), pp. 11–18.

14. There is considerable disagreement among exegetes concerning the structure of this "apostolic decree." What it comes down to ultimately is that there were probably two apostolic councils, but for theological reasons these were reported by Luke as one as far as their content was concerned. If this is so, then the first council must have been attended by all the apostles, including Paul, and the debate conducted under the leadership of Peter. The principal topic for discussion at this first council must have been the

significance of the Mosaic law for Christians, and especially the importance of circumcision (Acts xv. 1–12). A second council must have taken place within the community of Jerusalem, headed—in the absence of Peter—by James. The main topics for debate must have been the relevance to Christians of the dietary laws and *porneia* (Acts xv. 13–39). See, among other works, S. Giet, "L'assemblée apostolique et le décret de Jérusalem," *RSR*, 39 (1951), pp. 203–20; P. Benoit, "La primauté de saint Pierre selon le Nouveau Testament," *Ist*, 2 (1995), pp. 305–34; J. Dupont, "Pierre et Paul à Antioche et à Jérusalem," *RSR*, 45 (1957), pp. 42–60, 225–59. The consequence of this is that—in all probability—the apostolic decree came chronologically after Paul's first epistle to the Corinthians and also after that to the Galatians.

15. J. Dupont, *Mariage et divorce*, pp. 29 and 87.

16. As has already been indicated, this is no doubt the significance of the merging together by Matthew of what were originally two separate *logia* on Christ's part (Mt xix. 1–8 and xix. 9–12). See J. Dupont, *Mariage et divorce*, pp. 161–220. For a criticism of this, see M. Zerwick in *VD*, 38 (1960), pp. 193–212; M. Boismard in *RB*, 67 (1960), pp. 463–4.

17. A. Kuiters, "Kleine Dogmatiek van het huwelijk," *SC*, 35 (1960), especially pp. 111–50. The exegetical section of this appears under the name of A. Hulsbosch.

18. A. Kuiters, p. 125.

19. Well-known exegetes such as Vogt, Sickenberger, Allgeier, and others support this view. For a summary of their exegesis, see V. Holzmeister, "Die Streitfrage über die Ehescheidungstexte bei Mt.," *Bbl*, 26 (1945), pp. 133–46, and J. Dupont, *Mariage et divorce*, pp. 98 ff.

20. The text is nonetheless interpreted by almost all exegetes as a release from the bond of marriage. But not so long ago, besides several Protestant scholars, a Catholic exegete raised the question as to whether there is really any reference in 1 Cor vii. 12–16 to the "Pauline privilege: see P. Dulau, "The Pauline Privilege; is it promulgated in the first Epistle to the Corinthians?", *CBQ*, 13 (1951), pp. 146–52. In its defence of the Pauline privilege, the Catholic Church has never explicitly and directly based its teaching on 1 Cor vii. 15. See DS 768 and 778 (DB 405 and 408), and (*Casti Conubii*) DS 3712 (DB 2236). Only a declaration of the Holy Office, dated 11 July 1886, explicitly connects the "Pauline privilege" with this text of Paul. It will be necessary to examine how far this privilege is connected with the apostolic "power of the keys" in the synthesis that follows.

21. E. Hirsch, "Eine Randglosse zu 1 Kor. 7," *ZST*, 3 (1925–6), pp. 50–60. This point is dealt with very clearly.

22. Paul here disregards the question whether or not there is salvation for those who are not of the community of faith. Salvation comes from Christ, and salvation falls to the share of him who believes in Christ and is baptized in him. These formal statements do not therefore aim to deny the religious character of "Gentile" or "Jewish" marriage. Their further and more precise formulation is not the function of biblical exegesis, but of theology.

23. See A. Büchler, "The Levitical Impurity of the Gentile in Palestine before the Year 70," *JQR*, 17 (1926–7), pop. 1–81.

24. This is presupposed in Mt viii. 7; Jn xviii. 28; 1 Cor vii. 14 and Acts x. 28.

25. See J. Jeremias, *Infant Baptism in the First Four Centuries*, Philadelphia (Westminster, 1961); O. Cullmann, *Baptism in the New Testament*, Naperville, Ill. (Allenson, 1958).

26. See H. Braun, "Exegetische Randglossen zum 1. Korintherbrief," *TV*, 1 (1948–9), especially pp. 39 ff.

27. See Acts xvi. 30–34. The phrase "you and all your house" appears (with slight variations) in Acts xvi. 31; xvi. 34; xviii. 8; xi. 14; 1 Cor i. 16. In Acts xvi. 14–15, there is reference to a woman and "all her household."

28. It is not always easy for us to trace the motives for certain actions in apostolic times. An example of this is the practice alluded to in 1 Cor xv. 29—that of "being baptized on behalf of the dead." The idea of "family solidarity" appears to play a part here too.

29. For the idea of "zeal" in the faith, which is of such importance for Paul in the case of mixed marriages, see J. Jeremias, "Die missionarische Aufgabe in der Mischehe (1 Cor 7. 16)," *Neutestamentliche Studien für R. Bultmann*, Berlin (1957), pp. 255–60. The author does not accept the usual translation "Wife, how do you know whether you will save your husband?", but prefers, for philological reasons, the translation: "Perhaps (who knows!) you can, O wife, save your husband," Even though the eventual meaning may be the same, this translation fits far less well than the usual translation after the preceding verse.

30. See Col iii. 18–iv. 1, 5; Eph v. 22–vi. 9; 1 Tim ii. 8–15; v. 3–8; vi. 1–2; Tit ii. 1–10; 1 Pet ii. 13–iii. 7. These lists or "moral rules" have been called "household codes" (in German, *Haustafeln,* in dutch, *huisspiegels*). See E. G. Selwyn, *The First Epistle of St. Peter,* London (1946), pp. 419–39; K. H. Schelkle, *Die Petrusbriefe. Der Judasbrief,* Freiburg i. Br. (1961), especially pp. 96–8; H. Schlier, *Der Brief an die Epheser,* Düsseldorf (1959), pp. 250–52; 287–8.

31. Epictetus, *Dissert.* 2. 14. 8, Seneca, *Epist.* 94, 1, and Stobaios, *Anthologia,* 1. 3. 53, are especially typical, the last-named expressing the Stoic doctrine of civil duties.

32. That the immediate substratum in the New Testament "codes" (see note 30 above) is Judaeo-Hellenistic is clear from the Jewish element, the "fear of God." See, for example, Eph v. 21, 33.

33. 1 Pet ii. 13; ii. 17; ii. 20b; iii. 1–2; especially iii. 7; iii. 5–6; iii. 10–12.

34. There were, of course, many gradations within this relatively lowly position. Despite the authority of the *paterfamilias,* the Roman wife enjoyed a fairly privileged position, higher than that of the Jewish wife, or even than that of the Greek wife. See J. Leipoldt, *Die Frau in der Antike und im Urchristentum,* Gütersloh (1953).

35. On the other hand, however, Paul could say quite simply in his epistles to Titus: "They are to train the young women to love their husbands and their children" (Tit ii. 4), although the word used here is not *agapāin,* as for men, but the general and secular word *philandros.*

36. Douai version. Some translations (e.g., the RSV translation) have "her husband," which limits Paul's general assertion to the relationship of marriage and the family. See my critical examination of the text.

37. Josephus, *Contra Apionem,* 2. 24.

38. *Kyria,* "lady" or "madam," as the counterpart of *kyrios,* "lord" or "sir." See J. Leipoldt, *Die Frau,* p. 47. For the influence of the successive schools of Greek philosophy, see Fustel de Coulanges, *La cité antique,* Paris (n.d.), especially the chapter "Nouvelles croyances religieuses," pp. 136 ff.

39. See L. Cerfaux, *L'Eglise des Corinthiens,* Paris (1946).

40. See R. de Vaux, "Sur le voile des femmes dans l'Orient ancien," *RB,* 44 (1935), pp. 397–412.

41. This reference by Paul is clearly to something that had already for a long time been stripped of its ancient mythical elements. Since he is speaking here about religious meetings, it is obvious that he is thinking concretely of the angels who were present during prayer, an idea that recurs frequently in the first century A.D. and in the writings of the Fathers.

42. A very clear exposition of this can be found in E. A. Luyten's inaugural address, *Hoofd der echtvereniging. Enkele rechtsvergelijkende beschouwingen naar aanleiding van de pivaatrechtelijke emancipatie der gehuwde vrouw in de wetgeving van Nederland en enige andere Europese landen,* Nijmegen (1960) ("The head of the matrimonial union. Some considerations arising from the emancipation of the married woman in the legislation of private law in the Netherlands, compared with that in some other European countries").

43. Paul speaks of the obligations of the children towards the parents, and conversely of the obligations of the father—in the exercise of his authority—towards the children (Col iii. 20–21).

44. The Aristotelian idea that woman was "as a failed man" (*De generatione animalium,* II, 3) was taken over, along with many other of Aristotle's ideas, by the medieval Christians. Another fact that was well known was that *'ādhām,* originally a generic name meaning "mankind" (Gen i. 27–8), was later used as a proper name, without the article, and identified with the man (Gen iv. 25). The transition from the generic to the proper name is particularly striking in Gen v. 1, 3–5, where *'ādhām* is used as a proper name ("Adam"), and in Gen v. 2, where it is used in the generic sense.

45. The *'ādhām,* or human being, who was created consisted of two complementary and related beings, the *zākhār* (male), and the *neqêbhāh* (female), that is, man and woman. The derivation of these words is obscure, but it would seem that the first means the "sharp" one, that is, the being with the penis, and the second the "split" one, the being with the vagina. The *zākhār* is only called "man" (*'îš*) in contrast with the *neqêbhāh,* as *'iššāh* or woman.

46. See S. Bedale, "The Meaning of *kephalē* in the Pauline Epistles," *JTS,* 5 (1954), pp. 211–15.

47. Both the general statement, "the head of the woman is the man" (1 Cor xi. 3), and the particular statement, "the husband is the head of the wife" (Eph v. 23), are based on the same Yahwist account of the creation, in which the general and the particular intersect. In Rom vii. 2, *hupandros gunē* means a "woman

placed below the men," in other words, a married woman. This is certainly the main assertion, but the subordination of woman in general was at the same time undoubtedly in Paul's mind.

48. This view has clearly not yet penetrated to the sphere of legislation, which still aims to safeguard the separate personal rights of the husband and the wife.

49. See also V. Heylen, "Het hoofd van het gezin," *TT*, 1 (1961), pp. 309–28.

50. Although this was at the same time also conditioned by social factors in the hellenistic world. Widows who did not remarry enjoyed a high status in Hellenistic society.

51. In my anthropological analysis of the morality of married life I shall attempt to show how this distinction has not always been kept sufficiently in mind in connection with sexuality and marriage. An absolute ethical norm is above all an idea which is "open," pointing to the inalienable rights and duties connected with the dignity of the human person. An ethical "rule of behaviour" is, or may be, a concrete "moral obligation" which at the same time presupposes an appreciation of the actually existing situation, and which is also able to change if the situation itself changes. The ethical norm, the appreciation of human values, on the other hand, does not change, though it does develop. But this ethical norm only—and always—achieves authentic form *within* a concrete obligation and is therefore, even as norm, dynamic.

52. 1 Tim iii. 2 (the *episkopoi*); Tit i. 6 (the *presbuteroi*); 1 Tim iii. 12 (the *diakonoi*).

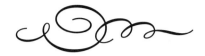

Marriage and Family in Christian History

7

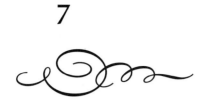

Augustine on the Nature of Marriage

Theodore Mackin

The historical setting of Augustine's thinking and writing on marriage was in great part his reaction to challenges to marriage coming from two sources that were almost polar opposites.[1] On the one side there was the Manichee condemnation of marriage, or at least of procreation, as essentially evil; on the other there was a charge against him personally coming from certain Pelagian Christians who insisted that his refutation of the Manichees was so qualified as to leave him in fundamental agreement with them.

The Manichee Christians with whom Augustine dealt were members of a worldwide religious movement that had infiltrated the Christian churches. The Manichees took their name from their prophet and founder, Mani, a Parthian born in Babylon in 216, who claimed to be as a youth the recipient of a divine revelation that disclosed to him the truth of the cosmos and of history, and that set him in a vocation to carry this disclosure to all the human race. At heart Manicheeism was Gnosticism reborn, since it proposed salvation through a perfect knowledge, or *gnosis,* and through the living out of the consequences of this knowledge.

Manichee doctrine proposed a dualistic structure of the universe. The dual and opposed elements are Good-Evil, or Light-Darkness. Behind these names it is spirit that is Light and goodness, matter in all its manifestations that is Darkness and evil. The doctrine divided the history of the universe into three epochs: the *initium,* when spirit and matter were separate, having been created by the respective good and evil deities, before the cosmic (and cosmogonic) conflict that introduced the second period, the *medium,* and formed the universe as it now exists; the *medium* is the epoch that witnessed the creation of Adam and the human race. During it spirit and matter are intermingled and are in constant conflict. But also during it the third and final epoch, the *finis,* is being prepared through the work of the Ambassadors of Light, who have succeeded one another since Adam. The *finis* will be the eschatological age, wherein the original separation of spirit and matter, of Good and Evil, will be repaired.

Meanwhile during the *medium* the entire cosmos is in struggle, and the struggle goes on in microcosm within every human being. Those who would emerge victorious from it into the Kingdom of Light must live a severely ascetic life. They are the demands of this asceticism that divide the human race into three classes of persons.

There is the tiny and elite group of the *electi,* who can live and must live the Manichee ascetic ideal in the highest degree. In its negative features this asceticism is abstention, withdrawal, separation from all that is evil in essence or leads to evil. Thus the *electi* must have nothing to do with wine, with meat, agriculture, hunting, business, sexuality, marriage. They must keep a triple guard over the person: by the *signaculum oris* (the seal over the mouth) they must avoid blasphemy and evil foods; by the *signaculum manus* (the seal on the hands) they must avoid work and the destruction of plants or animals, by the *signaculum sinus* (the seal on the duct) they must avoid any sexual activity.

The *auditores* make up the far more numerous sector of the Manichee church. Their asceticism, though obligatory, is less strict. They need fast only once a week, on Sunday. Marriage is tolerated for them, as is concubinage. But they must not procreate.

Outside the Manichee church all others are the damned, whose souls are fated to return by metempsychosis to this life after death in the bodies of animals, until eventually they end in hell for all eternity. These are the human beings who, among other kinds of evil conduct, procreate in their marriages.

The attack against Augustine from the opposite quarter came mainly from Pelagius' disciple, Julian. Again, it was that Augustine's defense of marriage against the Manichees was a half-hearted one. In truth Augustine was caught in a kind of cross-fire of twisted meanings. He insisted against the Manichees that marriages since the fall of the first parents (therefore since the dawn of creation) are not fundamentally evil. He based this insistence on evidence available to all. For even if the great majority of marriages are lived sinfully even by Christian spouses, the cause of this cannot be the state of marriage itself. Marriage can yield verifiable goods, and in fact does so among many Christian spouses.

But the Pelagians charged him with conceding too much to and even siding with the Manichees in acknowledging this fact of the sinfulness in almost all marriages. They acknowledged no real historical fall of mankind from original grace, and could thus see no fundamental difference between the human condition vis-à-vis sinfulness after the first sin and before it. Consequently by conceding the general sinfulness of marital conduct since the fall, Augustine had, they thought, acknowledged the fundamental sinfulness of marriage.

What Augustine did then, in order to counter both attacks, was to defend the fundamental goodness of marriage against the Manichees, and this on two levels, or at two moments in marriage's history. The first was marriage as God originally intended it, before its being damaged by the first sin. This was marriage as a kind of ideal institution, almost but not quite detached from its incarnation in real-life men and women. The second moment or level was marriage since the first sin, as it has been lived and will be lived in real life until the end of time. He claimed goodness for marriage in this "moment" too, but from different evidence than that supporting its pristine, ideal goodness.

The Goods of Marriage That Excuse Its Use

Augustine's claim for marriage against the Manichees was that it is good a priori because it is God's creation, and a posteriori because three observable goods are found in it. In the latter he seems to have had two meanings that are linked in marriage's history. As designed by God it is to contain these goods and can do so; and even after its being damaged by the first sin and by sinfulness ever since, many marriages (especially those of devout Christians) still contain them.

The goods he had in mind are three: fidelity (*fides*), offspring (*proles*) and the sacrament (*sacramentum*), which in his thought-system has many meanings, but seems in this case to designate persevering commitment. His first and briefest formulation of these is in *The Good of*

Marriage (Chapter 24, n. 30): "These are all the goods on account of which marriage [itself] is good: offspring, fidelity and the sacrament."[2]

He offered two other fuller formulations of these goods. In the *Commentary on the Literal Meaning of Genesis* (Book 9, Chapter 7, n. 12) he explains:

This [good] is threefold: fidelity, offspring, sacrament. Fidelity means that one avoids all sexual activity apart from one's marriage. Offspring means that a child is accepted in love, is nurtured in affection, is brought up in religion. Sacrament means that the marriage is not severed nor the spouse abandoned, not even so that the abandoner or the abandoned may remarry for the sake of children. This is a kind of rule set for marriage, by which nature's fruitfulness is honored and vicious sexual vagrancy is restrained.[3]

Yet a third formulation is in his treatise *On Original Sin* (Book 2, Chapter 39):

Marriage is therefore a good in all those elements that belong to marriage. And these are three: the orientation to procreation, the fidelity in chastity, and the sacrament of marriage. Because of the orientation to procreation it is written, "I want that the young widows should marry, bear children, become mothers of families." Because of the fidelity in chastity a wife has not authority over her body but her husband has it; as likewise a husband has not authority over his body but his wife has it. Because of the sacrament of marriage, what God has joined no man must separate.[4]

Augustine's logic in citing these goods that have been found in many marriages is that they cannot come from an essentially evil cause. But since he was pointing at evidence in real life, his claim of these three goods took on an inescapable apologetic stance. For he had elsewhere already admitted that because of the first parents' sin passed down to all succeeding generations, sexual intercourse even within marriage has been almost without exception an exercise in sinfulness. Thus these goods produced in marriage, that would otherwise have verified its goodness simply, now in Augustine's mind become excuses for marriage. Indeed if his supposition about the almost inevitable sinfulness of sexual intercourse even within Christian marriages is accurate, even these marriages need a justifying excuse. Such is his argument: even in sin-infected marriages the intent and the hope of realizing these goods provide the excuse for risking the sinfulness and even perpetrating it.

When Intercourse Is Sinful

The reasons for Augustine's thinking that sexual intercourse even within marriage is sin-infected since the fall of the first parents deserves a detailed explanation even at the cost of delaying the explanation of his understanding of the three goods. Let me borrow from Chapter 6 of *The Good of Marriage* to set out schematically his moral judgments on intercourse in different circumstances and for different motives.

1. Intercourse can be without sin only within marriage. It is in fact sinless even there if it is motivated only by the desire of conceiving a child, and provided that consent is given to no other pleasure than to that coming from anticipation of a possible conception. (It was the rare instances in which motivation is so confined and pleasure so carefully focused that produced Augustine's judgment that intercourse is almost never without sin.)

2. Intercourse is had with venial sin within marriage when a spouse engages in it impelled by concupiscent passion and/or if there is accompanying subsequent consent to the carnal pleasure attending the act. (Later, in Chapter 10, Augustine says that if one of the spouses no more than renders the marriage debt to the other passion-driven and therefore sinfully motivated spouse, he or she thereby saves the other from fornication and does not sin provided that there is no subsequent consent to the carnal pleasure in the act.)

3. Intercourse is had with mortal sin if it is with any person other than one's spouse; and it is mortally sinful also with one's spouse if it is done in any way that avoids the possibility of conception. (In Chapter 11 Augustine says that for the wife to do the latter is worse than her countenancing her husband's adultery.)

In effect, according to Augustine, since on the biblical record, as he interpreted it, Adam and Eve had intercourse for the first time only after their sin, the sole instances of sinless lovemaking with intercourse in the history of the race have been those of a married saint every century or so.

All this complex judgment follows as a necessary consequence of his theory of original sin, which I shall outline in a moment. But it is clear that Augustine saw a priori only three possible motives for lovemaking with intercourse: capitulation to concupiscent passion (sinful), conception (sinless) and consent to a spouse's concupiscent demand in order to protect him or her from worse sin (also sinless). Nowhere in his writings on the subject (in none of the titles listed in note 1 of this chapter) have I found a hint that he acknowledged a middle ground of motives for which men and women who love one another make love—among others the desire to show and to feel tenderness or gratitude, the desire to comfort and console, the simple celebration of happiness, the impulse for sheer fun, the desire to be known intimately and to know intimately.[5] Why he made no mention of these as possible motives may have been in part a consequence of the society in which he lived. The sexual arena in his twilight years of the Roman empire was as much an emotional slaughter-house as it is in our possibly twilight years of the post-Christian West. And men and women in his society did not ordinarily marry the persons they did out of love, but out of obedience to family arranging, often leaving their passion to wander elsewhere. Augustine's own experience with sexually expressed passion had for years been an agonizing struggle fought to less than a draw. Even while he was in Milan pondering baptism and had given up his mistress, taken when he was sixteen, to make way for an honorable marriage with the girl Monica had found for him, he took an interim mistress until the girl came of legal age. Somewhere in that bizarre sequence tenderness must have gotten lost and passion come to be despised.

But again his main reason for seeing almost inevitable sinfulness in marriage was his interpretation of original sin, the tragic event in the Garden of Eden and the tragic, history-long consequences of it; and joined with and doubly energizing this interpretation was that of the key portion of Chapter 5 of Paul's Epistle to the Romans.

Augustine's Interpretation of Original Sin

The narrative of the formation of the first man and woman, of their temptation and sin, contained in the second and third chapters of Genesis Augustine took without question to be a factual account of events that had transpired some four thousand years before the birth of Jesus, in a garden-like part somewhere in the Mesopotamian Valley. He would have rejected violently the suggestion that the narrative is a Hebrew parable composed in the ninth or tenth century

B.C., modeled literarily on the ancient Near Eastern creation myths, and intended by its author or authors to explain imaginatively the entry of evil and suffering into human experience—and differing from all earlier and contemporary explanations in that it insisted that this entry was by the free choice of the first human couple.

He did reject as ridiculous the opinion of some of his contemporaries that Adam's and Eve's sin was their having intercourse for the first time and prematurely against God's will, since it was clear in Genesis (he said in *De Genesi ad Litteram*, 11:41) that they had intercourse for the first time only after their sin. In countless places and in different ways he insisted that their sin was one of prideful disobedience to God's pointed command to not eat of the tree of the knowledge of good and evil. That was original sin the deed. What of original sin the inheritance, that with which every human being is infected as a consequence of his first parents' sin, and because of which Christians baptize their children? By a bitter irony that too, in Augustine's mind, is a kind of disobedience, but a disobedience carrying a sexual name. It is concupiscence.

His thinking, imagery and nomenclature for concupiscence shift focus constantly. I shall try to sort out their different meanings presently. For now a central element of his theology of original sin is to be noted. The anthropological part, so to speak, of the punishment coming to Adam and Eve was that, just as they had sinned by disobeying God's command and thereby upsetting the order of wills intended by him, so in just retribution their lower powers were always to disobey reason and will in them, thereby upsetting the order within their nature originally willed by God. Rather than obey reason and will, these lower powers are doomed to obey the stimulus of libido (the *incentivum libidinis*, as he named it).[6]

Augustine insisted on the hypothetical goodness and innocence of intercourse as God had originally intended it. He said that had Adam and Eve not sinned, and had every human being therefore lived in a paradisical state, there would indeed be intercourse, since that is the natural way for children to come into existence. But in such a situation intercourse would take place without concupiscence.[7] This means, as part of a striking religious psychology, that the genital organs of both men and women would be readied for intercourse only at the calm command of the will, itself drawn by a tranquil love.[8] These organs would obey as readily as the hand obeys the command of an artisan. They would not, as they do now, live a law of their own, defying the command of the will and moving into action impelled by a surge of passion.

Again, this disobedience of the genital organs to reason and will, which is a consequence of the one original, disobedient deed, is part of the punishment for that deed. It is the sinfulness that Adam and Eve carried about in their bodies until they died. Consequently only because of this concupiscence in their bodies did they have intercourse, and inevitably this intercourse itself was sinful. Consequently too their children, conceived by this sinful act, contract the sinfulness in their own bodies. Augustine said that the semen itself carries the corruption, the *vitium*, of sin.[9] This sinfulness is in every human being without exception, and would be there even if he or she were never to commit sin personally, because all are linked by flesh (genetically, we would say) with Adam's sinful flesh.[10]

What happened in Adam's and Eve's conceiving their children has been repeated in every conception since their time. Augustine explains this in his graphic way: "But when spouses come to the dutiful work of conceiving, the very licit and good act of intercourse, which ought to be the effect of reason in them, cannot take place without the heat of concupiscence (*ardor libidinis*). And certainly this heat, whether it follow upon one's choice or precede it, stirs one's member only by a command of its own, and shows itself too to be stirred not by a free choice but by a licentious stimulus. . . . From this concupiscence of the flesh as from the daughter of sin—which is also the mother of sin when surrendered to in shameful acts—any child that is born is itself bound by original sin."[11]

Original sin thus understood is a major ingredient in Augustine's theology of salvation. By their baptism Christians are gifted with the grace of Christ merited by his death. This grace's effect on original sin is a forgiving one in the sense of a healing. (Christ himself, despite having ordinary human flesh, was born free of sin-concupiscence because his conception was not the effect of sexual intercourse.[12]) Augustine explains that baptism forgives inherited original sin in such a way not that it ceases to exist in the baptized person, but that, though existing, it is not imputed to him as his guilt.[13] It remains sin in him in the mode of punishment. It does him no moral harm unless he consents to its stirring and enticement. Thus merely to feel concupiscence is not a sin,[14] though it does something to him even when he does not consent to it, and even though it does not go so far as to stir up his body. That is, it stirs up evil desires in him. Indeed it is sinful *libido* that causes erotic dreams and nocturnal emissions (although this is not a sinful fault) for men and women carry this sinfulness around in their bodies.[15] And though the guilt itself of this concupiscence is washed away by baptism, the concupiscence itself remains until a man's infirmity is healed by the continual, day-by-day renewing of the interior nature through prayer and good works, even as the exterior nature grows old and crumbles. But it does not die out in those who give in to it; old men can be moved by it insanely even though it can no longer stir their bodies.[16]

Augustine says that Christian marriage has this accessory good in it—that carnal concupiscence, which is bad in itself, is rescued and turned to a good use by the spouses' doing their duty of producing children. And in marriage this concupiscence is repressed by the *feeling* of parenthood when having intercourse.[17] In their intercourse Christian spouses are affected by sinful concupiscence in the measure in which they engage in it not for the motive of conceiving but in order to take pleasure in lascivious passion. Pleasure in intercourse is without sin only if it is pleasure in attaining intercourse's primary end, which is conception.[18]

Augustine was faced with the Pelagian objection asking how an infant born of baptized parents can contract original sin, since his parents have been cleansed from this sin by baptism. His answer is that even baptized persons, although their inherited sin is no longer imputed to them as guilt but is only a punishment, nevertheless pass on sin-carrying flesh to their child. This they do because their seed is sin-carrying. Baptism cleanses the soul. But it is not the soul of the child that is passed on by inheritance; it is rather the body.[19]

A baptized person who uses his concupiscence to conceive uses this evil for a good purpose.[20] Thus because of concupiscence in spouses it happens that even from the good and legitimate marriages of the children of God there are born into the world not children of God but children of this world. This happens because even the reborn (the baptized) who procreate do so not by that wherein they are children of God, but by that wherein they are still children of this world.[21]

The Nature of Concupiscence

I suggested at the beginning of this brief examination of Augustine's thought regarding sexuality that the words he uses to explain this thought exchange meanings rather freely. There is some profit in trying to do as exact a scrutiny as possible of the sexual interior of men and women that he describes. One point of profit is that since his influence on the moral theology of the centuries following him was so overpowering, we may better understand the mood he set and the details he supplied for what preachers said from thousands of pulpits and confessors advised penitents in thousands of confessionals. More than any man, more even than St. Paul, from whom he drew so much of his thought and mood, Augustine dictated the feeling of an entire civilization about sexuality. I think it is even accurate to say that the New Testament teaching about sexuality and marriage that was understood in Christendom from the fifth century onward was that teaching filtered through the mind—and certainly through the emotions—of Augustine. His nomenclature for sexual matters became the vocabulary of Christendom. And since in such large measure language determines at least popular thought, what the Christian populace has thought of sex until this century has been the thought conveyed to it in Augustine's vocabulary.

In those of his essays I have cited he uses three words quite freely as synonyms. These are *libido, concupiscentia* and *voluptas*. They are at one and the same time (1) the residual effect in men and women of Adam's sin, (2) the punishment in all of Adam's heirs for this sin, (3) this inherited sin itself, (4) the evidence of the presence of this sin, (5) a wound in everyone's nature, (6) a sickness or infection carried in this nature, and more exactly in its flesh, and (7) the cause within persons of their sinful sexual acts—which in the concrete means virtually all their sexual acts.

Libido he describes as the *indecens motus membrorum,* the unbecoming or shameful stirring of the sexual organs. Or equally, this indecent stirring is the manifestation of *libido*. What is indecent about it is that it is beyond the control of reason and will.[22] Said another way, *libido* is a kind of rebellious law of its own in genital anatomy stirring it to activity in disobedience to reason and will. An earthy phenomenon that Augustine reports again and again in descriptive definition of *libido* is this: that whereas a man's reason and will can command the performance of his hands, his feet, his tongue, his lips, even of his bladder, when it comes to the performance of conceiving a child—a good and holy duty—he loses command over the member that was created specifically for this task. He must wait patiently as it obeys its own law. Sometimes it refuses to stir when he wills it to; at other times it stirs when he wills it not to. And he laments, "Must not the freedom of human choice blush on finding that for having despised the commanding will of God it has now lost command over members that are in its own possession?" Echoing this lament is one of his incomparable epigrammatic lines: "*Ibi sumus veraciter liberi ubi non delectamur inviti*" ("Only there I am truly free where I take no pleasure against my will").[23]

Voluptas at least seems to be slightly different from *libido*. Augustine says that the semen of both men and women[24] is aroused and released by *voluptas* and with it; and *voluptas* is of course sinful. Again to the question how children could have been conceived sinlessly had Adam and Even not sinned, his reply is that both seminations would have taken place only at the command of the will.[25]

Concupiscentia seems to be the body's tendency to rebellion, its refusal to obey the command of the will. Therefore if one would categorize it, it is more in the domain of disobedience and perverted right order than of bodily urgency or emotional compulsion.[26]

Of what exactly does the sinfulness of *libido-voluptas-concupiscentia* consist? An answer here is possible only if one notes the distinction in Augustine's mind between two kinds or states of sinfulness. One is *reatus,* actual guilty fault which is the lasting consequence of one's own sinful choices. It is this by which one is an enemy of God; it is this for which one deserves punishment. Does repentance get rid of sin understood in this sense? Yes and no. After repentance the *reatus* is still there; one is still guilty before God. But the grace of Christ coming in baptism does not let the *reatus* prevail as a cause of sinful conduct if the person does not give in to this concupiscence.[27]

The other meaning of sinfulness is *supplicium*. This too is the consequence of one's sinful choices, but unlike *reatus* it is not fault remaining in oneself. By it one is not an enemy of God but an object of his pity and mercy. The persistence of *libido* in a person is part of this *supplicium*.

And what is peculiar about this part of the *supplicium* is that *libido* can become a source of subsequent sinful conduct and can again begin to rule reason and will. Of *concupiscentia* Augustine says pointedly that in those who have been baptized it is not a *reatus* if they do not consent to its "works" within their bodies. It is *called* a sin because it has been produced in persons by prior sinful conduct (Adam's) and because it in turn produces sin if it overpowers the person.[28]

He says that one of the ways in which a baptized person, a Christian husband otherwise good and faithful, lets *libido* overpower him is "to go to his wife intemperately." He offers only two criteria for the meaning here of "intemperately." One is that a man have intercourse for some other motive than to conceive. The other is that he not spare his wife even when she is pregnant.[29] He goes on to say that when a man has mastered *concupiscentia* in himself, he can use it for the one and only purpose which is to conceive.[30] Thus he is not used by his concupiscence, but on the contrary he uses it. A further step in this mastery is that he not ask his wife for the marriage debt at all, but that he no more than grant it to her when she requests it.[31]

Augustine passes a kind of summary judgment on sexuality early in *De Bono Coniugali*. When discussing the nature of the good that marriage is and does, he notes speculatively that some goods, such as wisdom, are good in themselves. Others are good for the sake of another good, as a means of attaining the latter. Marriage and intercourse are this second kind of good, since they provide the good that is friendship. But it is not friendship between the spouses that he has in mind. Rather it is friendship generally in the human race. Spouses make friendship possible by propagating the race. For this reason it is good to marry. But it is still better not to marry. Enough offspring are produced by the sinful to provide persons for friendship; God draws this good from their sin.[32] Augustine urges on Christians perfect continence even within marriage; it is even better than intercourse had for the motive of conceiving. Why? Because marriage will end with the end of mortal bodies, but continence will be the permanent condition of all after the resurrection.[33]

He goes willingly with the momentum of this thought. What if all men and women, even the married, practiced continence? His answer is that this would be good, since the end of time would be brought nearer. The city of God would be filled and perfected the more quickly—as, he says, St. Paul himself wished in 1 Corinthians 7.[34]

Augustine's Marriage Ethic in Principle

One should never underestimate the degree to which Augustine took his marriage ethic from St. Paul in 1 Corinthians and from his neo-Platonic Christian predecessors. But sources aside, a likely clue for understanding this ethic is in his concept of sexual immoderation within marriage. He says that a husband goes to his wife immoderately under two conditions, which are reducible to one. In the first he seeks intercourse with her if she is already pregnant or is for some reason sterile. In the second, in which she is neither pregnant nor sterile, he seeks intercourse not in order to conceive but in order to take pleasure. In either case the immoderation consists of the same defect: seeking intercourse not for conception but for pleasure, or rather for the wrong pleasure, because if a man sought only the pleasure of conceiving a child, he would not be immoderate.

But why is it immoderate to seek intercourse for the common pleasure that accompanies the act, apart from the unlikely pleasure of conceiving? One could say it is immoderate by extension, or *in causa*, because pleasure-seeking tends to lead a man into sexual vagrancy, into adultery and fornication. But a husband could keep his sexuality faithfully within his marriage and yet be immoderate, as Augustine understands this. So the nature of immoderation must be verifiable even within marital fidelity as this is commonly understood.

The understanding of this immoderation is drawn from the Stoic ethic. For a man to act with moral rightness he must act both reasonably and in accord with reason. He acts reasonably if within himself all other faculties or powers—his emotions (such as anger and joy), his feelings (such as fatigue and hunger), his compulsions (such as to relieve genital tension), his bodily parts (such as his genital organs)—are controlled by reason and by will. He thus keeps in himself a right because natural interior order; he suppresses the ever-threatening disorder, or inversion, of letting his conduct be produced and ruled by his sub-rational and sub-volitional powers. This would be to act like the brute beasts, or at best like children and infants.

A man acts with reason when he uses his faculties in such a way as to attain the natural goals of their use. For his genital anatomy the goal is conception. The natural goal of his *libido* is to stimulate his anatomy so that it can bring about conception. These goals have been set by the designer of nature—indwelling divine Reason for classic pantheist Stoicism, God the transcendent Creator for Christian Stoicism.

But how do we know that conception is the goal for the genital anatomy and for libido? The evidence yielding the Stoic answer is threefold. First, look to the effects coming from the use of the sexual anatomy and ask which is of greatest value. Verifying it—and what is of greater value among its effects than human life?—discovers what this anatomy is for. Second, consider its structure in action. All its parts are oriented to accomplishing the result that is conception. Third, consider for what goal sexuality functions in sub-human natures where (and this is a pivotal Christian Stoic point) nature has not been perverted by sinfulness. It is here that the Stoic quickly pointed to the sexual conduct of animals as unperverted and according to nature. He took for granted that they use their sexuality exclusively to procreate.[35]

Therefore the Stoic conclusion: it is the will of nature, of nature's Creator, that human beings use their genital anatomy for no other motive than to conceive. This is its only use that is according to nature; any other is unnatural. A man making love to his wife out of the desire for pleasure differs from a fornicator only in his degree of perversion. To recapitulate what Augustine considered a sad and undeniable fact: rarely can even a devout Christian confine his motivation exclusively to conception. Concupiscence, the wound in human nature caused by Adam's sin, has brought this about. Given this fact, what is expected of him is that he keep his sinfulness as venial as possible by suppressing his pleasure as firmly as possible even while going to his wife only in order to conceive. What is hoped of him, but probably unrealistically, is that self-denial will eventually subdue in him entirely the desire for pleasure, with the consequence that he will give up intercourse for good.

The Meaning of "The Goods of Marriage"

One can define a social relationship only if one can name the goods that it is meant to attain. Such a relationship is what it *is* in the sense of what it is *for*. This is true even if its goal lies wholly within itself, such as the safety or the happiness of its members. The goal of the relationship is the good that the parties to it seek in coming together. But if its goals lie outside itself, it is an instrumental relationship; as a society it is for something other than itself and its members.

When one abstracts Augustine's three goods of marriage from their polemic context in his essays as excuses sufficient for Christian spouses' risking sinful concupiscence, one can find them serving a defining function. He uses them to define only implicitly, but when he names the three goods he does define marriage in part as a self-contained society. The fidelity and persevering commitment make it this. He defines it also in part as an instrumental society in that procreation is a good that lies beyond marriage and is for the sake of the larger societies, the state and the Church.

It is not clear that he thought of the ends of marriage when naming these goods. Nowhere in the Latin of his essays does the word *finis* appear. It is true that the ends of marriage identified later by the Scholastics are drawn in part from the three goods, and in some degree coincide with them. But they are not Augustine's formulation.

Nevertheless his goods do imply finality. Since they are the advantages marriage can bring to private persons and to their societies, they are what a person may seek to realize in marrying. The beckoning logical step at this point is to conclude that they are the advantages that marriage according to its nature is intended to realize; and therefore (now the moral step) in marrying a person *ought* to be motivated by the desire for this realization. (Eventually Catholic marriage law was to add the final step—a philosophical-juridical one—that unless a person accepts these goals in his relationship, it cannot be a marriage.)

Is the establishment of procreation and nurture as the primary end of marriage traceable to Augustine? Again no, not if one looks for an express declaration. But he did claim a primacy for procreation and nurture among the goods of marriage. In the last of his essays on marriage, *On Adulterous Marriages* (*De Adulterinis Coniugiis*), Book 2, Chapter 12, he says, "Therefore the propagation of children is the first, the natural and the principal purpose of marriage." (The Latin noun that I have translated "purpose" is *causa*.) Earlier, in his essay *Against Faustus the Manichee* (*Contra Faustum Manichaeum*) Chapter 19, n. 26, he had seemed to make procreation the only good of marriage, or if not that, at least its only end. Only in his Latin can the near tautology he points to be seen: *Matrimonium quippe ex hoc appellatum est, quod non ob aliud debeat femina nubere quam ut mater fiat* ("For marriage is indeed called 'matrimony' from the fact that a woman ought to marry for no other reason than to become a mother").

To explain what Augustine means by each of the goods of marriage we may draw on his three statements quoted earlier in this chapter. The good that is offspring (*proles*) designates procreation, which includes not merely the bringing of children into the world but also their proper nurture. The good that is fidelity (*fides*) designates in a general way that the spouses will keep marital fidelity, but more particularly each one's honoring the other's exclusive right to the former's sexual acts. The good that is *sacramentum* designates the perseverance, the permanence of the marriage commitment, even the unbreakable character of the marital bond. (In using the word *sacramentum* Augustine did not mean to call marriage a sacrament of the New Law, a religious sign or manifestation in human conduct of God's grace-giving entry into the lives of the persons involved in this conduct. For one thing, he is here describing marriage as it is found among all human beings, pagans included. He predicates *sacramentum* of marriage according to various meanings in his essays. To date I have found that the term's principal meaning is that of a combined commitment and bond. What I have not yet found out clearly is the identity of the persons linked by the commitment-bond—whether spouse with spouse singly, or each spouse with God singly, or both spouses with God jointly while being themselves bonded to one another.)

Augustine's Secondary Goods of Marriage

However, it would be an incomplete and therefore inaccurate assessment of Augustine's understanding of marriage to say that he found no other goods in it than the three we have just examined. He found others. And as we shall see, they are, like fidelity and the *sacramentum,* goods internal to the relationship, advantages yielded to the spouses themselves.

In *The Good of Marriage,* Chapter 11, he offers a most general observation, that the husband-wife relationship is the first natural tie, or bond, of human society. Here he at least seems to set marriage in the context of friendship. He sees friendship as a primary datum, a given natural good in human association, because men and women are by nature social: "... because human nature is something social, because it possesses the capacity for friendship as a great and natural good."

He notes in this regard that the first man and woman did not come together as strangers. Taking the Garden of Eden parable as factual history he says that they were first of all blood relatives, since the woman was drawn from the man's body. He veers toward the Greek myth of the androgyne but reverses the path of etiological explanation in it. That is, he does not say that men's and women's craving for one another now is caused by their having been originally drawn from one another. He says rather that this attraction is evidence that the one was originally drawn from the other. He implies that Christians need invent no myths of origin to explain this power of attraction, because they have had revealed to them the history of an origin that explains it clearly. He adds that God drew all human beings from one set of parents just so that they might all be related by blood and thus might more readily take up the great natural good that is friendship.

But Augustine never takes the one more step, in developing this thought, of saying that what marriage is, is a form of friendship. On the contrary, he almost formally denies this. Later, in Chapter 9, he writes of two kinds of goods that God gives, one the instrumental good, the kind that is sought for the sake of something else that is good. The other is something good in itself, like wisdom, health and friendship. He says that marriage does not belong among the latter. It, along with sexual intercourse, is a good that is a necessary means for something else. Marriage's relationship to friendship is just this, that it is needed to provide children who may grow up to form friendships. Even so, he continues, a person does better not to wish for the (instrumental) good that is marriage. There is no danger that because of this the race will go out of existence. Illicit intercourse, given the actual state of human conduct, will assure enough human beings to form friendships. Besides, as I have noted earlier, he says in Chapter 10 that if all men and women remained continent, the sooner would come the end of history and the sooner would the City of God reach its consummation.

He does veer back toward calling marriage a friendship when, in replying to the Manichees' charge that marriage is evil, he says that it is not, because it produces good things. He says that it is valuable first of all because of its source. God created it; heterosexual attraction and union, whatever dismal things men and women have since done to them, exist by his design. (He adds a point he later repeats elsewhere, that when Jesus was invited to the wedding at Cana of Galilee, he did not turn down the invitation but accepted it. Presumably if he thought marriage were evil, Jesus would have declined.)

It is in Chapter 3 of *The Good of Marriage,* when he names the values internal to marriage making it good, that he glances again at friendship. Not the first, but the second value that marriage yields is the natural companionship of two persons of diverse sex. This is a natural good belonging in the domain of natural charity. It shows up in an especially helpful way in the care that elderly spouses, no longer capable of intercourse, can have for one another:

> One may ask justifiably why marriage is good. It seems to me to be good because of the procreation of children, but also because of even the natural association itself of the two different sexes. Otherwise one could not say that the elderly can be married, especially if they had lost their children or had simply never begotten any.

The same thought for the value of companionship appears in his essay, *On the Traditions of the Catholic Church* (*De Moribus Ecclesiae Catholicae*), Book 1, Chapter 30. He mentions there the simple association or companionship of domestic life as a good internal to marriage:

> You [the Catholic Church] subject women to their husbands in chaste and faithful obedience not for the satisfying of passion but for the procreating of children and for their sharing in family life. You set husbands over their wives not to demean the weaker sex, but themselves ruled by the law of genuine love.

Again, in his *Commentary on the Sermon on the Mount* (*De Sermone Domini in Monte*), Book 1, Chapter 15, n. 42, he distinguishes three values that a man and woman can seek for in their marriage. He all but expressly names these as motives they claim in marrying, all of them worthy. Without his taking note of it, in naming the second of these motives he touches also that good that he elsewhere identifies as marriage's (objective) primary end:

> Therefore a Christian man can live in peace with his wife. He can with her provide for the needs of the flesh—which the Apostle [Paul] sees as something permitted but not commanded. Or they can provide for the procreation of children, and this can be praiseworthy to some degree. Or they can provide a kind of brother-sister companionship, without any bodily commingling.

In these passages Augustine has enriched the source whence Catholic canonists and theologians will later draw one of their "secondary ends" of marriage, that one whose name least exactly describes its nature because the name can refer to so much—the *mutuum adiutorium* of the spouses, their mutual help, or support.

The other secondary end Augustine mentions in more than one place. It is obvious enough in Chapter 6 of *The Good of Marriage*, where he names a kind of mutual help spouses can give one another that could be deemed one of friendship's supports, but of a singular kind. They provide for one another an outlet for passion *within* fidelity, and therefore a licit outlet that protects them from fornication and adultery. Even more than this, by confining their intercourse within marriage they help one another by holding to the level of venial sin even that intercourse that is sought not for procreation but for the sinful motive of satisfying *libido*—a satisfying which outside marriage would be mortally sinful.

To return one last time to Augustine's judgment that procreation and nurture make up the principal value of marriage, and its principal reason for being chosen by men and women, I note again his axiomatic statement in Chapter 24 of *The Good of Marriage*: "These are all goods by reason of which marriage is good: offspring, fidelity, sacrament." This is a tauter summary of a looser formulation immediately preceding: two goods of marriage acknowledged among all nations and among all men are, first, that it is a source of procreation, and, second, that it is a place of faithful chastity. But among the people of God marriage has the added good that is the sanctity of the sacrament, which for them makes not only remarriage after divorce but divorce itself impossible.

Successively through the essay he advances on that formula along indirect paths. In Chapter 5 he implies that the intent to have children is so necessary to constitute a marriage that he does not see how a couple refusing to have them and taking contraceptive means to avoid conception can be married at all—although he acknowledges a marriage where the couple have the same intent against children but take no immoral means to avoid conception and therefore do not simply reject them.

In Chapter 6 he varies the earlier statement that marriage is the first association in the human race. Here he says that this association is fidelity in sexual intercourse for the purpose of procreating children. In Chapter 10 he says that that intercourse belonging to marriage is the intercourse needed for procreation. A couple having intercourse to gratify *libido* have intercourse that does not belong to marriage. In Chapter 11 he says ". . . the crown of marriage . . . is the chastity of procreation and faithfulness in rendering the carnal debt." In Chapter 17 he approximates the formula to come in Chapter 24 by offering anthropological information, saying that that which is common to marriage among all races is that it is for the one purpose of creating children; and then, going back to his biblical source, he says: ". . . marriage was instituted for this purpose, so that children might be born properly and decently." In Chapter 19 he offers another anthropological explanation: procreation is the good proper to marriage; and this is seen in the fact that men are led by an obligation, by a certain instinct of nature, to replace persons lost through death.

Such was Augustine's mind on the matter in 401, when he composed *The Good of Marriage*. As I have already pointed out, eighteen years later, when writing his *On Adulterous Marriages*, he had changed it not at all. There again in a formula he wrote, "Therefore the propagation of children is the first, the natural and the legitimate purpose of marriage."

Notes

1. Those of Augustine's treatises dealing formally with marriage are *The Good of Marriage* (*De Bono Coniugali*), written in 401; *On Marriage and Concupiscence* (*De Nuptiis et Concupiscentia*), in 418–420; *On Adulterous Marriages* (*De Adulterinis Coniugiis*), in 419. He had much to say about marriage also in his *Commentary on the Literal Meaning of Genesis* (*De Genesi ad Litteram*), a work to which he devoted himself intermittently from 401 to 414; and in *On Original Sin* (its full Latin title is *De Gratia Christi et de Peccato Originali*) written in 418.

2. "Haec omnia sunt bona, propter quae nuptiae bonae sunt: proles, fides, sacramentum" (PL 40:394).

3. "Hoc autem tripartitum est: fides, proles, sacramentum. In fide attenditur ne praeter vinculum coniugale, cum altera vel altero concubatur; in prole, ut amanter suscipiatur, benigne nutriatur, religiose educatur; in sacramento autem, ut coniugium non separetur, et dimissus aut dimissa nec causa prolis alteri coniungatur. Haec est tamquam regula nuptiarum, qua vel naturae decoratur fecunditas, vel incontinentiae regitur pravitas" (PL 34:397).

4. "Bonum ergo sunt nuptiae in omnibus quae sunt propria nuptiarum. Haec autem sunt tria, generandi ordinatio, fides pudicitiae, connubii sacramentum. Propter ordinationem generandi, scriptum est: Volo iuniores nubere, filios procreare, matresfamilias esse. Propter fidem pudicitiae: Uxor non habet potestatem sui corporis, sed vir; similiter et vir non habet potestatem sui corporis, sed mulier. Propter connubii sacramentum: Quod Deus coniunxit, homo non separet" (PL 44:404).

5. This is not to say that Augustine was blind to the possibility of dear and intimate love between a husband and wife. He speaks of this in *The City of God* where he accounts for both a reason and an effect of the first woman's being formed by being taken from her husband's side: "The fact that the woman was formed for Adam from his own side shows clearly enough how dear ought to be the union of husband and wife" (I, 12, 27). How overpowering was the bond between the first man and his wife Augustine suggests in his *Sermon* 51: "Even if it meant taking part in her sin he refused to be separated from her, his one companion." But still Augustine refuses to say that the most characteristic and strongest expression precisely of this union is sexual intercourse.

6. In *De Peccato Originali*, Lib. 2, Cap. 34.

7. *De Nuptiis et Concupiscentia*, Lib. 1, Cap. 1.

8. *De Peccato Originali*, Lib. 2, Cap. 35.

9. *De Nuptiis et Concupiscentia*, Lib. 2, Cap. 20.

10. *De Peccato Originali,* Lib. 2, Cap. 37.
11. *De Nuptiis et Concupiscentia,* Lib. 1, Cap. 24.
12. Op. cit., Lib. 2, Cap. 15.
13. Op. cit., Lib. 1, Cap. 25. The student of Reformation theology may recognize here a source of Luther's theory of forgiveness of sin by non-imputation of sin that remains nevertheless.
14. Op. cit., Lib. 1, Cap. 28.
15. *De Bono Coniugali,* Cap. 20, and *De Peccato Originali,* Lib. 2, Cap. 39.
16. *De Nuptiis et Concupiscentia,* Lib. 1, Cap. 25.
17. *De Bono Coniugali,* Cap. 3.
18. *De Peccato Originali,* Lib. 2, Cap. 38.
19. Ibid.
20. *De Nuptiis et Concupiscentia,* Lib. 2, Cap. 36.
21. Op. cit., Lib. 1, Cap. 18.
22. Op. cit., Lib. 1, Cap. 5.
23. Op. cit., Lib. 1, Cap. 6.
24. It was commonly accepted in the ancient and medieval understanding of the sexual anatomies that the lubricating secretion of the Bartholin's glands is a semination analogous to male ejaculation.
25. *De Nuptiis et Concupiscentia,* Lib. 2, Cap. 26.
26. Op. cit., Lib. 1, Cap. 6.
27. Op. cit., Lib. 1, Cap. 24.
28. Ibid.
29. *De Bono Coniugali,* Cap. 6.
30. *De Nuptiis et Concupiscentia,* Lib. 1, Cap. 8.
31. *De Bono Coniugali,* Cap. 13.
32. Op. cit., Cap. 9.
33. Op. cit., Cap. 7.
34. Op. cit., Cap. 10.
35. The ancients had no way of knowing what Jane Goodall would one day find out, that the most "intelligent" of the primates, those closest to man, the chimpanzees, engage commonly in masturbatory and incestuous conduct.

8

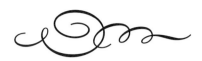

Sex, Marriage, and Family in Christian Tradition

Lisa Sowle Cahill

Faithfulness to New Testament criteria of moral discipleship should yield a sex and gender ethics which is also a social ethics, including and protecting society's judged, outcast, and vulnerable. Has Christian teaching and practice about sex, gender, marriage, and family enhanced appreciation of all persons' common humanity, the value of each, and the interdependence of all? Has it led to the construction of ecclesial and social institutions which give such appreciation stability and material expression? As on most other embodiments of discipleship, Christianity has on these issues a mixed record.

The pre-modern cultures which contributed to the first centuries of Christianity set a high priority on the *social* functions of marriage and family, and assumed gender to be both hierarchical and highly differentiated. According both to Roman law and to the traditions of the Germanic peoples who immigrated into Europe in the fourth century and later, sex was largely defined by its reproductive function, and parenthood and family by their socioeconomic functions. Sexual intimacy was structured patriarchally, and sexual pleasure was not linked to the mutual affection of the reproductive partners, so much as to the accomplishment of reproduction itself, whose requirements it always exceeded. Hence sex's reputation as unruly and dangerous to its own social role.

As we shall see, certain developments in the Christian theology and of marriage and in its regulation under ecclesiastical law worked to protect the dignity, freedom, equality, and affective relationship of spouses. The Middle Ages, especially through the Christian ban on divorce for both men and women and its requirement of personal consent in entering marriage, provide some precedents for the emphasis on personal relationships in marriage and family which gained full sway after the Enlightenment. Yet it was not until the modern period that theologies of marriage and church teaching about marriage presented its interpersonal dimensions as primary and overriding. Today, Christians in most cultures idealize the personal functions of marriage and family above the socioeconomic. Sex, interpreted in light of the individual's intersubjective experiences, is valued for allowing intimacy as reciprocity, and as supplying mutual pleasure which enhances intimacy. Parenthood too is valued for its affective rewards. In sex, marriage, and family, there is a proportionately low differentiation of female and male roles and increasing egalitarianism of gender, compared to most premodern societies.

The twentieth-century heirs of Western Christianity thus discern and resist in the received institutions of marriage and family a "regulation" of sex which seems to violate its personal and "covenantal" significance, taming sex in favor of institutional interests, and submitting it to bureaucracies which embody resentment and fear of sex's vitality, its irrepressibility, even its sacredness. The French historian Georges Duby plainly embarks on his study of medieval sexuality with an anti-juridical attitude: "Regulation, officialization, control, codification: the institution of marriage is, by its very position and by the role which it assumes, enclosed in a rigid framework of rituals and prohibitions."[1]

The historical accession of the individual to key importance in defining marriage and its purposes, as well as the modern ideal of equality across gender and class, have brought momentous changes in the understandings of sex. Only with the impact of these sea changes in human consciousness could the notion of marriage as a full commitment of individuals gain ascendancy, and the meaning of marriage take on the character of a personal covenant of woman and man. In the twentieth century, especially in the West, the interpersonal and affective replaced the institutional and economic aspects of marriage and family as paramount, leading to questions about the viability of the institutions themselves. These developments present modern interpreters with the problem of reinstating in relation to personal values the social and institutional realities, as well as the "sacramental" role of Christian marriage in mediating the "kingdom of God" in both the personal and the social spheres.

The present chapter will develop the dialectical, perennially uneasy relationship in Christian tradition among (1) the struggle to reflect radical discipleship by means of sexual teaching, and to use that teaching not just to delimit or reject family loyalties and hierarchies, but to transform them from within; (2) a persistent ambivalence toward both women and sexual pleasure; and (3) the newly enhanced personal and covenantal understandings of sex, marriage, and family, which exist in some tension with the biological and parental meanings so important in the past.

The interplay of these strands will be examined ... through the lenses of four contentious subjects: clerical celibacy, indissolubility, contraception, and reproductive technologies. Although the first three of these have been at issue more in Catholicism than in other Christian denominations,[2] they offer an occasion to look at the emergence in Christianity historically of sexual disciplines which resisted the sexual enforcement of status hierarchies but which tended eventually to be co-opted by lines of control in the church. All four issues also permit examination of the moral significance of sexual pleasure, the emergence of intimacy as a Christian sexual ideal, and the importance of procreation in defining the spousal relationship....

Celibacy

Although, as we have seen, sexual continence has been a Christian ideal since NT times, Roman Catholicism is unusual among the churches today in requiring a vow of permanent celibacy of all candidates for the priesthood. Although the Reformers were later to reject it, the discipline of clerical continence, having gathered momentum since the fourth century, was formally instituted for the whole church in 1123 (at the First Lateran Council). This regulation provided that priests who were already married must live continently with their wives. The Second Lateran Council (1139) went further and precluded ordination for anyone who did not observe strict celibacy, that is, who did not abandon married life entirely. The requirement of celibacy was reversed by the Reformers on the grounds both that marriage was instituted by God as most people's natural "estate," and that the rarity of a genuine celibate vocation had led to all kinds of abuse and vice among the supposedly virginal clergy.

The earliest legislation concerning celibacy dates to the Council of Elvira (c. 306), a local Spanish council, which decreed that bishops, priests, and deacons abstain from sexual relations with their wives; the Council of Arles concurred (314), and the practice was reaffirmed by Ambrose and Jerome. The ecumenical Council of Nicaea (325) decreed that men could not marry after they were ordained to the diaconate, though those who already had wives could still proceed through the levels of ordination to priesthood, remaining married but continent thereafter. The same practice was established by the Eastern Council of Ancyra (358), whose ruling was adopted as legislation for the Roman Empire (420). A similar practice continues today in the Orthodox churches. Married men can be ordained to the diaconate and priesthood, though bishops are chosen only from among celibates.[3]

In modern times, the Second Vatican Council of the Roman Catholic Church supported celibacy in its decree on priestly ministry (*Presbyterorum Ordinis*, 1965), and the 1967 encyclical *Sacerdotalis Celibatus* (1967) confirmed that the discipline would continue. The 1983 Code of Canon law states, "Clerics are obliged to observe perfect and perpetual continence for the sake of the kingdom of heaven and therefore are obliged to observe celibacy, which is a special gift of God, by which sacred ministers can adhere more easily to Christ with an undivided heart and can more freely dedicate themselves to the service of God and humankind" (Can. 277).

The currents of renewal in the church which led to and flowed from Vatican II included reconsideration among laity and theologians alike of almost all traditional Catholic sexual teachings, and clerical celibacy was no exception. Arguments in favor of change included the shortage of priests and consequent sacramental and eucharistic deprivation of the faithful; the centrality of marriage and fatherhood to male status in many countries of the world; a renewed appreciation of the goodness of sexuality and of marriage as a vocation in the church, with consequences for the "superiority" of virginity; the pastoral assets of a married clergy which could identify with the daily lives of their congregations; and the essential separability of celibacy and priestly ministry, as attested both in the New Testament (1 Tim. 3:2, 12; Tit. 1:6) and at least sporadically in church practice up to the Middle Ages. But perhaps the greatest focus was the personal plight of men who had complied with the celibacy requirement in order to enter the priesthood, yet had suffered as a result not only sexual frustration but deep loneliness. In the wake of the Council many have left the active ministry and married, but still yearn for a life in which one vocation does not have to be sacrificed for the other. Compounding the problem is the perception that many youthful candidates for the priesthood had in the past been ill-prepared for the demands and costs of sexual renunciation, and, indeed, had been trained to repress, rather than to live constructively with, their sexual drives and needs for intimacy.

The psychosexual well-being of individuals and the importance of freedom to choose celibacy as an "option" for priests thus moved to center stage in much of the debate about celibacy following Vatican II. Many felt that celibacy as a charism could only be appropriated in freedom, not legally imposed.[4] Arguments against mandatory celibacy frequently stressed the negative attitudes toward sex (and women) out of which it had seemed to emerge and which it continued to perpetuate. Although official documents spoke of celibacy for the sake of the kingdom, church practice seemed to many to amount to juridical control over the rank-and-file of priests and a sign of Christian misogynism and depreciation of sex.

Conversely, those who wanted to reconstrue celibacy positively, and who aimed at least to make the discipline not only bearable, but even attractive to priests and religious, focused on the goodness of sexuality, and the possibility of healthy psychosexual development even in the celibate state. Introducing his influential book, Donald Goergen avows, "*The Sexual Celibate* is based upon the growing conviction that friendship is not detrimental but central to celibate living, that celibate persons are also sexual persons, and that celibate life is a profound and rewarding way of living."[5] The eschatological witness of celibate life, as an embodiment of the radical nature of Christian love, and its availability for community service, did not drop out of sight, even among supporters of optional celibacy for priests.[6] But, especially with the continued decline of numbers of priests in those same cultures in which sex as embodying intimacy and love is prized, celibacy is more and more regarded in restrictive terms and suspected to be the bodily symbol of a repressive and highly controlling ecclesiastical hierarchy.

The truth behind this perception, as well as the possible renewal of celibacy's witness to the church, can be better appreciated in light of the ambivalent relation of celibacy to the ideals of early Christianity, as celibacy was gradually established to be the officially "higher vocation" in the mind of the church.

Peter Brown reviews the first centuries of Christian history in light of his thesis that Christian celibacy is a bodily symbol of resistance to the pagan state and family. Because young people, especially women, were still married off early by their parents in the first generations after Christ, virginity was not a decision that was likely to be undertaken as a life-long vocation. Brown surmises that Christian continence originated as a practice within marriage, and that the audience of moral exhortation regarding it was those whose spouses had died.[7] Widows were apparently more numerous in the early Christian communities than widowers, since women married much older men, and since the church discouraged women bereaved even in their twenties from re-entering the marriage market. Later New Testament materials reflect a special office of widows in the community (1 Tim. 2:11–15). Widows, many quite wealthy, thus made up an important and potentially influential constituency, and were seen as fulfilling an established and recognized role, often including patronage.

Following the example of the Hebrew prophets, sexual abstinence was associated with receptivity to the Spirit of God and to prophecy; and with martyrdom, which celibacy democratized as an analogous participation. By at least the second century, monastic communities began to withdraw into the hills and deserts to pray, to seek communion with God outside the social norms of home and family. Communities of consecrated women not only cultivated spirituality, but carried out a subtle revolt against cultural definitions of their roles in marriage and household.[8] Membership in the churches was, at the beginning of the third century, still dominated by married householders; continence served as an equalizing factor between men and women and between ordained ministers and laity. In particular, it allowed communities which had offended social mores by including women in religious leadership roles, and which constantly fell under pagan accusation of bizarre, demonic, or lascivious sexual behavior, to present male and female working relationships as above reproach. In this way then, celibacy in the early years narrowed the gap between priestly and lay status and facilitated the inclusion of women.[9]

Praise of virginity was not without converse effects on attitudes toward marriage and sex. Brown believes that sexual abstinence symbolizes for Origen (in the second century) a loosening of the bonds of kinship, and a freedom of the soul;[10] but even if so, this was certainly achieved at the price of a denigration of sex, marriage, and parenthood, and even the body, and amounted to the re-creation of a spiritual elite to which only the few could belong. For Tertullian sex was demeaning and impure. He insisted on strict control of the body, denounced sex as spiritually ennervating, and believed that it should be completely renounced after the death of a first spouse. Referring to women as "the Devil's gateway," Tertullian demanded that the holy observe continence in marriage, and maintain strictly the order of the patriarchal household. Both men and women could attain sanctity, however, by giving up sex.[11] In the third century, virginity or choice of the unmarried state by young men and women was acceptable and common. Yet the late second-century author Clement of Alexandria defended the married laity against "the rise of a dangerous mystique of continence"[12] by writing approvingly of sex in marriage, as long as it was ordered by the Stoic values of moderation, reason, and procreation. Moreover, Clement maintained that women and men were of the same moral nature, and were to be encouraged to similar virtues.[13]

By the beginning of the fourth century, celibacy as both a symbol of elitism and an instrument of control had made irreversible inroads. The "Desert Fathers" of the fourth century bore witness to the coming age by giving up the sort of immortality that could be achieved through offspring. The evil of sex was not for them a special focus; a strict asceticism about food was an even more important form of bodily control signifying their dedication to a new life. But by the time the synods of the early 300s began to legislate what was already no doubt well represented in practice, Christians thought in terms of "two ways" of life, highly differentiated both in terms of content and of value. In such a framework, virginity as a special vocation does not contribute much to solidarity among disciples. As Brown quotes Eusebius' account, those who forego marriage are "beyond common human living . . . Like some celestial beings, these gaze down upon human life."[14] It was the triumph of this point of view that seems to have backed the installation of clerical celibacy after 300.[15] The hardening compulsoriness of celibacy for clergy seemed to go hand-in-hand with a growing negativity about sex as such. It also served to protect clergy leadership against competition from married benefactors, thus accentuating hierarchies in the community, not overturning them.[16]

John Chrysostom, priest, theologian, and famed preacher of late fourth-century Antioch illustrates that neither the hierarchization of Christian identity, nor the ancillary regulation of celibate clergy, had yet poisoned fatally the transformations that were the Christian body's legitimate children. "His aim was to rob the city of its most tenacious myth—the myth that its citizens have a duty to contribute to the continued glory of their native Antioch by marrying."[17] Chrysostom permits marriage mostly as a compromise with the difficulty of sexual control. Yet he appeals to Christian households to remember the poor, daily collecting savings for them in a box beside the marriage bed. Austerity and almsgiving are a higher calling even than virginity. "For without virginity, indeed, it is possible to see the Kingdom, but without almsgiving this cannot be."[18]

Meanwhile, in the Latin Church, Ambrose and particularly Jerome preserved some of virginity's revolutionary effect by holding it forth to women as an avenue of equality with men. Ambrose insisted on the Christian equality of sexual standards for both men and women in marriage.[19] But he deprecated Roman noble families' pride in their fertility. In fact, he compared a virgin's being offered for marriage to being put up for sale in the slave market.[20] When one young girl sought refuge with the bishop from her family's pressure to marry, Ambrose reflected, "Conquer family-loyalty first, my girl: if you overcome the household, you overcome the world."[21] Upper class ascetic virgins, of whom Ambrose's elder sister was one, had an impact on the church as both patrons and companions of the clergy and theologians. Through their ecclesial dedication they achieved emancipation from matronly roles within the Roman household.

Like Origen, Jerome thought the sexual body required tight control, but refused to see it as a mirror of spiritual difference between the sexes. Two educated widows, Paula and Marcella, offered Jerome religious and financial support, and became his close colleagues. "Jerome, for all his fashionable misogyny and his sharp sense of sexual danger, would never for a moment have doubted that the minds of Paula or Marcella, and his other female allies and clients, did not have their full share of 'male' bone and muscle."[22]

Paradoxically, it is Augustine, the fourth-century bishop of Hippo in North Africa, to whom is attributed the most lasting influence both in defining Christianity's positive doctrine of marriage, and in surrounding sex with an aura of shame and danger from which celibacy serves as an escape. In Augustine's writing there culminate two tendencies which go back to Paul, and which also had characterized the emergence and interpretation of celibacy as a Christian option in the centuries leading up to Augustine. First, there was the ascetic tradition, always ready to erupt in extremist, gnostic forms, so strong in the first four centuries. Asceticism fed on a suspicion of sexual desire, on a resistance to marriage as a form of social control, and on a positive construal of virginity as offering both spiritual and social benefits. Second, there was a reinterpretation of Christian marriage, which affirmed the marital bond, sex, and family within certain defined structures, and which linked marriage with Christian symbols in a "sacramentalizing" trend. The transformation of marriage will be taken up in the subsequent section, on indissolubility; but it impinges on the discussion of celibacy insofar as approval of marriage as a sphere of sanctification has always furnished an important limit to Christian advocacy of celibacy.

Not only did Augustine stand at a historical point where Christian ambivalence toward sex, and all the social roles which channeled it, was practically unavoidable. His personal experience also positioned him perfectly to reflect and magnify the tension already expressed in the Christian differentiation of celibacy and marriage. Augustine invites biographical references in interpreting his theology, for he himself ties personal history, religious experience, and theological insight closely together in his *Confessions*. While it would be excessive to read Augustine's central theological proposals in light of his sexual history, his own experiences of sex and his relationships with women, as he himself reports them, can legitimately be brought to bear on his ideas about sex and gender.

Two women figured prominently in Augustine's life: his mother, and the woman with whom he lived for fifteen years and had a son. Only his mother, Monica, is mentioned by name and presented by Augustine as someone whose own aspirations, sorrows and loves are worthy in their own right. Augustine's *Confessions* are full of Monica's devotion to her son, her incessant prayers for his conversion away from Manicheanism, his long resistance and spiritual return to Catholicism, and his suffering upon her death.

Augustine's concubine was a woman of lower-class status, with whom a full Roman marriage would have been out of the question. As a young professor of rhetoric, from a respectable family but of scant means, Augustine might have been content to continue indefinitely in a "second-class" marriage, as other notable citizens had done.[23] However, his mother eventually intervened to arrange for Augustine a marriage with a young girl who could offer the son improved social standing and the prospect of an inheritance.[24] The concubine was sent away, back from Italy to Africa, though she vowed never to be united with any other man. Augustine kept their son. And, since he had to wait two years until his bride was of marriageable age, he promptly took another mistress, of whom he tells us almost nothing.[25]

Augustine mentions his concubine wholly in terms of his own desires and responses, and of those he focuses on a sexual need so acute and unrelenting that it binds him—according to his own testimony—in a sort of "slavery." Margaret Miles even describes Augustine as a sex addict,[26] although it is difficult to weigh his level of actual compulsiveness against his overwhelming revulsion in the face of sexual drives and reactions, especially in view of the fact that they represented to him a shameful lack of control.[27] Sex was much maligned by the religious sect (Manicheanism) to whose ideals he aspired. He once referred to "the shameful motions of the organs of generation," and went on to opine that in Eden sexual intercourse might fittingly have taken place without any sexual desire whatsoever, but rather by an act of sheer rationality.[28] Although Augustine says that "[t]o love and be loved was sweet to me," still, physical enjoyment of love turned friendship into "the hell of lustfulness."[29] Even though he describes his heart as "torn, wounded, and bleeding" at separation from his lover, he still looks back on their relationship as making him "a slave to lust."[30] He remembers himself as "enslaved with the disease of the flesh," captive to "an insatiable lust."[31] Of his son, who died as a youth, he also writes sparingly, though with emotion.[32] But, as Miles notes, Augustine never portrays his lover in a maternal role, reserving the honorifics of motherhood for Monica.[33]

Another factor in Augustine's view of sexuality must be the complex relations within his household of origin. His pagan father, Patricius, made enormous sacrifices to give his son an education, but was, in the latter's rather arrogant view, shallow in both intellect and paternal ambition.[34] Patricius' death is passed over almost in silence,[35] and in sharp contrast to the emotions lavished by his son on Monica. Augustine describes his parents' marriage—or at least his mother's role in it—in exactly the terms admired by Roman society in his day and in earlier times. His mother was given to a husband as soon as she was of marriageable age, served her husband "as her lord," and never began quarrels about his infidelities or his angry outbursts. She advised her friends to avoid beatings by considering their marriage contracts as "instruments whereby they were made servants." Against adversity and despite seemingly constant ill-treatment, she had honored her parents and mother-in-law, raised her children piously and governed her household well, and in widowhood had earned the Latin encomium *univira*, "wife of one man."[36] When one adds to all this the fact that Augustine's own prospect of marriage began with a political arrangement that promised perfectly to imitate the circumstances of his upbringing, one can hardly blame him for failing to perceive in the marital bond much potential for spiritual companionship and love.

Augustine came to see celibacy as his only hope for an integrated life, a life he heard praised in Ambrose's sermons, and to which he was eventually turned through a vision of Continence as a beckoning and reassuring mother.[37] His hope for friendship and progress in the love of God came to reside in a community of men, of close associates who would undistractedly share a way of life, intense conversation, prayer, and sexual sublimation. It is only male friendship which to Augustine finally seems noble, and he recalls mourning for a dead companion as for "a friendship that had grown sweet to me about all the sweetness of my life."[38] He is inspired to praise his mother as "in a woman's garb, but with masculine faith."[39] Margaret Miles remarks that Augustine "apparently has no fear of the 'glue of love' [iv. 4] when it connects his life with that of another man," even though "he cannot imagine loving a woman in a relationship in which each partner supported, encouraged, and provoked the other to self-knowledge and spiritual progress."[40] His spiritual life had to be focused with metaphors of sexual restraint, as well as with its physical reality.

No wonder that the works of this theologian transmit a certain negativity on sex and sexual pleasure. It was not in his emotional and imaginative range to discern in sex any potential for personal or spiritual enrichment. He had few models for mutual respect and a devotion in a marriage committed to Christian ideals. He was all too familiar with impermanent, only unintentionally procreative, sexual liaisons which ended badly, and which contributed to the demeaning both of a mistress's humanity, and of a lawful wife's position. Even sex in marriage for the wives of his acquaintance would have been the husband's prerogative and too often brutal or violent.

In the writings of the figure who has been most central to Roman Catholic ethics, we note a shift in perspective. Although, as far as we know, Thomas Aquinas lived an entirely celibate life himself, he was able to see sexual pleasure as a good if properly ordered within marriage; he also saw marriage as a friendship of the most intense sort, a friendship cemented by sexual intimacy. His view of marriage will be taken up further in the next section. No doubt this shift was enabled by the changes in the understanding of marriage which were already taking place in the Middle Ages, though Aquinas still quite definitely places women as the inferior sex. On celibacy, it is enough to say that Aquinas sees virginity as the higher way for a Christian without resorting to any crude denigration of marriage and sex.[41] Aquinas believes that virginity is preferable to marriage, since sex is a hindrance to the contemplative way of life.[42] Like the Fathers, Aquinas does think marriage "holier" if it remains without "carnal intercourse."[43] Virginity fosters a life hospitable to "thinking on the things of God" and thus to "the good of the soul."[44] Because Aquinas links virginity with contemplation, in contrast to an active life (which marriage serves), his theology diminishes the socially radical value of early Christian celibacy. He even characterizes the excellence of virginity as a "private good" in contrast to the common good of marriage.[45] He does, however, retain the equal accessibility of the celibate state to both men and women, and so it continues to serve as a path to spiritual equality in what was still a very gender unequal social world.

Although celibacy was institutionalized by church law in the twelfth century, it has never ceased to be disputed, whether more or less openly and vociferously. First of all, even in the second half of the twelfth century, clerical concubinage was still alive and well.[46] In the thirteenth and fourteenth centuries, some theologians, canonists, and even bishops, called for a repeal of mandatory celibacy; and the fourteenth and fifteenth centuries saw a resurgence of concubinage among the clergy, contributing to Luther's complaints. An extended debate at Trent (1545–63) produced a renewed insistence that priests and vowed religious could not contract valid marriages. This declaration was partly a reaction to the Reformers' challenge to church authority, as well as to the numbers of priests who were abandoning their Roman Catholic status and taking spouses.

The reaffirmation of celibacy was no doubt in some part a protective move on behalf of authority, and an exertion of control over clergy and religious. However, the exclusion for priests of sex, procreation, and even marriages without sex, also served the freedom of the clergy and of the church over against the medieval family. The children of married clergy stood to inherit church property; and not only a priest's own natal family, but also that of his wife (especially the children's maternal uncle) would customarily have taken an active interest in the social, economic, and political future of his offspring.[47]

It must be remembered as well that the association of continence with spiritual commitment still served to offer lay-people, especially women religious but occasionally married couples, the choice of a way of life outside the hierarchies and machinations of the feudal family. Communities of consecrated women had existed since the patristic period. In the "Dark Ages," women found a measure of independence from husband and family by entering convents and monasteries, sometimes after having raised a family. Widows often went to monasteries, and some women even left their spouses to do so. Noble women used their own resources (property received at marriage from their husbands, or inherited at the death of their fathers) to found religious communities, in which their daughters could be educated, and to which they themselves could later retire. Such houses, sometimes with separate accommodations for women and men, could become centers of learning. An example is Whitby, founded in Northumbria in the seventh century by Hild, a noblewoman baptized at the age of fourteen. Convents also served as a refuge for unmarriageable daughters, primarily of wealthy families, since entry required a dowry. This function contributed, predictable enough, to some scandalous violations of vows on the part of nuns who were personally less than fully committed to a religious vocation.[48] In the eleventh and twelfth centuries, a few men of means established religious communities which were open to persons, men and women, of any social standing, including repentant prostitutes.[49]

Continence in marriage, often at the urging of the wife, was another way to attain spiritual equality of men and women, clergy and laity, as well as to escape the heavy social determinations of family and parenthood. Augustine is reported by a fourth-century biographer to have commended a couple, who, at the woman's urging, had achieved self-discipline, replaced physical bonds with spiritual ones, and thus "passed from your own bodies into that of Christ."[50] Tracing the history of marital continence among laypersons in medieval times, Dyan Elliott notes that the great preponderance of women who instigated the practice, gaining not only freedom from standard domestic expectations but also the spiritual upper hand, represented a threat to male authority in the family and in public life. Continent lay married women, in particular, eventually presented a challenge to the spiritual superiority of the clergy. By the sixteenth century, after the appearance of a post-Reformation reinterpretation of the sanctity of married life, the custom of sexless marriage was in decline.[51]

Controversy about celibacy in the church today is sparked largely by its survival, primarily in Roman Catholicism, as a disciplinary requirement of priests, many of whom acquiesce to rather than embrace it. Vowed but nonordained members of religious orders, not all of which are Roman Catholic, are also obliged to celibacy; however, in such cases, it does not assume the form of so "extrinsic" a requirement as does priestly celibacy, since it is not attached to a state of life from which it is separable in principle, but to which there is no other ecclesially legitimate route of access. Groups of men or women living together in religiously consecrated community by definition choose to give up (or to avoid) marriage; there are other lay orders and even forms of communal life available to married couples. But in the Roman Catholic Church priests can be priests only by accepting celibacy, whether or not they live in community with other men. To choose the priesthood is to be made to choose celibacy. This has given debate about the value of celibacy much wider currency than would otherwise have been the case, and has forced a demand for consensus on the issue.

Sacerdotalis Celibatus (Paul VI's 1967 encyclical on priestly celibacy) praises celibacy without denigrating marriage, though it does see celibacy as manifesting the new reality initiated in Christ "in a clearer and more complete way" (.20). It portrays celibacy as a "support" for "the minister in his exclusive, definitive and total choice of the unique and supreme love of Christ," and in his offices of public worship and service to the Church (.14). It also commends "the free choice of sacred celibacy" as signifying "a love without reservations," and as stimulating "a charity which is open to all." One notes in *Sacerdotalis Celibatus* a tendency to portray celibacy as a heroic vocation in which the priest transcends earthly loves and takes on the likeness of Christ the eternal Priest (.26). The question remains whether the mandatory nature of what is legislated militates against its signification of solidarity in the body of Christ.

Schillebeeckx observes sensibly that as marriage is progressively re-evaluated as a fertile field for the kingdom's servants, religious fervor and enthusiasm which once found their outlet in virginity are able to energize Christian marriage. Of course, the embodiment of Christian ideals in marriage is facilitated today by increasing historical recognition of the equality and reciprocal contributions of all family members. Modern values distance family life more from the economic and political factors which have always determined its inner relations and social functions, and which were so objectionable to members of the early churches. This is not to say marriage and family should or even can be "freed" from their complex lines of connection to all levels of communal life. Individualism in the family is as unbalanced and pernicious as tyrannical social control. But the Christian family today, in nourishing the human capacity for compassion and solidarity, can provide a school for and support to Christian commitment which was once much more easily embodied in a renunciation of kin ties and of the bondedness to social structures represented by marital, procreative sexuality, or by other forms of sexuality (like concubinage, prostitution, and ancient homosexuality) which were just as bound to the enforcement of dominative gender roles.

The worth of celibacy itself, in Christianity today, must also be measured in communitarian terms, not in those either of personal perfectionism or of a new sexualization of the celibate state. Part of the value of celibacy is its witness to a transcendent fulfillment of all human strivings and the relativization of all human loves;[52] part of it is even a testimony that sexuality is not as deep and definitive a component of human identity as it seems for post-Freudian Westerners or was socially for premodern women. But surely another test, even a more important one, is its role in building up discipleship community. Seeing marriage and celibacy as interdependent gifts, William Spohn subjects celibacy to the tests of deeper intimacy and social fruitfulness. Drawing on Paul's corporate imagery, he rejects "an isolated or detached asceticism," in favor of celibacy as a "focused passion for the Kingdom," "ordered to building up the Body of Christ."[53] The test of consecrated celibacy is the concrete capacity of those who live it to magnify in the life of the community those values and relationships which Jesus held up as embodying the kingdom: compassion, mercy, forgiveness, and solidarity with the deprived and the "sinful."

Indissolubility

Another distinctive mark of Christian sexual ethics traditionally is its prohibition of divorce. This prohibition has had a long and tortuous career in church history and canon law. Since the Reformation, Protestant churches have, with varying degrees of leniency, permitted marriage to be dissolved in exceptional circumstances. The Anglican Church forbids divorce in theory, but sometimes permits pastorally the remarriage of persons divorced under civil law. But Roman Catholicism forbids the divorce of any two baptized persons whose marriage has been consummated sexually, and—at least in theory—excludes divorced and remarried persons from reception of the Eucharist. Indeed, dissolution of a valid marriage and consequent remarriage is viewed as ontologically impossible. The huge increase in the number of annulments after Vatican II, along with expansion of grounds on which declarations of nullity may be justified, have led to the perception (sometimes the accusation) that Catholic annulment amounts to a tacit form of divorce.[54]

The suffering of those who have experienced marital breakdown, who have established new relationships, and for whom religious identity is of immense importance, has led to many a call for a removal of the bar to remarriage or a relaxation of the penalties against those who transgress this line. (The prohibition of divorce is maintained more firmly in Roman Catholicism and Anglicanism than in many other communions.) A woman with long experience in ministry to divorced and remarried Catholics opens a collection of essays on the subject by asking, "How can we communicate the message of God's ever-present love to those who feel devastated and powerless in the wake of the loss of a marriage?" "How can we offer a support system in which hurting people can heal, learn from the past and have the hope of one day forming life-nurturing relationships?"[55]

This approach to divorce clearly represents the modern Western valuation of personal fulfillment and emotional welfare in marriage, and sees the alleviation of individuals' pain as a central part of the church's pastoral mission. Laws prohibiting divorce are perceived to injure and alienate those who are "powerless" in the face of church authority. Yet Christianity's stance against divorce was originally a stance against the manipulation of marriage, and of children and women, to serve family interests in power and property. A corollary was that permanency in marriage better served the growth of marital friendship and the nurturance of offspring. To understand the historical significance of the church's stand on indissolubility and divorce, one must return to some of the same considerations about social control of marriage and the family which bear on celibacy in primitive, patristic, and medieval Christianity. It is through the emergence of indissolubility as a mark of sacramental marriage that we may view the deepest transformations of Christian thinking about marriage as a relationship of equal persons who ideally unite their whole lives, and not only their bodies for procreation and their property for the formation of new households.

Virginity in the early church objected to institutions of marriage and kinship which made intimacy, reciprocity, and mutual responsibility for children virtually impossible. Yet, from primitive Christian times, marriage was respected as a realm in which a disciple could give practical expression to faith, and whose internal order could even be transformed by *agape*.[56] In the New Testament and in early teaching like the decrees of Elvira (which warned Christians away from adultery, but permitted men—not women—to remarry after divorcing an adulterous spouse[57]), Christians were instructed to adopt special marital behavior. Gradually marriage was taken over explicitly by the church as an arena of grace in its own right, with the implication that the social meaning of marriage, and not only the personal relationships of Christians within the standing institution, could be changed.

At the beginning of the fourth century, the assumption was that Christians would follow the marriage ceremonies and contracts of their pagan neighbors, according to Roman legislation. Marriage was a secular affair, arranged by families, celebrated in the home, and conformed to pagan traditions, though the baptized were expected to live in marriage, as in all relationships, by faith, hope, and love. In the fourth century, a priest's prayer and blessing begin to be associated with weddings, though not for second marriages. The first evidence of a nuptial mass and the solemnization by a priest of a marriage contracted civilly occurs in the fourth and fifth centuries. There was no obligation to receive such a blessing until the tenth century, around which time the church began to insist that the wedding ceremony be a public affair, in front of the church. The church was also assuming more jurisdictional power over marriage, not in the sense of legislating the contract, but in the sense of settling disputes about its validity, including the determination of impediments to marriage. Complete jurisdiction was to be in the hands of the church by the eleventh and twelfth centuries, and by the thirteenth, a developing theology of marriage's sacramentality had matured.[58]

From the end of the fourth century and on into the next three generations, Western Europe experienced a series of migrations of largely Germanic peoples, which were important to this process of church involvement in marriage and family practices. These migrations gradually displaced Roman institutions and government; by the beginning of the sixth century, the Roman Empire had been divided into a number of different states ruled by peoples with different tribal histories, for example, the Anglo-Saxons in Britain, the Franks in Gaul, and the Visigoths in Spain. The Roman population continued to observe its own customs alongside the newcomers. In a pluralistic situation, the Roman and "barbarian" ways influenced and modified one another, and Christian practices evolved partly as attempts to moderate both.[59] If anything, the Germanic influx accentuated the Greco-Roman proclivity to place authority over marriage in the hands of the kin group, represented by senior male members, and to determine the fate of young people and women in general according to the welfare of the family as a whole.

The law of the Germanic societies hinged on two archaic principles which made the Christianization of their marriage customs especially challenging: collective responsibility of the kindred for the actions of any members, and, derivatively, reciprocal revenge. Peace and security were valued and sought within the group, but the right of violence against outsiders was taken for granted if the interests of the kin group were at stake. For example, Germanic folklaw recognized three ways of contracting a marriage, one of which was by capture (abduction and rape). The less violent alternatives were purchase and consent. The latter was primarily an option when the groom and his family could not or would not come up with the price of a woman, but the woman agreed to marry. In such cases, the husband did not acquire the same legal rights over the wife as if he or his family had purchased her. Concubinage was also very widespread and involved longstanding unions (often polygynous) without full legal rights.[60] While divorce was almost exclusively a male prerogative, adultery was a crime of which virtually only women were accused.

Even by the time the migrations in Europe began, ancient assumptions had begun to undergo modification. However, the records of a few extreme cases—illustrating the effects of such practices on marriage and on the status of women, even after Christianization—survive to tell us that old attitudes die hard. Gregory of Tours relates a case from the early Middle Ages in which a family was humiliated by a daughter who had been taken as a priest's concubine. Imprisoning the priest, the family redeemed its honor by burning the woman alive. In another instance from the eighth century, a man abducted an engaged girl by force and raped her. The aggrieved fiancé obtained a court judgment by which both the victim and perpetrator were turned over to him. He spared their lives, sent the girl to a convent, then belatedly decided to marry her after all. Also reconsidering his pardon of the rapist, he killed him. As a result, half of his property and all of his bride's were confiscated by the king, who donated it to a monastery; the groom entered the same monastery, and "presumably" the woman had little alternative but to repair likewise to the cloister.[61]

Throughout the Middle Ages, church law attempted, with admittedly uneven results, to curtail sexual violence (for example, marriage by rape), to equalize sexual norms for men and women (no adultery or divorce), and to protect marriage as a personal relationship by making it contingent on the consent of the parties, not family negotiations or male prerogatives alone (Gratian's codification of church law, 1140). The legal definition of the "conjugal debt" as a claim right either party could exact from the other partly equalized the relationship of spouses, and protected their union from outside interference (for example, of parents or feudal lords controlling the movements of serfs).[62] The fact that by the time of Charlemagne (eighth century), the Western family had assumed the form of "a coresidential, primary descent group" also supported these trends, insofar as the quality of emotional relationships among family members had assumed a new domestic priority.[63]

Theologically, Augustine set the stage for the path the church was to follow in this gradual appropriation of marriage as a specifically Christian way of life. He wrote *On the Good of Marriage* in 401 as a rejoinder to the proposal of Jovinian that marriage was equal to virginity. However, he was also anxious to refute the teaching of the Manicheans that all sex and procreation were wrong. Augustine calls the union of "man and wife" "the first natural tie of human society," ideally "a kind of friendly and genuine union of the one ruling and the other obeying." He does not link sex directly to this relationship, for sexual passion seems inimical to the peaceful concord he envisions between spouses. Children "are the only worthy fruit" of sexual intercourse.[64] Although it would be better to refrain from sex entirely, by begetting children, "marital intercourse makes something good out of the evil of lust."[65] Sex outside of marriage is of course a mortal sin; even within marriage, it is a venial sin if sought for the purpose of pleasure. Only children or compliance with an undisciplined spouse who might fall to fornication save sex from sin.[66]

Children are not the only good of *marriage*, however; Augustine's enumeration of its three goods is the backbone of all later Christian teaching (which tended to convert them to "ends"[67]).

They are *fides* (sexual fidelity); *proles* (offspring); and *sacramentum* (the indissoluble bond). Although Augustine indicates that even natural marriage should be characterized by permanence, the "sacred bond" takes on a special significance for baptized persons. The bond is a mutual pledge of permanent fidelity. Christians, even if separated from their spouses, should not remarry as long as the spouse lives.[68] The permanence of Christian marriage is comparable to the union of Christ and church (Eph. 5:25), an analogy Augustine develops in *On Marriage and Concupiscence* (418).[69]

For several centuries after Augustine, the church wavered on indissolubility. From the time of the Fathers, adultery had been considered grounds for divorce, though not all presumed a right to remarry. Even when a marriage was unjustly terminated, the "adultery" of a remarriage was forgivable, and the second marriage was not necessarily considered invalid.[70] Although in the medieval theology of the sacrament, indissolubility came to be understood as an ontological reality that could not be dissolved, for the Fathers and their immediate heirs, the *sacramentum* of marriage was an obligation and task for Christian couples, a duty which they could fail to meet.[71]

As we have seen, divorce in the ancient world was generally to the disadvantage of women as individuals (even when legalized as a woman's "right"), and to the advantage of individual men and of powerful and wealthy families. This situation persisted through the Middle Ages, though early medieval women may have had considerable personal and economic freedom.[72] Marriage in feudal society was a social act which linked one blood line to another, and ensured that the eldest son of the eldest son would inherit the family patrimony. The virginity of women was a "saleable commodity," and their fidelity in marriage was paramount to the secure transmission of family wealth.[73] Women who were barren of male heirs could be divorced, abandoned or replaced by a fertile second wife. The upper classes in Europe also contracted mercenary child marriages—forbidden by the church but not declared invalid. The *Life of St. Hugh of Lincoln* tells of one child who was widowed by two noblemen and married to a third before she was eleven; Richard II of England was engaged to a seven-year-old daughter of the French king in 1395, and married to her the next year.[74]

The machinations required to protect property also had consequences for men, since younger sons were prevented from contracting legal marriages or setting up households. The conventions of courtly love, governing twelfth-century romantic liaisons between knights and married noblewomen, may be explained as a nonprocreative, non-kin-linked alternative both for men who found their marital opportunities to be virtually nonexistent and for women who found that marriage afforded little emotional fulfillment. Georges Duby conjectures that, in a military society, the ritualization of desire in courtly love reinforced "the rules of the ethics of vassalage," binding the knight to the lady's lord, and training the knight in submission, sublimation, and loyalty. Hence, it was at bottom a love between men, and in its own way misogynist.[75]

Three developments of church law in the Middle Ages were instrumental in fighting such abuses, although clearly not with total consensus behind them, nor success in attaining their aims. These remedies concerned the stability and permanence of a monogamous relationship, and centered on consent, indissolubility, and exogamy (enforced by "incest" laws). All of these developments reduced inequalities between rich and poor, and, to a perhaps lesser extent, those between men and women.

Going back to classical Rome, lawyers had debated whether consent or sexual consummation, or both, was necessary to bring marriage into being. From a Christian point of view, to require sexual intercourse threatened the perfection of the marriage of Mary and Joseph. Although Gratian's twelfth-century laws distinguished two stages of matrimony (as initiated by consent and confirmed by sexual union), the theological and canonical tide turned in favor of

Peter Lombard's opinion in favor of consent alone. Pope Alexander III, later in the same century, after having wavered between Gratian and Lombard, decreed that the consent of the marrying couple alone made their union valid and binding.[76] A contracted but unconsummated marriage could be dissolved under rare circumstances (such as the taking of religious vows by the bride), and only by special ecclesiastical dispensation. This had important consequences. The necessity and sufficiency of mutual consent to establish a marriage disrupted the authority of parents to trade or sell their offspring, especially those who were under the already-low legal age. The consent requirement also lent support to couples who desired to marry—or who had eloped—without parental consent. Not only did this deter the rich in their pursuit of wealth through arranged marriages, it refocused the meaning of marriage on the personal commitment of young women and men. Families were also less well-positioned to forbid marriage to sons in order to prevent division of the family estate. Indissolubility, realized haltingly over several centuries of developing church law, characterized the marriage of two baptized persons who had given their free and witnessed consent to the union, and only if that consent had been given. As in ancient Greece and Rome however, rapid repeat trading on the marriage-market was more a ploy of the higher classes than of the common people. Phillipe Ariés notes that rural communities no doubt depended on the stability of unions for their own stability and prosperity, and for the reliable continuance of the extensive and delicate negotiations necessary for the exchange of sons and daughters among families.[77]

Certain impediments to marriage—which would make consent ineffective—were also instituted by church law, and among these the one with the most serious consequences was the impediment of close relationship. Elite marriages within close degrees of relationship, between cousins for instance, were common in order to consolidate property, and had become more so after about 1100, with a reorganization of aristocratic inheritance to more strongly favor male lineages than they had even in the previous century.[78] The church unsettled the picture—in which there was less and less financial independence for women—by forbidding marriages within the seventh degree of kinship (eventually reduced to four), including relations by marriage and shared godparenting of a child. Legally mandated exogamy (marrying outside one's own kinship group), replacing endogamy (marrying kin), meant that wealthy households could no longer accumulate as many women or as much property, thus increasing the circulation of both in the less well-to-do population.[79] Perhaps predictably, those used to having their own way in the politics of marriage rebounded quickly by exploiting or creating loopholes in church regulations. Consanguinity at rather distant levels became a belated excuse for some divorces (as when Louis VII of France divorced Eleanor of Aquitaine). Betrothed couples could arrange to become co-godparents in order to break off the arrangements. Church bureaucrats, and even popes, were not above giving dispensations and legitimizing marriages for money, or in cooperation with figures allied with their own political interests.[80]

Accompanying the development of church law enhancing the permanence of Christian marriage, equalizing the obligations of the classes and sexes,[81] and carrying forward the personal meaning and mutuality of marriage by grounding it in consent, was an evolving theology of marriage as a sacrament. The special function of marriage as a sign and mediator of grace rested neither in sex nor in the production of children; both of these had long been manipulated by worldly "regimes" which undermined the gospel. Moreover, sex itself had been too lately identified by Christian thinkers as an unparalleled occasion of moral disgrace.

Since Augustine, it was the bond between spouses which was the sacramental analogue to redemption in Christ; and so consent was identified as establishing an indissoluble contract which becomes the bearer of sacramentality. Critics today rightly note the extrinsic and juridical nature of the virtual equation of consent with a contract, and the association of consent and indissolubility in canon law.[82] Yet it remains true that in opting for consent over familial financial negotiations or sexual consummation, the church enabled later sacramental theologies to magnify the personal meaning of marriage, gradually replacing contractual language with that of personal covenant. By the thirteenth century, a theology of marriage had emerged which combined the elements of personal commitment and union, sexual intercourse, and the education of children in a fitting social institution, albeit with a continuing gender imbalance. Although the majority saw sex as primarily for reproduction, a minority of thirteenth- and fourteenth-century theologians (like Hugh of St. Victor) stressed mutual love in their model of marriage.

The medieval theologians would have identified those things that make a marriage as the partners' mutual consent, primarily as spiritual communion and a desire for relationship, but open to and presuming sex, formulated legally in respect to both spouses equally as a "right to sexual intercourse."[83] The metaphysical bond of marriage existed from the moment of consent, and was irrevocable. The consent was the sacramental sign; the sacramental reality was the bond established by consent; and the grace caused by the sacrament created the unity and faithfulness represented legally and negatively as indissolubility.[84] The increased investment of the church in defending the goodness of legitimate marriage, and its lessening interest in placing moral capital in the perils of sexual intercourse, was prompted in part by the Catharist and Albigensian heresies. Their dualist and pessimistic views of the body and sex were condemned repeatedly in the twelfth century. Councils in the thirteenth through sixteenth numbered marriage among the seven sacraments. The indissolubility of Christian marriage, as obligatory and binding, was defined at Trent (1545–63).

The accomplishments and continuing ambivalences of the developing theology are well represented in Thomas Aquinas. Confirming the biases of his own culture with the philosophical explanations of Aristotle, Aquinas saw the female sex in pejorative terms, and as destined for a procreative role.[85] He takes a strongly communal view of marriage, subordinates wife to husband, sees the first purpose of sex in terms of the needs of the species, and defines marriage as a social and domestic partnership, rather than as a personally rewarding, mutual affective union.[86] Aquinas essentially follows Augustine and the *Sentences* of Peter Lombard in offering three purposes of marriage, among which he designates procreation as primary. The indissolubility of marriage, a natural property, is more directed to the proper education of children; to the need of the family for certain paternity; to harmonious familial relations; and to the fulfillment of the social obligations of the couple; than it is to their mutual self-dedication in love. However, the Christian couple's mutual fidelity is a sign to the church of Christ's presence.[87] And Aquinas shows some appreciation for the importance of mutuality in marriage when he objects that a husband's freedom to take many wives, or to send away an older wife who was no longer fertile or beautiful, would reduce wives to a state of servile inequality.[88]

Aquinas describes the love between husband and wife as the greatest sort of friendship, and as characterized by the highest intensity of all loves, because of their union "in the flesh."[89] Although Aquinas retains the Augustinian teaching that sex for pleasure's sake is a sin, he does not see the enjoyment of pleasure itself as wrong, as long as it is properly contained within the marital and procreative union. Aquinas has achieved a link between sexual intimacy, even sexual pleasure, and the intense love of spouses; his definition of marriage as a sacramental vehicle of Christ's presence in the church is not achieved over against or apart from sexual love and sexual pleasure.

For contemporary Christians, as for most members of modern society, the highest meaning of marriage, and its only really indispensable one, is love. In Catholic sacramental theology, the love union of the partners is associated with marriage's sacramentality, and mutually pleasurable sex and children are expressive and derivative of this union. In the words of Walter Kasper, "The love that exists between man and wife is . . . an epiphany of the love and faithfulness of God that was given once and for all time in Jesus Christ and is made present in the Church."[90] This reinterpretation undoubtedly owes much to Enlightenment and Romantic ideals of personal freedom and fulfillment outside the constraints of institutions. Also contributory are the Reformation affirmation of the equality of all persons in the sight of God; the presence of God in ordinary human vocations, including marriage; the strengthening of the idea that marriage is a social tie of which a key good is companionship; and the concomitant beginning of a deemphasis both on procreation and on juridical control over marriage.

Contemporary Roman Catholic thought about marriage has been shaped markedly by personalist philosophies growing out of the phenomenology of Edmund Husserl, Max Scheler, and Maurice Merleau-Ponty, and represented in relation to marriage by Dietrich von Hildebrand and Herbert Doms.[91] Personalism is a characteristically modern phenomenon in that it stresses the priority and the experience of the human subject. Intersubjective values become pre-eminently important in moral thinking. In the nineteenth and early twentieth centuries, Catholic moral theology had narrowed sexual morality to the act of sexual intercourse, especially its setting and structure, rather than considering the quality of the relationship in which sex occurred. Sex belonged in marriage; its form had to follow the requirements of conception. Marriage was in principle established by consent, and the conditions of consent could be juridically ascertained. Unconsummated marriages were in practice dissolvable, which led to theological and canonical inconsistencies, but to no great additional difficulty in the determination of the fact of a marriage. The universal moral relevance of the procreative end of sex was captured in crude if convoluted propositional form by any number of seminary manuals: all intentional acts resulting in "venereal pleasure" outside of marriage were illicit. And in marriage, all acts were required to follow the structure necessary to procreation. The "secondary ends" of marriage, mutual help and the avoidance of sexual sin, did not figure significantly when compared to procreation. Pregnancy could be avoided only by refraining from procreative acts; neither incomplete sexual acts (for example, withdrawal) nor artificial contraceptives were allowed.

Thus the moral theologians adopted the legalist approach of the canon lawyer, who determines validity and invalidity of unions; and of the confessor, who investigates degrees of sin and assigns penance. Moral casuistry did not adduce the quality of the couple's relationship as a measure of the morality of their sexual union. One moralist (who objected to the "personalist" reinterpretations) insisted that "[e]ven a marriage in which there is no mutual help, no life in common, hatred instead of love, and complete separation, both bodily and spiritually, remains a true marriage in the sense that the essence of marriage is still there."[92] To be fair, this man expressed some misgivings about such a conclusion, owning that it might seem an "affront" to the common sense of married people. It was a sign of the times that the latter consideration had no bearing at all on his final determination.

The casuistic approach took sex and marriage seriously as realms of moral striving and of social importance, about which the church was obliged to give guidance; but it was grievously inadequate to the human experiences of sex, marriage, parenthood, and family. In favor of the security of an instantaneous ontological change at the moment of consent, it abandoned the Fathers' vision of indissolubility as a "guiding ideal" realized only over the lifetime of a marriage.[93] It perpetuated enigmas such as the readiness of the church to dissolve unconsummated marriages (now even on the grounds of psychological nonconsummation), all the while maintaining that consent alone establishes the sacramental bond forever (compare new Cans. 1057 and 1055.2 with 1142).

It failed especially in identifying and nurturing the positive values that give these relationships their personal texture and might encourage moral excellence.

Whatever the medieval redefinition of marriage as a personal union of spouses had gained in human terms, or in terms of Christian compassion and upbuilding, had been submerged. The prevailing rigorist and "scientific" moral approach was sometimes "pastoral" about human failure, but created immense anxiety and guilt among the faithful and did little to encourage genuine sexual virtue. And yet, the personalist proposal that it is the actual love relationship of partners that constitutes marriage was already eroding the idea that an act of consent creates an ontological bond which cannot disappear, no matter what the real circumstances of the relationship which it supposedly grounds.

Another menace to the received definition of indissolubility was the move away from sexual acts as a tangible test of both the validity of the contract and the morality of married life. The 1917 Code of Canon Law had defined marriage as a contract in which spouses exchange the right over one another's bodies with a view to the acts apt for procreation (*ius in corpus*). As long as consent is given, the contract comes into being, the rights persist, and the specific bodily means of fulfilling the right can be used to supervise the couple. The actualization of the virtues of marital love are irrelevant to marriage's sacramental meaning.[94]

The 1983 Code replaces the definition of marriage as a contract to exchange sex acts with a combination of covenant and contract language, and indicates that that to which the partners consent is the partnership of the whole of life (*communio*).[95] This has so far meant no specific changes in magisterial teaching on sexual morality. Standard conclusions about sacramental marriage, indissolubility, and divorce, once derived from the notion of marriage as a contract, remain in place alongside the less congenial covenant and partnership language.

It is ironic that, despite the initial flood of objections and even incredulity directed at the personalists from the deputies of the magisterium, certain of the new recommendations were eventually to find their way into papal encyclicals, canon law, and other official teaching. Even while upholding the ban on contraception, Pius XI in 1930 (*Casti connubii*) already began to speak of marriage in terms of the fundamentality of the mutual love of spouses. Since Vatican II (*Gaudium et spes*, 1965) and the encyclical *Humanae vitae* (1968) the language of primary and secondary ends has been sidelined. And in the 1980s, John Paul II built an entire theology of sex and marriage around the concept that sex in marriage is first and foremost a total self-gift of spouses. Both Paul VI and John Paul II use personalist depictions of marital love to explain the immorality of artificial birth control. But the foundations of the edifice of tradition have been shaken.

The Christian normalization of permanency and sexual fidelity in marriage has, over the centuries, tended to equalize the relations of wife and husband, and to decrease the usefulness of marriage as a tool to secure political and economic goods. With these developments has come a proportionate rise in the companionate value of marriage. Especially since the Enlightenment, the distinction between passionate and romantic love outside marriage and loyal, domestic, procreative love in marriage has gradually diminished.[96] We (modern Westerners) expect from marriage and from our spouses a high degree of sexual and emotional fulfillment, as well as continuing to rely on marriage to supply household and family security. While the affective expectations of marriage present rich opportunities to overcome gender disparities, and to accomplish the sort of genuine friendship which supports and unites spouses in hardship and success, it also places new burdens and stresses on the marital relationship and on the family.

Divorce is no easy answer to difficulty, for it exacts a high psychological price from all involved, and usually places women and children at a consequent economic disadvantage.[97] Privatized sexual and marital decision-making, so often focused on the self-fulfillment of those individuals whose personal, economic, or social assets position them well to "trade up" in sexual partners, or to abandon the disappointments, sacrifices, and difficulties of an ongoing commitment to spouse and children, is a "liberal" version of the patriarchal socializations of sex against which Christianity originally reacted. Yet the painful exclusion of divorced and remarried persons who seek to mend their lives and make amends with the Christian community is neither a productive nor a compassionate method of countering marital breakdown. It offers no compelling alternate vision which can heal the ills of consumer sex and fragmented family ties.

The indissolubility of a personal, sexual union once served as an embodied sign of social solidarity, even if union in the Body of Christ has never been fully realized by any historical community. Indissolubility, as a canonical requirement of or limit on marital behavior, has since the Middle Ages become more and more marginal to, and even destructive of, a sense of communal transformation of spouses and families in Christ. New interpretations of marital love, consummated in pleasurable sexual intimacy; and of family, where shared parental love complements the love of woman and man, promise to renew Christianity's witness against the cynical, oppressive, and degrading transience too often seen in sexual relationships in modern societies. But this promise will not be realized if the agenda of renewal holds as its centerpiece the old machinery of constraint and condemnation; nor if it persists in continuing subtly to define women's identity in sexual terms.

At the bottom of some of the lingering paradoxes in Christian teaching on marriage may be the Augustinian anxiety that, while marriage is good, sex is dubious if not evil. A woman will wonder to what extent it is a male experience of sexuality, especially an experience of males struggling toward continence while shaping a normative theory and theology of sex, that has fostered this particular ambivalence. Male sexual drives are more genitally focused and urgent than those of most women; male sexual response may seem to have an autonomy and uncontrollability that accentuates sex's danger and easily represents all that is obsessive and addictive in human moral fault.[98] Marriage and family, as structured trainings and channelings of wild impulse, may appear to men, especially celibate men, as safe moral havens, as the counterbalancing sublimation of sexual gratification into socially constructive human relationships.

For women, on the other hand, sexual drives assume less importance on the landscape of identity. Although sexual pleasure may be a good and a goal, uncontrollability is rarely an issue.[99] Women's sexual dilemma focuses more on maternity—on the immediate and highly consequential potential of sexual acts to result in pregnancy and motherhood, and all that these realities socially entail. For women, it is precisely the social institutions that men find so consoling which, structured as a "male" solution, present personal and social perils for women. For men, sex is the locus of moral danger. For women, marriage and family are dangerous, at least as traditionally practiced. Women seek not so much a structuring of unruly sexual passion, as a mutually responsible and intimate human relationship in sex, including an experience of maternity that flows from and represents such reciprocity.

Male theologians early on praised virginity as a relief from the degradations of sex itself, as well as from women's ubiquitous subjection to husbands. For Christian women, sex was mostly an extrinsic demand to which one was subjected, requiring reluctant compliance, just as one was subjected to domestic structures dominated by, and at the service of, a "lord" and "master." The history of Christian teaching on marriage reveals the gradual ascendancy of the marital relationship as a covenant of spouses. Much of the ambiguity that remains is a symptom of the lasting influence of the perspective on sexual danger that has given form to most of the tradition.[100]

Procreation and Relationship in Tension: The Birth-Control Debate

The issue of birth control, especially artificial contraception, has been a nexus of the difficulties in reinterpreting procreation as "parenthood": a social relationship over time in which the emotional bonding of parents and child is as important as the physical realities of conception, birth, and kinship and the socioeconomic functions of the intergenerational family. Traditionally, birth control was forbidden both because procreation was seen as a duty to the family and species, not as a means of parental fulfillment, and because procreation was considered to be the ultimate purpose and sole real justification of sex. The protection of procreation as a divinely ordained reason for sex also counteracted religions and philosophies which saw the material world, the body, sex, or marriage as evil.[101]

In the early modern period, Catholic moral theology developed a rational, scientific casuistry, focused on clearly defined *acts,* isolable for analysis in terms of their empirical or material structure. The intentions behind the acts were also considered morally relevant, but the moralist's incisive logic and razor-thin distinctions were exercised nonetheless on fairly narrow slices of human sexual experience, from which the ambiguities and shadings of human emotions and relationships had been trimmed.

As the certainty and objectivity of the Enlightenment epistemologies have come under fire, the methods and conclusions of recent centuries of moral teaching have been re-established increasingly on church authority. A major consideration in the 1968 reassertion of Catholicism's condemnation of birth control—which many wanted withdrawn precisely in view of the total relation of spouses and the welfare of families—was consistency in authoritative church teaching. Thus have the stakes been raised.

Since the advent of personalism, relationship has become paramount in sexual ethics, even in Catholic theory. In accepting that couples could engage in sex acts while intentionally avoiding procreation, *Humanae vitae* envisioned a meaning of sex that was nonprocreative, that expressed the mutual commitment of the couple. Sex took on more meaning as part of the couple's intimate, loving relationship—but relationship remains disconcertingly hard to quantify. Current teaching and its backing theologies use the physical procreative structure of each sex act to test the personal intimacy of the union the acts express. The teachings are still put forward as genuine representations of human sexual experience. But the more relational and personal meanings of sex are not commensurate with a criterion of biological structure, and the insistence on interpreting experience this way seems more motivated by a desire to redeem the past than by a readiness to look carefully at what sex really means for couples today. The new values of interpersonal communion and sexual intimacy which receive such high magisterial praise, are already from the outset expected to carry the weight of the moral prescriptions whose originating "scientific" methodologies have fallen into disrepute.

A corollary problem is that "procreation" is often read in excessively individualist terms. The magisterium practically reduces it to a requirement of *sex acts;* the magisterium's critics usually move procreation out to the relation of the *couple* (and immediate family). But the meaning of parenthood, cross-culturally, historically, and experientially, is more *social* than either alternative. This at least was captured by Aquinas' (and the older tradition's) view that procreation is a service to the human race. The "procreative purpose" of sex cannot be adequately grasped, explained, or protected by the narrow access road of individual acts of sexual intercourse; to see parenthood as an undertaking of couples is an improvement, but does not go far enough. Parenthood makes sex (the couple's sexual relation) fully accountable for, and contributory to, human well-being and interdependence in communities beyond the couple. Although *sexual* couples can and should contribute to society and church in many ways, their union in parenthood is a specifically *sexual* mode of social participation. Not only the unity of love and procreation, but also the social implications of sex and its reproductive potential are at stake in the debate on contraception. Moreover, if women and men are to be equal partners in the conjugal relationship, their reproductive, familial, and social contributions must be seen in genuinely equal terms, and their control over family size must be shared.[102] This is poignantly evident in debates over population control in relatively poor countries where women are among the most disadvantaged. (We shall return to this question at the end of the chapter.)

Development of Church Teaching

In *Casti connubii* (*On Christian Marriage*, 1930), Pius XI calls marriage a "sacred partnership" (.9), of which children are the greatest blessing and fruit (.11, .12). The encyclical ranks procreation and fidelity as primary and secondary ends of sex and marriage (.17, .19, .54).[103] Any sex act which "is deliberately frustrated in its natural power to generate life is an offence against the law of God and nature" (.56). Procreation is completed in the education of offspring, in which parents give one another "mutual help" (.16). But the structure of the family, divinely instituted, is patriarchal: "This order includes both the primacy of the husband with regard to the wife and children [and] the ready subjection of the wife and her willing obedience" (.26). To say that the subjection of the wife is offensive to human dignity, or that rights of husband and wife are equal, is "a crime." A woman should devote her attention to children, husband, and family, and should not take up business or politics, or even be at liberty to "administer her own affairs." (.74).

On the other hand, the personalist philosophical trends which diminish procreation and enhance spousal reciprocity have already had a destabilizing effect on this procreation-centered hierarchy: "the love of husband and wife . . . holds pride of place in Christian marriage" (.23). "This mutual inward moulding of husband and wife . . . can in a very real sense be said to be the chief reason and purpose of matrimony" (.24). After the next half century, mutual love becomes dominant in Christian approaches to sex; in Roman Catholicism, it remains in uneasy alliance with the privileged role of procreation in defining sexual morality. The high praise accorded to marital love, coupled with an insistence that it be measured by its physical "openness" to conception, is symptomatic of this tension.[104]

Pope John Paul II is particularly energetic in pursuit of personalist as well as biblical themes, using the metaphor "language of the body," to play out sexuality's intersubjectivity.[105] The pope suggests that Adam's exclamation "This at last is bone of my bone and flesh of my flesh" (Gen. 2:23) recognizes the woman's human identity, realized bodily as "femininity" and in "the reciprocity and communion of persons" which sexual difference makes possible.[106] Moreover, the "finality" of "the life of the spouses-parents" is to make their "humanity" "subject, in a way" to "the blessing of fertility, namely, 'procreation,'" (Gen. 1:28).[107] Leaving aside the question whether or how these theological interpretations are linked to the original meanings of the biblical texts, one can still appreciate John Paul II's attempt to engage Catholic sexual morality with Scripture and to explore basic male-female relationships and their potential for mutual self-donation.

In *Familiaris Consortio* (Apostolic Exhortation *On the Family*, 1981), the pope elaborates sex as a language of totality. Adherence to *Humanae vitae*'s use of "each" sex act as final measure of the interpersonal and parental commitment of spouses is still demanded.[108] Every act of sexual intercourse is invested with the full weight of the couple's love and relationship, and that weight is pinned, not on the emotional or pleasurable aspects of the act, but on its procreativity, reduced to pristine biological format. "The total physical self-giving would be a lie if it were not the sign and fruit of a total personal self-giving" (.11). "When couples, by means of recourse to contraception, separate these two meanings [unitive and procreative] ... they ... degrade human sexuality and with it themselves and their married partner by altering its value of 'total' self-giving. Thus the innate language that expresses the total reciprocal self-giving of husband and wife is overlaid, through contraception, by an objectively contradictory language, namely, that of not giving oneself totally to the other" (.32).

On what basis is it affirmed that marital *experience* requires procreation as the completion of conjugal love (especially if tied to each sex act)?[109] The idea that each act is a total self-gift depends upon a very romanticized depiction of sex, and even of marital love. Certainly there will be times when an act of sexual sharing is hampered or disturbed by factors, intrinsically or extrinsically generated, which impinge, either temporarily or permanently, on the couple's relationship. They are stressed by economic difficulties, an ongoing disagreement about a family matter, blind spots in seeing one another's emotional needs, a crying child, lack of sleep, or an important project due at work. But even more than that, in the *most* ideal of circumstances, human beings rarely if ever accomplish "total self-gift." And the level of self-gift we do accomplish is rarely required to manifest itself, all or nothing, in a single action, much less in every one of a series of actions that we perform regularly. Would we subject the self-offering of the priest in the Eucharist to such a standard (under pain of mortal sin), even though the priest is supposedly standing in for Christ himself?

Couples need encouragement and support in nurturing a sex life which is indeed faithful to their full relationship, especially its interpersonal dimensions. Parenthood may well be a normative part of that relationship, and a part of which sex remains always a symbol and a bodily connection, even when sex acts are not individually fertile. A "positive refusal to be open to life" would certainly be wrong. But that refusal of or openness to "life" can be adequately tested in the way proposed, seems to me not only a preposterous but a harmful and even oppressive suggestion. This high and narrow standard militates against success in meeting the more practical demands of sexual, marital, and family life. When aligned with an "authoritative" overemphasis on procreation, an unreal idealization of sex acts can demean married persons' positive experiences of sexuality by labeling any so-called "compromise" of the ideal as dishonest, contradictory, false, and selfish.

As Rosemary Reuther observed early on in this debate, it is important to understand that, while the celibate cultivates sexual self-control and asceticism, that ethic should not dominate the sexuality of wives and husbands. Reuther insists rightly that a married person "has sublimated the sexual drive into a relationship with another person," the demands of which are "real and meaningful demands."[110] Yet one often finds couples who deviate from magisterial norms accused of a "lack of self-mastery."[111] The reality is that the sexual union of spouses needs at least as much to be encouraged, occasioned, and sustained, as to be mastered, limited, and scheduled.

Another critical issue is the assumptions about women which lie behind *Familiaris Consorti*'s delineation of the mutuality of sex. The pope deplores "machismo" as humiliating to women (.25), and declares that "the equal dignity and responsibility of men and women fully justifies women's access to public functions." However, the value of women's "maternal and family role" is supposed to exceed that of "all other public roles and all other professions;" women should not renounce their "femininity" or imitate masculine roles (.23). Apparently the full interpersonal and sexual reciprocity of women and men does not imply equality in all spheres of familial and social life. Therefore control of reproduction adequate to permit women as well as men to mesh family life with their contributions in other spheres is not a priority.

Indeed, the ideals of unity and mutual self-donation are presented with little attention to the social conditions which would make true reciprocity in sexuality, marriage, and parenthood a genuine possibility. The "mutual self-gift" language must be placed against the backdrop of gender roles, especially the pre-eminence of motherhood for women, which clearly color the picture John Paul II paints of sexual fulfillment in marriage.[112] One commends the pope for speaking out against injustice to women,[113] and giving attention to biblical evidence for the equality of women and for the sinfulness of their subordination to men.[114] Yet the practical consequences of biblical and personalist themes are far from receiving full recognition. One is struck by the coalescence of a sexual ethics of procreation and union represented in each and every sexual act, and a social context in which motherhood must constitute the primary identity of women.

In 1962, one author, in admittedly strong but not unrepresentative language, advanced the view that contraception is a bodily sign of "monstrous selfishness,"[115] and that it amounts to an unconscionable reversal of sex roles. "The woman who uses a diaphragm has closed herself to her husband. She has accepted his affection but not his substance. She permits him entrance but does not suffer him to be master." Thus sex as the "sign and symbol of wifely submission, of patriarchal authority, is made over covertly to serve the purposes of a weakly uxorious male and a domineeringly feminist wife."[116] One would expect that such florid language, enjoining in no uncertain terms the subordination of women and the equation of masculine identity with ejaculation of semen, would be unparalleled in theological writing over three decades later. Yet this essay was selected for publication in a major collection defending *Humanae vitae,* which appeared in 1993.[117] It seems not unreasonable to suppose therefore that fear of women's social equality with men and a tenacious grip on subordinating practices lie not far below the surface of readings of women's "dignity" which equate it with maternity and limit reliable control of pregnancy. Defenses of the magisterial view of sex rarely, if ever, explicitly envision a marital and familial situation in which both husband and wife serve in professions outside the home, and share equally in domestic responsibilities and rewards.

And yet the defenders of official Catholic teaching are not wrong in their uneasiness about the prevalence of social attitudes toward sex which, in divorcing sex from procreation, also seem to divorce it from commitment and responsibility.[118] Paul VI predicted "a general lowering of morality," and increasing disrespect for women as consequences of the contraception revolution (*Humanae Vitae,* .17). The status of women worldwide has certainly improved since 1968, partly due to increased access to education, health care, and family planning measures. Yet, at the same time, continuing permissiveness toward men's sexual behavior, combined with a greater social expectation that women will trade sex for relationship even without commitment, and the effective cultural dissociation of sex from responsibility for procreation, has contributed to widespread use of abortion as a means of birth control, and to the destabilization of families in industrialized nations. A result is that the psychological and economic needs of both women and children are often miserably neglected. Even progressive Catholics are likely to agree that "widespread unchastity has corrosive effects," and that a "contraceptive ethic" is rightly condemned, "if by that is meant a hedonistically inspired rejection of the deep and truly natural connection between making love and making babies."[119] I would only note that "permissiveness" and "hedonism" as cultural norms and realities are still gender-unequal.

The connection between sex, love, and babies cannot be apprehended, much less credibly advocated, in any individualist or act-oriented concept of sex, becoming a parent, or making a commitment. A strength of Catholic tradition is its strongly social vision of these realities.[120] They now require re-visioning toward a personalized and gender-equal paradigm, which recognizes the biographical and diachronic context of sexual and parental meaning and hence of sexual morality. To rehabilitate the parental significance of sexuality within such a paradigm, it may be necessary to give up specifying those purposes which fulfill sexual activity in the immediate experience of participants—where, in the event, procreation is rarely the dominant conscious aim—and to reposition reproduction in the social context which has for so long been so important in constituting its human meaning. The parenthood of the individual should be placed in the context of relationship to one's co-parent; conceiving, birthing, and parenting a child should be placed within the family, both nuclear and extended; and the family must be seen, neither as a "haven" from the world, nor as a nexus of social control, but as a school for critical contribution to the common good. To place parenthood in social context would also mean, from a Christian standpoint, to ask how Christian values transform the family, and shape the family's contribution to society.

Family as Domestic Church

One resource of renewal for a Christian theology of the family is the metaphor of "domestic church," harking back to writings of the Fathers. Currently enjoying a resurgence in Roman Catholic writings, this metaphor may be of general use in meshing social context with personal vocation and fulfillment in marriage and family. Indeed, an exclusively Roman Catholic exposition of this new theology might suffer from the gender imbalance in ecclesial roles (the exclusion of women from priestly ordination) which makes "church" an unhappy model for the Christian family and an inadequate foundation for the family's social mission. But important assets of this metaphor as developed in Catholicism to date are its vision of the family's transformative commitment to society, and its presupposition that the family as a community of social service can by virtue of that very function be a locus of its members' happiness and fulfillment.

The phrase "the domestic church," goes back to Irenaeus and Augustine; and other patristic writers also referred to religious devotion in the home.[121] "Domestic Church" appears in the documents of Vatican II (*Lumen gentium*, 11). In *On the Family* (.21, .49), it is linked to the reciprocal roles of men and women in the family, to the indissolubility and sacramentality of marriage, as well as to the nurture and education of children, and the contributions of families to church and society. "The Christian family constitutes a specific revelation and realization of ecclesial communion, and for this reason too it can and should be called 'the domestic church'" (.21). The purpose of this community, however, is not to enclose its members or Christian values for safety in a hostile world. The family should serve, in the words of *Gaudium et spes* (.52), as "a school of deeper humanity." "This happens where there is care and love for the little ones, the sick, the aged; where there is mutual service every day; when there is a sharing of goods, of joys and of sorrows" (*Familiaris Consortio*, .21).

In John Paul II's 1994 *Letter to Families*, in honor of the United Nation's Year of the Family, the family is defined as a community with a social vocation. The letter makes repeated use of the phrase "domestic church" (.3, .15, .16, .19), and defines the family as "a firmly grounded social reality," and "an institution fundamental to the life of every society" (.17). Contraception (2.1), broken families (.13), and abortion (.13, .21) are mentioned more with an eye to social dangers than to condemnation of individuals. Probably the major shortcomings of the letter are that the family's social mission is still focused on overcoming practices which contradict the magisterium's sexual teaching, rather than on social and economic injustices; and that the letter is not much attuned to the shapes and circumstances of families around the globe. The author seems much more to address dangers that are perceived to exist in consumerist societies where the standard family form is nuclear, with some intergenerational extension, and where various new technologies of birth control and reproduction are commanding social acceptance and medical and funding support. Not much encouragement and counsel are provided in this letter even to families in the assumed cultural setting who for a variety of reasons do not fit the standard model. However, given the model that the letter assumes, the family is expected to be socially engaged, and especially to focus on the humanization and "civilization" of relationships in the larger communities in which the family participates.[122]

The Christian family's "true vocation" is "the transformation of the earth and the renewal of the world, of creation and of all humanity" (.18; cf. .15). The interior solidarity of the family flows outward in a "civilization of love" for humanity and the common good, in country, state, and world (.15). Civilizing love, gift of self, and the social role of the family are directly linked to Jesus' commands to provide food, drink, clothing, and welcome to the needy (Matt. 25:34–36); and to his warning of judgment on those who turn the needy away (Matt. 25:41–43). These commands are given application in terms of problems besetting families and family members, however, not directly in terms of the family's contribution to wider justice concerns. Christlike action is exemplified in welcome to the unborn child; adopting abandoned or orphaned children and raising them as one's own; helping pregnant women under pressure; and assisting large families and families in difficulty. Judgment falls on families, social institutions, governments, and international organizations which cannot identify with the vulnerable and rejected, exemplified in the conceived "child" or the abandoned husband or wife (.22). Moreover, "[m]otherhood, because of all the hard work it entails, should be recognized as giving the right to financial benefits at least equal to those of other kinds of work undertaken in order to support the family during such a delicate phase of its life." (.17).

New attention to the family as a theological and ethical *topos* in Roman Catholic teaching and theology thus represents a social and relational appreciation of marriage, now informed by more egalitarian and personalist insights. It engages not only the spouses' personal commitment, but also the parental, intergenerational, and communal relationships out of which it flows and which it in turn augments. Whether Roman Catholic rhetoric about family as domestic church will succeed in rising above well-meaning but ineffectual piety will depend on overcoming Catholicism's recent history of approaching both sex and marriage with a regulatory mentality, infected by fear and ignorance of the sexual lives of its audience. It will also depend on whether, in practice, it can escape being dogged by the sexism that shadows official presentations, with their expectations about women's roles.[123] Local episcopacies have often been more responsive to the social causes and symptoms of sexism, like domestic violence;[124] realities of family life in the more prosperous countries, like nontraditional families, economic pressures on the family, and gender stereotyping and working parents;[125] and the effects of economic deprivation and political repression on the family in the Third World.[126]

The family as a bounded kinship group is ever an occasion of temptation to sublimate self-interest into dedication to one's mate, offspring, or kinship group, using these objects of devotion to justify callousness toward outsiders. The Christian meaning of parenthood takes biological kinship as a base, but not as a limit. Children fulfill a couple and link their sexuality and commitment to intergenerational embodiment of human bondedness and community. The community which is family can be a place in which to nurture spiritual ideals, and to transmit a sense of the "unconditional love" which Christ promises the church. The Christian family may be seen as a biologically-based sphere of special affections, "a school of virtue" in which we learn what love means.[127] But the specifically Christian meaning of family does not stop with biology, mutual love, or even religious practices and cultivation of spirituality within the family.

If the family is truly a community of disciples, then it reflects the transforming power of kingdom life. It educates in solidarity and compassion for those excluded from the social, material, psychological and spiritual conditions of human flourishing. The specifically Christian contribution of the family is sublimation of kinship loyalty into identity with all those who suffer or are in need, as "God's children" or our "brothers and sisters in Christ." "As the gospel parables indicate, the church of God is to be a leaven in society, deeply transforming the world, God's instrument in the completion of God's kingdom or reign. If this is how we understand church, then to invite families to see themselves as domestic church will help families move more fully into the world rather than retreat from it."[128]

POPULATION, BIRTH CONTROL, AND GENDER

Birth control is a social as well as a personal and marital problem. The issue of population control demonstrates quite clearly the inadequacy of act-oriented moral analysis to address the transformative effect Christianity should have on social practices in which sexual behavior and gender roles are entwined with inequities of political and economic power. This was evident during the September, 1994 United Nations International Conference on Population and Development, which met in Cairo. Two earlier UN population conferences met in Bucharest in 1974 and in Mexico City in 1984, but the Cairo conference much more explicitly set population in the context of worldwide distribution of resources. The primary thrust of the draft document was development, especially health care and the education of women.

The Vatican affirmed these social objectives, and did not make condemnation of artificial means of birth control an agenda item. Yet Vatican representatives clashed with other delegates, especially from the US, over the inclusion of abortion as part of health services. The final conference document (a 113–page "Program of Action") was changed to exclude abortion as a means of family planning. Any suggestion that legal abortion should be a legal right for women was eliminated in favor of a statement that simply prescribed that where abortion is in fact legal, it should be safe. But church representatives still approved only the sections on development. Several Third World delegates, mostly from Muslim countries and from Latin America, sided with Vatican concerns.

Three aspects of this incident have particular bearing on the church's vision of sex and gender, and on its role as a public moral voice. First, both the Vatican and its "liberal" opponents contributed to polarization of the debate in terms of issues which they see both as sexual and as symbolic of their general social commitments. Both employed the rhetoric of power struggle in depicting their interaction on population issues, rather than that of cooperation toward consensus. One reporter for the *New York Times* saw the Vatican representatives, described as "the legalistic warriors of the Roman Catholic Church," as "unable to prevent" the mention of legal abortion, and pronounced that they had capitulated in "a total denial of Roman Catholic doctrine."[129] This characterization of the Vatican's situation was not only inaccurate but inflammatory and prejudicial. On the other side, Archbishop Renato R. Martino, head of the Vatican delegation, referred to the changed abortion wording as "a great victory," while a fellow delegate relished it as "a great gain, a great success" that "made the feminists angry."[130]

Second, both the Vatican and its counterparts in fact modified their positions in order to produce more mutually agreeable wording. So, despite the verbal and political polarization, practical engagement "around the table" did result in movement. As the Catholic News Service reported, the "verbal battles overshadowed the fact that 90 percent of the 'Program of Action' has drawn widespread support—including the Vatican's—for its promotion of women's health, improved education, reduction of child and maternal mortality, and greater international economic balance."[131]

Some of the most effective promoters of women's health and women's agency in family planning are women in poor countries themselves. Just before the Cairo conference convened, ten developing nations with successful family-planning programs announced a cooperative partnership formed to share experience with other Third World countries. All emphasize the role of women as agents of change, and most rely on the leadership of local religious leaders, whether Christian, Muslim, or Buddhist.[132] Bangladesh, still one of the poorest countries, has achieved a cut in birth-rate among rural, illiterate women by the use of female health workers, who sometimes must brave the insults and criticism of fellow Muslims who link women's control over fertility with women's abandonment of traditional wifely and maternal roles, and with sexual permissiveness in general. Zimbabwe similarly has managed a steady decline in population growth through the work of over 800 women who are bicycle-riding "community based distributors," and a government-sponsored male awareness campaign.

Many population experts concur in seeing the reduction of infant mortality and women's literacy as the key factors in reducing population growth, and these are usually associated with economic development. What the Vatican fails to appreciate, however, is that abortion functions for many as a symbol of women's rights; to effectively promote other means of limiting family size, the Vatican must also demonstrate strong, practical support for women. Archbishop Renato R. Martino, head of the Vatican delegation, in fact drew attention on the third day of the Cairo conference to the fact that Catholic agencies and donors worldwide support a range of health and education services, "with special attention to women and children, especially the poor."[133] However, undisguised hostility toward "feminists," and greater apparent expenditures of energy and activism on abortion than on maximizing opportunities for women, undercut the Catholic Church's social commitment. Chief Bisi Oguuley of the Country Women Association of Nigeria expressed the fundamental problems of justice which were almost lost in the Cairo duel: "What is more clearly seen in Africa is hunger, poor health, even the lack of the recognition that women are people. Our program is: 'Allow people to count, do not count people.'"[134]

The lesson to be drawn is that the moral significance of sex's procreative power can be adequately captured neither with a criterion of biological structure, nor with a personalist one which does not extend much further than the spousal relationship. The social conditions in which marriage, family, and gender relations are realized are an inalienable dimension of sexual morality, including the proper use of procreativity. The welfare and flourishing of spouses, families, and communities may require the limitation of births, but the question of fertility and its limits must be addressed in light of economic and political justice, including justice for women. Considerations of personal, marital, familial, and social justice will be more important in determining times and means of fertility regulation than a truncated version of their human context, as a reproductive structure. By the same token, calls for the global slowdown of population growth, urging contraceptive availability, must be assessed in light of the fairness of geopolitical resource distribution and in terms of the interdependence of family size and other social factors in disadvantaged populations.

Conclusions

Procreation is an important meaning of human sexuality, as Catholic representatives rightly perceive, and its value should be institutionalized in family forms which are stable and beneficent toward children. Abortion as a "means of birth control" is a threat to social support of pregnancy, birth, and childrearing in the family. And when promoted individualistically as a "woman's right," it also detracts from public awareness of the much broader and deeper economic and political supports needed to ensure equality and full moral agency for women. However, Catholicism has not gone nearly as far in implementing responsibility for women cross-culturally as it has in establishing itself as a foe of what to many Western or educated women has become the banner of their liberation from patriarchal gender stereotypes and dependence on men for economic survival. Many Third World countries would align themselves against the individualist "rights" rhetoric with which Western feminists can seem to denigrate the importance of motherhood for women in traditional societies, where kin and community are much more definitive of any person's identity than individual achievement. Unfortunately, women's community-oriented roles are still very often placed at relatively low levels of the family and community hierarchy, and this is a social problem in which "official" Roman Catholicism has as yet a seemingly slim interest at the concrete level.

Since at least the 1960s, contraception has functioned as a status-marker in the church, defining "orthodoxies" on both sides, and fueling division, attack, and self-satisfied defense. Abortion is an issue on which most Catholics are in much more general agreement with one another, and are sympathetic to Catholicism's positive valuation of unborn life, if not always to the absoluteness of the prohibitions their church derives from it. Yet abortion has become another weapon of division, now between the church and the larger public order which it ought to influence constructively by building reasonable consensus about the values of sex, commitment, and parenthood. Although Christianity, including Catholicism, is gradually coming to recognize the value and equality of women, and interprets marriage and the family in "personalist," nonhierarchical terms, it still has not registered the range of ecclesial, familial, and social change which women's equality requires. Catholicism's inability to recognize and come to terms with the reasons why so many Western women advocate "abortion rights" is emblematic of this failure.

The failure is played out tragically when a Christian church addresses women in dreadful situations of poverty, violence, and devaluation by investing most of its public capital in the anti-abortion campaign and in scoring political victories over "feminists." The "language" of the sexual body for women in acutely deprived circumstances is not romantic mutuality, spiritual union, or a celebration of women's reproductively oriented, nurturing psychology. It is submission, exhaustion, poor health, a continual struggle to provide materially for one's young, and the probability of early death. The personalist potentials of sex and marriage are in fact being destroyed for poor women because the biological meaning of sex as reproduction is culturally not only primary, but often a means of constraint and even oppression, even as, through motherhood, it can be poor women's only source of social prestige and personal joy.

The Christian social message of reciprocity and inclusion must begin by transforming the family—and women's sexual roles as mothers and wives—if it is to be a genuine school of Christian values, and if it is to redefine biological connection in Christian terms. The role of Christian disciples, and of the Christian family as a kinship group whose interests and actions are transformed by Christian values, is to work to overcome every inequity of race, class, or gender. The way to this end is not condemnation of the sexual sinfulness of those who are already on society's bottom rung, or who are already devalued even by their own family members and religious communities. Jesus never addressed his warnings of perdition to the prostitutes and tax collectors, but to their "righteous" oppressors. The Christian way of participation in public, intercultural efforts toward social change is to constantly refocus attention on those who are most excluded from the process, gradually enabling their greater contribution to the common good, and their equal share in the benefits flowing from it.

Notes

1. Georges Duby, *Love and Marriage in the Middle Ages,* trans. Jane Dunnett (University of Chicago Press, 1988), 3–4.

2. That is to say, official Roman Catholic insistence on strict observance has been sharpest, and ecclesiastical sanctions against dissenters most aggressive.

3. See Donald J. Goergen, O.P., "Celibacy," in Joseph A. Komonchak, Mary Collins, and Dermott A. Lane, *The New Dictionary of Theology* (Wilmington DL: Michael Glazier, Inc., 1987), 174–76; Eduard Schillebeeckx, O.P., trans. C. A. L. Jarrott, *Celibacy* (New York: Sheed and Ward, 1968), 19–50; and John T. Noonan, Jr., "Celibacy in the Fathers of the Church: The Problematic and Some Problems," in George H. Frein, ed., *Celibacy: The Necessary Option* (New York: Herder and Herder, 1968), 420. Schillebeeckx remarks that the law of continence was "a dead letter" for married clergy before the twelfth century, because the practice of living "like brother and sister" was humanly abnormal and in fact regularly resulted in the births of additional children (41–42).

4. Schillebeeckx, *Celibacy,* 116–17.

5. Donald Goergen, *The Sexual Celibate* (New York: Seabury, 1974), v. See also, Mary Anne Huddleston, I.H.M. ed., *Celibate Loving: Encounter in Three Dimensions* (New York and Ramsey NJ: Paulist Press, 1984).

6. See Karl Rahner, S.J., "The Theology of Renunciation," *Theological Investigations III;* essays by Jerome Murphy-O'Connor, O.P. ("Celibacy and Community") and David M. Knight ("Will the New Church Need Celibates?") in Huddleston, *Celibate Loving,* 198–225; and especially, William C. Spohn, S.J., "St. Paul on Apostolic Celibacy and the Body of Christ," *Studies in the Spirituality of Jesuits* 17/1 (1985).

7. Peter Brown, *Body and Society: Men, Women, and Sexual Renunciation in Early Christianity* (New York: Columbia University Press, 1988), 149–50.

8. Jo Ann McNamara, *A New Song: Celibate Women in the First Three Christian Centuries* (New York: The Hawthorne Press, 1983).

9. Brown, *Body and Society,* 148–50.

10. Ibid., 170.

11. Ibid., 78–79, 153. See also McNamara, *A New Song,* 110–11.

12. Ibid., 138.

13. McNamara, *A New Song,* 94–98. (Citing Stromata 4.8.)

14. Brown, *Body and Society,* 205. (Brown cites Eusebius, *Demonstratio Evangelica* 1.8.).

15. See also Gerard Sloyan, "Biblical and Patristic Motives for Celibacy of Church Ministers," in William Bassett and Peter Huizing eds., *Celibacy in the Church, Concilium* 78 (NY: Herder and Herder, 1972), 29.

16. Brown, *Body and Society,* 144.

17. Ibid., 307.

18. Ibid., 311. (Citing, *Hom in Matt.* 47:4.).

19. Jo Ann McNamara, "Sexual Equality and the Cult of Virginity in Early Christian Thought," *Feminist Studies* 3/3–4 (1976) 149. (Citing *De Abraham,* 1, 35).

20. Ibid., 150–51. (Citing *De Virginibus,* 1, 56.).

21. Brown, *Body and Society,* 344. (Citing Ambrose, *de Virginibus* 1.11.65–66.).

22. Ibid., 385.

23. Peter Brown, *Augustine of Hippo: A Biography* (New York: Dorset Press, 1967), 62. Such liaisons were common and socially acceptable for young men who could not yet afford to marry.

24. *Confessions,* VI.11, 13. (Hal M. Helms, trans., *The Confessions of St. Augustine: A Modern English Version* [Paraclete Press, 1986]).

25. Ibid., VI.15.

26. Margaret R. Miles, "The Erotic Text: Augustine's Confessions," *Continuum* 2/1 (1992) 134.

27. Lack of control and need for external constraint are common themes in Augustine's views of sin and ethics generally. See Brown, *Augustine,* 238.

28. Augustine, *City of God,* trans. Henry Bettenson, ed. David Knowles (New York: Penguin Books, 1972), XIV.19, 21, 23–24.

29. *Confessions*, III.1.
30. Ibid., VI.15.
31. Ibid., VI.12.
32. Ibid., IX.6.
33. Miles, "Erotic Text," 145.
34. *Confessions*, II.3.
35. Ibid., III.4.
36. Ibid., IX.9.
37. Ibid., VIII.11.
38. Ibid., IV.4.
39. Ibid., IX.4.
40. Miles, "Erotic Text," 143.
41. *ST*, II-11.152, 155.
42. *ST*, II-11.152.4; suppl. 49.1
43. *ST*, suppl., 42.4.
44. *ST*, II-11.152.4.
45. Ibid., 152.4.
46. James A. Brundage informs us that "Bishop Arnulf of Lisieux (d. 1184) reported to Pope Alexander III (1159–81), for example, that he had banished no less than seventeen concubines from the chambers of his cathedral canons in a single day" (*Law, Sex and Christian Society in Medieval Europe* [Chicago and London: University of Chicago Press, 1987] 314–15).
47. Schillebeeckx, *Celibacy*, 60–61.
48. Angela M. Lucas, *Women in the Middle Ages: Religion, Marriage and Letters* (New York: St. Martin's Press, 1983) 30–42. See also Brundage, *Law, Sex, and Christian Society*, 151.
49. Ibid., 47–50.
50. McNamara, "Sexual Equality," 154. (Citing Palladius, *The Lausiac History*, 132).
51. Dyan Elliott, *Spiritual Marriage: Sexual Abstinence in Medieval Wedlock* (Princeton University Press, 1993).
52. Philip S. Keane, S.S., *Sexual Morality: A Catholic Perspective* (New York, Ramsey, Toronto: Paulist Press, 1977), 151.
53. Spohn, "St. Paul on Apostolic Celibacy," 21.
54. Consult Ladislas Orsy, S.J., "Annulment," in Komonchak et al., eds., *Dictionary of Theology*, 19–21; and "Questions Concerning Matrimonial Tribunals and the Annulment Process," in William P. Roberts, *Divorce and Remarriage: Religious and Psychological Perspectives* (Kansas City: Sheed and Ward, 1991), 138–55.
55. Paula Ripple, "Remarriage: Shaping the Pastoral Questions That Facilitate Life," in Roberts, *Divorce and Remarriage*, 6. See Gerald D. Colman, S.S., *Divorce and Remarriage in the Catholic Church* (New York and Mahwah: Paulist, 1988), which discusses the "internal forum" solution by which a couple unable to obtain a church annulment may view themselves in conscience as free to remarry and receive the sacraments.
56. Eduard Schillebeeckx, O.P., trans. N. E. Smith, *Marriage: Human Reality and Saving Mystery* (New York: Sheed and Ward, 1996), 137.
57. Theodore Mackin, S.J., *Divorce and Remarriage* (New York/Ramsey NJ: Paulist Press, 1984), 172–74.
58. Ibid., 255, 275–76, 280. See also Michael G. Lawler, *Secular Marriage, Christian Sacrament* (Mystic CT: Twenty-Third Publications, 1985).
59. Brundage, *Law, Sex and Christian Society*, 124–25.
60. Ibid., 128–29.
61. Ibid., 151, 148, n. 102, respectively.
62. Charles J. Reid, Jr., "History of the Family," in Lisa Sowle Cahill and Dietmar Mieth, eds., *The Family* (Maryknoll NY: Orbis, 1995), *Concilium* 1995/4, 10–17. Reid offers an overview of the medieval history of the Christian family, emphasizing effects on barbarian customs.
63. Ibid., 134–35.
64. "The Good of Marriage", in Roy J. Deferrari, ed., *The Fathers of the Church*, Vol. 15, *St. Augustine: Treatises on Marriage and Other Subjects* (New York: Fathers of the Church, Inc., 1955), ch. 1. In *The City*

of God, Augustine says that to multiply the human race is the purpose for which God instituted marriage from the beginning (XIV.22).

65. "Good of Marriage," ch. 3.

66. Ibid., ch. 6–7.

67. See Lawler, *Secular Marriage*, 44–46.

68. Ibid., ch. 15, 24.

69. For a detailed discussion of and substantial quotations from Augustine's works on marriage and divorce, see Mackin, *Divorce and Remarriage*, 194–221.

70. Mackin, *Divorce and Remarriage*, 170.

71. Schillebeeckx, *Marriage*, 141, 284.

72. David Herlihy, *Medieval Households* (Cambridge MA and London: Harvard University Press, 1985), 100.

73. Lucas, *Women in the Middle Ages*, 85.

74. Ibid., 89–90.

75. Duby, *Love and Marriage*, 62–63.

76. Herlihy, *Medieval Households*, 81; Schillebeeckx, *Marriage*, 294–95; Theodore Mackin, S.J., *The Marital Sacrament* (New York/Mahwah NJ: Paulist, 1982), 291.

77. Phillipe Ariés, "The Indissoluble Marriage," in Phillipe Ariés and André Béjin, eds., *Western Sexuality: Practice and Precept in Past and Present Times* (Oxford and New York: Basil Blackwell, 1985), 153.

78. Ibid., 108.

79. Herlihy, *Medieval Households*, 136; Duby, *Love and Marriage*, 124.

80. In a late fourteenth-century romance which enjoyed wide popular circulation, an emperor obtains a papal dispensation to marry his own beautiful daughter (who voices disgust and dismay at the prospect). "It must have been thought in some quarters that a king could be permitted to do exactly what he likes" (Lucas, *Women in the Middle Ages*, 93).

81. The church's equalizing of sexual morality across social classes is a large part of Herlihy's thesis (*Medieval Households*, 61); but certainly people with money were better able to manipulate the system as they still are in the case of annulments. A parallel situation exists with the sexes. The more rigorous laws about adultery and divorce were applied with increasing stringency to men as well as women, but men remained the more equal among equals in sex and marriage. At the root of the problem is the gender inequity to the analogy of Ephs. 5:25. See Margaret A. Farley, R.S.M., "Divorce and Remarriage: A Moral Perspective," in Roberts, *Divorce*, 109.

82. Schillebeeckx, *Marriage*, 297, 301; Peter Huizing, S.J., "Canonical Implications of the Conception of Marriage in the Conciliar Constitution *Gaudium et Spes*," in William P. Roberts ed., *Commitment to Partnership: Explorations of the Theology of Marriage* (New York/Mahwah NJ: Paulist, 1987), 122–23, 125.

83. Ibid., 303.

84. Martos, "Marriage," 54–55.

85. *ST*, I.92.

86. *ST*, II.153; Suppl. 49, 65, 67.

87. *ST*, Suppl. 49. especially 3; 67.1; *ST*, II-11.153.2; *Summa Contra Gentiles*, 3/II.123, 126.

88. *SCG*, 3/II.123–124.

89. *ST*, II-11.26.11–12; *SCG* 3/II.123.

90. Walter Kasper, *Theology of Christian Marriage* (New York: Crossroad, 1981), 30. The residual patriarchal bias of the wording is also representative of much theological idealization of love, especially in magisterial writings.

91. Herbert Doms, *The Meaning of Marriage* (New York: Sheed and Ward, 1939): originally *Vom Sinn and Zweck der Ehe* (Breslau: Ostdeutsche Verlagsanstalt, 1935); and Dietrich von Hildebrand, *Marriage* (New York: Longmans, 1942); originally Die Ehe (Munich: Kosel-Pustet, 1929). For a history, see Theodore Mackin, S.J., *What Is Marriage?* (New York/Ramsey: Paulist, 1982), 225–31.

92. John C. Ford, S.J., "Marriage: Its Meaning and Purposes," *Theological Studies* 3 (1942) 348.

93. Bernard Cooke, "Indissolubility: Guiding Ideal, or Existential Reality?" in Roberts, *Commitment to Partnership*, 64–75; Huizing, "Canonical Implications," 123, 126. In 1977, the International Theological

Commission, sponsored by the Congregation for the Doctrine of the Faith, met to study marriage, and focused much of its attention on indissolubility, which it reaffirmed. For its conclusions and a set of supportive theological essays mostly by members of the Commerce, see Richard Malone and John R. Connery, S.J., *Contemporary Perspectives on Christian Marriage: Propositions and Papers from the International Theological Commission* (Chicago: Loyola University Press, 1984).

94. Ford, "Marriage," 345, 360.

95. The 1983 Code of Canon Law provides that:

The matrimonial covenant, by which a man and a woman establish between themselves a partnership of the whole of life, is by its nature ordered toward the good of the spouses and the procreation and education of offspring; this covenant between baptized persons has been raised by Christ the Lord to the dignity of a sacrament.

For this reason a matrimonial contract cannot validly exist between baptized persons unless it is also a sacrament by that fact.

The essential properties of marriage are unity and indissolubility, which in Christian marriage obtain a special firmness in virtue of the sacrament.

Marriage is brought about by the consent of the parties...

Matrimonial consent is an act of the will by which a man and a woman, through an irrevocable covenant, mutually give and accept each other in order to establish marriage. (Cans. 1055–1057).

96. Philippe Ariés, "Love in Married Life," in *Western Sexuality*, 133–34.

97. Jack Dominian, "The Consequences of Marital Breakdown," in Roberts, *Divorce and Remarriage*, 128–37; Sylvia Ann Hewlitt, *When the Bough Breaks: The Cost of Neglecting Our Children* (New York: Harper-Collins, 1991), 110–17, 135–47; Pamela D. Couture, *Blessed Are the Poor? Women's Poverty, Family Policy, and Practical Theology* (Nashville: Abingdon, 1991).

98. Explains Augustine, "the genital organs have become as it were the private property of lust, which has brought them so completely under its sway that they have no power of movement if this passion fails. If it has not arisen spontaneously or in response to a stimulus. It is this that arouses shame; it is that makes us shun the eyes of beholders in embarrassment" (*City of God*, XIV.19).

99. Mary D. Pellauer, "The Moral Significance of Female Orgasm: Toward Sexual Ethics That Celebrates Women's Sexuality," in James B. Nelson and Sandra P. Longfellow, eds., *Sexuality and the Sacred: Sources for Theological Reflection* (Louisville KY: Westminster/John Knox Press), 149–68.

100. On distrust of sexual pleasure as in competition with the "personal aspect" that should center sacramentality, see Wilhelm Ernst, "Marriage as Institution and the Contemporary Challenge to It," in Malone and Connery, *Contemporary Perspectives on Christian Marriage*, 53–55.

101. For a fine historical analysis of procreation and birth control in Christianity, see John T. Noonan, Jr., *Contraception: A History of Its Treatment by the Catholic Theologians and Canonists* (enlarged edn.: Cambridge: Harvard University Press, 1986; original edn., 1965).

102. See Susan A. Ross, "The Bride of Christ and the Body Politic: Body and Gender in Pre-Vatican II Marriage Theology," *Journal of Religion* 71 (1991), 345–61.

103. The primacy of procreation was repeated in several subsequent documents prior to Vatican II, including, "The Order of the Purposes of Matrimony," Holy Roman Rota, January 22, 1944; Address of Pope Pius XII to the Italian Medical-biological Union of St. Luke, November 12, 1944; Address of Pope Pius XII to Delegates at the Fourth International Congress of Catholic Doctors, September 29, 1949; Address of Pope Pius XII to Midwives, October 29, 1951. Excerpts from all these, as well as *Castii connubii*, are included in Odile M. Liebard, *Official Catholic Teachings: Love and Sexuality* (Wilmington NC: McGrath Publishing Company, 1978).

104. For a detailed analysis of developments in Catholic sexual theology during this period, including the debate over contraception, see my "Catholic Sexual Ethics and the Dignity of the Person: A Double Message?," *Theological Studies* 50/1 (1989), 120–50.

105. The idea that sex could be viewed as a "language" had already been offered by Paul Ricoeur, "Wonder, Eroticism and Enigma," *Cross Currents* 14 (1964), 133–41; and André Guindon, *The Sexual Language: An Essay in Moral Theology* (Ottawa: University of Ottawa, 1976). However, Ricoeur and Guindon use the metaphor to reconsider sexual meaning, and Guindon in particular suggests that a linguistic understanding

of sex implies changes in moral norms; the pope keeps it firmly attached to the ban on contraception. The "Theology of the Body" is the theme of the Pope's Wednesday afternoon general audience talks in 1979–81. The series is published in three volumes by the Daughters of St. Paul (Boston). They are *Original Unity of Man and Woman: Catechesis on the Book of Genesis* (1981); *Blessed are the Pure of Heart: Catechesis on the Sermon on the Mount and Writings of St. Paul* (1983); *Reflections on Humanae Vitae: Conjugal Morality and Spirituality* (1984). An apology for the tradition which the pope represents is Rev. Ronald Lawler, O.F.M. Cap., Joseph Boyle, Jr. and William E. May, *Catholic Sexual Ethics: A Summary, Explanation, & Defense* (Huntington IN: Our Sunday Visitor, 1985).

106. Original Unity of Man and Woman, 109–10.

107. Ibid., 111.

108. The ban on contraception is affirmed vehemently in *Familiaris Consortio,* no. 32; and in *Reflections on Humanae Vitae.*

109. The pope has claimed that "lack of direct personal experience" is "no handicap" at all to celibate authors, who can rely on experience which is "second-hand, derived from their pastoral work." See Karol Wojtyla, *Love and Responsibility* (New York: Farrar, Straus, Giroux, 1981), 15, originally in Polish (Krakow: Wydawnicto, Znak, 1960).

110. Rosemary Radford Reuther, "Birth Control and the Ideals of Marital Sexuality," in *Contraception and Holiness: The Catholic Predicament,* ed. Thomas D. Roberts, S.J. (New York: Herder and Herder, 1964), 87.

111. The term "self-mastery" appears as a separate index entry in Janet E. Smith, ed., *Why Humanae Vitae Was Right: A Reader* (San Francisco: Ignatius Press, 1993). The reader is referred to two essays by Smith and one by John Crosby.

112. See, for instance, the general audience talk of March 12, 1980, "Mystery of Woman Revealed in Motherhood," *Original Unity of Man and Woman,* 153–161; *Familiaris Consortio,* no. 23; and *Mulieris Dignitatem* (September 30, 1988), *Origins* 18/17 (October 6, 1988) nos. 17–19, especially 18.

113. *Familiaris Consortio,* no. 24; *Mulieris Dignitatem,* no. 14; and John Paul's June 1995 "Letter to Women" in preparation for the September 1995 Fourth World Conference on Women In Beijing. In this letter, he recognizes for the first time that working women make vital contributions to culture, apologizes for church culpability for discrimination against women, and commends women's fight "for basic social, economic, and political rights" (.6). Yet he also holds up Mary in her maternal role as "the highest expression of the "feminine genius," and insists that men's and women's roles are different and complementary (.10). This allows the pope to reaffirm the exclusion of women from the ministerial priesthood (.11).

114. See *Mulieris Dignitatem,* no. 10, on Gen. 3:16 as a consequence of sin; and no. 16 on Mary Magdalene as the first witness to the resurrection and " 'apostle to the apostles.'"

115. Paul M. Quay, S.J., "Contraception and Conjugal Love," 40.

116. Ibid., p. 35.

117. It appears in *Why Humanae Vitae Was Right,* 19–43. It is presented as a "superb defense" of church teaching, and especially of the "human and spiritual meaning" of sexuality and marriage.

118. Janet E. Smith, "Paul VI as Prophet," in *Why Humanae Vitae Was Right,* 521–23.

119. Editorial, "It Still Doesn't Scan," *Commonweal* 121/13 (1994) 4. The editors were responding to, and in large part in agreement with, a defense of Natural Family Planning which appeared in the same issue: Paul Murray, "The Power of 'Humanae Vitae,'" ibid., 14–18.

120. As one presentation of Catholic teaching states it, "Marriage is one of the most profound and important aspects of human social existence." "Since marriage is an institution for the procreation and education of children, marital consent involves a commitment to this worthy enterprise" (Rev. Ronald Lawler, O.F.M., Cap., Joseph Boyle, Jr., and William E. May, *Catholic Sexual Ethics: A Summary, Explanation, & Defense* [Huntington IN: Our Sunday Visitor, 1985] 134, 137).

121. For a historical survey of the function of the concept "domestic church," see Norbert Mette, "The Family in the Official Teaching of the Church," and Michael Fahey, S.J., "The Christian Family as Domestic Church at Vatican II," in Lisa Sowle Cahill and Dietmar Mieth, eds., *The Family, Concilium* 1995/4 (Maryknoll NY: Orbis, 1995).

122. For a largely sympathetic but also critical discussion of the Catholic ideology of the family, see Margaret Farley, "The Church and the Family," *Horizons* 10 (1983) 49–71; Mitch and Kathy Finley, *Christian Families in the Real World: Reflections on a Spirituality for the Domestic Church* (Chicago: The Thomas More Press, 1984); James and Kathleen McGinniss, "Family as Domestic Church," in John Coleman, S.J., ed., *One Hundred Years of Catholic Social Thought* (Maryknoll NY: Orbis, 1991), 120–34; Toinette M. Eugene, "African American Family Life: An Agenda for Ministry Within the Catholic Church," *New Theology Review* 5 (1992) 33–47; and the articles in Cahill and Mieth, *The Family*.

123. Egalitarian themes and messages are now astoundingly common, if compared to the official rhetoric of less than a generation ago. But the social mission of Christianity, to create ecclesial and human solidarity with "the poor," will never be fulfilled in Catholic teaching as long as it is tainted by the residue of sexism. The same year, 1994, that saw the promulgation of John Paul II's new letter on the family also saw the publication of an encyclical insisting on women's inability to represent Christ in priestly ministry; and the much-delayed publication of the English version of the *Universal Catechism*, which had to undergo a second translation from the French in order to extirpate gender-inclusive language.

124. US Bishops' Committee on Women in Society and in the Church and Committee on Marriage and Family Life, *When I Call for Help: A Pastoral Response to Domestic Violence*, in *Origins* 22 (November, 1992), 353, 355–58.

125. US National Conference of Catholic Bishops, *Putting Children and Families First: A Challenge for Our Church, Nation and World*, *Origins* 21 (1991), 393, 395–404; US National Conference of Catholic Bishops, *Follow the Way of Love: Pastoral Message to Families*, *Origins* 23 (1993), 433, 435–448; Australian Catholic Bishops Conference, "Families: Our Hidden Treasure," *Catholic International* 5 (1994), 315–28.

126. Peruvian Bishops' Conference, "The Family: Heart of the Civilization of Love," *Catholic International* 5 (1994), 270–72.

127. Gilbert Meilaender, "A Christian View of the Family," in David Blankenhorn, Steven Bayme, and Jean Bethke Elshtain, eds., *Rebuilding the Nest: A New Commitment to the American Family* (Milwaukee: Family Services America, 1990), 145.

128. James and Kathleen McGinnis, "Family as Domestic Church,": in John Coleman, S.J., *One Hundred Years of Catholic Social Thought* (Maryknoll NY: Orbis, 1991), 125. See also William P. Roberts, "The Family as Domestic Church: Contemporary Implications," in Roberts, ed., *Christian Marriage and Family: Contemporary Theology and Pastoral Perspectives* (Collegeville MN: Liturgical Press, 1996). Roberts maintains that "the domestic church of family serves the cause of justice." As examples, he mentions that family members learn equity in their own relationships; they contribute time and money to the poor; they lobby to change sinful social structures.

129. Alan Cowell, "How Vatican Views Cairo: Damage Control Seen in the Talks' Details," *New York Times*, September 18, 1994, 25.

130. John Thavis, "U.N. Conference Struggles With Abortion Issue," *Arlington Catholic Herald*, September 15, 1994, 12. The second Vatican delegate is an Australian, Msgr. Peter Elliott.

131. Thavis, "U.N. Conference," 1.

132. Barbara Crossette, "A Third-World Effort on Family Planning," *New York Times*, September 7, 1994, A8. The countries are Bangladesh, Colombia, Egypt, Indonesia, Kenya, Mexico, Morocco, Thailand, Tunisia and Zimbabwe.

133. Renato Martino, "Population and Development: The Issues, the Context," *Origins* 24/25 (September 22, 1994) 261.

134. As quoted by David S. Toolan, "Hijacked in Cairo," *America* 171/9 (1994) 4. Toolan was present at the conference and his assessment seems right on target:

Somehow the deeper symbolism of the event was missed—that this was another threshold in the historic march to give women, especially poor women, a decent share in the world's goods, a say in shaping their own destiny. From the outset, the Vatican had put the worst possible interpretation on the drafters (and their motives). And then, rallying conservative Islamic patriarchalists to its side, it had committed the mistake of positioning itself, at least in the eyes of the Western press, as hostile to the cause of women. In a strange way, a penchant for the perfect text became the enemy of the good, and any chance of strengthening the Program of Action in the area of development vanished into the smoggy Cairo air. (3)

9

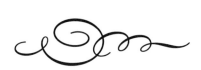

The Family in Early Christianity: "Family Values" Revisited

Carolyn Osiek, R.S.C.J.

For several years now, "family values" have come to represent a volatile substance deposited at the crossroad between American politics and religion, with the Bible as the fuel waiting to be ignited.[1] "Biblical" family values, sometimes also known as "the American way of life," convey an aura of tranquility, respectability, and moral rectitude: everyone knows where *he* belongs and what God wants *him* to do, and everyone is therefore content, as go the lines of a familiar chorale, "God's in his heaven, all's right with the world." But we know that all is not right with the world, least of all in families, with talk of orphanages instead of foster care and withdrawal of welfare to mothers and children, and with slogans of "children having children" and "children killing children" which have become familiar. In Chicago, for instance, the *Chicago Tribune* for two years ran a front-page series called "Killing Our Children," which chronicled the violent deaths of children in the city.

Can we as Catholic biblical scholars make any contribution to this anguished situation from our own expertise? In view of the massive upheavals and uncertainties about family life today, it is not surprising that some would prefer a return to what is perceived to be a traditional, and supposedly safer, ethic.[2] But are the so-called biblical family values that are promised as a remedy really all that biblical? Which is more biblical, "Wives be submissive to your husbands as to the Lord" (Eph 5:21) or "Whoever loves father or mother or son or daughter more than me is not worthy of me" (Matt 10:37)?

I

There is a fundamental tension in the NT portrait of the family. The famous household codes are the lightning rod for an ethos of peaceful domestic existence in which all members acknowledge their position and responsibilities in an atmosphere of mutual love and deference.[3] Since this harmony is based on Hellenistic teaching and Roman sensibilities about the ordering of domestic life as model for public life, the ethos of the private household extends to church community life and civic responsibility as well. Thus, all are to reverence one another as fathers, mothers, sisters, and brothers (1 Tim 5:1; 1 Pet 5:5), and ecclesial authority is to be exercised in paternal style, as one would rule one big, happy household (1 Tim 3:2–7).[4]

On the other hand, the sayings and deeds attributed to Jesus about family life are not very reassuring for those who would hold the above picture as normative. In Luke, a precocious twelve-year-old Jesus begins the pattern by seemingly being totally insensitive to parental worry while he fledges his theological wings in the temple (Luke 2:41–51). Early in Mark's Gospel, Jesus' relatives come to fulfill their responsibility to care for an ailing member, to take him home because he was believed to be out of his mind (ἐξέστη, Mark 3:20).[5] He responds by accusing them of the sin against the Holy Spirit, the deliberate misjudgment of the spirits (Mark 3:28–30).[6] When they try again, his answer is a rejection of the demands of blood ties: "Whoever does the will of God is my brother, sister, and mother."[7] This is enough to drive the family away, for in the Synoptics they never appear again, in spite of the fact that they are well known in the locality (Matt 13:55–56 par. Mark 6:3; Luke 4:22; John 6:42). Luke, by giving Jesus' answer to the woman in the crowd who pronounces a blessing on his mother: "Rather, blessed are those who hear the word of God and keep it" (Luke 11:27–28 par. *Gos. Thom.* 79),[8] even adds to Jesus' lack of enthusiasm for his family.

In John, Jesus' family is present at Cana, where, according to some interpreters, he publicly rebuffs maternal authority, even though he accedes to his mother's request.[9] His brothers appear again five chapters later (John 7:3–5)—as unbelievers, which coheres with the Synoptic image. John's death scene features a rare moment of Jesus' concern for his otherwise rejecting family; here, his mother is present, and he is faithful to the end in his responsibility to provide for a widowed mother (John 19:25–27).

It is not that Jesus is portrayed as being insensitive to the religious requirements with regard to family. He quotes the fourth commandment to religious experts who would dodge its requirements (Matt 15:3–6 par. Mark 7:10–12) and considers it fundamental to a man who seeks to do more than the commandments require (Matt 19:19 par. Mark 10:19; Luke 18:20). He is aware of the kinds of situation that arise in family and household (two distinct terms for us that would translate the same words in Greek, Hebrew, Aramaic, or Latin), and he uses them in his teaching. He understands the household dynamics of slaves who are both debtors and creditors in the story of the unmerciful servant (Matt 18:23–35), of slaves who make wise and foolish choices when their master is away (Matt 24:45–51 par. Luke 12:41–46), and of domestic slaves entrusted with a *peculium*, a sum of money to manage, in the parable of the talents or pounds (Matt 25:14–30 par. Luke 19:11–27). He uses the competitive dynamic between sons vying for a father's attention in two parables about two sons, one about their differing responses to the father's wishes (Matt 21:28–31), and the other about the dissolute son and his unforgiving elder brother (Luke 15:11–24).[10] He also has to fend off an ambitious mother, "Mrs. Zebedee," who tries to broker patronage for the eschatological social advancement of her two sons (Matt 20:28–31).[11]

The sayings on divorce attributed to Jesus have brought untold difficulties to the Christian community.[12] They are so ubiquitous and varied and so distinct from their context that their basic content must be taken with utmost seriousness as historical. Here the authority of Jesus intrudes directly and in a startling way into family life.

Nor is Jesus portrayed as lacking in sensitivity to family suffering. In an age of high infant mortality he demonstrates compassion for distraught parents of sick children: the synagogue official with a dying daughter (Matt 9:18–26 par. Mark 5:21–43; Luke 8:40–56), a royal official with a sick son (John 4:46–53), the widow at Nain (Luke 7:11–17) to whose plight Jesus responds without having to be asked (καὶ ὁ κύριος ἐσπλαγχνίσθη ἐπ' αὐτῇ, v. 13); the Syrophoenician or Canaanite woman with a sick daughter (Matt 15:21–28 par. Mark 7:24–30), and the father of an epileptically possessed boy (Matt 17:14–20 par. Mark 9:14–28; Luke 9:37–42). In Mark's version of this last story Jesus even inquires about the symptoms and is spurred on by the father's insistent and increasingly pitiful pleas. The scenes in which Jesus sets a child as example of qualifications for entry into the kingdom (Matt 18:1–5 par. Mark 9:36–37; Luke 9:48; *Gos. Thom.* 22) must be seen in light of the social situation of children at the time. The scene in which he takes children into his arms with blessing (Matt 19:13–15 par. Mark 10:13–16; Luke 18:15–17), long interpreted with reference to the baptism of children, should rather be seen over against the common practice of abandonment of infants, and with reference to the Jewish and Christian prohibition of this custom.[13]

So it would seem that Jesus is portrayed as a person who takes an interest in the family life of others, in spite of the way he seems to give up on his own. Yet the Synoptic passage Matt 19:27–29 par. Mark 10:28–30; Luke 18:28–30 encourages the disciples in their renunciation of "houses, brothers, sisters, father, mother, children, and fields" (Luke: "house, wife, brothers, parents, and children") for the sake of Jesus and the gospel, with the promise of an abundance in return. To be a disciple includes imitation of this pattern of Jesus to separate from family.

But the most difficult sayings about family that are attributed to Jesus in the Gospels warn of deep divisions within the family itself over the issue of discipleship. In the discourse on apostolic mission, Matthew's Jesus warns of persecutions and trials that could be seen as partly historical, partly eschatological. In that context, brother will betray brother, father child, and children parents (Matt 10:21), a dire prediction that Mark saves for his apocalyptic discourse (Mark 13:12).

Jesus' presence will inevitably bring divisiveness that strikes at the heart of household relationships, as he brings not peace but the sword (Matthew), or divisions (Luke). Micah 7:6 had lamented the breakdown of family loyalties, so that the enemy lay within the household. Echoing Micah, the Q passage has Jesus say without the slightest sign of regret that it is part of his mission to set son and father, daughter and mother, bride and mother-in-law against each other (Matt 10:34–36 par. Luke 12:51–53).[14] Not only does his mission pit members of a household against each other but Jesus pits family love and loyalty against discipleship in a disturbing either/or dichotomy: whoever loves father, mother, son, or daughter more than Jesus is not worthy of him (Matt 10:37), or, in the rendition of Luke and *The Gospel of Thomas*, whoever does not hate father, mother, wife, children, brothers and sisters, and even one's own self cannot be Jesus' disciple (Luke 14:25–26 par *Gos. Thom.* 55, 101).[15] The one called to discipleship is not to look back to say good-bye (Luke 9:61) or even to bury a dead father, one of the most sacred duties of a son (Matt 8:21–22 par. Luke 9:59–60).

This deprioritizing of family for the sake of the gospel is to be seen within the tradition of a higher loyalty to philosophy in Graeco-Roman context, and to God in Jewish intertestamental literature, where a fear is manifested that for the sake of familial affection, the clear-sighted will be seduced into security, softness, and betrayal of their higher truth.[16] This prioritization no doubt reflects the experience of many an early Christian, and not only in times of persecution, but the possibility cannot be excluded that within early Christian groups the attitude was fueled by their memory of it as a reflection of Jesus' own attitude toward the members of his family as well as theirs toward him. That Christian churches admitted to baptism on an individual basis persons, particularly married women, who were subordinate members of households is already documented in 1 Cor 7:13–16 and 1 Pet 3:1. Quite likely, some of the suffering for the sake of Christ alluded to elsewhere in 1 Peter (3:16–17; 4:1–4, 13–19) is related to this very point rather than to some outside source of persecution.[17]

But a comparison of 1 Pet 3:1–2 ("Wives, submit to your husbands, so that those who are not persuaded by the word will be won over without a word by your reverent and chaste behavior") with Mark 10:29–30 ("Anyone who has left house, brothers, sisters, mothers, children, and fields . . . will receive now a hundredfold of houses, brothers, sisters, mothers, children, and fields along with persecution, and eternal life in the next world") illustrates well the built-in tension. The wives of 1 Peter are told to "hang in there." The disciples of Mark are presumed already to have left.[18]

This is the fundamental tension of the biblical witness: does discipleship consist of the promotion of harmonious relationships within recognized social structures, even in the face of suffering, or does it consist in the jolting challenge that overturns and rejects our most cherished human relationships and structures, whether social or conceptual? It is not the conventional cleavage between law and spirit that we are talking about here, for there are claims to freedom in the Spirit and fulfillment of law on both sides. Nor is it adequate to pit the radical challenge attributed to Jesus and the Gospels against the seemingly more prosaic admonitions of the NT letters—give or take a historical Paul somewhere in the middle—because the potential for disruption of household order is also present, for example, in 1 Peter's reflection of a community's willingness to admit wives and slaves independently of patriarchal compliance (1 Pet 2:18; 3:1–2), and the tendency to harmony is implied in such passages as the Johannine love commandment (John 13:34–35; 15:12) or the Matthean exhortation to multiple forgiveness (Matt 18:21–22) and to reluctance to denounce a personal offender to the community, except as a last resort (Matt 18:15–17).[19]

Nearly the entire weight of modern NT scholarship assigns the final redaction of the Gospels to the period roughly contemporary with the production of the Deuteropauline letters and 1 Peter, which contain the best of the "family values" material of the NT. At the same time when some Christian authors are advocating harmonious family life conformable to patriarchal hierarchy, others attribute to Jesus seeming rejection of basic family loyalties and allegiances. The question must have presented itself to the first Christian generations after Jesus: How were they to be family in the Lord? By being living examples of *pietas,* or by following the example of Jesus and defying societal expectations of domestic harmony? Both messages must have been coming at them simultaneously, and the Gospel allusions to the breaking up of families must be taken seriously as a reflection of what was happening to many.

II

To approach an understanding of this problem, we must acquire some knowledge of the Christian experience of family in this period. To do that, we must also know something of family life in the world in which Christianity took root. Study of the Jewish family of the Greco-Roman period is still in its infancy,[20] as is direct study of the Christian family (except for study of the household codes and the house church, where good progress has been made).[21] Study of the Roman family has been a major scholarly pursuit among ancient historians for some years. There is, of course, a huge discrepancy in the amount and character of the surviving evidence. In the case of the Roman family, there is an abundance of literary texts, not only prescriptive but also descriptive of the experience of specific individuals. The weakness of this evidence is that it reveals primarily the life of the elite. In addition to literary evidence, however, there is the spectacular archaeological evidence of such sites as Pompeii, Herculaneum, Ostia, and Ephesus, while the published inscriptions of funerary dedications from family members number in the many thousands. If we take Roman family life in the broadest sense to mean family life, not specifically Jewish or Christian, across the empire in the Roman period, the evidence includes vast papyrological resources and wider epigraphical collections.

For the Jewish family of the Greco-Roman period, there is a good amount of inscriptional and papyrological material, and an abundance of literary texts that describe, prescribe, and debate matters of family life—depending, of course, on the value of mishnaic texts for earlier years. But when it comes to the Christian family, we are at a distinct disadvantage in terms of the amount of available material. What we can know of the Christian family in its first two centuries must be inferred from a few literary texts of various genres, mostly prescriptive, and from the Greco-Roman domestic life which Christians must have shared with others. Only in the latter part of the third century does the evidence furnished by specifically Christian art, epigraphy, and papyrology begin to appear.[22]

III

What did "family" mean to the inhabitants of the Mediterranean shores in the imperial period? Historians agree that whatever the term meant, it did not mean what it means to most modern Westerners. Hebrew בית, Greek οἶκος and οἰκία, and Latin *domus* can all mean the physical structure of the house, but more frequently what they designate is the household as a broader horizontal concept including slaves and material goods, or immediate family related by blood but not necessarily living under one roof, or the vertical dimension of lineage or family tree. Compare, for instance, these three uses of οἶκος in 1 Corinthians: Paul baptizes the οἶκος of Stephanas (1 Cor 1:16); Aquila and Prisca hold an ἐκκλησία in their οἶκος (1 Cor 16:19); but women are told to ask their husbands their questions ἐν οἴκῳ (1 Cor 14:35). In the first passage, all the persons of the household are signified; in the second, the physical place with its furnishings and personnel; in the third, not only the physical location but the social construct of private space, which, in more conservative circles, was the context in which it was appropriate for dominant males to recognize the existence of women.

Further, the Latin *familia* means predominantly one of two things: those under the authority of the *paterfamilias*, or those related as *agnati*, that is, through the male line. The first meaning caused great ambiguity about the status of the *materfamilias*, who by imperial times usually came into her husband's family by marriage *sine manu*, that is, without passing over legally from her father's to her husband's *familia*. She was thus not legally under her husband's authority, though she was by tradition subject to him; nor was she in his line of inheritance, because she was not a member of his *familia*. The second meaning of *familia* could include lateral relatives who stood in the line of inheritance, as well as children, both by blood and by adoption, but again, not the wife.[23] In practice, husbands and wives increasingly disregarded the legal strictures and willed property to each other, but the legal ambiguity continued, because it was economically and socially advantageous to a woman's *familia* to keep her as a member.

Two conclusions can be drawn. First, lest we think that Roman usage had little to do with the first Greek-speaking Christians, let us remember that Roman law, including family law, applied to all Roman citizens anywhere in the empire, and that although many of the probable freedmen and freedwomen in the Pauline and other early communities spoke Greek, they must have been Roman citizens, especially in Roman colonies like Philippi and Corinth. Thus, they may have been in real cross-cultural situations in which legal and social expectations differed a great deal. Second, the inevitable conclusion must be drawn that none of the ancient terms to which we assign the meaning "family" had what is for us the first and most obvious meaning of "family," the nuclear family. Though the nuclear family certainly existed, it does not seem to have functioned as a social unit in isolation, and therefore, it had no nomenclature. This realization alone should endow us with proper caution in our investigations.

Households and family units included children, slaves, unmarried relatives, and often freedmen and freedwomen or other renters of shop or residential property. The easy access between commercial and domestic space in the surviving archaeological material attests to this, as does the literary evidence. All, including slaves, seem to have participated in family religious festivals. Household ownership and management was not restricted to a single nuclear group and its dependencies; there are known examples of houses owned and occupied by brothers, for instance, presumably each with his own dependents.[24] Women headed households, too, both singly and with other women.[25] Therefore, it would seem that, in spite of the strictly patriarchal legal structure of families, there was a great deal of variety in the composition of actual households (οἰκίαι, *domus*). Family and household in our meanings of the words are not necessarily to be equated with their ancient counterparts.

Formal dining was a regular activity for those with both a spacious house and some level of social prominence, and it was an important occasion for cementing bonds of friendship, loyalty, and patronage with influential guests and hosts. Among both the elite and those who emulated them, the association of dining with political and social status markers was strong.[26]

However, the vast majority of urban dwellers lived not in the spacious *domus* seen at Pompeii or Herculaneum but in more crowded surroundings. The multistoreyed apartment houses (*insulae*) of the imperial period were a common and growing phenomenon in all major cities. In some cases, they had comfortable, spacious apartments at lower levels, while the low-rent crowd climbed to their lodgings. But these buildings' shabby construction, crowded conditions, and vulnerability to fire were notorious.[27] Many others lived behind and above shops, in one or two dark and poorly ventilated rooms. Only those with spacious houses could afford the luxury of kitchens. The rest prepared food on portable grills or ate regularly at the local "fast food" shop in the neighborhood (*caupona, taverna,* or *thermopolium*). The rich ate in, the poor ate out.[28] For the poor, a formal meal was had only for special occasions sponsored by a civic benefactor or a benefactor of some other kind; thus the regular Christian community meal would have had far greater significance than a meal would among the wealthy. In both cases, however, the daily family meal as locus for social and moral development, an important piece in the myth of the American family, has no apparent ancient counterpart.

Nor can we imagine the distinction between public and private to have worked in the way we experience it, as a sharp division between the public sphere of work and the privacy of family life. Vitruvius lists the public areas of the Roman house of an important person to which anyone had access by right (*suo jure*) and uninvited: the vestibules, the atria, and the peristyles (*vestibula, cava aedium, peristylia*).[29] Off of these areas lay all the "private" areas like the *cubicula, triclinia,* and *balneae* for sleeping, eating, and bathing, those areas to which one had access only with invitation. The same areas that served for entertaining in the afternoon and evening were spaces for children's play and domestic work in the morning. The house was one of the most important places both for conducting business and for the production of salable goods. The house was not the place to escape from work but the place where much of the work was done; it was not the place to be free of a public role but the place to enhance that role by hospitality.[30] The modern idea of the sacred privacy of the home does not apply.

Christian families were just like all others in many respects, yet different in others. Diognetus says Christians are not different in language, customs, or habitation, but they have an allegiance of citizenship elsewhere—a theme echoed in other Christian writers, and one that must have caused a great deal of suspicion to outsiders who heard of it.[31] Tertullian says they did not frequent games, circus, theater, or gymnasium,[32] which must have made them seem like pretty sober types (but then again, he wrote an entire treatise, *De spectaculis,* to prove *why* Christians should not attend these activities, which would seem to indicate that not every Christian agreed with him). They followed an ethical system inherited from Judaism through the Scriptures; to the extent that they were serious about following it,[33] they must have been known and admired for their honesty and reliability. Like the Jews, they were forbidden to abort or expose unwanted children;[34] rather, they were to raise all children, which must have made them seem foolhardy. They were rigidly monotheistic, which must have made them, like the Jews, seem odd. They frequented the markets, the baths, the shops, the neighborhood streets. Their children continued to attend the same schools and to learn from the same Greco-Roman literary models. Christians kept up their relationships with nonbelieving neighbors and friends.[35] Yet a clear sense of a distinct identity was emerging, an identity that found expression in such ideas as heavenly citizenship,[36] new race,[37] and the analogy of soul (Christians) to body (world).[38]

IV

Acceptance of new members into the church happened in two different ways: by entire households and by individuals. When large households joined together, on the authority of their male or female head, it is impossible to know how well many of the members knew what they were doing, in the case of the household of Stephanas (1 Cor 1:16), for example, or of the stories of Cornelius' household at Caesarea (Acts 10:24, 44–48), or Lydia's and the jailer's households at Philippi (Acts 16:15, 33); in each case, all were baptized together—in the last case, in the middle of the night! Perhaps these whole Christian households were more prone to welcome teaching about family harmony in structured submission than would be those households divided by different beliefs.

When all the members of a large household had accepted baptism, they could presumably become a self-contained "house church," which may have welcomed others if space allowed, but which could also function on its own. In this case, *familia* or οἶκος coincided with ἐκκλησία, as did family leadership and church leadership. Such a situation would have been a laboratory for what was to be the next development in church structure: to see the church as one large extended family and to extend household mores to the whole church.

The other conversion pattern was that of admitting individuals to baptism apart from any family structure in which they belonged; an example is Paul's baptism of Crispus and Gaius, mentioned almost in the same breath as his baptism of the whole household of Stephanas, a different kind of procedure (1 Cor 1:14–16).[39] Paul's listing of wives and dependents as individuals, if they were married, implies that they could make their own decisions. It is clear from 1 Cor 7:12–16 and 1 Pet 2:18–3:6 that this was the case for wives;[40] 1 Peter suggests the same for slaves, which is corroborated by other evidence.[41] Even if Crispus and Gaius, two men with Roman names, were not married, they may still have been legally under the authority of their father, if he was still alive. If they were adult and fatherless, they were legally independent, *sui juris*. But we do not know what effect their conversion may have had on others in their households.

How did family life work in the case of households and extended families divided by different beliefs? Roman domestic religion emphasized the integral role of all household members, including children and slaves, but especially of the *paterfamilias* and *materfamilias*, in daily, monthly, and other regular sacrifice together to the *lares*, *penates*, and other *numina* of the particular house, worshipped at the household *lararium*, of which many examples are preserved at Pompeii.[42] It is probably for this reason that Plutarch counsels that at marriage, a bride should cease to worship any other gods than those of her husband, so that there will be unity and conformity in worship as in everything else, for, he adds, no god encourages secret rituals done by a woman.[43] Family members were free to pursue other devotions alongside those of the family, but conservative opinion was against it. When individual family members converted to Judaism or Christianity, the exclusivity of their religious claims must have constantly caused tense situations that threatened the harmonious ordering of the *domus*.

Tertullian, trying to convince North African Christian women of the late second century to marry Christians, describes such a situation. The unbelieving husband is not likely to tolerate his wife joining a vigil (*statio*) at daybreak (he will tell her to meet him at the baths), or fasting (he will schedule an important dinner), or visiting the poor for the sake of charity (he will have urgent family business that she must attend to with him), or attending meetings at night, especially the all-night paschal celebration, or visiting martyrs in prison, or offering hospitality to visiting Christian strangers in their home. On the contrary, she will have to smell the incense of family festivals and go through a door hung with laurels and lanterns for monthly and New Year celebrations in which she no longer wishes to participate.[44] In the cases where this situation was full of tension, the acerbic antifamily sayings of the Synoptics must have provided beleaguered Christians with meaning and with the consolation that they were not alone in this experience.

V

The existence of individual Christians in unbelieving households raises for our prevailing "house church" model the question where these individuals went for regular worship and other religious activities. They must have belonged to groups that met in someone else's house or apartment, in a place, and among people, approved perhaps by the head of their own household, and perhaps not. This means that, while we envision house churches made up of families coming together, many house churches must also have had a good number of such individual Christians as well—adult freeborn and freed men and women, single and married, perhaps with their children but without spouses, as well as male and female slaves, perhaps also with children, but without their owners. The idea that everything was done in family or household units is not supported by the evidence.[45] When such groups had a patron or patroness in whose house they met, the assembly may have appeared to an outsider somewhat like a patron's dinner for his or her clients, except that unattached freeborn women and slaves not of the household would not likely belong to such a group. The indiscriminate mixing of persons of every age, sex, and social status without proper supervision by appropriate patriarchal authority was perennially suspect, for it threatened to undermine the social hierarchy by which power was maintained.[46]

The Christians' regular ritual meal on the first day of the Jewish week took place either in a *domus* or in an apartment complex, but under private auspices. When the venue was a *domus*, the host and (or) hostess, with their closest friends or the most important members, must have occupied the *triclinium*, one of the most conspicuous rooms in the house and the one with the best view. In it were dining couches usually arranged for nine persons to recline in a three-sided arrangement. The rest of the assembly must have spilled out into the peristyle, on either portable couches or chairs, within earshot of a speaker in the *triclinium* who would want to be heard. A visiting apostle or teacher would be placed in the *triclinium* in the position of guest of honor. Thus, in spite of what was said of partaking of the one bread (1 Cor 1:17) at the common table, some hierarchy of importance was inevitably present. Pliny the Younger speaks of a reprehensible dinner host who set out three different classes of food and drink, one for his inner circle of guests, another for his "lesser friends" (clients), and a third for the freedmen. Pliny disapproves of the practice and says that he sets the same fare before all—but implicit in his description is an accepted seating arrangement in which the three groups are separated.[47] This was presumably the practice to which all were accustomed. Vitruvius comments that people could wander uninvited into the atrium and peristyle of a *domus*;[48] this suggests that Christians may not have been alone at their meetings. This is perhaps what Paul means by the ἰδιώτης who cannot understand tongues without an interpreter (1 Cor 14:16).

Whether men and women ate together is uncertain; it probably depended on place, time, and occasion. The traditional custom was for men and women to dine separately on formal occasions; in more intimate situations with family or close friends, the custom was for women and children to sit on chairs by the couches on which men reclined. In the classic symposium, women customarily left after the meal, before the heavy drinking and philosophical discussion began, though they might stay for lighter entertainment following the meal. Exceptions, of course, were ἑταῖραι and other women of questionable reputation.

Among Romans, however, these customs were changing at the beginning of the Christian era. Vitruvius states explicitly that one of the differences between the Greek house and the Roman house was the Greek house's separation of the women's quarters in the back from the men's entertainment area in the front.[49] The Roman house, on the contrary, did not separate space by gender or by a distinction of public and private function. The same rooms that could be used for entertaining guests in the afternoon could also be used for family activities in the morning. The ideal of women secluded within the doors of the house, held by the Eastern elite,[50] differed distinctively from Roman practice.

At the beginning of the Roman era, women were beginning to attend men's dinner parties and even to recline with them.[51] Cornelius Nepos, writing from Rome about 35 B.C.E., remarks that Roman men are not ashamed to take their wife to a dinner party, and that matrons take part in all the festivities of their houses, in contrast to the Greek custom, still in force, of allowing women to attend dinner parties only with relatives, and of confining them usually to the women's quarters.[52] Valerius Maximus remarks that dining positions differentiated by sex are now observed more in civic religious banquets than in private ones—which just goes to show that goddesses care more for discipline than real women do.[53] Indeed, Livia reclined with Octavian at their wedding, but for the banquets following military triumphs and other public events, she held separate dinners for the women.[54] The compromise custom seems to have been for women to be present at men's dinners, but to recline on separate couches.[55] In view of these comments, the archaeological evidence for separate dining rooms in Roman houses of the period must be assessed with care. They *may* be men's and women's dining rooms, or they may be simply alternatives, offering different views or exposure to different breezes.[56]

So the alternatives for women's participation in house church meals seem to be the following: reclining or sitting in separate dining areas, sitting next to reclining men, or reclining alongside men. The picture is complicated even more by the known examples of women heads of households and the lack of comparative data by which to get an idea of the way they functioned socially.[57] Among Roman elites and their imitators at many different social levels, probably by the late first century, women were reclining alongside men in both West and East. It is difficult to imagine that this would be the case among more traditional and less romanized groups, especially in a movement with Eastern roots, but it is equally difficult to imagine that women would be completely excluded from the men's activities at a house church meal; nothing in the sources suggests this. Rather, in more traditional groups, especially in the East, women and children probably either sat or reclined in separate groups in the peristyle or sat next to men's couches. In those houses both sufficiently affluent and sufficiently traditional to have a parallel women's dining room, the *materfamilias* probably hosted the most important women there. At any given time, there were probably several different ways in which people were grouped for the weekly festive meal, different even at different places in the same city, depending on physical arrangements, status identification, and degree of romanization.

In more traditional settings, it is highly unlikely that families were grouped together. The presence of individual converts without families in any large numbers would also facilitate gender and status groupings at the assembly rather than family units. The image of the family at Sunday worship together does not fit the ancient pattern.

The other likely venue for a gathering of the Christian community is the *insula* or apartment building, the place of the so-called tenement church. While it is fairly certain that such Christian groups existed, we know even less about *how* they existed than we do about house churches in a *domus*. References to Christian groups not identified with a house (e.g., Chloe's people, 1 Cor 1:11) may be to such groups. They may have met in someone's apartment room, under very crowded circumstances, or in a shop on the first floor, or in an available meeting room, perhaps rented for the occasion. A second phase of development, parallel to the transition from *domus* to *domus ecclesiae* in house churches, may have been permanently to secure a particular room of an apartment house, as Mithraists took over a ground-floor room of the so-called House of Diana at Ostia in the second or third century. Both archaeological and literary evidence indicate that something like this happened at the sites which later became the churches of San Clemente, San Crisogono, and Santi Giovanni e Paolo at Rome.[58]

In the original form of "tenement church," meetings and dining arrangements must have been less formal than in a *domus*. Leadership, too, must have taken more flexible forms, since the pattern of patronage was not automatic. It is interesting to speculate that in such meetings more collegial forms of both participation and leadership were possible than in meetings under the patronage of a prominent figure. At the same time, such an organization would necessarily be more dependent on the full cooperation of all its members.[59] These are the gatherings that may more closely have resembled meetings of *collegia*, which constitute one of the suggested models of Christian assemblies. Most *collegia*, however, seem to have sought wealthy patrons, so that the hierarchical pattern based on social status re-emerges.

But how did the weekly Christian assembly affect family life at home? The earliest sources are nearly silent on this question, except in prescriptive terms which give us little indication of the way things really were. One thing is clear, however: the church began very early to see itself as surrogate family, with its male leadership modeled on ideals of civic leadership, in keeping with a long tradition that saw the household as a microcosm of the state and that tied effective public leadership to proven effective family management.[60] This development may have contributed to undermining patriarchal household authority, since by the middle of the third century it did succeed in undermining the authority of individual patrons in favor of the more centralized patronage of the bishop.[61] Yet ironically, Christianity in the long run enhanced patriarchy rather than undermining it, in spite of certain opposite tendencies present from the beginning.[62] It was given a special boost by the absolute fatherhood of the monotheistic God "after whom all fatherhood in the heavens and on earth is named" (Eph 3:15). Not that God was presented as a stern and fearful disciplinarian;[63] rather, early Christian writers tend to stress mercy and compassion in contrast to severity in their description of God. Punishment was only that of a wise father who must discipline his children.[64] Yet the image of the male authority was inevitably reinforced.[65]

The local house church or apartment church provided, among other things, a sense of communal life and individual commitment, theological pluralism, a base for mission, and a model of the universal church.[66] Its communal life must have been less attractive to those from large Christian households, and more attractive to those without large families, those who were members without their families, and the poorer members who lacked other means of social incorporation in a wider context. The appeal to the sense of extended family that the church provided must have been approved and fostered especially by members of these kinds.

The multiplication of different worshiping groups had necessarily to foster theological pluralism. That this happened is evident from Paul's letters to such places as Galatia, Corinth, and Rome in the first generation, and in Rome, Alexandria, and Gaul in the course of the second century. The responses to excessive pluralism, otherwise called heresy, have been much studied; they include centralization of teaching leadership and the canonization of Scripture.

House churches were the nurturing ground for missionaries, both local and visiting. Here local members would hear the call and respond by putting their efforts into evangelization, whether in the neighborhood (Acts 10:24; Col. 4:5–6; Heb 12:14), in their own homes (1 Tim 6:1; 1 Pet 3:1), or abroad (Acts 13:1–3). In these groups, too, visiting missionaries received support, encouragement, and material assistance (Acts 20:7; Rom 15:24; 16:1–2).

Local church groups also understood themselves to be smaller units of a larger body. In the local groups, people learned to be aware of what was happening in other parts of the Roman world to those who shared their faith (Acts 14:26–27; 1 Thess 1:7–9; 2:14–16; Col 4:8, 16). Increasingly, church leadership was modeled on familiar forms of government, though the transition to imperial modeling was to take several centuries.

VI

To return to the problem posed at the beginning, what was the reception of the very different messages coming through to families in the earliest Christian writings about family life? It might seem that those portrayals of family life that stress unity, harmony, and patriarchal structures had greater appeal, and perhaps even originated in house churches which were composed of one or more households that were completely Christian, whether they met in a *domus* or in an *insula* in which they lived as small family groups. Here all the values represented in the general paraenesis of the NT letters could be extolled, and perhaps even lived.

By contrast, the biting pessimism about family members being worthy of trust that is characteristic of many of the traditions attributed to Jesus would not have been well received in such homogeneous circles. Since family leadership and church leadership were so closely associated, such criticism of family would have been seen as a questioning of legitimate authority. We know what happened in some of the cases in which church leadership was questioned: Galatians, 1 and 2 Corinthians, and *1 Clement* tell us that every attempt was made to suppress the questioning. Other unspecified incidents of encouragement to unity in the Pauline letters may be not only about petty disagreements but about crises of local leadership.[67]

It would seem that the criticism of family and the urging to outside loyalties would have expressed better the experience of individual converts who had made the difficult decision to act alone in joining a Christian community. They must often have found it to be true that family members could not be relied upon for support, and that, ultimately, loyalties had to be chosen and sides taken, sometimes against family and friends.

This would be a neat picture—in fact, too neat. The pebble that shatters the picture is 1 Peter, in which the paraenesis to wives, and probably also to slaves, is addressed to persons who do not belong to households that are all Christian—quite the contrary, for wives are explicitly told that their virtuous behavior may convert their husbands. Slaves are told to be obedient even to unjust owners, after the example of Christ who suffered unjustly.[68] Thus, with many students of the household codes we must conclude that those codes were intended to allay fears of Christian subversion of the social order, whether they are primarily addressed to a suspicious outside audience or to insiders for their instruction.[69] Part of the propaganda present in paraenetic discourse is that good example will win people over. Not only honest traders and conscientious craft workers but also submissive wives, obedient children, and slaves were living advertisements for the truth of the faith; they were home missionaries. Whether the household codes are heard primarily by insiders or outsiders, they bolster the defensive posture of the church, which seeks to protect vulnerable members, and thus ultimately the whole church, from attack by outsiders, especially by authoritative unbelieving family members who resent the church's exclusive claims over the thoughts and lifestyle of believers.

What, then, are we to make of the other side of the picture, the portrait of the skeptical Jesus who has nothing good to say about family and who direly predicts that family members cannot be counted upon? One major import of these sayings is that the group of disciples must now function as a family: family is not abolished but extended. The boundaries of kinship are not removed but reset. Those who will fulfill the role of true family members are those bound together not so much by blood or social structures as by Baptism and Eucharist.

Seen this way, the two semantic worlds of household paraenesis and sayings about discipleship are not as diametrically opposed as we may have thought. The tradition of radical discipleship exemplified by the Synoptic Gospels warned Christians not to set down roots in a fickle set of relationships that might reject the demands of the gospel. On the other side, 1 Peter and the Pastorals deliberately portray the church as a household. Colossians and Ephesians draw the reader into a vision of a universal church in which the interests and concerns of Christians must be as wide as those of Christ.[70] Church structures of the next few centuries would attempt to make the church into a kind of welfare state in which, from birth to grave, all essential needs are taken care of, education, marriage, pastoral care, relief from hunger, health care, and burial. Each tradition, each in a different way, issued a challenge to widen one's perspective, to go beyond the narrow expectations of family for the sake of a greater mission. Seen this way, the early Christian agenda *did* set out to undermine the foundations of society and create a new social order of wider horizons.

If biblical scholars can make any contribution to the present debate about "family values," perhaps it can be to bring an awareness that the mid-twentieth-century nuclear family is not normative, that the golden age of biblical families was not all it is cracked up to be, but that the family is a very strong social structure, strong precisely because it is so flexible. It was in fact more flexible in early Christianity that in its contemporary idealized version. Its forms are changing, as they always have been. The family must look outward and be part of something greater than itself. Only then will it achieve its end of fostering the most basic qualities of faith, hope, and love. These are the family values worth striving for.

Notes

This article is the presidential address delivered at the Fifty-eighth General Meeting of the Catholic Biblical Association of America, held at Siena College, Loudonville, NY, August 12–15, 1995.

I am deeply grateful to the Religion, Culture, and Family Project of the University of Chicago for much of the funding for the research undertaken for this address, made possible by a generous grant from the Lilly Endowment. The address is dedicated to Kathryn Sullivan, R.S.C.J., first woman elected to active membership in the CBA (in 1948), first woman elected vice-president (in 1958), compiler of the decennial index of the CBQ in 1949, 1959, and 1969, and the person who first awakened in me the interest to do graduate biblical studies.

1. See "Whose Family Values Are They, Anyway?" *New York Times*, Sunday, August 6, 1995, 4. 1, 3. Some moderate attempts to address the situation at the level of public policy are D. Browning, "Re-Building the Nest: Families and the Need for a New Social Agenda," *Just Reading* 3 (Melbourne: Catholic Commission for Justice, Development and Peace, 1994) 1–12; D. Browning and C. Browning, "Better Family Values," *Christianity Today* 39 (1995) 29–32; J. Wall, "The New Middle Ground in the Family Debate: A Report on the 1994 Conference of the Religion, Culture, and Family Project," *Criterion* 33/3 (1994) 24–31.

2. Such nostalgia is hardly new. Tacitus (*Dial.* 28) laments that "in the good old days" (*pridem*), every child was legitimate and raised by its mother, who "could have no higher praise than that she managed the house and gave herself to her children" (W. Peterson's translation, *Tacitus: Dialogus, Agricola, Germania* [LCL; Cambridge, MA: Harvard University Press, 1946] 89).

3. Col 3:12–4:6; Eph 5:21–6:9; 1 Pet 2:13–3:7; also 1 Tim 2:8–15, passim; Titus 2:2–10.

4. The literary relationship of the NT household codes to the Hellenistic topos on household management is now well known. See D. L. Balch, *Let Wives Be Submissive: The Domestic Code in 1 Peter* (SBLMS 26; Chico, CA: Scholars, 1981); idem, "Household Codes," *Greco-Roman Literature and the New Testament: Selected Forms and Genres* (SBLSBS 21; ed. D. E. Aune; Atlanta, GA: Scholars, 1988); idem, "Neophythagorean Moralists and the New Testament Household Codes," *ANRW* 2/26/1. 380–411.

5. H. Wansbrough ("Mark iii. 21—Was Jesus Out of His Mind?" *NTS* 18 [1971–72] 233–35, taken up by D. Wenham, "The Meaning of Mark iii.21," *NTS* 21 [1975] 292–300) argues that it is not Jesus but the crowd that is out of its mind. This suggestion has not been widely accepted.

6. That the Beelzebul controversy applies to the family as well is rejected by some, but others agree. S. C. Barton (*Discipleship and Family Ties in Mark and Matthew* [SNTSMS 80; Cambridge: Cambridge University Press, 1994] 75–77) gives "a qualified affirmative."

7. Mark 3:31–35 par. Matt 12:46–50; Luke 8:19–21; *Gos. Thom.* 99; *Gos. Eb.* (Epiphanius *Pan.* 30.14.5). Note the softening of the rebuke in Luke 8:19–21; yet contrast Matt 10:37 and Luke 14:26, where Luke's language is stronger. An understandable reluctance to attribute historicity to this motif is noticeable, e.g., on the part of J. Gnilka, *Das Evangelium nach Markus* (EKKNT 2; Zurich: Benziger; Neukirchen-Vluyn: Neukirchener Verlag, 1978) 1. 146, 152–53. I. Ellis, "Jesus and the Subversive Family," *SJT* 38 (1985) 173–88 defends Jesus' interest and participation in family, considering the supposed tension to be a misinterpretation. Most commentators, e.g., W. Grundmann, *Das Evangelium nach Markus* (THKNT 2; 7th ed.; Berlin: Evangelische Verlagsanstalt, 1977) 86–87; D. E. Nineham, *The Gospel of St. Mark* (Pelican Gospel Commentaries; New York: Penguin, 1963) 122–23, stress the focus on the disciples as the new community. Mark's portrayal of Jesus' family rejection is widely considered to be Marcan redaction, e.g., by J. D. Crossan, "Mark and the Relatives of Jesus," *NovT* 15 (1973) 81–113. J. Lambrecht, "The Relatives of Jesus in Mark," *NovT* 16 (1974) 241–58 revises some of Crossan's argument but still holds that Mark "changed a possible pre-Markan tension between Jesus and his relatives into explicit opposition" (p. 244); for Lambrecht, as for many, the passage is staged to highlight the teaching on discipleship. Whether the passage is historical or has been developed as contrast to the new family of disciples is not the point here; the point is rather the impact of the *portrayal* of Jesus on the next generations. On later traditions about the family of Jesus as believers, see H. Koester, *Introduction to the New Testament 2: History and Literature of Early Christianity* (Hermeneia; Philadelphia: Fortress, 1982) 200; B. L. Mack, *A Myth of Innocence: Mark and Christian Origins* (Philadelphia: Fortress, 1988) 91 n. 11.

8. Another way to read this exchange is the traditional reluctance to draw public attention to a respectable woman, who should be talked about in public only in praise after her death (cf. Plutarch *De mul. vir.* 242). But given the rest of the pattern of Jesus' treatment of his own family, this motivation does not seem primary.

9. C. K. Barrett, *The Gospel according to St. John* (2d ed.; Philadelphia: Westminster, 1978) 191; D. A. Carson, *The Gospel according to John* (Grand Rapids: Eerdmans, 1991) 170–71; C. R. Koester, *Symbolism in the Fourth Gospel: Meaning, Mystery, Community* (Minneapolis: Fortress, 1995) 11, 78, 215; F. J. Moloney, *Belief in the Word* (Minneapolis: Fortress, 1993) 81. Biblical references and discussion of the unusual form of address can be found in R. Schnackenburg, *The Gospel according to St. John* (New York: Seabury, 1980) 1. 328.

10. Through an analysis of Greco-Roman literature on household management, W. Pöhlmann (*Der Verlorene Sohn und das Haus: Studien zu Lukas 15, 11–32 im Horizont der antiken Lehre von Haus, Erziehung, und Ackerbau* [WUNT 68; Tübingen: Mohr (Siebeck), 1993]) argues that the story is meant to be a sweeping challenge to the orderly world of the household, for the father acts totally inappropriately and thus signals a change in the social order.

11. For the role of the (elite) mother in pushing her sons' social advancement, see S. Dixon, *The Roman Mother* (London / New York: Routledge, 1988) esp. pp. 168–209.

12. Matt 5:31–32; 19:3–12; Mark 10:2–12; Luke 16:18; 1 Cor 7:10–16; Herm. *Man.* 4.1.6; cf. Mal 2:13–16. Cf. J. A. Fitzmyer, "The Matthean Divorce Texts and Some New Palestinian Evidence," *TS* 37 (1976) 197–226; W. J. Harrington, "The New Testament and Divorce," *ITQ* 39 (1972) 178–87; P. Hoffmann, "Jesus' Saying about Divorce and Its Interpretation in the New Testament Tradition," *The Future of Marriage as an Institution* (*Concilium* 5/6; ed. F. Böckle; New York: Herder and Herder, 1970) 51–66; G. MacRae, "New Testament Perspectives on Marriage and Divorce," *Divorce and Remarriage in the Catholic Church* (ed. L. G. Wrenn; New York: Newman, 1973) 1–13; L. Sabourin, "The Divorce Clauses (Mt. 5:32; 19:9)," *BTB* 2 (1972) 80–86; B. Vawter, "Divorce and the New Testament," *CBQ* 39 (1977) 528–42; J. S. Kloppenborg, "Alms, Debt and Divorce: Jesus' Ethics in Their Mediterranean Context," *Toronto Journal of Theology* 6 (1990) 182–200.

13. A. van Aarde, "The *Evangelium Infantium*, the Abandonment of Children, and the Infancy Narrative in Matthew 1 and 2 from a Social Scientific Perspective," *God-With-Us: The Dominant Perspective in Matthew's Story and Other Essays* (Hervormde Teologiese Studies, Supplementum 5; Pretoria: Nederduitsch Hervormde Kerk van Afrika, 1994) 261–76. On children in the ancient Mediterranean world, see J. Pilch, "'Beat His Ribs While He Is Young' (Sir 30:12): A Window on the Mediterranean World," *BTB* 23 (1993) 101–13; B. Rawson, "Children in the Roman *Familia*," *The Family in Ancient Rome: New Perspectives* (ed. B. Rawson; Ithaca, NY: Cornell University Press, 1986) 170–200 (esp. on *alumni/ae* and *vernae*); T. Wiedermann, *Adults and Children in the Roman Empire* (London: Routledge, 1989); O. L. Yarbrough, "Parents and Children in the Letters of Paul," *The Social World of the First Christians: Essays in Honor of Wayne A. Meeks* (ed. L. M. White and O. L. Yarbrough; Minneapolis: Augsburg Fortress, 1995) 126–41.

14. But see Luke 1:17, where an allusion to Mal 3:24 (4:6) suggests that part of John the Baptist's mission is to turn fathers' hearts to their sons—but not vice versa as the MT (but not the LXX) goes on to say. A. Milavec ("The Social Setting of 'Turning the Other Cheek' and 'Loving One's Enemies' in Light of the *Didache*," *BTB* 25 [1995] 131–43) suggests family intergenerational conflict as the historical setting for Matt 5:38–48; Luke 6:27–38; *Did.* 1.3–4.

15. U. Luz (*Das Evangelium nach Matthäus* [EKKNT 1; Zurich: Benziger; Neukirchen-Vluyn: Neukirchener Verlag, 1990] 2. 140–42) speaks of reluctant priorities. D. A. Hagner (*Matthew 1–13* [WBC 33A; Dallas, TX: Word, 1993] 292) links Matt 10:37 to the family divisions in vv 35–36, so that v 37 means that neither the people nor the divisions can get in the way of discipleship. J. D. Crossan (*The Historical Jesus: The Life of a Mediterranean Jewish Peasant* [San Francisco: HarperSanFrancisco, 1991] 299–302, but more strongly in *Jesus: A Revolutionary Biography* [San Francisco: HarperSanFrancisco, 1994] 58–60) tries to make the case that the family divisions are deliberately intergenerational, so that the attack is on the exercise of hierarchical power in the family. But as Crossan acknowledges, Mark 3:35; 6:3; *Gos. Thom.* 55; *2 Clem.* 9.11 also speak of siblings. On intergenerational conflict, cf. *Jub.* 23.16, 19.

16. See e.g., 4 Macc 2:10–13 "The Law takes precedence over benevolence to parents and will not betray virtue for their sake; it takes precedence over love for a wife and reproves her for transgression; it overrules love for children and punishes them for wrongdoing; and it exercises its authority over intimate relationships with friends and rebukes them for evil" (tr. H. Anderson, *OTP* 2. 546). Cf. *Jos. and Asen.* 11.4–6. Already Deut. 13:6–11 had warned in the strongest terms against letting family ties seduce into pagan worship. For Philo, Josephus, Qumran, Cynics, and Stoics (cf. esp. Epictetus 3.3.5–10), see Barton, *Discipleship and Family Ties*, 23–56; for further discussion of the Cynics, see A. J. Droge, "Call Stories in Greek Biography and the Gospels," *SBLSP, 1983* (Chico, CA: Scholars, 1983) 245–57; F. G. Downing, *Christ and the Cynics: Jesus and Other Radical Preachers in First-Century Tradition* (JSOT Manuals 4; Sheffield: JSOT Press, 1988); idem, *Cynics and Christian Origins* (Edinburgh: T. & T. Clark, 1992).

17. M. Y. MacDonald ("Early Christian Women Married to Unbelievers," *SR* 19 [1990] 221–34) stresses both the importance of the household as mission center and the vulnerability of such wives if they were

divorced by their husbands: if poor, they would be destitute and in need of church support; if prominent, they would be under outside social pressure to remarry.

18. One might question whether sexism is at work here: wives must grin and bear it, but no disciples in Mark's passage leave husbands. Within a century or so, however, that is exactly what the wives in the apocryphal acts are doing.

19. For further discussion, see Barton, *Discipleship and Family Ties,* 224–25.

20. A fine early example is *The Jewish Family in Antiquity* (BJS 289; ed. S. J. D. Cohen; Atlanta: Scholars, 1993).

21. See P. A. Foulkes, "Images of Family Life in the Scriptures," *The Way* 32 (1992) 83–92 (on both Testaments); L. A. Hennessey, "Sexuality, Family, and the Life of Discipleship: Some Early Christian Perspectives," *Chicago Studies* 32 (1993) 19–31; P. Lampe, "'Family' in Church and Society of New Testament Times," *Affirmation* (Union Theological Seminary in Virginia) 5 (1992) 1–20.

22. The only two locations in which pre-Constantinian Christian epitaphs occur in noticeable accumulations are Rome and central Anatolia. On Rome, see A. Ferrua, "L'epigrafia cristiana prima di Costantino," *Atti del IX Congresso internazionale di archeologia cristiana, Roma, 21–27 Settembre 1975* (Studi di antichità cristiana 32; Città del Vaticano: Pontificio Istituto di Archeologia Cristiana, 1978) 1. 583–613. On Anatolia, see G. J. Johnson, *Early Christian Epitaphs from Anatolia* (SBLTT 35; Early Christian Literature Series 8; Atlanta: Scholars, 1995), who observes (p. 1) that "the surviving Christian funerary monuments with engraved epitaphs simply number several tens of thousands fewer than the non-Christian."

23. R. P. Saller, "*Familia, Domus,* and the Roman Conception of the Family," *Phoenix* 38 (1984) 336–55; idem, *Patriarchy, Property, and Death in the Roman Family* (Cambridge Studies in Population, Economy, and Society in Past Time 25; Cambridge: Cambridge University Press, 1994) 74–101.

24. For instance, the well-known House of the Vettii at Pompeii was owned by two freedmen brothers, Aulus Vettius Restitutus and Aulus Vettius Conviva.

25. Among aristocrats, Ummidia Quadratilla ran her own household to the age of seventy-nine, with her grandson at one time in residence; Pliny the Younger (*Ep.* 7.24) was critical of her dinner entertainment. Matidia, great-aunt of Marcus Aurelius, had a house outside Rome where Marcus' daughters were staying in the year 161; after her death, Fronto was involved in a dispute over inheritance (*The Correspondence of Marcus Cornelius Fronto* [2 vols.; LCL; ed. C. R. Haines; London: Heinemann, 1919–20] 1. 301; 2. 94–97). At more modest social levels, examples besides Nympha (Col 4:15), the mother of John Mark (Acts 12:12), and Lydia (Acts 16:14–15, 40) are women mentioned in Ign. *Smyrn.* 13.2 and Ign. *Pol.* 8:1–2; probably the Jewish Rufina of Smyrna (*CII* 741; discussion by D. Martin, "Slavery and the Ancient Jewish Family," *Jewish Family in Antiquity,* 124–25); several women, Roman citizens, who made their own tax declarations in Egypt (R. S. Bagnall and B. W. Frier, *The Demography of Roman Egypt* [Cambridge Studies in Population, Economy, and Society in Past Time 23; Cambridge: Cambridge University Press 1994] 11–13); and several other examples from the papyri mentioned in *New Documents Illustrating Early Christianity* (ed. G. H. R. Horsely; Sydney: Ancient History Documentary Research Centre, Macquarie University, 1982) 2. 25–32, esp. Didymaion (P. Wisc. 72).

26. J. D'Arms ("The Roman *Convivium* and the Idea of Equality," *Sympotica: A Symposium on the Symposion* [ed. O. Murray; Oxford: Clarendon, 1990] 308–20) concludes that in spite of the rhetoric of equality and social leveling, social hierarchy prevailed. Cf. Pliny *Ep.* 9.5.3: there is nothing more unequal than the "equality" of not preserving distinctions of *ordo* and *dignitas.*

27. Seneca *De ira* 3.35.5; Juvenal *Sat.* 3.5–9, 190–202; Martial *Epig.* 1.117.7; 7.20.20.

28. I owe this insight and its wording to Dr. Caroline Dexter of George Washington University.

29. Vitruvius *De arch.* 6.5.1.

30. A. Wallace-Hadrill, "The Social Structure of the Roman House," *Papers of the British School at Rome* 56 (1988) 43–97; idem, *Houses and Society in Pompeii and Herculaneum* (Princeton: Princeton University Press, 1994) 10–12, 17–37; M. Peskowitz, "'Family/ies' in Antiquity: Evidence from Tannaitic Literature and Roman Galilean Architecture," *Jewish Family in Antiquity,* 9–36 [26–28].

31. *Diogn.* 5.

32. Tertullian *Apol.* 38.4–5 and *De spec.* passim.

33. Pliny, in his famous letter to Trajan, says that they took an oath not to steal, rob, or commit adultery, not to betray a trust or withhold a deposit when it was called for (*Ep.* 10.96.7). Yet other texts suggest that not every Christian was perfectly law-abiding, e.g., 1 Pet 4:15; Hippolytus *Ref.* 9.12 on the checkered career of Callistus (which could be largely concocted).

34. Jews do not, according to Tacitus, *Hist.* 5.5; Diodorus Siculus 40.3; Philo. *Spec.* 3.110 and *Virt.* 131–32; Josephus *Ap.* 2.20.2; Pseudo-Phocylides 184–85; but to the contrary, see a tax register of 73 C.E. from Arsinoe (*Corpus Papyrorum Judaicarum* 421) cited by R. Kraemer, "Jewish Mothers and Daughters in the Greco-Roman World," *Jewish Family in Antiquity*, 108 n. 51. Christians do not, according to *Did.* 2.2; 5.2; *Barn.* 19.5; 20.1–2; Justin *Apol.* 1.27; *Ad Nat.* 1.15; *Diogn.* 5.6; Minucius Felix, *Oct.* 30.2. On ancient child abandonment generally, see A. Cameron, "The Exposure of Children and Greek Ethics," *Classical Review* 46 (1932) 105–14; J. Boswell, *The Kindness of Strangers: The Abandonment of Children in Western Europe from Late Antiquity to the Renaissance* (New York: Pantheon, 1988) 53–179. On ancient abortion and contraception, see R. Crahey, "Les moralistes anciens et l'avortement," *L'Antiquité classique* 10 (1941) 9–23; J. H. Waszink, "Abtreibung," *RAC* 1. 55–60; M. Drury, "Les femmes et le vin," *Revue des études latines* 33 (1995) 1–13; K. Hopkins, "Contraception in the Roman Empire," *Comparative Studies in Society and History* 8 (1965) 124–51; E. Eyben, "Family Planning in Graeco-Roman Antiquity," *Ancient Society* 11–12 (1980–81) 5–82.

35. They accepted dinner invitations in temples and private houses (1 Cor 8:10; 10:27), and they continued to value social standing (Herm. *Man.* 10.1.4; Herm. *Sim.* 8.9.1; 9.20.2).

36. Phil 3:20; Heb 11:9–16; Herm. *Sim.* 1; *Diogn.* 5.4–5,9.

37. *Diogn.* 1.

38. *Diogn.* 6.

39. Crispus, a previous *archōn* of the synagogue (Acts 18:8–9), and Gaius, a host of the church (Rom 16:23), were probably, with Stephanas, among the most prominent members of the Corinthian community (G. Theissen, *The Social Setting of Pauline Christianity: Essays on Corinth* [Philadelphia: Fortress, 1982] 55).

40. Compare Justin 1 *Apol.* 2.2; *Acts of Perpetua and Felicitas*. In the latter, Perpetua's father is not Christian and is anguished by her fate. No information is provided about the belief of the rest of her family, including a husband. Compare, too, *Acts of Paul and Thecla* and many of the apocryphal acts, in which women's defiance of familial authority to become Christian is a major theme. According to Hippolytus *Ap. Trad.* 41 (B. Botte, *La Tradition apostolique de saint Hippolyte: Essai de reconstitution* [Liturgiewissenschaftliche Quellen und Forschungen 39; Münster: Aschendorf, 1963] 93), Christian couples are to rise for prayer at midnight. If a Christian husband has an unbelieving wife, he is not excused but must go to another room to pray.

41. Still in the early third century, for example, Hippolytus *Ap. Trad.* 15 (Botte, *Tradition apostolique*, 32–34) prescribes that a slave catechumen must have the endorsement of the owner, if the owner is Christian; if he is not Christian, the slave will be taught to please him in order to avoid scandal.

42. See D. P. Harmon, "The Family Festivals of Rome," *ANRW* 2/16/2. 1592–1603; D. G. Orr, "Roman Domestic Religion: The Evidence of the Household Shrine," *ANRW* 2/16/2. 1557–91.

43. Plutarch *Conj. praec.* 19 (*Mor.* 140d).

44. Tertullian *Ad uxor.* 2.4,6.

45. Lampe's comment (twice, "'Family' in Church and Society," 8, 13) that in the first two centuries the church did not exist alongside households but "exclusively *in* them" cannot be taken to mean that it was composed only of household units.

46. Compare Livy's description of the suppression of the Bacchanalian cult in Rome (39.8–18, esp. 39.8.6–7 and 39.13.10); Minucius Felix *Oct.* 9:6; Tertullian *Apol.* 7:1.

47. Pliny *Ep.* 2.6. See Theissen, *Social Setting*, 153–63. On the importance of Greco-Roman dining customs for early Christian worship, see D. E. Smith, "Table Fellowship as a Literary Motif in the Gospel of Luke," *JBL* 106 (1987) 613–38; idem, "Social Obligation in the Context of Communal Meals: A Study of the Christian Meal in 1 Corinthians in Comparison with Graeco-Roman Communal Meals" (Th.D. diss., Harvard University, 1980).

48. Vitruvius *De Arch.* 6.5.1.

49. Ibid., 6.7.

50. According to Philo *Spec.* 3.169, 171–77 and *Flac.* 2.89, married women were to remain within the outer doors, girls within the middle door (*mesaulon*), that is, in the women's section at the back of the house; see also 4 Macc 18:7; Ps. Phocylides 215–18. All these texts reflect earlier Greek ideals (K. J. Dover, "Classical Greek Attitudes to Sexual Behavior," *Arethusa* 6 [1973] 59–73).

51. The threat that this represented to tradition-minded men is shown in the assaults on the reputation of women who did so; see Balch, *Wives Be Submissive*, 66–76; K. E. Corley, *Private Women, Public Meals: Social Conflict in the Synoptic Tradition* (Peabody, MA: Hendrickson, 1993) 24–79. Even in the "liberated" atmosphere of imperial Rome, the best way to discredit a woman was to raise questions about her chastity.

52. Nepos *De vir. illust.* preface 6–7.

53. Valerius Maximus 2.1.2 (early first century C.E.).

54. Dio Cassius 48.44.3; 55.2.4,8.2; 57.12.5.

55. Athenaeus *Deipn.* 14.644d; Lucian *Symp.* 8–9; perhaps Petronius *Sat.* 76–69.

56. Examples of apparent double dining rooms at Pompeii include the House of the Vettii, the Labyrinth, and the House of Meleager. L. Richardson, Jr. (*Pompeii: An Architectural History* [Baltimore: Johns Hopkins University Press, 1988] 322, 398, and passim) assumes that in each case, a double dining room indicates that one part is a "ladies' dining room" in a house owned by people who had not yet adopted the new way. Wallace-Hadrill ("Social Structure of the Roman House," 93 n. 147) explicitly disagrees with Richardson on this point. Richardson adduces as a supporting text Petronius *Sat.* 67, in which Trimalchio's wife Fortunata is not present at the first part of the meal and is called for. The reason for her absence is not propriety, however, but managerial duties for the dinner, and when she enters, she reclines where Scintilla, a woman guest, is already reclining. The other example usually brought forward is Cicero *Verr.* 2.1.26,65–68, where Verres' agent Rubrius, at his instigation, disgraces both of them at Lampsacus in Asia Minor by calling for the presence of the host's young unmarried daughter at the drinking bout after a dinner. The host refuses, saying that it is not the Greek custom (compare Vitruvius *De arch.* 6.7.4). On the whole issue, see Corley, *Private Women*, 24–52.

57. Acts 12:12; 16:14–15; Col. 4:15; maybe 1 Cor 1:11 and Rom 16:1–2. See the references at n. 25 above.

58. B. Blue, "Acts and the House Church," *The Book of Acts in Its First Century Setting 2: The Book of Acts in Its Graeco-Roman Setting* (ed. D. W. J. Gill and C. Gempf; Grand Rapids: Eerdmans, 1994) 119–222; J. S. Jeffers, *Conflict at Rome: Social Order and Hierarchy in Early Christianity* (Minneapolis: Fortress, 1991) 63–89; L. M. White, *Domus Ecclesiae-Domus Dei: Adaptation and Development in the Setting for Early Christian Assembly* (2 vols.; Ph.D. diss., Yale University, 1982), idem., *Building God's House in the Roman World: Architectural Adaptation among Pagans, Jews, and Christians* (ASOR Library of Biblical and Near Eastern Archaeology; Baltimore: Johns Hopkins University Press, 1990).

59. See R. Jewett, "Tenement Churches and Communal Meals in the Early Church: The Implications of a Form-Critical Analysis of 2 Thessalonians 3:10," *BR* 38 (1993) 23–43.

60. Aristotle *Pol.* 1.2.1252b and *Eth. Nic.* 8.12.7–8; Isocrates *Ad Nic.* 19; Pseudo-Isocrates *Ad Dem.* 35; Seneca *Ep.* 5.4.14; Cicero *Off.* 1.54; *Fin.* 5.65: Philo *Praem.* 113; 1 Tim 3:4–5; Titus 1:6; M. Dibelius and H. Conzelmann, *The Pastoral Epistles* (Hermeneia; Philadelphia: Fortress, 1972) 53; Lampe, "'Family' in Church and Society," 20 n. 54; Balch, "Neopythagorean Moralists," 394, 403–4; idem, "Household Codes," 32–33.

61. L. W. Countryman, *The Rich Christian in the Church of the Early Empire: Contradictions and Accommodations* (Texts and Studies in Religion 7; New York/Toronto: Mellen, 1980); C. A. Bobertz, "The Role of Patron in the *Cena Dominica* of Hippolytus' *Apostolic Tradition*," *JTS* ns 44 (1993) 170–84.

62. E. Schüssler Fiorenza, *In Memory of Her: A Feminist Theological Reconstruction of Christian Origins* (New York: Crossroad, 1983) esp. 105–59; 251–84; idem, "'You Are Not to Be Called Father': Early Christian History in a Feminist Perspective," *Discipleship of Equals: A Critical Feminist Ekklesia-logy of Liberation* (New York: Crossroad, 1993) 151–79.

63. It is the thesis of Saller (*Patriarchy*, 102–32) that the modern stereotype of the stern Roman father is greatly exaggerated for modern polemical purposes.

64. Pilch, "'Beat His Ribs,'" 101–13.

65. Tertullian *Marc.* 2:13; Cyprian *Laps.* 35; Novatian *Trin.* 3:1; Clement of Alexandria *Paed.* 1.7,8. I owe these references to Jerry Andrews.

66. Lampe, "'Family' in Church and Society," 8–12; D. W. Riddle, "Early Christian Hospitality: A Factor in the Gospel Transmission," *JBL* 57 (1938) 141–54.

67. Especially Phil. 2:1–18; 4:2–3.

68. It is not out of the question that abusive Christian owners are envisioned. On the topos of the advantages of slavery, see D. Kyrtatas, "Slavery as Progress: Pagan and Christian Views of Slavery as Moral Training," *International Sociology* 10 (1995) 219–34.

69. J. H. Elliott, *A Home for the Homeless: A Social-Scientific Criticism of 1 Peter, Its Situation and Strategy, with a New Introduction* (Minneapolis: Fortess, 1990); Balch, *Wives Be Submissive*.

70. 1 Pet 2:5,18; 4:10,17; 1 Tim 3:15; 2 Tim 2:20–21; Eph 2:11–22; Col 1:15–23.

10

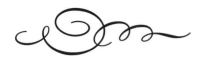

The Theory and Practice of Marriage on the Eve of the Reformation

H. J. Selderhuis

Marriage in Canon Law

In the course of many centuries there originated in the Catholic Church an elaborate system of rules and laws in which all aspects of marriage were treated.[1] The church had drawn all marriage legislation under its aegis, first to offer certainty concerning the material and procedural rules governing the formation of marriages, later also on the ground that marriage was regarded as a sacrament. The possibilities for this development were handed to the church by the civil authorities who at a certain stage in history simply left the regulation of marriage legislation to the church. This development occurred under the enormous influence the church had acquired but also because it suited the convenience of the civil authorities to have the church bear this burden and so to be relieved of it.

The manner in which canonical marriage law, as we encounter it at the end of the fifteenth century, developed is far from even. Whereas in the early centuries the church hardly had the elbow room to implement its view of marriage, this situation underwent a radical change with the conversion of Emperor Constantine in the year 312 A.D. Along with a great measure of freedom the church gained a chance to give shape to its views in the matter of marriage and divorce. Still this opportunity was not unlimited inasmuch as at many points the church had to come to terms with the wishes of the emperors who based their legislation in part on the Bible but mostly on Roman law. However seriously the emperors took account of the norms presented by the church, jurisdiction over marriage remained in the hands of the secular authorities.[2]

But whereas the unity of the empire presently broke down in favor of the rise of national states, the transnational unity of the church and its body of laws remained. Still, the church gained exclusive jurisdiction in matters of marriage only toward the end of the ninth century, many centuries later than is often assumed. At this point, free from the influence of secular authorities, the study of canon law and the associated jurisprudence began to flourish, a process in which the study of marriage law occupied a significant position. The study of canon law enjoyed its "golden age" from the twelfth to the middle of the sixteenth century, the works of Peter of Lombard (d. 1160) and Master Gratian (d. 1158),[3] which appeared in the twelfth century, being pivotal.

Although this is not the place for a comprehensive historical survey of the development of canon law, for a good understanding of the place and significance of Martin Bucer's views on marriage it is nevertheless essential for us to offer a brief account of the state of affairs in this area on the eve of the Reformation. The definitive conclusion of this development, meanwhile, only occurred at the Council of Trent (1545–1563).

Canon law strongly emphasized the indissolubility of marriage. It was, of course, first of all the words of Christ that led to this emphasis; nevertheless, in addition it was especially the sacramental character of marriage that brought the church to this position. Tertullian (d. 223) was the first to speak of marriage as being sacrament-like.[4] He employs the term "sacrament" in the sense of a *figura*, a symbol of the indissoluble bond between Christ and the church. On the basis of this image he is also opposed to permission for a second marriage. Also in Augustine (354–430) we find a direct link between "sacrament" and "indissolubility," but in his thinking, too, the sacrament is still a sign, not a means, of grace.[5] Sacraments, to him, are actions that can function as signs of the work of God's love and in light of this he also views marriage as a God-given sign of the mystery of salvation. It is not until Thomas Aquinas (1225–1274) that—with an appeal to Augustine—marriage is subsumed under the heading of sacraments that convey grace. It is also Augustine who further defines the nature and purpose of marriage.[6] To this end he employs three concepts that have since then become determinative for the whole body of canonical marriage legislation: the concerns of *proles* (progeny), *fides* (trust), and *sacramentum* (sacrament).

The primary purpose of marriage is *proles* offspring, procreation. The natural motivation for this is that, as long as people die, marriage and offspring are necessary. In addition, and on a higher level, is a spiritual motive: through natural progeny the number of God's children is made full and the world can attain the eschaton.[7] Second, marriage must be characterized by *fides;* that is, a relation of trust and love that should exist between spouses. Just as God is faithful, so also a husband and wife should be faithful to each other, and that to the extent that a faithful partner must again accept an unfaithful partner if the latter wants to return to the chastity of marriage. But most essential is that marriage is a sacrament. This means it is a mirror of the marriage between Christ and the church. It is especially this last aspect that explains indissolubility. The relation between a man and a woman in marriage is no less unbreakable than the relation between Christ and the church. Still, also in Augustine, a chaste unmarried life is on a higher level than married life. Marriage, after all, is for those who cannot control themselves and therefore serves as a means of avoiding unchaste relations (*remedium concupiscentiae*). Tertullian, too, praises those women who, instead of marrying a man, enter into marriage with God.

Augustine is committed to the same view, though in his case it does not lead to a condemnation of marriage.[8] The reason for this overvaluation of the unmarried state is Augustine's negative assessment of sexuality.[9] Sexual intercourse is a shameful activity, one that leads to sin and should be restricted to occasions of utmost necessity. A true Christian will as much as possible attempt to resist and overcome his or her sex drives. Only when sexual intercourse is expressly intended for the procreation of children can it take place without sin. It is hardly surprising that this view of marriage and sexuality finally issued into a prohibition of marriage for the clergy.[10] A further consequence is that the Catholic view of marriage is characterized by a remarkable ambivalence: on the one hand, it views virginity as the ideal and, on the other, it believes marriage is a sacrament.

Up until the heyday of canon law little is added to these views of Augustine. A growing consensus about the indissolubility of marriage develops. The sacramental character of marriage means that husband and wife can no more be separated than Christ and the church. In this position the church distinguishes itself from Roman and Jewish law where possibilities for divorce are in fact left open.

An extensive discussion arose about the question at what moment a marriage comes into being. In fact, Peter Lombard is of the opinion that an indissoluble marriage originates the moment a man and woman mutually agree to be married to each other.[11] The formula in Roman law for this is: "Consensus, not copulation, makes a marriage."[12] This implies that mutual consent is definitive for marriage. In this connection he does make a distinction between the different wordings in which promises are couched. If we are looking at words that indicate that the partners promise to marry each other (*verba de futuro*), the promise can still be broken. But if the words indicate that the partners are aiming at concluding a marriage that is immediately effective and the words serve as the actual equivalent of marital consent (*verba de praesenti*), then we are looking at a sacrament and therefore at an indissoluble marriage bond, even if no sexual intercourse has as yet taken place and no witnesses have been present. In contrast, Gratian affirmed that physical intercourse is essential to the legitimacy of a marriage. While for him, too, the consent is the essential element in marriage, he only considers the marriage complete and indissoluble when after consensus also coitus has followed. He, accordingly, makes a distinction between a *matrimonium initiatum*, a marriage that has been formed by verbal consent, and a *matrimonium consummatum*, which is the result of the intercourse that followed verbal consent. Inasmuch as the marriage bond is indissoluble only after the initial act of sexual intercourse, one can only then speak of a valid marriage (*matrimonium ratum*).

After years of discussion between the two schools, Pope Alexander III in 1559 decided on a compromise.[13] A marriage was considered valid when there had been verbal consent to it, but it was not completed until after sexual intercourse had taken place. As long as this was not yet the case there still existed a few grounds for the dissolution of the marriage bond. Such a dissolution could still take place after mutual consent, or on the basis of a few other grounds such as the existence of a marriage bond with another person, entry into a spiritual order, the fiancé(e)'s departure to another country without the knowledge or the consent of the other, serious illness, or the unexpected origination of consanguinity by the marriage of mutual family members before one's own marriage had been consummated. The moment at which the *verba de praesenti* are pronounced is sometimes also called the "betrothal."[14]

Although clear conditions were attached to a marriage formed in this manner—such as the presence of witnesses and the consent of the parents—the marriage was not considered invalid when these words were spoken outside of the presence of witnesses. This presence was prescribed, to be sure, as was the ecclesiastical blessing, but these were not absolutely necessary for the validity of the marriage. The definition of the marriage sacrament implies that by making the right promise of fidelity, the one partner administers the sacrament of marriage to the other as a result of which an indissoluble relation originates. This implies a fundamental change with respect to the folk tradition in which the father of the bride and the bridegroom effect the marriage. In fact, the marriage is now no longer a matter of the village and family community,[15] but only of the two persons involved. The church might indeed punish abuses, but in virtue of its own rules it was powerless to alter the fact that, when a man and a woman, or even a boy and a girl, had uttered the *verba de praesenti*, a marriage had come into being. This ambiguous legislation led to numerous lawsuits over (spoken or unspoken) marriage vows. Also as a result of this legislation there originated so-called clandestine marriages, marriages concluded outside of the presence of witnesses, yet permanently valid.[16] These marriages were given the name *Winkelehen*.[17] Existing marriages could be nullified if someone could present a persuasive plea that at the beginning the wrong words were used or that legal marriage vows had already been made to someone else. Since no witnesses were required for the administration of this sacrament, the possibilities for abuse and injustice were increased. It was finally the Council of Trent that, partly in response to the criticism of the Reformation, took steps against these "clandestine marriages" by deciding that promises of fidelity intended as *verba de praesenti* had legal effect only when pronounced in the presence of at least three witnesses, one of whom must be a priest.[18]

A problem that now surfaced was whether or not the marriage between Joseph and Mary had been a true marriage.[19] Whereas church fathers like Chrysostom (d. 407) and Ambrose (d. 397) denied it, Augustine maintained that in the relation between Joseph and Mary the three elements essential to marriage, viz. *fides, proles,* and *sacramentum,* were present, conveniently overlooking the fact that in virtue of the conception of the Holy Spirit and the virgin birth there was no progeny (*proles*) in the original sense of the word. Peter Lombard, as a result of his theory that a marriage was effected by the spoken consent of the two partners, had no difficulty whatever in recognizing the marriage between Joseph and Mary as having full legal validity. Things were different for Gratian who, as the reader will remember, deemed the *copula carnalis* necessary for a complete marriage. But in the case of Joseph and Mary he did not dare to draw this conclusion.

In this entire discussion it was self-evident to all that even after the birth of the Savior there was no sexual intercourse between Joseph and Mary, with the result that Jesus had no siblings. The Scripture passages in which mention is made of Jesus' brothers were interpreted to the effect that these men could not have been sons of Joseph and Mary and were presumably cousins or spiritual brothers.

It will be clear to the reader that this complicated body of marriage theories led in turn to a detailed system of laws designed to counter abuses. It became an obligation to make a marriage known to the church so that it could be determined whether there were impediments to the marriage. This was done in part by announcing the names of prospective marriage partners in church, thereby involving the local population in checking the legitimacy of the marriage.

On what grounds could a marriage vow be dissolved? In attempting to answer this question we need to realize that the dissolution of a fully valid marriage was not really possible. A marriage relation could indeed be terminated by nullifying it on certain grounds but that is synonymous with saying that there really had been no marriage. The connection was only called a marriage. In this connection it is necessary carefully to define the concept of "divorce," since even medieval canonists sometimes used the words "divortium" and "separatio" interchangeably, while we are really dealing with dissimilar concepts. *Separatio,* then, means the invalidation of a marriage that is not a genuine marriage. If, on the other hand, the marriage is genuine, a separation from bed and board can take place, but the marriage bond remains and there is no divorce. A divorce is in effect only when a fully valid marriage is dissolved in such a way that there is no longer a marriage bond and remarriage (under certain conditions) becomes a possibility. Then we have what is called *divortium a vinculo matrimonii* (a separation from the bond of marriage) or sometimes also *divortium plenum* (a full separation). When in the remainder of this book [the author's *Marriage and Divorce in the Thought of Martin Bucer*] we speak of divorce, it is always in this latter sense.

In the assessment of the legal validity of marriages a distinction was made between *impedimenta dirimentia* (diriment impediments) and *impedimenta prohibitiva* (prohibitive impediments). In the first class of impediments we are speaking of causes that have an invalidating effect, i.e. on these grounds a concluded commitment can be declared null and void. But there are also prohibitive impediments. In that case we are dealing with grounds that prohibit a man and a woman from entering a marriage. If the parties in question take no notice of these impediments, they will, to be sure, have to submit to an ecclesiastical punishment, but the marriage is not considered invalid. While this class of grounds prohibit a marriage, they are not sufficient to invalidate a prohibited marriage. In that case we are dealing, not with an invalid marriage, but an illicit marriage.

A brief overview of the most important concepts follows. In this connection the reader must bear in mind that people increasingly appealed to Rome for a papal dispensation from certain laws.

Grounds That Invalidate a Marriage (Diriment Impediments)

Disabilities

Under this heading the reference is to the lack—in at least one of the partners—of one of the necessary conditions for a valid and completed marriage.

1. Age. The minimum age for a valid marriage was twelve for girls and fourteen for boys. Despite this law there was a stipulation that when a marriage had nevertheless been concluded before the attainment of this age and the underage partner was sexually mature and conscious of what he or she had done by pronouncing the *verba de praesenti,* the marriage was nevertheless valid. If these conditions were not fulfilled, the *verba de praesenti* were treated as *verba de futuro.* Vows made by children under the age of seven lacked legal validity. But since sexual intercourse completed the marriage, sexual maturity was decisive and marriages at a younger age were in principle possible.

2. Unbelief (Disparity of Cult). Although the church fathers and especially Augustine were more flexible on this point, in canon law it had become a rule that marriage to an unbeliever who had not been baptized was invalid. The fact of not being baptized makes it impossible for the person to administer the sacrament of marriage to the other, with the result that the baptized person cannot receive the sacrament. Especially Gratian strove for legislation in which the marriages of Catholics to heretics, pagans, and Jews would be invalidated. The situation was different in case of mixed religion (*religio mixta*), that is, the situation in which a Catholic marries a member of a schismatic group or church. Although such a marriage was prohibited, if it had nevertheless been contracted, it could not be invalidated.

3. Impotence (Incapacity for the Marital Act). As long as no sexual intercourse had taken place, there existed a *matrimonium initiatum, nondum consummatum,* i.e. an as yet unconsummated marriage. If sexual intercourse was impossible, there was a three-year period of probation in which qualified judges had to determine in which partner the cause was present and whether the impotence was permanent. If the latter was the case, the marriage was invalid, provided the impotence was antecedent to the marriage.[20] If intercourse had occurred at the beginning and the impotence arose later, the marriage was valid and indissoluble. If the marriage was invalidated but the man later proved capable of sexual intercourse with another woman, there existed a condition of temporary impotence (*frigiditas*) and the church had erred. As a result, the first marriage was now in fact valid and the divorced partners had to reunite. If the impotence was permanent and therefore also in effect in other relations, the condition was called a *maleficium* (defect).

4. A Preexisting Marriage Obligation. The principle of monogamy ruled out the possibility of concluding a valid marriage when a preexisting marriage obligation existed. Such a marriage bond disappeared only at the death of the partner. An obligation assumed during an existing marriage resulted in bigamy and had to be annulled. In connection with this condition the question arose whether the prolonged absence of a spouse on account of war, say, and the suspicion that he had been killed, did not dissolve the marriage bond. Although a large number of canonists demanded written proof of death for the fulfillment of this condition, there were also others who deemed a well-founded suspicion that the other partner had died sufficient. But the canonists were unanimous in the conviction that if a new marriage had been concluded but the spouse who had been presumed dead returned, the first marriage had to be restored and the second invalidated.

5. *A Vow of Chastity.* The ideal of virginity and the negative appraisal of sexuality coupled with it resulted in the declaration that a vow of chastity was a ground for the dissolution of a marriage. A distinction was made between two kinds of vows. The first was called a solemn vow (*votum solemne*). This was a vow solemnly made in the presence of a properly authorized clergyman. This vow rendered a marriage invalid, for a vow made to God and a vow made to a human, though equally irrevocable, were not on the same level and the former certainly has priority over a marriage to a human. The other vow—the so-called *votum simplex*—meant that someone had decided to live a life of chastity but without making and registering an official vow. This vow implied the prohibition of marriage, but did not render an existing marriage invalid.

6. *Reception of Sacred Orders.* An invalidating impediment is also present in the case of a person who has received one of the so-called higher orders. A person who has been consecrated as subdeacon, deacon, priest, or bishop cannot enter a valid marriage.

Lack of Consent

Since a marriage had essentially been concluded the moment a man and a woman exchanged the words of consent, the lack of such consent on the part of one of the partners was a ground for invalidating the marriage.[21] It was impossible, therefore, to enter into marriage with a mental patient. A marriage did remain valid when it concerned a person who had become mentally ill after the conclusion of the marriage and was therefore of a sound mind at the time the *verba de praesenti* were pronounced.[22]

The necessary consent was also lacking if someone had—either physically or mentally—been forced into a marriage. If a woman had been violently abducted against her will with the intent to force her into marriage the marriage was self-evidently invalid.[23] These stipulations were particularly relevant in view of the marriages concluded for the purpose of consolidating or expanding political or financial positions.

It is noteworthy that in the fifteenth century the absence of parental consent was no longer viewed as a hindrance to a valid marriage.

Error

Peter Lombard and Master Gratian distinguished the following four types of error:

1. *An Error Concerning the Person.* A marriage is invalid if the partner proves to be other than the person intended and expected, as happened in the case of Jacob and Leah. This stipulation also applies when someone assumes a false public identity for the purpose of entering a marriage by deception.

2. *An Error in (Social) Position.* There is an error that invalidates a marriage when someone thinks he is married to a free person who afterwards proves to be a slave. This stipulation stems from Roman times when a slave was not yet considered a legal agent. In contrast to imperial law,[24] canon law did not prohibit a marriage between a slave and a free person, provided the free person had advance knowledge of the status of the prospective marriage partner.

3. *An Error of Fortune.* Not being informed of a partner's financial capacity or—more likely—incapacity is not an error that invalidates a marriage. The same is true of the following error.

4. *An Error in Quality.* This error concerns a situation in which the partner exhibits characteristics other than those expected or hoped for.

Kinship

1. *Blood Relationship.* In the determination of degrees of consanguinity the method of counting was a problem. Whereas first the Roman method was followed, in the eleventh century the Germanic method was introduced into canon law. The Germanic computation coincided with double the number of the Roman system. The seventh degree of the canonical computation now in force was equal to the thirteenth or fourteenth degree of the Roman system in force earlier. After years of discussion the fourth Lateran Council (1215) decreed that in the collateral line, hence the line pertaining to brothers, sisters, their children, and grandchildren, marriages were forbidden to the fourth degree. True, on good grounds and for payment a dispensation could be obtained, but for the majority of the population this stipulation continued to mean that in the closed communities of the time it was sometimes very difficult to find a marriage partner who did not belong to the prohibited members of the family.

For those who had become blood relations by adoption (*cognatio legalis*), consanguinity was an impediment only between the natural and the adopted children. Those who had become part of a family through marriage (*affinitas*) were fully counted as members of the family. Inasmuch as married partners became one flesh the two related families also became one. In the last case the blood relationship only counted after sexual intercourse.[25]

The resulting complex ramifications were a constant source of lawsuits concerning the legitimacy of marriages.

2. *Spiritual Relationship.* Spiritual relationship (*cognatio spiritualis*) originated because, on receiving a sacrament, a person becomes spiritually related to another. This kinship arises from baptism and confirmation but also from the catechesis given to adults who still have to be baptized. The reference is to a spiritual relationship between the catechist and the person receiving baptism. As a result of baptism there arises as it were a new spiritual life that is valued more highly than the natural life. A consequence is that a special relationship has come into being between the person baptized and the one baptizing as well as between the person baptized and the baptismal sponsors. This results in a direct paternity (*paternitas directa*), which is the relationship between the godfather and godmother on the one hand and the child that is baptized on the other. Indirect paternity (*paternitas indirecta*) exists in reference to the relation that exists between the baptized child and the marriage partner of the sponsor and between the child baptized and the children of the sponsor(s).

Confirmation as the completion of baptism has the same effects. The extent and opacity of precisely this form of "kinship" were constant sources of much misunderstanding among canonists.

3. *Public Decency.* No one can enter a valid marriage with a blood relation of his or her betrothed. This impediment is present also in the case of a person's marriage to a blood relation of the partner with whom he or she lives in an invalid marriage or in concubinage.

Crime

In the case of adultery and a subsequent attempt to dissolve one's own marriage by homicide for the purpose of clearing the way for a new marriage, this new marriage is invalid. The reference here, therefore, is to criminal actions that aggravate the sin of adultery.[26]

Grounds That Prohibit Marriage (Prohibitive Impediments)

By comparison with the extensive treatment of the diriment impediments the treatment of the prohibitive impediments recedes into the background. The lists of prohibitive impediments we encounter among the canonists also in no small measure differ among themselves.

The grounds that prohibited marriage, but did not invalidate a concluded marriage, generally pertained to the same issues that could dissolve a betrothal. A number of canonists further added the so-called church prohibition (*vetitum ecclesiae*) and "the time of feast days" (*tempus feriarum*). The former refers to a special and incidental prohibition, occasioned by the suspicion that there are obstacles to the marriage, though they cannot be proven to exist. The second is a prohibition against organizing marriage festivities at certain times in the church year and completing the necessary communion.[27] Making marriage vows, on the other hand, is not prohibited on those days.

Generally speaking, the prohibitive impediments only play a subordinate role, particularly because they cannot render void an established marriage.

Divorce

In all the above cases we are not really dealing with divorce because the reference is to the invalidation of a relationship that only bore the name of marriage. But in reality there was no marriage and therefore no dissolution of a marriage, or divorce.

For a divorce in the sense of the dissolution of a marriage, the possibilities in canon law were much more limited. In this connection one must make a careful distinction between the nullification of the marriage bond and the termination of married life. Only in the former case are we dealing with divorce in the sense that an existing and valid marriage is dissolved. In the latter case we are speaking of the termination of connubial communion though the marriage bond remains intact. In light of the view that a marriage bond is twofold, viz. a sacramental bond that is indissoluble and a natural bond that embraces physical communion and can be dissolved, the idea of separation from bed and board (*divortium quoad torum et mensam*) arose. Also without communion of bed and board the marriage continues to exist on account of its sacramental character.

Dissolution of Marriage

Just as in the determination of the moment a marriage is concluded, so also in the matter of the breakup of the marriage, the schools of Peter Lombard and Master Gratian took opposing positions. Gratian considered a marriage that had been concluded but not yet consummated dissolvable, because the critical component of indissolubility essential to a complete marriage, viz. sexual intercourse (*copula carnalis*) was not yet present. Peter Lombard, who considered a marriage valid from the moment of verbal consent, believed that even if sexual intercourse had not yet occurred, the marriage was indissoluble.

An essential element of the views of Gratian was established in canon law. In cases where no sexual intercourse has occurred, a marriage is dissoluble only when a condition of impotence is present that originated after the formation of the marriage, or one of the married partners makes a monastic vow, or the pope grants a dispensation. In any of the above cases the marriage can be dissolved and a new marriage may be undertaken. If sexual intercourse has taken place, however, the above-mentioned three grounds for the dissolution of the marriage bond no longer apply. Then the only remaining ground for divorce is the Pauline privilege (*privilegium paulinum*). At stake here is what Paul writes in 1 Corinthians 7 about the marriage between a believer and an unbeliever. According to canon law, a marriage between two unbelievers, though genuine, is—in contrast to a Christian marriage—still dissoluble even after sexual intercourse. If one of the two partners becomes a believer, that believer cannot end the marriage. But if the unbelieving partner no longer wishes to be married to the believer, the marriage can be dissolved and the believer can contract a new marriage. Should the believer prefer to live apart from the unbeliever, the marriage bond continues intact. If the two partners continue to live together but the unbeliever blasphemes the name of God or leads the believer into serious sin, a divorce can still be arranged (affront to God dissolves the right of matrimony).

Separation From Bed and Board

The possibility of separation from bed and board is not introduced until the twelfth century and means that marital communion ends while the marriage bond continues. No dissolution of the marriage takes place so that there can be no new marriage as long as the other partner is alive. As the result of the separation from bed and board the partners are exempt from the duty of rendering the marital service of sexual intercourse and at the same time from the obligation to live together and the obligations that flow from it. At the same time they must abstain from sexual intercourse with others. Only the death of the partner cancels the still-existing marriage bond. Separation from bed and board is permitted in the following cases:

1. *Physical Adultery*. If the innocent party consents to continued cohabitation, this can only occur after the guilty party has done penance.

2. *Spiritual Adultery*. Spiritual adultery occurs when one of the two partners lapses from the faith, falls into heresy, leads or forces the partner into this, or other grave sins.

3. *Entry into a Monastery by Mutual Consent of the Partners*. The reference here is to a decision to live a chaste life in isolation from the world that stops short of making solemn monastic vows.

4. *Abuse*. The reference here is only to very grave offenses, for it was not unusual and quite widely accepted that a husband could beat his wife if he judged it necessary.

The Position of Husband and Wife

In canon law, as opposed to Roman law, the wife gains as many rights as the husband.[28] For example, neither partner can make monastic vows or vows to live a chaste life without the knowledge and consent of the other. True, the wife is obligated to follow her husband, but if the latter continually moves from one place to another without settling down or decides to go on a crusade or pilgrimage, she is relieved of this obligation unless she was privy to these facts prior to the marriage.

Husband and wife are equally obligated to mutual fidelity and the performance of the marriage vows, whereas in Roman law the husband was much less bound to these obligations.[29] A husband nevertheless has the right to punish his wife, but only on good grounds and in moderation.

A Second Marriage

A second marriage is permitted only after divorce—a fact by which the marriage bond has disappeared in every respect—or after the death of the other marriage partner. An illegitimate second marriage is usually described as bigamy.[30]

The rule for every second marriage is that the marriage blessing cannot be received again, not even when this is the first marriage for the partner. The mystical union between Christ and the church is only depicted in the first marriage. Once that marriage has been broken the surviving partner cannot depict that unity a second time. The marriage blessing, accordingly, is unrepeatable and, given this reality, a church wedding has become impossible.

Similarly, the person who marries a second time is no longer qualified to make monastic vows. This last point is based on the—mistakenly interpreted—stipulation in 1 Timothy 3:2, which states that officebearers must be the husband of one wife. As a result, second marriages generally became seriously suspect. If the purpose of marriage is the procreation of progeny and a person has achieved this purpose in his first marriage, then what can be the motives for a second marriage? Is the motive the avoidance of fornication? That, too, is suspect, for what kind of person is still troubled by sexual desires after a first marriage? If marriage per se is a sign of weakness, then how much more a second marriage! This at the same time explains why books of penance prescribe a certain period of penance for everyone who enters on a new marriage.[31]

*   *   *

As we look back on this section it is clear that at the end of the fifteenth and the beginning of the sixteenth century canon law developed into a system that was virtually impenetrable to the laity. Precisely because of the multiplicity and opacity of its laws it gave rise to much conscious and unconscious abuse. The difficulty and scope of the stipulations are evident from the fact that, for ease of memorization, they were reduced to verse. Although in a theologian like Thomas Aquinas one senses a growing appreciation for marriage, most medieval publications display a low estimate of marriage, sexuality, and women. The church viewed marriage as a sacrament, thereby bringing marriage law under its own jurisdiction. The de facto lack of the option of divorce forced people who nevertheless wanted to leave their partner and to enter a new marriage to secure a declaration in which their marriage was invalidated. Thus laws designed to prevent divorce (*divortium*) furnished countless ways, via a nullification, of achieving the breakup of their marriage (*separatio*). Many persons entered marriage without being aware of having violated one or more of the diriment impediments. For some of them the violation then proved highly convenient later inasmuch as, when divorce was impossible, there was still a ground for the annulment of their marriage. In practice, however, ecclesiastical courts prove to have precisely investigated whether in fact there had been a diriment impediment.[32] All in all the canon law of marriage in many ways served as a barrier both to the formation and the dissolution of a marriage. The Council of Trent later made only a few cosmetic changes in this legislation. It expressly rejected the Reformational view of marriage as ungodly and worthy of condemnation.

The Practice of Marriage

In the late Middle Ages, contrary to what we would expect from the complex canonical marriage legislation, we encounter a rather uncomplicated and free marriage practice. In addition this marriage legislation resulted in countless and frequently terribly complex lawsuits. The data—also those recorded by Catholic scholars—show that the criticism by Reform-minded writers of the lifestyle of clergy as well as laity, though sometimes one-sided, was by no means incorrect. The abstinence recommended by Augustine had turned into its opposite and issued in widespread sexual degeneracy. The number and nature of the cases that marriage courts in evangelical cities had to adjudicate illustrate the kind of practices to which the population had become accustomed.[33]

The focal point of the criticism is celibacy, which in the lives of many occasioned a double morality of preached chastity and practiced immorality. Already at the beginning of the thirteenth century there is fierce criticism of this theory and the consequent lifestyle of the clergy. At the time there lived in and around Strasbourg a large group of Waldensians who, with the help of Dominicans from Italy, were opposed by Rome. They were regarded as heretics because they taught that the clergy could marry and that marriage is better than the degenerate lifestyle of the clergy as that manifested itself at the time.[34] Three hundred years later the Dominican Bucer, rather than oppose the views of the Waldensians, would adopt them and even put them in practice. His criticism was also directed against celibacy, which, to him, was the source of ecclesiastical and social misery. People who lack the gift of abstinence but still have to practice abstinence will satisfy their natural needs in immoral ways so that not only their office, work, and church, but also society as a whole is adversely affected. In making these assertions Bucer reflects the charges of the Strasbourg humanist Jacob Wimpheling (like Bucer, born in Schlettstadt) who in 1505 published a small book entitled *De integritate* in which he exposes the immorality of the clergy.[35] The following year a new work containing the same indictments makes its appearance. The priests have their wives sitting at home, expensively dressed and all made up, and on all sorts of occasions occupying the front seats. Just like the laity, the priests marry off their daughters and arrange their inheritance for the benefit of their sons. Such priests, says Wimpheling, should be disciplined, but it will not happen because the bishop himself has a wife and children as well. Wimpheling asks whether the people must hand over the tithes of their hard-earned money to that end. By putting his finger on the financial aspect Wimpheling touched a sensitive nerve, thereby getting the people on his side and the clergy against him.

Of especial importance in this connection was the heavy criticism and mordant satire of Erasmus (d. 1536). In his writings he makes a plea for a fundamental purification of the priestly apparatus and the abolition of compulsory celibacy, but he does it cautiously, i.e. by ridicule and questioning.[36] Also the common people mocked the clerical class. Public opinion came through unambiguously in the popular saying: "If you wish to keep your house pure, then leave clerics and monks at the door" ("Willst du rein behalten dein Haus, so lass Pfaffen und Mönche draus").[37] But despite all this criticism hardly anything changed. During these centuries church leaders did indeed make attempts at raising the moral standard of the clergy and at combating abuses, but no discussion was possible on the subject of the marriage of priests. In addition these leaders were largely blind to the social and societal consequences of the lifestyle of the clerics.

Money, sexuality, and theology were uniquely intertwined. Though there were ecclesiastical penalties for the violation of church laws, it was possible, after all, to buy off these penalties. A theology that was conducive to the externalization of the religious life therefore, in turn, favored the rise of more abuses so that an economic relation of almost complete interdependence arose between the church and the brothel. Many a clergyman who had to but could not live a life of celibacy sought refuge in a brothel. Since frequenting a brothel was still consistently deemed less sinful than marriage, the clerics in question felt properly covered. For many people the brothel was in any case already an acceptable institution that was of benefit to the whole community. Unmarried young men could meanwhile pick up some experience there; married men found in it a substitute for an unhappy marriage; and women could walk the streets more safely since men could satisfy their lusts at reasonable prices in the brothel and would therefore not have to lay violent hands on respectable women.[38] Priests did not really belong there and therefore had of course to be penalized if caught going there. Fortunately, by paying the church a fine they could buy off the penalty. The pope badly needed this money for conducting wars to maintain and strengthen his position, and for building churches. Thus both the brothel and the church had a financial interest in maintaining celibacy and the church indirectly lived off prostitution. The clergy hardly considered the fact that the money the priest paid to the prostitute and the pope came out of the pockets of poor folks—poor in more than one respect—who both by what they gave and what they saw increasingly lost their respect for celibacy and priests.[39]

But even when a priest lived a morally cleaner life and kept only one woman with whom he lived as though they were married, this practice served as an important source of revenue for the church. In 1521 the bishop of Constanz, Hugo von Landenberg, collected approximately 6,000 guilders in fines that were paid as penance for the birth of 1,500 "papist children" in his diocese that year. Hence the attack on celibacy was at the same time an attack on an important source of income for the church. In view of the above situation it is not surprising, therefore, that when the Reformation aimed its criticism at celibacy it found so much resonance among the common people.

It was not only the common people, however, but also the civil authorities who had increasing problems with the church, even though in the case of the latter this was due especially to the great power that the church had accumulated. And to the degree that princes and cities gained more insight into the political and societal importance of marriage and family, their interest in what the Reformation had to say on these subjects also increased.

In light of the entrenched abuses described above Bucer's sharp attacks on celibacy make sense. Whereas Rome appealed to Scripture and tradition, Bucer asserted that the prohibition of marriage, as Rome at a certain stage in history introduced it for the clergy, was completely contrary to Scripture and the church fathers.[40]

Another serious abuse arising from canonical marriage law was the existence of the so-called *Winkelehen*, marriages contracted in secret. Many church trials were conducted over the precise wording used in making the vows.[41] The marriage vows of children—vows sometimes made with the parents standing by to prompt them—had to be recognized as valid. The same was true of vows made between a boy and a girl without the knowledge and often against the will of the parents. Though the church might berate such a state of affairs, the marriage could no longer be nullified. Thus, according to the proceedings of diocesan marriage courts, it frequently happened that a girl had allowed herself to be sweet-talked into sexual intercourse after the boy had promised to marry her. But in the absence of witnesses it was a rather simple thing for the boy to deny he made the promise and he was then as a rule found innocent.[42] The immediate result of this state of affairs was a high number of unmarried mothers and abandoned children.

Marriage law additionally offered an abundance of opportunities for escaping one's promises and obligations. By an appeal to, say, the complexity of the laws pertaining to the degrees of spiritual relationship, a (concluded) marriage could still be invalidated years later.[43]

Thus, though there was a strong canonical focus on the formation of a marriage, there was but little interest in the conditions for a good married life.[44] By way of reaction, a number of books came out that did address this need. The best-known work was that of Albrecht von Eyb, entitled *Ob einem manne sey zunemen ein eelichs weyb oder nicht* (*Whether it is Advisable for a Man to Marry or Not*).[45] Albrecht was of the opinion that it was, and proceeded to sketch for his readers what a good marriage should be like. Proof of the need for and of interest in such a book at the time is that this little work, which was published in 1472, enjoyed eleven reprints up until 1540 alone. Other books discussed marriage-related issues as well and found readers among the common people.[46] All these books, nevertheless, remained rooted in the traditional view that the unmarried life was superior to and less sinful than the married life. Moveover, hardly any attention was given to marriage as a personal relationship in which affection and openness played an essential role.[47] Marriage as an institution remained necessary for weak believers and was, accordingly, discussed with little appreciation. A number of church fathers, following a highly questionable exegetical practice, drew from the parable of the sower the conclusion that the virginal state would bear fruit and yield a hundredfold. Sixty-fold was the yield of widowhood and hence a reason not to remarry. The spiritual yield of marriage, however, was only thirtyfold. This exegesis was at the time still frequently repeated. Also among the people in general it was quite commonly thought that, aside from sporadic sexual pleasure, marriage merely brought with it a multiplicity of burdens. For the husband they were the burdens of wife and children, and for the wife the burdens of putting up with the whims of her husband and the bearing and taking care of many children, half of whom would not live past the age of ten. In addition there was the example of the clergy that prompted also many of the laity to visit brothels and to commit adultery, all the more where it concerned sins that could be bought off for a small fine. It is clear from many sources that the state of matrimony enjoyed but little esteem and was frequently ridiculed.[48]

The rules framed by the church were mainly limited to sexual intercourse and in this area, too, life was constricted by doctrine. The most radical restriction of conjugal intercourse was inherent in the dogma that it was permitted only for the purpose of procreation. Since certain days—Wednesday, Friday, and Saturday—were special, it was prohibited on these days. Intercourse was further forbidden during daylight hours and pregnancy. Opportunity was further reduced when—in light of the carnal nature of the sex act—it was forbidden on Sundays and feast days, for on those days the body of Christ was received in holy communion. In view of the enormous number of feast days, one gathers that conjugal intercourse was in fact hardly possible at all. In violent contrast to all these restrictions is the comprehensiveness with which—in the confessional, confessional books, and (wedding) sermons—the sex act was elaborated.[49] In minute detail people were told what was permitted and—predominantly—what was not permitted in the conjugal act.

Among the critics of this system of canon law was Martin Bucer. To understand his attempts at reforming marriage law it is essential for us to listen to his criticism and to note its pastoral character. Bucer knew—from his own experience—that people experienced canonical marriage legislation as a very heavy burden. This prompted him to speak of the "tyranny" of the canons.[50] The consciences of the married and the unmarried alike were oppressed and put to the test.[51] He denied to the Catholic church the right to treat matrimonial cases and, accordingly, launched the indictment that the church drew marriage under its jurisdiction by violence.[52] Nor did it stop here but, in view of many other matters as well, one can say that the church usurped dominion over the souls of humans.[53] Bucer is not prepared to accept this situation: the fact that it is so does not mean it ought to be so.

In a brief survey he describes the course of these developments in his large opus on marriage.[54] By expanding the number of the sacraments and making them necessary for salvation the church enlarged its power, while all the while the civil authorities willingly abdicated it. If in the course of time all kinds of divine institutions thereby fall into decay, it is no wonder that this decay also strikes marriage.[55] The truth is that the church sought to be more rigorous than God and this meant that whereas God had commanded that a minister of the church should have only one wife, the church simply decreed that it was better that he should have no wife at all. "And what is the result? The result is that there are no people on earth who live more unchaste and luxurious lives than these holy papists."[56] This is also how things went with the laws for divorce and remarriage. The church "did not want to be as irresponsible as God," with the result that irresponsibility now reigns supreme. Bucer especially stresses that it is the poor who are suffering under the tyranny of these laws, for the rich can always obtain dispensation in exchange for money. When a rich man is fed up with his wife he has no problem—in exchange for a large sum of money—getting a divorce and permission to remarry and "in that way the church can certainly excuse him." But for a poor man the situation is very different. He must submit to the laws of the canon and remain in his situation, however wretched it may be. Rich folk can afford to sin in a big way but a poor man is immediately punished by the church.[57] Like his predecessors Wimpheling and Gailer von Kaisersberg, Bucer, in his criticism, appealed to the people and put into words what many of them had been thinking for centuries.

For the wife traditional theology spelled degradation. In consequence of celibacy—a requirement for priests who dispense salvation—and on account of the sinfulness of sexuality a woman was per se a threat. Genesis 3 already designated her as the cause of the fall and ever since that time it has been natural for her to bring about the fall of men or to lure them into a trap. These notions—reinforced by misogynous preaching—created fertile soil for belief in and the suppression of witches. Every woman was a potential witch, and was approached accordingly.[58] Public opinion held that a husband had the right to beat his wife.[59] Beatings with a stick or rod or—for gentler men—house arrest were generally accepted methods of punishing wives. Wives had no legal basis from which to make a solid case against abusive husbands and the church acquiesced in this by referring the wife to the submission required of her by God. The clergy at most offered her suggestions on how best to deal with such husbands. More than any other Reformer, Bucer saw that it was the women who were being victimized by the existing marriage legislation. He, accordingly, speaks of the "poor oppressed wives."[60] Many wives, according to him, are burdened by having to live with "heartless, evil husbands."[61]

Other sources indicate that there was also official acknowledgement of the fact that at least some of the marriage laws were not working. The numerous dispensations requested and granted in the fifteenth and the beginning of the sixteenth century for marriages between persons who on the basis of the law on degrees of consanguinity had entered scandalous and even incestuous relationships are proof that not only the people but also the clergy had changed their minds.[62]

Bucer cannot imagine why, on the one hand, the church is extremely rigorous in its divorce legislation and, on the other, makes ample room for immoral conduct by priests and parishioners alike.

> It is simply incredible that in all sorts of matters we have been struck blind and everyone therefore dreads a legal and beneficial divorce that opens the door to a second marriage, while people at the same time shut their eyes to the adulterous affairs and scandalous deeds of bishops, and even wink at them. We approve of divorces, but prohibit second marriages, and this is done by people who themselves are regularly involved in fornication and nurture and encourage the commission of every possible outrage. Nowadays you hear people rage against the marriages of priests but they are the same people who the moment it somewhat touches themselves in the matter of affairs and scandals know no indignation whatever.[63]

The very laws that were supposedly designed for the protection of marriage now serve as excuses for immorality, states Bucer in his commentary on Ephesians 5.[64] Since we have replaced God's laws with human laws there has come about a legal disparity in virtue of which the adulterous are not punished but innocent people are denied the marriage they need.[65] Of these laws it can be said that they prompt people of ill will to sin and force those of good will to sin as well. In the interest of building a Christian society Bucer will attempt to develop new marriage legislation and a biblical view of marriage. He wants to do this by listening to what the Word of God and imperial law—which in this matter is fully biblical, according to him—have to say about marriage and divorce. "The pope has ruled so long that Christian, imperial law which agrees with the divine law has long ago disappeared."[66] Now that papal law has collapsed, imperial law can again become effective. The reformation Bucer has in mind[67] is one in which people are no longer guided by pagan or papal rules but only by divine law.

Notes

1. For the history of canonical marriage law, see J. A Brundage, *Law, Sex and Christian Society in Medieval Europe* (Chicago: University of Chicago Press, 1987); A. Esmein, *Le Mariage en Droit Canonique*, 2 vols. (Paris: Librairie du recueil Sirey, 1929, 1935); J. Freisen, *Geschichte des Canonischen Eherechts bis zum Verfall der Glossenliteratur* (Paderborn, 1893); G. H. Joyce, *Die christliche Ehe* (Leipzig: J. Hegner, 1934; Dutch trans., Haarlem, 1940); W. M. Plöchl, *Geschichte des Kirchenrechts*, vol. 2, 2d ed. (Vienna: Herold, 1962); and E. Schillebeeckx, Het huwelijk: Aardse werkelijkheid en heilsmysterie, vol. 1 (Bilthoven: H. Nelissen, 1963), 160–272.

2. "Comme la législation, l'Etat avait conservé la juridiction sur le mariage: les tribunaux de l'état étaient seuls compétents pour statuer sur les causes matrimoniales. . . ." Esmein, *Mariage*, 1:7.

3. See Brundage, *Law*, 229–55, and Plöchl, *Das Eherecht des Magister Gratianus* (Leipzig: F. Deuticke, 1935) (hereafter cited Plöchl, *Gratianus*).

4. L. Brink, *De taak van de kerk bij de huwelijkssluiting* (Nieuwkoop: Heuff, 1977), 7.

5. "Mais c'est vraiment dans saint Augustin que l'on voit établie pour la première fois une relation logique et nécessaire entre le sacrement et l'indissolubilité." Esmein, *Mariage*, 1:69. Cf. also Schillebeeckx, *Huwelijk*, 193–98.

6. For Augustine see especially M. Müller, *Die Lehre des hl. Augustinus von der Paradiesehe und ihre Auswirkung in der Sexualethik des 12. und 13. Jahrhunderts bis Thomas von Aquin* (Regensburg: F. Pustet, 1954); J. van Oort, "Augustinus, Mani en de sexuele begeerte," in idem, Augustinus: Facetten van leven en werk (Kampen: Kok, 1989), 92–103; J. Peters, Die Ehe nach der Lehre des hl. Augustinus (Paderborn, 1918); and E. Schmitt, *Le mariage chétien dans l'oeuvre de Saint Augustin* (Paris: Etudes Augustiniennes, 1983).

7. Brink, *Taak van de Kerk*, 14.

8. "Ook in De sancta virginitate oordeelt hij zo, als hij zegt dat de maagdelijkheid de voorkeur verdient boven het huwelijk, maar niet in die zin, als zou het huwelijk iets verkeerds zijn, vant de keuze voor hogere gaven mag niet leiden tot veroordeling van lagere." Brink, *Taak van de Kerk*, 23.

9. Van Oort, "Augustinus," 92, speaks in this connection of "een donkere schaduwkant van zijn denken en invloed."

10. For a critical survey of the history of celibacy, see R. Gryson, *Les origines du célibat ecclésiastique du premier au septième siècle* (Gembloux: J. Duculot, 1970), and U. Ranke-Heinemann, Eunuchen voor het hemelrijk (Baarn, 1990).

11. "Die durch einen consensus per verba de praesenti, das heisst eine auf unmittelbaren Abschluss der Ehe gerichtete übereinstimmende Willenserklärung zustande gekommene Ehe war demgemäss, gleichgültig, ob vollzogen oder nicht, sacramental une unauflöslich." Plöchl, *Geschichte*, 307. For a historical survey of these developments, see R. Sohm, *Das Recht der Eheschliessung aus dem deutschen und kanonischen Recht geschichtlich entwickelt* (Weimar, 1875).

12. Dig. 50.17.30.

13. "Die kirchliche Gesetzgebung ging auch hier die via media." Plöchl, *Geschichte*, 307.

14. Whenever "betrothal" is mentioned hereafter, it always refers to the situation established by verbal consent. A betrothal had the legal force of a marriage. Hence the term betrothal had a different meaning

in that time than it does in our own. If one wishes to understand the way in which Bucer dealt with this whole problem, one must keep in mind the original meaning of this concept.

15. See I. Schwarz, *Die Bedeutung der Sippe für die Öffentlichkeit der Eheschliessung* (Tübingen: E. Fabian, 1959).

16. "For nearly half a millennium European marriage law wrestled with this tension between the insistence of preserving the couple's right to contract freely by simple consent and society's interest in requiring persons to marry openly." Brundage, *Law*, 415.

17. Loosely translated as "marriages contracted in a dark corner."

18. See Joyce, *Christliche Ehe*, 118–24, and R. Lettmann, *Die Diskussion über die klandestinen Ehen und die Einführung einer zur Gültigkeit verpflichtenden Eheschliessungsform auf dem Konzil von Trient* (Münster: Aschendorff, 1966).

19. See Freisen, *Geschichte*, 83–90.

20. "Unfruchtbarkeit und Unvermögen, die erst nach Vollzug der Ehe auftraten, waren für die Frage der Auflösung der Ehe nicht bestimmend." Plöchl, *Geschichte*, 318.

21. "Da die Grundlage der Ehe der freie Konsens der Nupturienten war, konnte durch erzwungene Konsenserklärung eine Ehe nicht geschlossen werden." Plöchl, *Geschichte*, 315.

22. "Nach der Eheschliessung erst auftretende Geisterkrankheit war nicht eheauflösend, weil sie beim Abschluss nicht vorhanden war." Plöchl, *Geschichte*, 314.

23. "La violence viviait le consentement et était un empêchement dirimant du mariage." Esmein, *Mariage*, 1:334.

24. "Dans le droit de Justinien le mariage n'est jamais valable entre personnes libres et personnes esclaves." Esmein, *Mariage*, 1:363.

25. "L'affinité ne provenait pas du mariage lui-même, mais de la copula carnalis." Esmein, *Mariage*, 1:418.

26. "Das Hindernis des Verbrechens . . . entstand aus einer rechtlichen Qualification erschwerender Umstände des Ehebruchs." Plöchl, *Geschichte*, 325.

27. "Unter *tempus feriarum* (geschlossene Zeit) verstand man das Verbot besonderer Hochzeitsfeierlichkeiten, des Hochzeitmahls und des Vollzugs der Ehe während bestimmter Zeiten." Plöchl, *Geschichte*, 327.

28. "Die mittelalterliche Kanonistik und das Kirchenrecht haben die natürlichen Gleichberechtigung von Ehemann und Ehefrau weit mehr Ausdruck verliehen als das weltiche Recht." Plöchl, *Geschichte*, 328.

29. Esmein, *Mariage*, 1:97.

30. Plöchl, *Gratianus*, 65.

31. R. Phillips, *Putting Asunder: A History of Divorce in Western Society* (Cambridge: Cambridge University Press, 1988), 28–29.

32. Phillips, *Putting Asunder*, 10–12.

33. "Immerhin lassen die Ehegerichtsprotokolle einen Einblick tun in eine Ungebundenheit sittlicher Verhältnisse, die dem primitiven Triebleben in weitestem Masse Raum gab." Köhler, *Zürcher Ehegericht*, 1:445. For a description of the situation at the beginning of the sixteenth century and the Reformation reactions to it, see W. Kawerau, *Die Reformation und die Ehe* (Halle, 1892).

34. J. Adam, *Evangelische Kirchengeschichte der Stadt Strassburg biz zur französischen Revolution* (Strasbourg, 1922), 5.

35. Adam, *Evangelische Kirchengeschichte*, 12. On abuses in the area of celibacy and concubinage, see W. Andreas, *Deutschland vor der Reformation* (Stuttgart: Deutsche Verlags-Anstalt, 1948), 111–15.

36. K. Koebner, "Die Eheauffassung des ausgehenden deutschen Mittelalters." *Archiv für Kulturgeschichte* 9 (1911): 73, speaks of "das rhetorische Beweismittel des Erasmus."

37. Cited in Kawerau, *Reformation*, 5.

38. L. Roper, *The Holy Household: Women and Morals in Reformation Augsburg* (Oxford: Clarendon Press, 1989), 91–93.

39. "Der Zölibat wurde weithin nicht mehr vom Allgemeinbewusstsein des christlichen Volkes getragen, weil sein Sinn durch die Praxis entstellt war." A. Franzen, *Zölibat und Priesterehe* (Munich: Aschendorff, 1969), 22.

40. *BDS* 17:98: "Die Ehe haben sie auch wider das offenbare wort Gottes und lehr der Alten verpotten...."

41. K. M. Lindner, "Courtship and the Courts: Marriage and Law in Southern Germany 1350–1550" (Th.D. diss., Harvard University, 1988), demonstrates from case documents that the majority of lawsuits were related to this problem.

42. Lindner, "Courtship and the Courts," 12.

43. Plöchl, *Geschichte*, 324. On the difference between secret marriages and clandestine marriages, see Lindner, "Courtship," 119–23.

44. "Nowhere was their indifference more marked than in matters concerning reproduction and family life," Brundage, *Law*, 587.

45. Albrecht von Eyb, *Ob einem manne sey zunemen ein eelichs weyb oder nicht* (Reprint, Darmstadt, 1990).

46. *Ain rückliche lere und predig wie sich zwey menschen in dem sakrament der heiligen ee halten süllen* (1472), and *Spigell des ehelichen ordens* (1487)—both mentioned by Koebner, *Eheauffassung*, 9, 11.

47. "Der Gedanke, daß auch eine geistige Germeinschaft und ein persönliches Verstehen den Inhalt der Ehe bilden können, liegt Geistlichen und Laien gleichmässig fern." Koebner, *Eheauffassung*, 317.

48. Kawerau, *Reformation*, 49–50.

49. Koebner, *Eheauffassung*, 25; see esp. T. N. Tentler, *Sin and Confession on the Eve of the Reformation* (Princeton: Princeton University Press, 1977), 186–223.

50. *BDS* 17:407.

51. "innumeras conscientias, partim excarnificari, partim periclitari...." *Ev.*, 152D.

52. *DRC*, 153.

53. "Non solum enim multa quae sunt magistratus profani, sibi illi vendicarunt, sed plurima etiam Christi, dum omne fere in animas sibi imperium usurparunt et fidem sub suas leges coegerunt." *Ev.*, 151B.

54. *EE*, 2b–5b.

55. "wie solte die Eh frey blibenn sein?" *EE*, 3a.

56. *EE*, 3b.

57. *EE*, 4b–5. Bucer further remarks concerning the poor: "mit denen die welt nit gern fil zuthun hat...." He knows how to put his theology to use in a social-critical way.

58. See, inter alia, "The Witch as a Focus for Cultural Misogyny," in *The Politics of Gender in Early Modern Europe*, ed. J. R. Brink, A. P. Coudert, and M. C. Horowitz (Kirksville, Mo.: Sixteenth Century Journal Publishers, 1989), 13–90.

59. See Koebner, *Eheauffassung*, 162–68.

60. *EE*, 41a, 42a.

61. *EE*, 42a. Brundage, *Law*, 549, concludes from his extensive study of medieval law codes that "women were generally handicapped by the law, not favored by it, and this was notably true in the law concerning sexual behavior."

62. C. Seeger, *Nullité de Mariage: Divorce et Séparation de corps à Genève au temps de Calvin* (Lausanne: Meta-Editions, 1989), 37–38. Plöchl, *Geschichte*, 328, calls the increase in the number of dispensations "ein deutliches Zeichen des Verfalls."

63. *Ev.*, 152B.

64. *Eph.* (1551), 173A: "Nam leges ... quod autem praetexunt curam matrimonialis honestatis et iuventutis, falso id dicunt, cum potius aperiant quasi publicas scholas omnis impuritatis et inhonestatis."

65. *Ev.*, 153A.

66. *EE*, 4a–b.

67. *Antwort*, 168a: "unser furgenommen reformatio...."

11

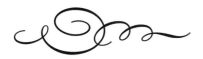

From Secular to Ecclesiastical Marriage

Joseph Martos

With the coming of the dark ages in Europe after the fall of the Roman empire, churchmen were called upon more and more to decide marriage cases. Centuries before, Constantine had given them authority to act as judges in certain civil matters, and now that authority grew as the regular judicial system collapsed. Bishops also began to issue canonical regulations about persons who should not marry because they were too closely related. Initially the churchmen simply adopted the prevailing Roman customs, although they sometimes added prohibitions that were found in the Old Testament. Later they incorporated the customs of the invading Germanic peoples into the church's laws. These customs varied somewhat from tribe to tribe, but generally speaking persons who were more closely related than the seventh degree of kinship (for example, second cousins) were not allowed to marry legally.

Moreover, just as the bishops had earlier accepted Roman wedding customs, so they now also accepted the marriage practices of the Germanic peoples who settled within the old Roman provinces. Again these varied from tribe to tribe, although they, too, followed a general cultural pattern. Marriages were basically property arrangements by which a man purchased a woman from her father or some other family guardian to be his wife. The arrangement involved a mutual exchange of gifts, spoken and sometimes written agreements between the groom and the bride's guardian. In many places brides were betrothed ahead of time in return for a token of earnestness such as a small sum of money or a ring from the prospective husband, which would be forfeited if the marriage did not take place as agreed. On the wedding day the guardian handed over the woman and her dowry of personal possessions to her new husband, and received the bride price as compensation for the loss her family incurred by allowing her to leave it. After the wedding feast that was celebrated by the relatives and other witnesses to the marriage, the bride and groom entered a specially prepared wedding chamber for their first act of intercourse, which formally sealed the arrangement.

Throughout this early period, then, marriage was still a family matter similar to what it had been in the Roman empire, and the clergy were not involved in wedding ceremonies except as guests. Bishops in their sermons and letters tried to impress their people with the Christian ideal of marriage found in the New Testament, and they sometimes urged them to have their marriages blessed by the clergy, but again this blessing was not essential to the marriage itself. In some places it was given during the wedding feast, in others it was a blessing of the wedding chamber, and in others it was a blessing during a mass after the wedding. Some bishops in southern Europe also suggested that the Roman custom of veiling the bridal couple should be done by a priest, but it was not a very common practice.

Just as churchmen were not officially involved in weddings, so also they were not officially involved in divorces when they occurred. However, some divorces ran counter to accepted Christian practices, and when they occurred those who were responsible for them had to confess their sin and do penance for it. The penitential books from the early Middle Ages show that divorce was more accepted in some places than others, but almost all allowed husbands to dismiss unfaithful wives and marry again. An Irish penitential book written in the seventh century instructed that if one spouse allowed the other to enter the service of God in a monastery or convent, he or she was free to remarry. The penitential of Theodore, archbishop of Canterbury in the same century, gave the following prescriptions: a husband could divorce an adulterous wife and marry again; the wife in that case could remarry after doing penance for five years; a man who was deserted by his wife could remarry after two years, provided he had his bishop's consent; a woman whose husband was imprisoned for a serious crime could remarry, but again only with the bishop's consent; a man whose wife was abducted by an enemy could remarry, and if she later returned she could also remarry; freed slaves who could not purchase their spouse's freedom were allowed to marry free persons. Other penitential books on the continent contained similar provisions.

The penitential books contained only unofficial guidelines to be followed in the administration of private penance, but conciliar and other church documents contained more official regulations. Again here these were not uniform, and ecclesiastical practices during this period ranged from extreme strictness to extreme laxness, but at least they show that there was no universal prohibition against divorce. In Spain the third and fourth councils of Toledo in 589 and 633 invoked the "Pauline privilege" in allowing Christian converts from Judaism to remarry. Irish councils in the seventh century allowed husbands of unfaithful wives to remarry, and although the council of Hereford in England advised against remarriage it did not forbid it. In eighth-century France the council of Compiègne allowed men whose wives committed adultery to remarry, and it allowed women whose husbands contracted leprosy to remarry with their husband's consent. In 752 the council of Verberie enacted legislation which allowed both men and women to remarry if their spouses committed adultery with a relative, and it prohibited those who committed the sin from marrying each other or anyone else. It also permitted a man to divorce and remarry if his wife plotted to kill him, or if he had to leave his homeland permanently and his wife refused to go with him. Pope Gregory II in 725 advised Boniface, the missionary bishop to Germany, that if a wife were too sick to perform her wifely duty it was best that her husband practice continence, but if this was impossible he might have another wife provided that he took care of the first one. Boniface himself recognized desertion as grounds for divorce, as well as adultery and entrance into a convent or monastery. Other popes of the period, however, protested against what they considered to be unlawful divorces, and the Italian council of Friuli in 791 strictly forbade divorced men to remarry even if their wives had been unfaithful.

One reason why churchmen became involved in marriage and divorce cases, especially after the popes started sending missionaries into northern Europe, was the difference between Roman and Germanic marriage customs. According to Roman tradition marriage was by consent, and after the consent was given by either the spouses or their guardians the marriage was considered legal and binding. In the Frankish and Germanic tradition, however, the giving of consent came at the betrothal, and the marriage was not considered to be completed or consummated until the first act of intercourse had taken place. Moreover, it was customary for parents to consent to the marriage of their children months and even years before they would begin to live together as husband and wife. This was particularly prevalent among the nobility, who often arranged such marriages as a means of securing allies or settling territorial disputes between them. But it sometimes happened that one of the betrothed spouses would undermine the parental arrangement by marrying someone else before the arranged marriage could be consummated. Bishops who were asked to settle these and similar cases could follow either the Roman or the Germanic tradition in coming to their decision. Under Roman law the arranged marriage was the binding one and the subsequent marriage was adultery, but according to Germanic custom the arrangement between the parents was only a nonbinding betrothal and the second marriage was the real one. Even before any marriage was arranged young people might consent to each other in marriage and then claim that they were not free to marry the partners their parents picked out for them, whereupon the parents might appeal to the episcopal court for a decision. In still other cases people sought to rid themselves of unwanted spouses by claiming that they had secretly contracted a previous marriage, which would make their present marriage unlawful. The legal question that had to be decided in each case was: Which marriage was the real marriage? And underlying the practical matters was the more theoretical question: Are marriages ratified by consent or by intercourse? For a long time there was no uniform answer to that theoretical question, and both episcopal and royal courts decided the practical matters according to which tradition they were accustomed to follow.

As Charlemagne initiated legal reforms in his European empire, both church and civil governments made an effort to impose stricter standards for marriage. Late in the eighth century the regional council of Verneuil decreed that both nobles and commoners should have public weddings, and a similar council in Bavaria instructed priests to make sure that people who wanted to marry were legally free to do so. In 802 Charlemagne himself passed a law requiring all proposed marriages to be examined for legal restrictions (such as previous marriages or close family relationships) before the wedding could take place. When the false decretals of Isidore were "discovered" in the middle of the ninth century, they contained documents purportedly from the patristic period aimed against the practice of secret marriage. A decree attributed to Pope Evaristus in the second century read, "A legitimate marriage cannot take place unless the woman's legal guardians are asked for their consent, . . . and only if the priest gives her the customary blessing in connection with the prayers and offering of the mass." Another decree represented the third-century pope Calixtus as saying that a marriage was legal only if it was blessed by a priest and the bride price was paid. The proponents of reform in the Frankish empire used these spurious documents to support their efforts to outlaw secret marriages, and they were partially successful. Laws were passed making marriages legal only if guardians gave their consent and were present at the wedding.

In the meanwhile, however, Rome continued to follow its own tradition. In 866 Pope Nicholas I sent a letter to missionaries in the Balkans who had asked about the Greek church's contention that Christian marriages were not valid unless they were performed and blessed by a priest. In his reply Nicholas described the wedding customs that had become prevalent in Rome: the wedding ceremony took place in the absence of any church authorities and consisted primarily in the exchange of consent between the partners; afterward there was a special mass at which the bride and groom were covered with a veil and given a nuptial blessing. In Nicholas' opinion, however, a marriage was legal and binding even without any public or liturgical ceremony: "If anyone's marriage is in question, all that is needed is that they gave their consent, as the law demands. If this consent is lacking in a marriage then all the other celebrations count for nothing, even if intercourse has occurred" (*Letters* 97). According to Rome, then, it was the couple's consent, not their betrothal by their parents or their blessing by a priest, which legally established the marriage.

Charlemagne had wanted Roman practices to become normative in his empire, and in the years that followed, a Roman-style nuptial liturgy sometimes began to be included in the festivities that followed a wedding, though it was never very prevalent. Moreover, the pope's insistence that only consent constituted a marriage was initially ignored or largely unknown in the rest of Europe. Hincmar, the bishop of Rheims during this period, decided a number of marriage and divorce cases among the Frankish nobility, and he generally followed the opinion of the false decretals that legal marriages had to be publicly contracted. He also followed the Germanic tradition in ruling that marriages had to be consummated by sexual intercourse, and he allowed that people who had been given in marriage but who had not yet lived together could be legally divorced.

For a while, divorce regulations in northern Europe became more stringent under the impetus of ecclesiastical reform. As early as 829 a council of bishops at Paris decreed that divorced persons of both sexes could not remarry even if the divorce had been granted for adultery. By the end of the century a number of other councils in France and Germany passed similar prohibitions, and the penitential books were revised accordingly. But at the same time in Italy, popes and local councils continued to allow divorce and remarriage in certain circumstances, especially adultery and entering the religious life. Then in the next two centuries the trend in northern Europe reversed itself, and councils at Bourges, Worms, and Tours again allowed remarriages in cases of adultery and desertion.

During this same period, moreover, ecclesiastical courts were slowly gaining exclusive jurisdiction over marriage and divorce cases. As Charlemagne's short lived empire dissolved into a disunited array of local principalities, more and more marriage cases were appealed to church tribunals. Eventually the secular courts came to be bypassed altogether, and by the year 1000 all marriages in Europe effectively came under the jurisdictional power of the church.

There was as yet no obligatory church ceremony connected with marriage, but in the eleventh century this began to change. In order to insure that marriages took place legally and in front of witnesses, bishops invoked the texts of Popes Evaristus and Calixtus in the false decretals to demand that all weddings be solemnly blessed by a priest. It gradually became customary to hold weddings near a church, so that the newly married couple could go inside immediately afterward to obtain the priest's blessing. Eventually this developed into a wedding ceremony that was performed at the church door and was followed by a nuptial mass inside the church during which the marriage was blessed. At the beginning of this development the clergy were present at the ceremony only as official witnesses and to give the required blessing, but as the years progressed priests began to assume some of the functions once relegated to the guardians and the spouses themselves, and many of the once secular customs in the wedding ceremony became part of an ecclesiastical wedding ritual.

By the twelfth century in various parts of Europe there was an established church wedding ceremony that was conducted entirely by the clergy, and although there were numerous local variations it generally conformed to the following pattern. At the entrance to the church the priest asked the bride and groom if they consented to the marriage. The father of the bride then handed his daughter to the groom and gave him her dowry, although in many places the priest performed this function instead. The priest then blessed the ring which was given to the bride, after which he gave his blessing to the marriage. During the nuptial mass in the church itself the bride was veiled and blessed, after which the priest gave the husband the ritual kiss of peace, who passed it to his wife. In some places the priest also pronounced an additional blessing over the wedding chamber after the day's festivities had concluded.

Along with the church's liturgical and legal involvement in marriage came a growing body of ecclesiastical laws about premarriage kinship, the wedding ceremony itself, and the social consequences of marriage and divorce. The medieval system of government and inheritance emphasized property rights and blood relationships arising from marriage, making it important for ecclesiastical judges to know who was legally free to marry, who was married to whom, and who could have their marriage legally dissolved. In the eleventh century the discovery and circulation of the Code of Justinian led to increasing acceptance of the idea that marriage came about by the consent of the partners, and this idea was reflected in the new rituals for church weddings in which the priest asked the bride and groom, not their parents, for their consent to the marriage. But the growth of the consent theory also led to an increase in the number of secret marriages, which brought legal difficulties about the legitimacy of children and their right to inherit their father's property, as well as pastoral difficulties when women and children were deserted by men who claimed they had never intended to establish a marriage.

In response to these difficulties some church lawyers defended a different theory about when a marriage legally took place, based on the old Germanic notion that intercourse was needed to ratify a marriage. As it was taken up and developed by the law faculty at the University of Bologna, this theory proposed that a real marriage did not exist unless and until the couple had sexual relations. But the opposing theory, that consent alone made a marriage, also had its staunch defenders, mainly at the University of Paris.

Around 1140 Francis Gratian in Bologna published his collection of canonical regulations known as the *Decree* in which he tried to bring some order into the sometimes conflicting decrees and decisions of popes and councils dating back to the patristic era. He was aware of the two schools of thought about what constituted a marriage, and he tried to harmonize them by suggesting that the consent of the spouses or their parents (in the case of betrothal) contracted a marriage and that sexual intercourse completed or consummated it. His opinion was that a marriage could be legally dissolved before it was consummated but not afterward, and in this respect he sided with the Bologna school. But he also agreed with the Paris school's contention that a binding marriage could be made in secret, without any public ceremony or priestly blessing. In his opinion such a marriage would be illicit or illegal because it flouted the laws of the church, but it would nonetheless be a real marriage, initiated by consent and consummated by intercourse.

Gratian's work clarified but did not settle the issue. In Italy, for example, church courts continued to dissolve marriages if it could be proven that no sexual relations had taken place, but in France the courts refused to dissolve any marriage once the partners' consent had been given. It was not until later in the twelfth century, when a noted canon lawyer of the period became Pope Alexander III, that a definitive solution was worked out and legislated for the whole Latin church. Because it offered a clearer criterion of an intended marriage between two individuals, Alexander sided with the ancient Roman practice that was defended by the Paris school, and he decreed that the consent given by the two partners themselves was all that was needed for the existence of a real marriage. This consent was viewed as an act of conferring on each other the legal right to marital relations even if they did not occur, and so from the moment of consent there was a true marriage contract between the two partners. In and of itself it was an unbreakable contract, but since the church had jurisdiction over it by the power of the keys, it could also be nullified or annulled by a competent ecclesiastical authority if sexual relations between the spouses had not yet taken place.

The decision of Alexander III became the legal practice of the Catholic church. It was reinforced by further papal decrees in the thirteenth century and has remained in effect in canon law through the twentieth century. With the exception of the "Pauline privilege" by which non-Christian marriages could be dissolved if one of the spouses converted to Catholicism, henceforward the church would grant no divorces whatever. Henceforward the marriage bond would be considered indissoluble not only as a Christian ideal but also as a rule of law. Henceforward if Catholics wanted to be freed from their spouses they would have to prove that their marriage contract could be nullified, declared to be nonexistent, either for lack of intercourse or for some other canonically acceptable reason.

But the pope's decision and the support it received in subsequent centuries did not rest only on the practical needs of ecclesiastical courts. Rather, the indissolubility of Christian marriage in the mind of Alexander and later churchmen rested also on a firm theological ground, the sacramentality of Christian marriage. For it was precisely around this time—the late twelfth century and the early thirteenth century—that marriage came to be viewed as one of the church's seven official sacraments.

What Francis Gratian did for canon law in his *Decree*, Peter Lombard did for theology in his *Sentences*. Lombard's collection of theological texts did not solve many of the theological problems of the Middle Ages but it did go a long way toward defining what they were and how they should be treated. Marriage was treated in the section on the sacraments, for by this time in mid-twelfth-century France there was an established Christian ritual for marriage which was not unlike the other rituals that Lombard classified as sacramental.

When the book of *Sentences* was first published, however, many theologians still had difficulty in accepting the idea that marriage was a sacrament in the strict sense which was then being developed, and Lombard himself believed that it was different from the other six sacraments in that it was a sign of something sacred but not a cause of grace. One reason for the difficulty was that marriages involved financial arrangements, and if marriage was counted as a sacrament like the others it looked as though grace could be bought and sold. Another reason they hesitated to call marriage a sacrament was that it obviously existed before the coming of Christ, and so it could hardly be said to be a purely Christian institution like the others. But the third reason was the most crucial, and it was that marriage involved sexual intercourse.

Throughout the early Middle Ages most churchmen held virginity in higher esteem than marriage. On the one hand Christians could not deny that God had told Adam and Eve to increase and multiply, and so marriage itself had to be good. But on the other hand marriage, as Paul said, distracted one from the things of the Lord, and he seemed to suggest that people should marry only if they could not quench the fire of sexual desire. So marriage in the Middle Ages was often viewed negatively as a remedy against the desires of the flesh rather than positively as a way to become holy, and those desires themselves were viewed as sinful or at best dangerous. Some bishops who blessed newly married couples recommended that they abstain from intercourse for three days out of respect for the blessing; others told them not to come to church for a month after the wedding, or a least not to come to communion with their bodies and souls still unclean from intercourse. Most of the writers held that sexual activity which was motivated by anything but the desire for children was sinful, but most of them also believed that even here children could not be conceived without the stain of carnal pleasure.

So the western theological tradition through the eleventh century taught that marriage was good even though sexual activity was usually sinful. Three things in that century, however, forced them to reexamine that view. The first was the rise of a religious sect in southern France which, like the Manichaeans in the patristic period, taught that matter was evil and so marriage was sinful because it brought new material beings into the world. The Albigensians (so named because many lived around the town of Albi) did not accept the Christian concept of God, they denied the value of church rituals, and their leaders attacked the Catholic clergy as corrupt, so they were first denounced and later burned as heretics. And in combating the Albigensian view of marriage Christian writers began to propose more strongly than before that intercourse for the sake of having children was positively good. The second thing that happened during this century was the development of a Christian wedding ritual which, by the presence of the clergy and the blessing they gave, implied that the church officially sanctioned sexual relations in marriage. And the third thing was the rediscovery of the writings of Augustine on marriage in which he developed the idea that marriage was a *sacramentum*. To the early schoolmen it seemed to suggest that marriage was a sacrament in the same way that baptism and the eucharist were sacraments.

Augustine had taught that marriage was a *sacramentum* in two ways. It was a sign of the union between Christ and his church, and it was also a sacred pledge between husband and wife, a bond of fidelity between them that could not be dissolved except by death. It was something like a character on the souls of the spouses which permanently united them, and it was this permanence of their union which symbolized the eternal union of Christ and the church. It seemed to the schoolmen, therefore, that the Christian marriage ritual should be open to the same kind of analysis that they gave to the other sacraments, namely that in marriage there was a *sacramentum*, a sacred sign, a *sacramentum et res*, a sacramental reality, and a *res*, a real grace that was conferred in the rite. It took most of the twelfth century for the scholastics to satisfactorily fit marriage into this scheme, but by the time they did it the Catholic concept of sacramental marriage had become the theological basis for the canonical prohibition against divorce.

But what was the *sacramentum*, the sacramental sign in marriage? At the beginning it seemed to many of the schoolmen that it should be the priest's blessing since in the wedding ritual it corresponded to the part that was played by the priest in the other sacramental rites. Later, others suggested that it should be the physical act of intercourse between the spouses since this physical union could be taken as a sign of the spiritual union between the incarnate Christ and his spouse, the church. Still others felt it should be the spiritual unity of the married couple since this union of wills was closer to the actual way that Christ and the church were united with each other. However, each of these suggestions met with difficulties and had to be abandoned. It was objected that the priest's blessing could not be the sacramental sign because some people were truly married even though they never received the blessing, for example, people who married in secret. The schoolmen who still believed that sexual relations even in marriage were venially sinful objected to intercourse's being considered the sign because this would paradoxically raise a sinful act to the dignity of a sacrament. And it was objected that the union of wills in the married life could not be the sacramental sign because sometimes this spiritual unity was minimal at the beginning of a marriage and altogether lacking later on.

Eventually, because of the growing acceptance of the consent theory of the canon lawyers, the *sacramentum* in a sacramental marriage came to be viewed as the consent that the spouses gave to each other at the beginning of their married life. This mutual consent was something that had to be present in all canonically valid marriages, even those that were unlawfully contracted in secret. Both the canonists in Paris and Pope Alexander in Rome insisted that a real marriage existed from the moment that the consent was given, and theologians such as Hugh of St. Victor argued that a real marriage would have to be possible even without consummation in intercourse since according to tradition Joseph and the Virgin Mary had been truly married even though they had never had sexual relations. In addition, locating the *sacramentum* in the mutual consent kept it within the wedding ritual for most Christian marriages, and it made it possible to look upon the union of wills in a happy married life as a "fruit" of the sacrament even if it was not the sacrament itself.

But the greatest theological consequence of seeing the act of consent as the *sacramentum* in marriage was that it made it possible to regard the marriage contract or bond as the *sacramentum et res*. According to canon law the bond of marriage was a legal reality which came into existence when the two spouses consented to bind themselves to each other in a marital union. Now, in theology, the bond of marriage could also be understood as a metaphysical reality which existed in the souls of the spouses from the moment that they spoke the words of the sacramental sign. Following the lead of Augustine, the scholastics argued that this metaphysical bond was unbreakable since it was a sign of the equally unbreakable union between Christ and the church. It was not, as in the early church, that marriage as a sacred reality *should* not be dissolved; now it was argued that the marriage bond as a sacramental reality *could* not be dissolved. According to the church fathers the dissolution of marriage was possible but not permissible; according to the schoolmen it was not permissible because it was not possible. Thus the absolute Catholic prohibition against divorce arose in the twelfth century both as a canonical regulation supported by sacramental theory, and as a theological doctrine buttressed by ecclesiastical law. The two came hand in hand.

Even through the beginning of the thirteenth century, however, many theologians found it hard to admit that marriage as a sacrament conferred grace like the other sacraments. The traditional view of marriage was that it was more of a hindrance than a help toward holiness, a remedy for the sin of fornication rather than a means of receiving grace. Many theologians accepted Augustine's idea that original sin was transmitted from one generation to the next through the act of intercourse, and so even sexual relations for the sake of having children were often seen as a mixed blessing. Alexander of Hales was the first medieval theologian to reason that since marriage was a sacrament and since all the sacraments bestowed grace, then marriage must do so as well. But William of Auxerre believed that if any grace came from marriage it must be only a grace to avoid sin, not a grace to grow in holiness. William of Auvergne and Bonaventure both agreed that the effect of the sacrament must be some sort of grace, but both of them also held that the grace came through the priest's blessing.

Nevertheless, under the influence of reasoning like Alexander's and the desire to fit all the sacraments into a single conceptual scheme, theologians from Thomas Aquinas onward admitted that the sacrament gave a positive assistance toward holiness in the married state of life. That grace was first of all a grace of fidelity, an ability to be faithful to one's marriage vow, to resist temptation to adultery and desertion despite the hardships of married life. It was also even more positively a grace of spiritual unity between the husband and the wife, enabling him to love and care for her as Christ did the church, and enabling her to honor and obey him as the church did her Lord. It was true, of course, that even non-Christians could be faithful to one another and achieve marital harmony, but for Aquinas Christians were called to an ideal of constant fidelity and perfect love which could not be attained without the supernatural power of God's grace.

Aquinas also realized as did the other scholastics that marriage existed long before the coming of Christ, but for him this was no different from the fact that washing existed before the institution of baptism or that anointing existed before the sacraments that used oil. It was thus, like the other sacraments, something natural that had been raised in the church to the level of a sacramental sign through which grace might be received. But this also meant for Aquinas that the *sacramentum* in marriage was not just the act of mutual consent in the wedding ritual but the marriage itself, which came into existence through the giving of consent, was sealed by the act of intercourse, and continued for the remainder of one's life. As a sacramental sign it was therefore permanent, as was the sacramental reality of the marriage bond which was created by consent and made permanent through consummation. As a natural institution marriage was ordered to the good of nature, the perpetuation of the human race, and was regulated by natural laws which resulted in the birth of children. As a social institution it was ordered to the good of society, the perpetuation of the family and the state, and was regulated by civil laws which governed the political, social, and economic responsibilities of married persons. And as a sacrament it was ordered to the good of the church, the perpetuation of the community of those who loved, worshipped, and obeyed the one true God, and was regulated by the divine laws which governed the reception of grace and growth in spiritual perfection. The "matter" of the sacrament was therefore the human reality of marriage as a natural and social institution since this was the natural element, like water or oil, out of which it was made. And the "form" of the sacrament consisted of the words of mutual consent spoken by the spouses, since these were what signified the enduring fidelity which would exist between them, just as it existed between Christ and the church.

Most of the other things that Aquinas had to say about marriage—and this was true of the other schoolmen as well—had to do with the ecclesiastical regulation of marriage, with the laws governing who may and may not lawfully marry, with regulations regarding betrothal and inheritance, and so on. For marriage in the Middle Ages was viewed not so much as a personal relationship but as a social reality, an agreement between persons with attendant rights and responsibilities. Thus Aquinas and the other thirteenth-century scholastics occasionally spoke of marriage as a contract, and in the centuries that followed the legal terminology of canon law was further incorporated into the sacramental theology of marriage.

John Duns Scotus, for instance, conceived of marriage as a contract which gave people a right to have sexual relations for the purpose of raising a family, and from this he drew the inference that intercourse in marriage was legitimate not only for begetting children but also for protecting the marriage bond. A woman was bound in justice to give her husband what was his by right, he reasoned, and so she had to grant his requests lest he be tempted to bring discord into the marriage by satisfying his desires with someone else. Other theologians in the fourteenth and fifteenth centuries also came to accept this argument, and by the sixteenth century it was commonly taught that not every act of intercourse had to be performed with the intention of having children. Married people could ask for sex without blame, provided they did it not out of lust but only to relieve their natural needs.

Scotus was also the first theologian to teach that the minister of the sacrament was not the priest but the couple that was getting married. According to canon law people who wed without a priest were validly married even thought they went about it illegally, and according to theology people who were validly married received the sacrament. It followed, therefore, that the bride and groom had to be the ones who administered the sacrament to each other when they gave their consent to the marriage. In the fourteenth and fifteenth centuries this view became more widely accepted, but even in the sixteenth century some theologians still maintained that the priest was the minister of the sacrament, for in many places the priest not only handed over the bride to the groom during the wedding ceremony but he also said, "I join you in the name of the Father and of the Son and of the Holy Spirit."

One thing that did not change, however, was the official prohibition against divorce. In the decree that was drawn up for the Armenian Christians during the Council of Florence in 1439, marriage was listed among the seven sacraments of the Roman church and explained as a sign of the union between Christ and the church. It adopted Augustine's summary of the goods of marriage as the procreation and education of children, fidelity between the spouses, and the indissolubility of the sacramental bond. It granted that individuals might receive a legal separation if one of them was unfaithful, but denied that either one of them could marry again "since the bond of marriage lawfully contracted is perpetual."

Nonetheless, Christians in certain cases did separate and remarry. The hierarchy no longer allowed divorces but ecclesiastical courts were now empowered to grant annulments to those who could prove that their present marriage was invalid by canonical standards. If a married person could show, for example, that he had previously consented to marry someone else, the court could decide that the first marriage was valid even though unlawful and that the present marriage was therefore null and void. Marriage within certain degrees of kinship was also regarded as grounds for annulment even after years of marriage. But the closeness of prohibited relationships varied in different parts of Europe, and so a marriage that might be upheld in one country might be annulled in another. And if the blood relationship or secret marriage was difficult to prove, ecclesiastical courts were sometimes open to being persuaded by financial considerations, generously but discreetly offered.

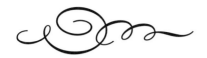

Marriage and Family in the Teaching of the Church

12

Gaudium et Spes: Promoting the Dignity of Marriage and the Family

Vatican II

47. (*Marriage and the family in the modern world*). The wellbeing of the person and of human and christian society is intimately connected with the healthy state of the community of marriage and the family. That is why Christians and all who value this community derive real satisfaction from the various supports being developed today in promoting this community of love and caring for its life as well as in helping married couples and parents in their outstanding task. They also look for further benefits and desire to encourage them.

The dignity of this institution, however, is not in evidence to the same degree everywhere, being obscured by polygamy, the plague of divorce, free love and other deformities. And married love is often demeaned by selfishness, pleasure-seeking and wrongful practices against having children. In addition, modern economic, socio-psychological and public conditions are seriously disrupting families, and in some regions the problems arising from increasing population are causing anxiety. All these factors are disturbing the consciences of people. And yet the power and vigour of marriage and the family are also to be seen in the fact that, whatever difficulties the profound changes in modern society may entail, they also frequently bring to light in various ways the true character of this institution.

Accordingly, by highlighting some major features of the church's teaching, the council aims to enlighten and encourage Christians and all people who are working for the protection and fostering of the inherent dignity and the noble and sacred significance of the state of matrimony.

48. (*The holiness of marriage and the family*). The covenant, or irrevocable personal consent, of marriage sets up an intimate sharing of married life and love as instituted by the creator and regulated by God's laws. Thus, the human action in which spouses give themselves to each other and accept each other results in an institution which is stable by divine ordinance and also in the eyes of society. This sacred bond, aimed at the good of the couple and their children and of society, does not depend on human decision. It is God who is the author of marriage and its endowment with various values and purposes,[1] all of which are of such vital importance for the continuance of the human race, the personal development and eternal destiny of the individual members of the family, and the dignity, stability, peace and prosperity of the family itself and of human society as a whole. The institution of marriage and married love are, of their nature,

directed to the begetting and upbringing of children and they find their culmination in this. Thus it is that a man and a woman, who "are no longer two but one flesh" (Mt 19, 6) in their marital covenant, help and serve each other in their intimate union of persons and activities, and from day to day experience and increase their sense of oneness. Such intimacy, as a mutual giving of two persons, as well as the good of their children require complete faithfulness between the partners, and call for their union being indissoluble.[2]

Christ the Lord has richly blessed this varied love, which has sprung from the divine fountain of love, to be a reflection of his union with the church. As God once approached his people with a covenant of love and faithfulness,[3] so now the saviour of women and men, and husband of the church,[4] comes to meet Christian couples through the sacrament of matrimony. God abides with them so that, as he loved the church and gave himself for it,[5] likewise marriage partners may love each other with everlasting fidelity in their dedication to each other. Genuine married love is taken up into the divine love and is directed and endowed by the redeeming power of Christ and the saving action of the church, so that married couples may be successfully led to God and be helped and strengthened in their noble task as father and mother.[6] For this reason christian partners are fortified and in a sense consecrated for the duties and dignity of their state by a special sacrament,[7] by virtue of which they fulfil their marital and parental tasks, imbued with the Spirit of Christ who fills their whole life with faith, hope and love, and increasingly attain to their own perfection, their mutual sanctification and their joint glorying of God.

With parents leading them by example and family prayer, children and all who live within the family circle will more readily discover the way to humanity, salvation and holiness. And married couples, honoured with the dignity and duty of parenthood, will diligently discharge their responsibility of education, especially in religion, which belongs to them before anyone else.

As active members of the family, children contribute in their own way to the sanctification of their parents. They will respond with gratitude, respect and trust to what their parents do for them and will help them, as children should, in their difficulties and the loneliness of old age. Widowhood accepted bravely as an extension of the vocation of marriage will be respected by all.[8] The family will generously make its spiritual resources available to other families. And the christian family, springing as it does from marriage as reflecting and sharing in the covenant of the love of Christ and the church,[9] will reveal to all people the active presence of the Saviour in the world and the genuine nature of the church, in the love, the generous fruitfulness, the unity and the faithfulness of husband and wife, and the loving cooperation of all the members.

49. (*Married love*). The word of God regularly invites engaged and married couples to nurture and cherish their betrothal with a love which is chaste, and their marriage with a devotion which is undivided.[10] And many people today value true love between husband and wife as this finds expression in various ways according to the honourable practices of different peoples and times. Fully human as it is, in being willed by one person for another, such a love embraces the good of the entire person and is therefore capable of endowing human expressions with a particular dignity and of ennobling them as special features and manifestations of married friendship. The Lord deigned to heal, perfect and raise this love by a special gift of grace and charity. Such love, bringing together the human and the divine, leads couples to a free and mutual self-giving shown in tender feelings and actions, and permeates the whole of their lives,[11] being itself also perfected and increased by its own generosity. Thus it is vastly more than mere eroticism which is selfishly stimulated and quickly and disappointingly vanishes.

This devoted love finds its unique expression and development in the behaviour which is proper to marriage. The acts by which married couples are intimately and chastely united are honourable and respectable, and when they are carried out in a truly human way they express and encourage a mutual giving in which a couple gladly and gratefully enrich each other. This love sincerely confirmed by mutual fidelity, and made especially sacrosanct by the sacrament of Christ, is indissolubly faithful physically and mentally in prosperity and adversity, and is therefore far removed from all adultery and divorce. The unity of matrimony confirmed by the Lord is also clearly apparent in the equal personal dignity of the wife and the husband which is recognizable in mutual and full love. Outstanding virtue, however, is needed to fulfil the duties of this christian vocation with constancy. This is why married couples, strengthened by grace for a holy life, will perseveringly practise, and gain through prayer, endurance in love, generosity of heart and a spirit of sacrifice.

Real marital love will be thought of more highly and held in public esteem if christian married couples are noted for the witness of faithfulness and harmony in their love and for their concern to bring up their children, and if they contribute to the cultural, psychological and social renewal which is required for marriage and the family. Young people should be instructed suitably and in good time on the dignity, duty and details of married love, especially within the family, so that they may acquire the practice of chastity and at a suitable age can make the transition through honourable engagement to marriage.

50. (*The fruitfulness of marriage*). Of their nature marriage and married love are directed towards the begetting and bringing up of children. Children are the supreme gift of a marriage and they contribute greatly to the good of their parents. God who said "it is not good that the man should be alone" (Gn 2, 18) and who "from the beginning made them male and female" (Mt 19, 4), wished to give them a special share in the divine work of creation and blessed the man and woman, saying, "be fruitful and multiply" (Gn 1, 28). Thus the true practice of marital love and the whole dimension of family life which results from it, without prejudice to the other purposes of marriage, point towards married couples being courageously prepared to cooperate with the love of the creator and saviour who is daily increasing and enriching his family through them.

In the office of transmitting and bringing up human life, which should be considered their special mission, married couples know that they are cooperators with the love of God the creator and in a sense its interpreters. They will accordingly discharge their task with human and christian responsibility, and will reach a right decision for themselves in humble reverence for God and by shared counsel and endeavour, with an eye to their own good and that of their children, whether those already born or those foreseen, discerning the material and spiritual conditions of the times and of their conditions of life, and bearing in mind the good of the family community, of human society and of the church. Ultimately married couples ought to make this decision themselves before God. In reaching it, however, christian couples should be aware that they cannot just do as they please, but ought always to be ruled by a conscience in conformity with the divine law, and be attentive to the church's teaching authority which officially interprets that law in the light of the gospel. That divine law shows the full meaning of marital love, it protects it and encourages it toward its truly human perfection. Thus christian couples who trust in divine providence and practise a spirit of sacrifice[12] are glorifying their creator and advancing towards perfection in Christ when they discharge their office of procreating with generous, human and christian responsibility. Among the couples who fulfil the task given them by God in this way, special recognition should be accorded those who prudently and jointly decide with open hearts to have a large family which they will bring up in a suitable manner.[13]

Marriage, however, was not instituted just for procreation; the very nature of an unbreakable covenant between persons and the good of the offspring also demand that the mutual love of the partners should be rightly expressed and should develop and mature. And therefore even if children, often longed for, are not forthcoming, marriage remains as a sharing and communion for the whole of life and retains its goodness and indissolubility.

51. (*Reconciling married love with respect for human life*). The council is aware that in living their married life harmoniously, couples can often be restricted by modern living conditions and find themselves in circumstances in which the number of their children cannot be increased, at least for a time, and the constant expression of love and the full sharing of life are maintained only with difficulty. When the intimacy of married life is broken off, the value of fidelity can frequently be at risk and the value of children can be undermined; and then the bringing up of the children and the readiness to have further children are endangered.

Some people take it upon themselves to solve these difficulties by dishonourable solutions, and do not even shrink from killing. But the church reiterates that there cannot be a true contradiction between the divine laws of transmitting life and of promoting genuine married love.

For God, the lord of life, has entrusted to women and men the outstanding service of watching over life and of fulfilling this in a manner worthy of human beings. Therefore from the time of conception life is to be safeguarded with the greatest of care; abortion and infanticide are abominable crimes. The sexual nature of man and woman and the human faculty of reproduction are wonderfully superior to what is possessed in the lower stages of life; consequently those acts which are proper to married life and directed in accordance with true human dignity are to be treated with great respect. When there is, therefore, a question of reconciling marital love with the responsible transmission of life, the moral character of the behaviour does not depend simply on good intention and evaluation of motives, but ought to be determined by objective criteria, derived from the nature of the person and its acts, which take account of the whole meaning of mutual giving and human procreation in the context of true love; and this cannot be achieved if the virtue of marital chastity is not sincerely practised. It is not permitted to daughters and sons of the church who rely on these principles to take steps for regulating procreation which are rejected by the teaching authority in its explanation of the divine law.[14]

All should be aware that the life of human beings, and the office of transmitting that life, cannot be restricted just to this world or be measured and understood by the criterion, but always look to the eternal destiny of humanity.

52. (*Promoting marriage and the family as the concern of all*). The family is a school for a richer humanity. For it to find fulfilment in its life and mission, it needs openness and collaboration on the part of husband and wife and their committed cooperation in raising their children. The involvement of the father can contribute greatly to their formation, and the care of the mother in the home which younger children especially need must be safeguarded, without prejudice to the legitimate advancement of woman in society. Children should be educated in such a way that on reaching adulthood they can exercise full responsibility in following their calling, including a sacred vocation, and in choosing a state of life in which, if they marry, they can found their own family under suitable moral, social and economic conditions. It is for parents or educators to act as guides to young people establishing a family, by their prudent advice which should be willingly listened to, while taking care not to drive them directly or indirectly into marriage or the choice of a partner.

In this way the family, where different generations meet and help each other to increase in wisdom and to reconcile the rights of persons with other requirements of social life, constitutes the basis of society. Therefore all who have influence in communities and social bodies ought to contribute effectively to encouraging marriage and the family. Public authority should consider it its sacred duty to recognise, protect and advance the true nature of marriage and the family, to safeguard public morality and to promote family prosperity. The right of parents to have children and to bring them up in the home should be protected. Legal provision and other initiatives should also protect and provide suitable assistance for those who unfortunately do not have the benefit of a family.

The faithful, redeeming the present time[15] and distinguishing between eternal verities and their changeable expressions, should constantly further the values of marriage and the family, both by the witness of their own lives and by acting in concert with others of good will, and in this way they will overcome difficulties and provide the family with the supports and helps which are suited to our changing times. To this end the christian sense of the faithful, the correct moral conscience of people, and the wisdom and expertise of those who are versed in the sacred disciplines, will be of great help.

Those who are learned in the sciences, especially in the biological, medical, social and psychological fields, can be of considerable service to the good of marriage and the family, and to peace of conscience, if they collaborate in trying to throw more light on the various conditions which favour the virtuous control of procreation.

It is for priests, duly informed in family matters, to foster the vocation of married couples in their married and family life by various pastoral means—preaching God's word, the liturgy, and other spiritual helps—and to strengthen them gently and patiently in their difficulties, and to encourage them in love to produce families which are truly shining examples.

Various bodies, especially family associations, should take steps by their teaching and action to encourage young people and couples, especially those recently married, and to prepare them for family, social and apostolic life.

Married couples themselves, made in the image of the living God and established with the true status of persons, should be united in equal regard, similarity of mind and mutual holiness[16] so that, following Christ the beginning of life[17] in the joys and sacrifices of their vocation, they may become through their faithful love witnesses to that mystery of devoted love which the Lord in his death and resurrection revealed to the world.[18]

Notes

1. See Augustine, *De bono coniugali* (*The good of marriage*), PL 40, 375–376 and 394; Thomas Aquinas, *Summa Theol.* (*Summa of Theology*), Supplementary question 49, art. 3, to 1; *Decree for the Armenians*: D 702 (1327); Pius XI, Encyclical *Casti Connubii*: AAS 22 (1930), pp. 543–555; D 2227–2238 (3703–3714).

2. See Pius XI, Encyclical *Casti Connubii*: AAS 22 (1930), pp. 546–547; D 2231 (3706).

3. See Hos 2; Jer 3, 6–13; Ez 16 and 23; Is 54.

4. See Mt 9, 15; Mk 2, 19–20; Lk 5, 34–35; Jn 3, 29; 2 Cor 11, 2; Eph 5, 27; Ap 19, 7–8; 21, 2 and 9.

5. See Eph 5, 25.

6. See Vatican council II, Dogmatic constitution on the church, *Lumen Gentium*: AAS 57 (1965), pp. 15–16, 40–41, 47.

7. See Pius XI, Encyclical *Casti Connubii*: AAS 22 (1930), p. 583.

8. See 1 Tm 5, 3.

9. See Eph 5, 32.

10. See Gn 2, 22–24; Pro 5, 18–20; 31, 10–31; Tb 8, 4–8; Sg 1, 1–3; 2, 16; 4, 16–5, 1; 7, 8–11; 1 Cor 7, 3–6, Eph 5, 25–33.

11. See Pius XI, Encyclical *Casti Connubii*: AAS 22 (1930), pp. 574–548; D 2232 (3707).

12. See 1 Cor 7, 5.

13. See Pius XII, Allocution *Tra le visite*, 20 Jan. 1958: AAS 50 (1958), p. 91.

14. See Pius XI, Encyclical *Casti Connubii*: AAS 22 (1930), pp. 559–561; D 3716–3718; Pius XII, Allocution to the Congress of the Italian Union of Obstetricians, 29 Oct. 1951: AAS 43 (1951), pp. 835–854; Paul VI, Allocution to their Eminences, 23 June 1964: AAS 56 (1964), pp. 581–589. Some questions requiring further and closer investigation have been remitted by command of the supreme pontiff of the commission for the study of population, the family and birth, so that when it completes its task the supreme pontiff can

deliver a judgment. This being the position of the teaching of the magisterium, the council is not aiming immediately to propose specific solutions.

15. See Eph 5, 16; Col 4, 5.
16. See *Gregorian Sacramentary*: PL 78, 262.
17. See Rm 5, 15 and 18; 6, 5–11; Gal 2, 20.
18. See Eph 5, 25–27.

13

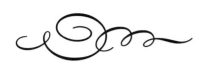

Familiaris Consortio (On the Family)

Pope John Paul II

PART TWO: THE PLAN OF GOD FOR MARRIAGE AND FAMILY

11. Man, the image of the God who is love

God created man in his own image and likeness:[1] calling him to existence through love, he called him at the same time for love.

God is love[2] and in himself he lives a mystery of personal loving communion. Creating the human race in his own image and continually keeping it in being, God inscribed in the humanity of man and woman the vocation, and thus the capacity and responsibility, of love and communion.[3] Love is therefore the fundamental and innate vocation of every human being.

As an incarnate spirit, that is, a soul which expresses itself in a body and a body informed by an immortal spirit, man is called to love in his unified totality. Love includes the human body, and the body is made a sharer in spiritual love.

Christian revelation recognizes two specific ways of realizing the vocation of the human person, in its entirety, to love: marriage and virginity or celibacy. Either one is in its own proper form an actuation of the most profound truth of man, of his being "created in the image of God."

Consequently sexuality, by means of which man and woman give themselves to one another through the acts which are proper and exclusive to spouses, is by no means something purely biological, but concerns the innermost being of the human person as such. It is realized in a truly human way only if it is an integral part of the love by which a man and a woman commit themselves totally to one another until death. The total physical self-giving would be a lie if it were not the sign and fruit of a total personal self-giving, in which the whole person, including the temporal dimension, is present: If the person were to withhold something or reserve the possibility of deciding otherwise in the future, by this very fact he or she would not be giving totally.

This totality which is required by conjugal love also corresponds to the demands of responsible fertility. This fertility is directed to the generation of a human being, and so by its nature it surpasses the purely biological order and involves a whole series of personal values. For the harmonious growth of these values a persevering and unified contribution by both parents is necessary.

The only "place" in which this self-giving in its whole truth is made possible is marriage, the covenant of conjugal love freely and consciously chosen, whereby man and woman accept the intimate community of life and love willed by God himself,[4] which only in this light manifests its true meaning. The institution of marriage is not an undue interference by society or authority, nor the extrinsic imposition of a interference by society or authority, nor the extrinsic imposition of a form. Rather, it is an interior requirement of the covenant of conjugal love which is publicly affirmed as unique and exclusive in order to live in complete fidelity to the plan of God, the creator. A person's freedom, far from being restricted by this fidelity, is secured against every form of subjectivism or relativism and is made a sharer in creative wisdom.

12. Marriage and communion between God and people

The communion of love between God and people, a fundamental part of the revelation and faith experience of Israel, finds a meaningful expression in the marriage covenant which is established between a man and a woman.

For this reason the central word of revelation, "God loves his people," is likewise proclaimed through the living and concrete word whereby a man and a woman express their conjugal love. Their bond of love becomes the image and the symbol of the covenant which unites God and his people.[5] And the same sin which can harm the conjugal covenant becomes an image of the infidelity of the people to their God: Idolatry is prostitution,[6] infidelity is adultery, disobedience to the law is abandonment of the spousal love of the Lord. But the infidelity of Israel does not destroy the eternal fidelity of the Lord, and therefore the ever faithful love of God is put forward as the model of the relations of faithful love which should exist between spouses.[7]

13. Jesus Christ, bridegroom of the Church, and the sacrament of matrimony

The communion between God and his people finds its definitive fulfillment in Jesus Christ, the bridegroom who loves and gives himself as the savior of humanity, uniting it to himself as his body.

He reveals the original truth of marriage, the truth of the "beginning,"[8] and, freeing man from his hardness of heart, he makes man capable of realizing this truth in its entirety.

This revelation reaches its definitive fullness in the gift of love which the word of God makes to humanity in assuming a human nature, and in the sacrifice which Jesus Christ makes of himself on the cross for his bride, the church. In this sacrifice there is entirely revealed that plan which God has imprinted on the humanity of man and woman since their creation,[9] the marriage of baptized persons thus becomes a real symbol of that new and eternal covenant sanctioned in the blood of Christ. The Spirit which the Lord puts forth gives a new heart, and renders man and woman capable of loving one another as Christ has loved us. Conjugal love reaches that fullness to which it is interiorly ordained, conjugal charity, which is the proper and specific way in which the spouses participate in and are called to live the very charity of Christ, who gave himself on the cross.

In a deservedly famous page, Tertullian has well expressed the greatness of this conjugal life in Christ and its beauty: "How can I ever express the happiness of the marriage that is joined together by the church, strengthened by an offering, sealed by a blessing, announced by angels and ratified by the Father?!!! How wonderful the bond between two believers, with a single hope, a single desire, a single observance, a single service! They are both brethren and both fellow servants; there is no separation between them in spirit or flesh. In fact they are truly two in one flesh, and where the flesh is one, one is the spirit."[10]

Receiving and meditating faithfully on the word of God, the church has solemnly taught and continued to teach that the marriage of the baptized is one of the seven sacraments of the new covenant.[11]

Indeed by means of baptism, man and woman are definitively placed within the new and eternal covenant, in the spousal covenant of Christ with the church. And it is because of this indestructible insertion that the intimate community of conjugal life and love, founded by the creator,[12] is elevated and assumed into the spousal charity of Christ, sustained and enriched by his redeeming power.

By virtue of the sacramentality of their marriage, spouses are bound to one another in the most profoundly indissoluble manner. Their belonging to each other is the real representation, by means of the sacramental sign, of the very relationship of Christ with the church.

Spouses are therefore the permanent reminder to the church of what happened on the cross; they are for one another and for the children witnesses to the salvation in which the sacrament makes them sharers. Of this salvation event marriage, like every sacrament, is a memorial, actuation and prophecy:

"As a memorial, the sacrament gives them the grace and duty of commemorating the great works of God and of bearing witness to them before their children. As actuation, it gives them the grace and duty of putting into practice in the present, toward each other and their children, the demands of a love which forgives and redeems. As prophecy, it gives them the grace and duty of living and bearing witness to the hope of the future encounter with Christ."[13]

Like each of the seven sacraments, so also marriage is a real symbol of the event of salvation, but in its own way.

"The spouses participate in it as spouses, together, as a couple, so that the first and immediate effect of marriage (*res et sacramentum*) is not supernatural grace itself, but the Christian conjugal bond, a typically Christian communion of two persons because it represents the mystery of Christ's incarnation and the mystery of his covenant. The content of participation in Christ's life is also specific: Conjugal love involves a totality, in which all the elements of the person enter—appeal of the body and instinct, power of feeling and affectivity, aspiration of the spirit and of will. It aims at a deeply personal unity, the unity that, beyond union in one flesh, leads to forming one heart and soul; it demands indissolubility and faithfulness in definitive mutual giving; and it is open to fertility (cf. *Humanae Vitae*, 9). In a word, it is a question of the normal characteristic of all natural conjugal love, but with a new significance which not only purifies and strengthens them, but raises them to the extent of making them the expression of specifically Christian values."[14]

14. *Children, the precious gift of marriage*

According to the plan of God, marriage is the foundation of the wider community of the family, since the very institution of marriage and conjugal love is ordained to the procreation and education of children, in whom it finds its crowning.[15]

In its most profound reality, love is essentially a gift; and conjugal love, while leading the spouses to the reciprocal "knowledge" which makes them "one flesh,"[16] does not end with the couple, because it makes them capable of the greatest possible gift, the gift by which they becomes cooperators with God for giving life to a new human person. Thus the couple, while giving themselves to one another, give not just themselves but also the reality of children, who are a living reflection of their love, a permanent sign of conjugal unity and a living and inseparable synthesis of their being a father and a mother.

When they become parents, spouses receive from God the gift of a new responsibility. Their parental love is called to become for the children the visible sign of the very love of God, "from whom every family in heaven and on earth is named."[17]

It must not be forgotten however that, even when procreation is not possible, conjugal life does not for this reason lose its value. Physical sterility in fact, can be for spouses the occasion for other important services to the life of the human person, for example, adoption, various forms of educational work, and assistance to other families and to poor or handicapped children.

15. *The Family, a communion of persons*

In matrimony and in the family a complex of interpersonal relationships is set up—married life, fatherhood and motherhood, filiation and fraternity—through which each human person is introduced into the "human family" and into the "family of God," which is the church.

Christian marriage and the Christian family build up the church: for in the family the human person is not only brought into being and progressively introduced by means of education into the human community, but by means of the rebirth of baptism and education in the faith the child is also introduced into God's family, which is the church.

The human family, disunited by sin, is reconstituted in its unity by the redemptive power of the death and resurrection of Christ.[18] Christian marriage, by participating in the salvific efficacy of this event, constitutes the natural setting in which the human person is introduced into the great family of the church.

The commandment to grow and multiply, given to man and woman in the beginning, in this way reaches its whole truth and full realization.

The church thus finds in the family, born from the sacrament, the cradle and the setting in which she can enter the human generations and where these in their turn can enter the church.

16. *Marriage and virginity or celibacy*

Virginity or celibacy for the sake of the kingdom of God not only does not contradict the dignity of marriage but presupposes it and confirms it. Marriage and virginity or celibacy are two ways of expressing and living the one mystery of the covenant of God with his people. When marriage is not esteemed, neither can consecrated virginity or celibacy exist; when human sexuality is not regarded as a great value given by the creator, the renunciation of it for the sake of the kingdom of heaven loses its meaning.

Rightly indeed does St. John Chrysostom say:

"Whoever denigrates marriage also diminishes the glory of virginity. Whoever praises it makes virginity more admirable and resplendent. What appears good only in comparison with evil would not be particularly good. It is something better than what is admitted to be good that is the most excellent good."[19]

In virginity or celibacy, the human being is awaiting, also in a bodily way, the eschatological marriage of Christ with the church, giving himself or herself completely to the church in the hope that Christ may give himself to the church in the full truth of eternal life. The celibate person thus anticipates in his or her flesh the new world of the future resurrection.[20]

By virtue of this witness, virginity or celibacy keeps alive in the church a consciousness of the mystery of marriage and defends it from any reduction and impoverishment.

Virginity or celibacy, by liberating the human heart in a unique way,[21] "so as to make it burn with greater love for God and all humanity,"[22] bears witness that the kingdom of God and his justice is that pearl of great price which is preferred to every other value no matter how great, and hence must be sought as the only definitive value. It is for this reason that the church throughout her history has always defended the superiority of this charism to that of marriage, by reason of the wholly singular link which it has with the kingdom of God.[23]

In spite of having renounced physical fecundity, the celibate person becomes spiritually fruitful, the father and mother of many, cooperating in the realization of the family according to God's plan.

Christian couples therefore have the right to expect from celibate persons a good example and a witness of fidelity to their vocation until death. Just as fidelity at times becomes difficult for married people and requires sacrifice, mortification and self-denial, the same can happen to celibate persons, and their fidelity, even in the trials that may occur, should strengthen the fidelity of married couples.[24]

These reflections on virginity or celibacy can enlighten and help those who, for reasons independent of their own will, have been unable to marry and have then accepted their situation in a spirit of service.

Part Three: The Role of the Christian Family

17. Family, become what you are

The family finds in the plan of God the creator and redeemer not only its identity, what it is, but also its mission, what it can and should do. The role that God calls the family to perform in history derives from what the family is; its role represents the dynamic and existential development of what it is. Each family finds within itself a summons that cannot be ignored and that specifies both its dignity and its responsibility: Family, become what you are.

Accordingly, the family must go back to the "beginning" of God's creative act if it is to attain self-knowledge and self-realization in accordance with the inner truth not only of what it is, but also of what it does in history. And since in God's plan it has been established as an "intimate community of life and love,"[25] the family has the mission to become more and more what it is, that is to say, a community of life and love in an effort that will find fulfillment, as will everything created and redeemed, in the kingdom of God. Looking at it in such a way as to reach its very roots, we must say that the essence and role of the family are in the final analysis specified by love. Hence the family has the mission to guard, reveal and communicate love, and this is a living reflection of and a real sharing in God's love for humanity and the love of Christ the Lord for the church, his bride.

Every particular task of the family is an expression and concrete actuation of that fundamental mission. We must therefore go deeper into the unique riches of the family's mission and probe its contents, which are both manifold and unified.

Thus, with love as its point of departure and making constant reference to it, the recent synod emphasized four general tasks for the family:

I. Forming a community of persons;
II. Serving life;
III. Participating in the development of society;
IV. Sharing in the life and mission of the church.

I. Forming a Community of Persons

18. Love as the principle and power of communion

The family, which is founded and given life by love, is a community of persons: of husband and wife, of parents and children, of relatives. Its first task is to live with fidelity the reality of communion in a constant effort to develop an authentic community of persons.

The inner principle of that task, its permanent power and its final goal, is love: Without love the family is not a community of persons and, in the same way, without love the family cannot live, grow and perfect itself as a community of persons. What I wrote in the encyclical *Redemptor Hominis* applies primarily and especially within the family as such: "Man cannot live without love. He remains a being that is incomprehensible for himself, his life is senseless, if love is not revealed to him, if he does not encounter love, if he does not experience it and make it his own, if he does not participate intimately in it."[26]

The love between husband and wife and, in a derivatory and broader way, the love between members of the same family—between parents and children, brothers and sisters and relatives and members of the household—is given life and sustenance by an unceasing inner dynamism leading the family to ever deeper and more intense communion, which is the foundation and soul of the community of marriage and the family.

19. The indivisible unity of conjugal communion

The first communion is the one which is established and which develops between husband and wife: By virtue of the covenant of married life, the man and woman "are no longer two but one flesh"[27] and they are called to grow continually in their communion through day-to-day fidelity to their marriage promise of total mutual self-giving.

This conjugal communion sinks its roots in the natural complementarity that exists between man and woman and is nurtured through the personal willingness of the spouses to share their entire life project, what they have and what they are: For this reason such communion is the fruit and the sign of a profoundly human need. But in the Lord Christ God takes up this human need, confirms it, purifies it and elevates it, leading it to perfection through the sacrament of matrimony: the Holy Spirit who is poured out in the sacramental celebration offers Christian couples the gift of a new communion of love that is the living and real image of that unique unity which makes of the church the indivisible mystical body of the Lord Jesus.

The gift of the spirit is a commandment of life for Christian spouses and at the same time a stimulating impulse so that every day they may progress toward an ever richer union with each other on all levels—of the body, of the character, of the heart, of the intelligence and will, of the soul[28]—revealing in this way to the church and to the world the new communion of love, given by the grace of Christ.

Such a communion is radically contradicted by polygamy: This, in fact, directly negates the plan of God which was revealed from the beginning, because it is contrary to the equal personal dignity of men and women, who in matrimony give themselves with a love that is total and therefore unique and exclusive. As the Second Vatican Council writes: "Firmly established by the Lord, the unity of marriage will radiate from the equal personal dignity of husband and wife, a dignity acknowledged by mutual and total love."[29]

20. An indissoluble communion

Conjugal communion is characterized not only by its unity, but also by its indissolubility: "As a mutual gift of two persons, this intimate union, as well as the good of children, imposes total fidelity on the spouses and argues for an unbreakable oneness between them."[30]

It is a fundamental duty of the church to reaffirm strongly, as the synod fathers did, the doctrine of the indissolubility of marriage. To all those who in our times consider it too difficult or indeed impossible to be bound to one person for the whole of life, and to those caught up in a culture that rejects the indissolubility of marriage and openly mocks the commitment of spouses to fidelity, it is necessary to reconfirm the good news of the definitive nature of that conjugal love that has in Christ its foundation and strength.[31]

Being rooted in the personal and total self-giving of the couple and being required by the good of the children, the indissolubility of marriage finds its ultimate truth in the plan that God has manifested in his revelation: He wills and he communicates the indissolubility of marriage as a fruit, a sign and a requirement of the absolutely faithful love that God has for man and that the Lord Jesus has for the church.

Christ renews the first plan that the creator inscribed in the hearts of man and woman, and in the celebration of the sacrament of matrimony offers "a new heart": thus the couples are not only able to overcome "hardness of heart,"[32] but also, and above all, they are able to share the full and definitive love of Christ, the new and eternal covenant made flesh. Just as the Lord Jesus is the "faithful witness,"[33] the "yes" of the promises of God[34] and thus the supreme realization of the unconditional faithfulness with which God loves his people, so Christian couples are called to participate truly in the irrevocable indissolubility that binds Christ to the church, his bride, loved by him to the end.[35]

The gift of the sacrament is at the same time a vocation and commandment for the Christian spouses, that they may remain faithful to each other forever, beyond every trial and difficulty, in generous obedience to the holy will of the Lord: "What therefore God has joined together, let not man put asunder."[36]

To bear witness to the inestimable value of the indissolubility and fidelity of marriage is one of the most precious and most urgent tasks of Christian couples in our time. So, with all my brothers who participated in the Synod of Bishops, I praise and encourage those numerous couples who, though encountering no small difficulty, preserve and develop the value of indissolubility: Thus in a humble and courageous manner they perform the role committed to them of being in the world a "sign"—a small and precious sign, sometimes also subjected to temptation, but always renewed—of the unfailing fidelity with which God and Jesus Christ love each and every human being. But it is also proper to recognize the value of the witness of those spouses who, even when abandoned by their partner, with the strength of faith and of Christian hope have not entered a new union: These spouses too give an authentic witness to fidelity, of which the world today has a great need. For this reason they must be encouraged and helped by the pastors and the faithful of the church.

21. The broader communion of the family

Conjugal communion constitutes the foundation on which is built the broader communion of the family, of parents and children, of brothers and sisters with each other, of relatives and other members of the household.

This communion is rooted in the natural bonds of flesh and blood and grows to its specifically human perfection with the establishment and maturing of the still deeper and richer bonds of the spirit: The love that animates the interpersonal relationships of the different members of the family constitutes the interior strength that shapes and animates the family communion and community.

The Christian family is also called to experience a new and original communion which confirms and perfects natural and human communion. In fact the grace of Jesus Christ, "the firstborn among many brethren,"[37] is by its nature and interior dynamism "a grace of brotherhood," as St. Thomas Aquinas calls it.[38] The Holy Spirit, who is poured forth in the celebration of the sacraments, is the living source and inexhaustible sustenance of the supernatural communion that gathers believers and links them with Christ and with each other in the unity of the church of God. The Christian family constitutes a specific revelation and realization of ecclesial communion, and for this reason too it can and should be called "the domestic church."[39]

All members of the family, each according to his or her own gift, have the grace and responsibility of building day by day the communion of persons, making the family "a school of deeper humanity":[40] This happens where there is care and love for the little ones, the sick, the aged; where there is mutual service every day; when there is a sharing of goods, of joys and of sorrows.

A fundamental opportunity for building such a communion is constituted by the educational exchange between parents and children,[41] in which each gives and receives. By means of love, respect and obedience toward their parents, children offer their specific and irreplaceable contribution to the construction of an authentically human and Christian family.[42] They will be aided in this if parents exercise their unrenounceable authority as a true and proper "ministry," that is, as a service to the human and Christian well-being of their children and in particular as a service aimed at helping them acquire a truly responsible freedom, and if parents maintain a living awareness of the "gift" they continually receive from their children.

Family communion can only be preserved and perfected through a great spirit of sacrifice. It requires, in fact, a ready and generous openness of each and all to understanding, to forbearance, to pardon, to reconciliation. There is no family that does not know how selfishness, discord, tension and conflict violently attack and at times mortally wound its own communion: Hence there arise the many and varied forms of division in family life. But, at the same time, every family is called by the God of peace to have the joyous and renewing experience of "reconciliation," that is, communion re-established, unity restored. In particular, participation in the sacrament of reconciliation and in the banquet of the one body of Christ offers to the Christian family the grace and the responsibility of overcoming every division and of moving toward the fullness of communion willed by God, responding in this way to the ardent desire of the Lord: "that they may be one."[43]

22. *The rights and role of women*

In that it is, and ought always to become, a communion and community of persons, the family finds in love the source and the constant impetus for welcoming, respecting and promoting each one of its members in his or her lofty dignity as a person, that is, as a living image of God. As the synod fathers rightly stated, the moral criterion for the authenticity of conjugal and family relationships consists in fostering the dignity and vocation of the individual persons, who achieve their fullness by sincere self-giving.[44]

In this perspective the synod devoted special attention to women, to their rights and role within the family and society. In the same perspective are also to be considered men as husbands and fathers, and likewise children and the elderly.

Above all it is important to underline the equal dignity and responsibility of women with men. This equality is realized in a unique manner in the reciprocal self-giving by each one to the other and by both to the children which is proper to marriage and the family. What human reason intuitively perceives and acknowledges is fully revealed by the word of God: The history of salvation, in fact, is a continuous and luminous testimony to the dignity of women.

In creating the human race "male and female,"[45] God gives man and woman an equal personal dignity, endowing them with the inalienable rights and responsibilities proper to the human person. God then manifests the dignity of women in the highest form possible, by assuming human flesh from the Virgin Mary, whom the church honors as the mother of God, calling her the new Eve and presenting her as the model of redeemed woman. The sensitive respect of Jesus toward the women that he called to his following and his friendship, his appearing on Easter morning to a woman before the other disciples, the mission entrusted to women to carry the good news of the resurrection to the apostles—these are all signs that confirm the special esteem of the Lord Jesus for women. The apostle Paul will say: "In Christ Jesus you are all children of God through faith . . . There is neither slave nor free, there is neither male nor female; for you are all one in Christ Jesus."⁴⁶

23. Women and society

Without intending to deal with all the various aspects of the vast and complex theme of the relationships between women and society and limiting these remarks to a few essential points, one cannot but observe that in the specific area of family life a widespread social and cultural tradition has considered women's role to be exclusively that of wife and mother, without adequate access to public functions, which have generally been reserved for men.

There is no doubt that the equal dignity and responsibility of men and women fully justifies women's access to public functions. On the other hand the true advancement of women requires that clear recognition be given to the value of their maternal and family role, by comparison with all other public roles and all other professions. Furthermore, these roles and professions should be harmoniously combined if we wish the evolution of society and culture to be truly and fully human.

This will come about more easily if, in accordance with the wishes expressed by the synod, a renewed "theology of work" can shed light upon and study in depth the meaning of work in the Christian life and determine the fundamental bond between work and the family, and therefore the original and irreplaceable meaning of work in the home be recognized and respected by all in its irreplaceable value.⁴⁷

This is of particular importance in education: For possible discrimination between the different types of work and professions is eliminated at its very root once it is clear that all people in every area are working with equal rights and equal responsibilities. The image of God in man and in woman will thus be seen with added luster.

While it must be recognized that women have the same right as men to perform various public functions, society must be structured in such a way that wives and mothers are not in practice compelled to work outside the home, and that their families can live and prosper in a dignified way even when they themselves devote their full time to their own family.

Furthermore, the mentality which honors women more for their work outside the home than for their work within the family must be overcome. This requires that men should truly esteem and love women with total respect for their personal dignity, and that society should create and develop conditions favoring work in the home.

With due respect to the different vocations of men and women, the church must in her own life promote as far as possible their equality of rights and dignity: and this for the good of all, the family, the church and society.

But clearly all of this does not mean for women a renunciation of their femininity or an imitation of the male role, but the fullness of true feminine humanity which should be expressed in their activity, whether in the family or outside of it, without disregarding the differences of customs and cultures in this sphere.

24. Offenses against women's dignity

Unfortunately the Christian message about the dignity of women is contradicted by that persistent mentality which considers the human being not as a person but as a thing, as an object of trade, at the service of selfish interest and mere pleasure: The first victims of this mentality are women.

This mentality produces very bitter fruits, such as contempt for men and women, slavery, oppression of the weak, pornography, prostitution—especially in an organized form—and all those various forms of discrimination that exist in the fields of education, employment, wages, etc.

Besides, many forms of degrading discrimination still persist today in a great part of our society that affect and seriously harm particular categories of women, as for example childless wives, widows, separated or divorced women, and unmarried mothers.

The synod fathers deplored these and other forms of discrimination as strongly as possible. I therefore ask that vigorous and incisive pastoral action be taken by all to overcome them definitively so that the image of God that shines in all human beings without exception may be fully respected.

25. Men as husbands and fathers

Within the conjugal and family communion-community, the man is called upon to live his gift and role as husband and father.

In his wife he sees the fulfillment of God's intention: "It is not good that the man should be alone; I will make him a helper fit for him,"[48] and he makes his own the cry of Adam, the first husband: "This at last is bone of my bones and flesh of my flesh."[49]

Authentic conjugal love presupposes and requires that a man have a profound respect for the equal dignity of his wife: "You are not her master," writes St. Ambrose, "but her husband; she was not given to you to be your slave, but your wife.... Reciprocate her attentiveness to you and be grateful to her for her love."[50] With his wife a man should live "a very special form of personal friendship."[51] As for the Christian, he is called upon to develop a new attitude of love, manifesting toward his wife a charity that is both gentle and strong like that which Christ has for the church.[52]

Love for his wife as mother of their children and love for the children themselves are for the man the natural way of understanding and fulfilling his own fatherhood. Above all where social and cultural conditions so easily encourage a father to be less concerned with his family or at any rate less involved in the work of education, efforts must be made to restore socially the conviction that the place and task of the father in and for the family is of unique and irreplaceable importance.[53] As experience teaches, the absence of a father causes psychological and moral imbalance and notable difficulties in family relationships, as does, in contrary circumstances, the oppressive presence of a father, especially where there still prevails the phenomenon of "machismo," or a wrong superiority of male prerogatives which humiliates women and inhibits the development of healthy family relationships.

In revealing and in reliving on earth the very fatherhood of God,[54] a man is called upon to ensure the harmonious and united development of all the members of the family: He will perform this task by exercising generous responsibility for the life conceived under the heart of the mother, by a more solicitous commitment to education, a task he shares with his wife,[55] by work which is never a cause of division in the family but promotes its unity and stability, and by means of the witness he gives of an adult Christian life which effectively introduces the children into the living experience of Christ and the church.

26. The rights of children

In the family, which is a community of persons, special attention must be devoted to the children by developing a profound esteem for their personal dignity and a great respect and generous concern for their rights. This is true for every child, but it becomes all the more urgent the smaller the child is and the more it is in need of everything, when it is sick, suffering or handicapped.

By fostering and exercising a tender and strong concern for every child that comes into this world, the church fulfills a fundamental mission: for she is called upon to reveal and put forward anew in history the example and the commandment of Christ the Lord, who placed the child at the heart of the kingdom of God: "Let the children come to me, and do not hinder them, for to such belongs the kingdom of heaven."[56]

I repeat once again what I said to the General Assembly of the United Nations Oct. 2, 1979:

"I wish to express the joy that we find in children, the springtime of life, the anticipation of the future history of each of our present earthly homelands. No country on earth, no political system can think of its own future otherwise than through the image of these new generations that will receive from their parents the manifold heritage of values, duties and aspirations of the nation to which they belong and of the whole human family. Concern for the child, even before birth, from the first moment of conception and then throughout the years of infancy and youth, is the primary and fundamental test of the relationship of one human being to another. And so, what better wish can I express for every nation and for the whole of mankind, and for all the children of the world than a better future in which respect for human rights will become a complete reality throughout the third millennium, which is drawing near."[57]

Acceptance, love, esteem, many-sided and united material, emotional, educational and spiritual concern for every child that comes into this world should always constitute a distinctive, essential characteristic of all Christians, in particular of the Christian family: Thus children, while they are able to grow "in wisdom and in stature, and in favor with God and man,"[58] offer their own precious contribution to building up the family community and even to the sanctification of their parents.[59]

27. The elderly in the family

There are cultures which manifest a unique veneration and great love for the elderly: Far from being outcasts from the family or merely tolerated as a useless burden, they continue to be present and to take an active and responsible part in family life, though having to respect the autonomy of the new family, above all they carry out the important mission of being a witness to the past and a source of wisdom for the young and for the future.

Other cultures, however, especially in the wake of disordered industrial and urban development, have both in the past and in the present set the elderly aside in unacceptable ways. This causes acute suffering to them and spiritually impoverishes many families.

The pastoral activity of the church must help everyone to discover and to make good use of the role of the elderly within the civil and ecclesial community, in particular within the family. In fact, "the life of the aging helps to clarify a scale of human values; it shows the continuity of generations and marvelously demonstrates the interdependence of God's people. The elderly often have the charism to bridge generation gaps before they are made: How many children have found understanding and love in the eyes and words and caresses of the aging! And how many old people have willingly subscribed to the inspired word that the 'crown of the aged is their children's children' (Prv. 17:6)!"[60]

II. Serving Life

A. The Transmission of Life

28. Cooperators in the love of God the creator

With the creation of man and woman in his own image and likeness, God crowns and brings to perfection the work of his hands: He calls them to a special sharing in his love and in his power as creator and Father through their free and responsible cooperation in transmitting the gift of human life: "God blessed them, and God said to them, 'be fruitful and multiply, and fill the earth and subdue it.'"[61]

Thus the fundamental task of the family is to serve life, to actualize in history the original blessing of the creator—that of transmitting by procreation the divine image from person to person.[62]

Fecundity is the fruit and the sign of conjugal love, the living testimony of the full reciprocal self-giving of the spouses: "While not making the other purposes of matrimony of less account, the true practice of conjugal love, and the whole meaning of the family life which results from it, have this aim: that the couple be ready with stout hearts to cooperate with the love of the creator and the savior, who through them will enlarge and enrich his own family day by day."[63]

However, the fruitfulness of conjugal love is not restricted solely to the procreation of children, even understood in its specifically human dimension: It is enlarged and enriched by all those fruits of moral, spiritual and supernatural life which the father and mother are called to hand on to their children, and through the children to the church and to the world.

29. The church's teaching and norm, always old yet always new

Precisely because the love of husband and wife is a unique participation in the mystery of life and of the love of God himself, the church knows that she has received the special mission of guarding and protecting the lofty dignity of marriage and the most serious responsibility of the transmission of human life.

Thus, in continuity with the living tradition of the ecclesial community throughout history, the recent Second Vatican Council and the magisterium of my predecessor Paul VI, expressed above all in the encyclical *Humanae Vitae,* have handed on to our times a truly prophetic proclamation, which reaffirms and reproposes with clarity the church's teaching and norm, always old yet always new, regarding marriage and regarding the transmission of human life.

For this reason the synod fathers made the following declaration at their last assembly:

"This sacred synod, gathered together with the successor of Peter in the unity of faith, firmly holds what has been set forth in the Second Vatican Council (cf. *Gaudium et Spes,* 50) and afterward in the encyclical *Humanae Vitae,* particularly that love between husband and wife must be fully human, exclusive and open to new life (*Humanae Vitae,* 11: cf. 9, 12)."[64]

30. The church stands for life

The teaching of the church in our day is placed in a social and cultural context which renders it more difficult to understand and yet more urgent and irreplaceable for promoting the true good of men and women.

Scientific and technological progress, which contemporary man is continually expanding in his dominion over nature, not only offers the hope of creating a new and better humanity, but also causes ever greater anxiety regarding the future. Some ask themselves if it is a good thing to be alive or if it would be better never to have been born; they doubt therefore if it is right to bring others into life when perhaps they will curse their existence in a cruel world with unforeseeable terrors. Others consider themselves to be the only ones for whom the advantages of technology are intended and they exclude others by imposing on them contraceptives or even worse means. Still others imprisoned in a consumer mentality and whose sole concern is to bring about a continual growth of material goods, finish by ceasing to understand, and thus by refusing, the spiritual riches of a new human life. The ultimate reason for these mentalities is the absence in people's hearts of God, whose love alone is stronger than all the world's fears and can conquer them.

Thus an anti-life mentality is born, as can be seen in many current issues: One thinks, for example of a certain panic deriving from the studies of ecologists and futurologists on population growth, which sometimes exaggerate the danger of demographic increase to the quality of life.

But the church firmly believes that human life, even if weak and suffering, is always a splendid gift of God's goodness. Against the pessimism and selfishness which cast a shadow over the world, the church stands for life: In each human life she sees the splendor of that "yes," that "amen," who is Christ himself.[65] To the "no" which assails and afflicts the world, she replies with this living "yes," thus defending the human person and the world from all who plot against and harm life.

The church is called upon to manifest anew to everyone, with clear and stronger conviction, her will to promote human life by every means and to defend it against all attacks in whatever condition or state of development it is found.

Thus the church condemns as a grave offense against human dignity and justice all those activities of governments and other public authorities which attempt to limit in any way the freedom of couples in deciding about children. Consequently any violence applied by such authorities in favor of contraception or, still worse, of sterilization and procured abortion must be altogether condemned and forcefully rejected. Likewise to be denounced as gravely unjust are cases where in international relations economic help given for the advancement of peoples is made conditional on programs of contraception, sterilization and procured abortion.[66]

31. *That God's design may be ever more completely fulfilled*

The church is certainly aware of the many complex problems which couples in many countries face today in their task of transmitting life in a responsible way. She also recognizes the serious problem of population growth in the form it has taken in many parts of the world and its moral implications.

However, she holds that consideration in depth of all the aspects of these problems offers a new and stronger confirmation of the importance of the authentic teaching of birth regulation reproposed in the Second Vatican Council and in the encyclical *Humanae Vitae*.

For this reason, together with the synod fathers I feel it is my duty to extend a pressing invitation to theologians, asking them to unite their efforts in order to collaborate with the hierarchical magisterium and to commit themselves to the task of illustrating ever more clearly the biblical foundations, the ethical grounds and the personalistic reasons behind this doctrine. Thus it will be possible, in the context of an organic exposition, to render the teaching of the church on this fundamental question truly accessible to all people of good will, fostering a daily more enlightened and profound understanding of it. In this way God's plan will be ever more completely fulfilled for the salvation of humanity and for the glory of the Creator.

A united effort by theologians in this regard, inspired by a convinced adherence to the magisterium, which is the one authentic guide for the people of God, is particularly urgent for reasons that include the close link between Catholic teaching on this matter and the view of the human person that the church proposes: Doubt or error in the field of marriage or the family involves obscuring to a serious extent the integral truth about the human person in a cultural situation that is already so often confused and contradictory. In fulfillment of their specific role theologians are called upon to provide enlightenment and a deeper understanding, and their contribution is of incomparable value and represents a unique and highly meritorious service to the family and humanity.

32. In an integral vision of the human person and of his or her vocation

In the context of a culture which seriously distorts or entirely misinterprets the true meaning of human sexuality because it separates it from its essential reference to the person, the church more urgently feels how irreplaceable is her mission of presenting sexuality as a value and task of the whole person, created male and female in the image of God.

In this perspective the Second Vatican Council clearly affirmed that "when there is a question of harmonizing conjugal love with the responsible transmission of life, the moral aspect of any procedure does not depend solely on sincere intentions or on an evaluation of motives. It must be determined by objective standards. These, based on the nature of the human person and his or her acts, preserve the full sense of mutual self-giving and human procreation in the context of true love. Such a goal cannot be achieved unless the virtue of conjugal chastity is sincerely practiced."[67]

It is precisely by moving from "an integral vision of man and of his vocation, not only his natural and earthly, but also his supernatural and eternal vocation,"[68] that Paul VI affirmed that the teaching of the church "is founded upon the inseparable connection willed by God and unable to be broken by man on his own initiative between the two meanings of the conjugal act: the unitive meaning and the procreative meaning."[69] And he concluded by re-emphasizing that there must be excluded as intrinsically immoral "every action which, either in anticipation of the conjugal act, or in its accomplishment, or in the development of its natural consequences, proposes, whether as an end or as a means, to render procreation impossible."[70]

When couples, by means of recourse to contraception, separate these two meanings that God the creator has inscribed in the being of man and woman and in the dynamism of their sexual communion, they act as "arbiters" of the divine plan and they "manipulate" and degrade human sexuality and with it themselves and their married partner by altering its value of "total" self-giving. Thus the innate language that expresses the total reciprocal self-giving of husband and wife is overlaid, through contraception, by an objectively contradictory language, namely, that of not giving oneself totally to the other. This leads not only to a positive refusal to be open to life, but also to a falsification of the inner truth of conjugal love, which is called upon to give itself in personal totality.

When, instead, by means of recourse to periods of infertility, the couple respect the inseparable connection between the unitive and procreative meanings of human sexuality, they are acting as "ministers" of God's plan and they "benefit from" their sexuality according to the original dynamism of "total" self-giving, without manipulation or alteration.[71]

In the light of the experience of many couples and of the data provided by the different human sciences, theological reflection is able to perceive and is called to study further the difference, both anthropological and moral, between contraception and recourse to the rhythm of the cycle: It is a difference which is much wider and deeper than is usually thought, one which involves in the final analysis two irreconcilable concepts of the human person and of human sexuality. The choice of the natural rhythms involves accepting the cycle of the person, that is, the woman, and thereby accepting dialogue, reciprocal respect, shared responsibility and self-control. To accept the cycle and to enter into dialogue means to recognize both the spiritual and corporal character of conjugal communion and to live personal love with its requirement of fidelity. In this context the couple comes to experience how conjugal communion is enriched with those values of tenderness and affection which constitute the inner soul of human sexuality in its physical dimension also. In this way sexuality is respected and promoted in its truly and fully human dimension and is never "used" as an "object" that, by breaking the personal unity of soul and body, strikes at God's creation itself at the level of the deepest interaction of nature and person.

33. The church as teacher and mother for couples in difficulty

In the field of conjugal morality the church is teacher and mother and acts as such.

As teacher, she never tires of proclaiming the moral norm that must guide the responsible transmission of life. The church is in no way the author or the arbiter of this norm. In obedience to the truth which is Christ, whose image is reflected in the nature and dignity of the human person, the church interprets the moral norm and proposes it to all people of good will without concealing its demands of radicalness and perfection.

As mother, the church is close to the many married couples who find themselves in difficulty over this important point of the moral life: She knows well their situation, which is often very arduous and at times truly tormented by difficulties of every kind, not only individual difficulties but social ones as well; she knows that many couples encounter difficulties not only in the concrete fulfillment of the moral norm but even in understanding its inherent values.

But it is one and the same church that is both teacher and mother. And so the church never ceases to exhort and encourage all to resolve whatever conjugal difficulties may arise without ever falsifying or compromising the truth: She is convinced that there can be no true contradiction between the divine law on transmitting life and that on fostering authentic married love.[72] Accordingly, the concrete pedagogy of the church must always remain linked with her doctrine and never be separated from it. With the same conviction as my predecessor, I therefore repeat: "To diminish in no way the saving teaching of Christ constitutes an eminent form of charity for souls."[73]

On the other hand, authentic ecclesial pedagogy displays its realism and wisdom only by making a tenacious and courageous effort to create and uphold all the human conditions—psychological, moral and spiritual—indispensable for understanding and living the moral value and norm.

There is no doubt that these conditions must include persistence and patience, humility and strength of mind, filial trust in God and in his grace, and frequent recourse to prayer and to the sacraments of the eucharist and of reconciliation.[74] Thus strengthened, Christian husbands and wives will be able to keep alive their awareness of the unique influence that the grace of the sacrament of marriage has on every aspect of married life including, therefore, their sexuality: The gift of the Spirit, accepted and responded to by husband and wife, help them to live their human sexuality in accordance with God's plan and as a sign of the unitive and fruitful love of Christ for his church.

But the necessary conditions also include knowledge of the bodily aspect and the body's rhythms of fertility. Accordingly, every effort must be made to render such knowledge accessible to all married people and also to young adults before marriage through clear, timely and serious instruction and education given by married couples, doctors and experts. Knowledge must then lead to education in self-control: Hence the absolute necessity for the virtue of chastity and for permanent education in it. In the Christian view, chastity by no means signifies rejection of human sexuality or lack of esteem for it: Rather it signifies spiritual energy capable of defending love from the perils of selfishness and aggressiveness, and able to advance it toward its full realization.

With deeply wise and loving intuition, Paul VI was only voicing the experience of many married couples when he wrote in his encyclical: "To dominate instinct by means of one's reason and free will undoubtedly requires ascetical practices, so that the affective manifestations of conjugal life may observe the correct order, in particular with regard to the observance of periodic continence. Yet this discipline which is proper to the purity of married couples, far from harming conjugal love, rather confers on it a higher human value. It demands continual effort, yet thanks to its beneficent influence husband and wife fully develop their personalities, being enriched with spiritual values. Such discipline bestows upon family life fruits of serenity and peace, and facilitates the solution of other problems; it favors attention for one's partner, helps both parties to drive out selfishness, the enemy of true love, and deepens their sense of responsibility. By its means, parents acquire the capacity of having a deeper and more efficacious influence on the education of their offspring."[75]

34. The moral progress of married people

It is always very important to have a right notion of the moral order, its values and its norms; and the importance is all the greater when the difficulties in the way of respecting them become more numerous and serious.

Since the moral order reveals and sets forth the plan of God the creator, for this very reason it cannot be something that harms man, something impersonal. On the contrary, by responding to the deepest demands of the human being created by God, it places itself at the service of that person's full humanity with the delicate and binding love whereby God himself inspires, sustains and guides every creature toward its happiness.

But man, who has been called to live God's wise and loving design in a responsible manner, is an historical being who day by day builds himself up through his many free decisions; and so he knows, loves and accomplishes moral good by stages of growth.

Married people too are called upon to progress unceasingly in their moral life with the support of a sincere and active desire to gain ever better knowledge of the values enshrined in and fostered by the law of God. They must also be supported by an upright and generous willingness to embody these values in their concrete decisions. They cannot, however, look on the law as merely an ideal to be achieved in the future: They must consider it as a command of Christ the Lord to overcome difficulties with constancy. "And so what is known as 'the law of gradualness' or step-by-step advance cannot be identified with 'gradualness of the law,' as if there were different degrees or forms of precept in God's law for different individuals and situations. In God's plan, all husbands and wives are called in marriage to holiness, and this lofty vocation is fulfilled to the extent that the human person is able to respond to God's command with serene confidence in God's grace and in his or her own will."[76] On the same lines, it is part of the church's pedagogy that husbands and wives should first of all recognize clearly the teaching of *Humanae Vitae* as indicating the norm for the exercise of their sexuality, and that they should endeavor to establish the conditions necessary for observing that norm. As the synod noted, this pedagogy embraces the whole of married life. Accordingly, the function of transmitting life must be integrated into the overall mission of Christian life as a whole which, without the cross, cannot reach the resurrection. In such a context it is understandable that sacrifice cannot be removed from family life, but must in fact be wholeheartedly accepted if the love between husband and wife is to be deepened and become a source of intimate joy.

This shared progress demands reflection, instruction and suitable education on the part of the priests, religious and lay people engaged in family pastoral work: they will all be able to assist married people in their human and spiritual progress, a progress that demands awareness of sin, a sincere commitment to observe the moral law and the ministry of reconciliation. It must also be kept in mind that conjugal intimacy involves the wills of two persons, who are thereby called to harmonize their mentality and behavior, requiring much patience, understanding and time. Uniquely important in this field is unity of moral and pastoral judgment by priests—a unity that must be carefully sought and ensured in order that the faithful may not have to suffer anxiety of conscience.[77]

It will be easier for married people to make progress if, with respect for the church's teaching and with trust in the grace of Christ, and with the help and support of the pastors of souls and the entire ecclesial community, they are able to discover and experience the liberating and inspiring value of the authentic love that is offered by the Gospel and set before us by the Lord's commandment.

35. Instilling conviction and offering practical help

With regard to the question of lawful birth regulation, the ecclesial community at the present time must take on the task of instilling conviction and offering practical help to those who wish to live out their parenthood in a truly responsible way.

In this matter, while the church notes with satisfaction the results achieved by scientific research aimed at a more precise knowledge of the rhythms of women's fertility, and while it encourages a more decisive and wide-ranging extension of that research, it cannot fail to call with renewed vigor on the responsibility of all—doctors, experts, marriage counselors, teachers and married couples—who can actually help married people to live their love with respect for the structure and finalities of the conjugal act which expresses that love. This implies a broader, more decisive and more systematic effort to make the natural methods of regulating fertility known, respected and applied.[78]

A very valuable witness can and should be given by those husbands and wives who, through the joint exercise of periodic continence, have reached a more mature personal responsibility with regard to love and life. As Paul VI wrote: "To them the Lord entrusts the task of making visible to people the holiness and sweetness of the law which unites the mutual love of husband and wife with their cooperation with the love of God the author of human life."[79]

B. Education

36. The right and duty of parents regarding education

The task of giving education is rooted in the primary vocation of married couples to participate in God's creative activity: By begetting in love and for love a new person who has within himself or herself the vocation for growth and development, parents by that very fact take the task of helping that person effectively to live a fully human life. As the Second Vatican Council recalled, "Since parents have conferred life on their children, they have a most solemn obligation to educate their offspring. Hence, parents must be acknowledged as the first and foremost educators of their children. Their role as educators is so decisive that scarcely anything can compensate for their failure in it. For it devolves on parents to create a family atmosphere so animated with love and reverence for God and others that a well-rounded personal and social development will be fostered among the children. Hence, the family is the first school of those social virtues which every society needs."[80]

The right and duty of parents to give education is essential, since it is connected with the transmission of human life; it is original and primary with regard to the educational role of others on account of the uniqueness of the loving relationship between parents and children; and it is irreplaceable and inalienable and therefore incapable of being entirely delegated to others or usurped by others.

In addition to those characteristics, it cannot be forgotten that the most basic element, so basic that it qualifies the educational role of parents, is parental love, which finds fulfillment in the task of education as it completes and perfects its service of life. As well as being a source, the parents' love is also the animating principle and therefore the norm inspiring and guiding all concrete educational activity, enriching it with the values of kindness, constancy, goodness, service, disinterestedness and self-sacrifice that are the most precious fruit of love.

37. Educating in the essential values of human life

Even amid the difficulties of the work of education, difficulties which are often greater today, parents must trustingly and courageously train their children in the essential values of human life. Children must grow up with a correct attitude of freedom with regard to material goods, by adopting a simple and austere lifestyle and being fully convinced that "man is more precious for what he is than for what he has."[81]

In a society shaken and split by tensions and conflicts caused by the violent clash of various kinds of individualism and selfishness, children must be enriched not only with a sense of true justice, which alone leads to respect for the personal dignity of each individual, but also and more powerfully by a sense of true love, understood as sincere solicitude and disinterested service with regard to others, especially the poorest and those in most need. The family is the first and fundamental school of social living: As a community of love, it finds in self-giving the law that guides it and makes it grow. The self-giving that inspires the love of husband and wife for each other is the model and norm for the self-giving that must be practiced in the relationships between brothers and sisters and the different generations living together in the family. And the communion and sharing that are part of everyday life in the home at times of joy and at times of difficulty are the most concrete and effective pedagogy for the active, responsible and fruitful inclusion of the children in the wider horizon of society.

Education in love as self-giving is also the indispensable premise for parents called to give their children a clear and delicate sex education. Faced with a culture that largely reduces human sexuality to the level of something commonplace, since it interprets and lives it in a reductive and impoverished way by linking it solely with the body and with selfish pleasure, the educational service of parents must aim firmly at a training in the area of sex that is truly and fully personal: for sexuality is an enrichment of the whole person—body, emotions and soul—and it manifests its inmost meaning in leading the person to the gift of self in love.

Sex education, which is a basic right and duty of parents, must always be carried out under their attentive guidance whether at home or in educational centers chosen and controlled by them. In this regard, the church reaffirms the law of subsidiarity, which the school is bound to observe when it cooperates in sex education, by entering into the same spirit that animates the parents.

In this context education for chastity is absolutely essential, for it is a virtue that develops a person's authentic maturity and makes him or her capable of respecting and fostering the "nuptial meaning" of the body. Indeed Christian parents, discerning the signs of God's call, will devote special attention and care to education in virginity or celibacy as the supreme form of that self-giving that constitutes the very meaning of human sexuality.

In view of the close links between the sexual dimension of the person and his or her ethical values, education must bring the children to a knowledge of and respect for the moral norms as the necessary and highly valuable guarantee for responsible personal growth in human sexuality.

For this reason the church is firmly opposed to an often widespread form of imparting sex information dissociated from moral principles. That would merely be an introduction to the experience of pleasure and a stimulus leading to the loss of serenity—while still in the years of innocence—by opening the way to vice.

38. The mission to educate and the sacrament of marriage

For Christian parents the mission to educate, a mission rooted as we have said in their participation in God's creating activity, has a new specific source in the sacrament of marriage, which consecrates them for the strictly Christian education of their children: that is to say, it calls upon them to share in the very authority and love of God the Father and Christ the shepherd, and in the motherly love of the church, and it enriches them with wisdom, counsel, fortitude and all the other gifts of the Holy Spirit in order to help the children in their growth as human beings and as Christians.

The sacrament of marriage gives to the educational role the dignity and vocation of being really and truly a "ministry" of the church at the service of the building up of her members. So great and splendid is the educational ministry of Christian parents that St. Thomas has no hesitation in comparing it with the ministry of priests: "Some only propagate and guard spiritual life by a spiritual ministry: This is the role of the sacrament of orders, others do this for both corporal and spiritual life, and this is brought about by the sacrament of marriage, by which a man and a woman join in order to beget offspring and bring them up to worship God."[82]

A vivid and attentive awareness of the mission that they have received with the sacrament of marriage will help Christian parents to place themselves at the service of their children's education with great serenity and trustfulness, and also with a sense of responsibility before God, who calls them and gives them the mission of building up the church in their children. Thus in the case of baptized people, the family, called together by word and sacrament as the church of the home, is both teacher and mother, the same as the worldwide church.

39. First experience of the church

The mission to educate demands that Christian parents should present to their children all the topics that are necessary for the gradual maturing of their personality from a Christian and ecclesial point of view. They will therefore follow the educational lines mentioned above, taking care to show their children the depths of significance to which the faith and love of Jesus Christ can lead. Furthermore, their awareness that the Lord is entrusting to them the growth of a child of God, a brother or sister of Christ, a temple of the Holy Spirit, a member of the church, will support Christian parents in their task of strengthening the gift of divine grace in their children's souls.

The Second Vatican Council describes the content of Christian education as follows: "Such an education does not merely strive to foster maturity... in the human person. Rather, its principal aims are these: that as baptized persons are gradually introduced into a knowledge of the mystery of salvation, they may daily grow more conscious of the gift of faith which they have received; that they may learn to adore God the Father in spirit and in truth (cf. Jn. 4:23), especially through liturgical worship; that they may be trained to conduct their personal life in true righteousness and holiness, according to their new nature (Eph. 4:22–24), and thus grow to maturity, to the stature of the fullness of Christ (cf. Eph. 4:13), and devote themselves to the upbuilding of the mystical body. Moreover, aware of their calling, they should grow accustomed to giving witness to the hope that is in them (cf. 1 Pt. 3:15), and to promoting the Christian transformation of the world."[83]

The synod too, taking up and developing the indications of the council, presented the educational mission of the Christian family as a true ministry through which the Gospel is transmitted and radiated, so that family life itself becomes an itinerary of faith and in some way a Christian initiation and a school of following Christ. Within a family that is aware of this gift, as Paul VI wrote, "all the members evangelize and are evangelized."[84]

By virtue of their ministry of educating, parents are through the witness of their lives the first heralds of the Gospel for their children. Furthermore, by praying with their children, by reading the word of God with them and by introducing them deeply through Christian initiation into the body of Christ—both the eucharistic and the ecclesial body—they become fully parents, in that they are begetters not only of bodily life but also of the life that through the Spirit's renewal flows from the cross and resurrection of Christ.

In order that Christian parents may worthily carry out their ministry of education, the synod fathers expressed the hope that a suitable catechism for families would be prepared, one that would be clear, brief and easily assimilated by all. The episcopal conferences were warmly invited to contribute to producing this catechism.

40. Relations with other educating agents

The family is the primary but not the only and exclusive educating community. Man's community aspect itself—both civil and ecclesial—demands and leads to a broader and more articulated activity resulting from well-ordered collaboration between the various agents of education. All these agents are necessary, even though each can and should play its part in accordance with the special competence and contribution proper to itself.[85]

The educational role of the Christian family therefore has a very important place in organic pastoral work. This involves a new form of cooperation between parents and Christian communities and between the various educational groups and pastors. In this sense, the renewal of the Catholic school must give special attention both to the parents of the pupils and to the formation of a perfect educating community.

The right of parents to choose an education in conformity with their religious faith must be absolutely guaranteed.

The state and the church have the obligation to give families all possible aid to enable them to perform their educational role properly. Therefore both the church and the state must create and foster the institutions and activities that families justly demand, and the aid must be in proportion to the families' needs. However, those in society who are in charge of schools must never forget that the parents have been appointed by God himself as the first and principal educators of their children and that their right is completely inalienable.

But corresponding to their right, parents have a serious duty to commit themselves totally to a cordial and active relationship with the teachers and school authorities.

If ideologies opposed to the Christian faith are taught in the schools, the family must join with other families, if possible through family associations, and with all its strength and with wisdom help the young not to depart from the faith. In this case the family needs special assistance from pastors of souls, who must never forget that parents have the inviolable right to entrust their children to the ecclesial community.

41. Manifold service to life

Fruitful married love expresses itself in serving life in many ways. Of these ways, begetting and educating children are the most immediate, specific and irreplaceable. In fact, every act of true love toward a human being bears witness to and perfects the spiritual fecundity of the family, since it is an act of obedience to the deep inner dynamism of love as self-giving to others.

For everyone this perspective is full of value and commitment, and it can be an inspiration in particular for couples who experience physical sterility.

Christian families, recognizing with faith all human beings as children of the same heavenly Father, will respond generously to the children of other families, giving them support and love not as outsiders but as members of the one family of God's children. Christian parents will thus be able to spread their love beyond the bonds of flesh and blood, nourishing the links that are rooted in the spirit and that develop through concrete service to the children of other families, who are often without even the barest necessities.

Christian families will be able to show greater readiness to adopt and foster children who have lost their parents or have been abandoned by them. Rediscovering the warmth of affection of a family, these children will be able to experience God's loving and provident fatherhood witnessed to by Christian parents, and they will thus be able to grow up with serenity and confidence in life. At the same time the whole family will be enriched with the spiritual values of a wider fraternity.

Family fecundity must have an unceasing "creativity," a marvelous fruit of the Spirit of God, who opens the eyes of the heart to discover the new needs and sufferings of our society and gives courage for accepting them and responding to them. A vast field of activity lies open to families: Today even more preoccupying than child abandonment is the phenomenon of social and cultural exclusion, which seriously affects the elderly, the sick, the disabled, drug addicts, ex-prisoners, etc.

This broadens enormously the horizons of the parenthood of Christian families: These and many other urgent needs of our time are a challenge to their spiritually fruitful love. With families and through them, the Lord Jesus continues to "have compassion" on the multitudes.

III. Participating in the Development of Society

42. The family as the first and vital cell of society
"Since the Creator of all things has established the conjugal partnership as the beginning and basis of human society," the family is "the first and vital cell of society."[86]

The family has vital and organic links with society since it is its foundation and nourishes it continually through its role of service to life: It is from the family that citizens come to birth and it is within the family that they find the first school of the social virtues that are the animating principle of the existence and development of society itself.

Thus, far from being closed in on itself, the family is by nature and vocation open to other families and to society and undertakes its social role.

43. Family life as an experience of communion and sharing
The very experience of communion and sharing that should characterize the family's daily life represents its first and fundamental contribution to society.

The relationships between the members of the family community are inspired and guided by the law of "free giving." By respecting and fostering personal dignity in each and every one as the only basis for value, this free giving takes the form of heartfelt acceptance, encounter and dialogue, disinterested availability, generous service and deep solidarity.

Thus the fostering of authentic and mature communion between persons within the family is the first and irreplaceable school of social life, an example and stimulus for the broader community of relationships marked by respect, justice, dialogue and love.

The family is thus, as the synod fathers recalled, the place of origin and the most effective means for humanizing and personalizing society: It makes an original contribution in depth in building up the world, by making possible a life that is, properly speaking, human, in particular by guarding and transmitting virtues and "values." As the Second Vatican Council states, in the family "the various generations come together and help one another to grow wiser and to harmonize personal rights with the other requirements of social living."[87]

Consequently, faced with a society that is running the risk of becoming more and more depersonalized and standardized and therefore inhuman and dehumanizing, with the negative results of many forms of escapism—such as alcoholism, drugs and even terrorism—the family possesses and continues still to release formidable energies capable of taking man out of his anonymity, keeping him conscious of his personal dignity, enriching him with deep humanity and actively placing him, in his uniqueness and unrepeatability, within the fabric of society.

44. *The social and political role*

The social role of the family certainly cannot stop short at procreation and education even if this constitutes its primary and irreplaceable form of expression.

Families therefore, either singly or in association, can and should devote themselves to manifold social service activities, especially in favor of the poor or at any rate for the benefit of all people and situations that cannot be reached by the public authorities' welfare organization.

The social contribution of the family has an original character of its own, one that should be given greater recognition and more decisive encouragement, especially as the children grow up, and actually involving all its members as much as possible.[88]

In particular, note must be taken of the ever greater importance in our society of hospitality in all its forms, from opening the door of one's home, and still more of one's heart, to the pleas of one's brothers and sisters, to concrete efforts to ensure that every family has its own home as the natural environment that preserves it and makes it grow. In a special way the Christian family is called upon to listen to the apostle's recommendation. "Practice hospitality,"[89] and therefore, imitating Christ's example and sharing in his love, welcome the brother or sister in need: "Whoever gives to one of these little ones even a cup of cold water because he is a disciple, truly, I say to you, he shall not lose his reward."[90]

The social role of families is called upon to find expression also in the form of political intervention: Families should be the first to take steps to see that the laws and institutions of the state not only do not offend, but support and positively defend the rights and duties of the family. Along these lines families should grow in awareness of being "protagonists" of what is known as "family politics" and assume responsibility for transforming society; otherwise families will be the first victims of the evils that they have done no more than note with indifference. The Second Vatican Council's appeal to go beyond an individualistic ethic therefore also holds good for the family as such.[91]

45. *Society at the service of the family*

Just as the intimate connection between the family and society demands that the family be open to and participate in society and its development, so also it requires that society should never fail in its fundamental task of respecting and fostering the family.

The family and society have complementary functions in defending and fostering the good of each and every human being. But society—more specifically the state—must recognize that "the family is a society in its own original right,"[92] and so society is under a grave obligation in its relations with the family to adhere to the principle of subsidiarity. The public authorities should take care not to take from families the functions that they can just as well perform on their own or in free associations; instead it must positively favor and encourage as far as possible responsible initiative by families. In the conviction that the good of the family is an indispensable and essential value of the civil community, the public authorities must do everything possible to ensure that families have all those aids—economic, social, educational, political and cultural assistance—that they need in order to face all their responsibilities in a human way.

46. *The charter of family rights*

The ideal of mutual support and development between the family and society is often very seriously in conflict with the reality of their separation and even opposition.

In fact, as was repeatedly denounced by the synod, the situation experienced by many families in various countries is highly problematical if not entirely negative: Institutions and laws unjustly ignore the inviolable rights of the family and of the human person; and society, far from putting itself at the service of the family, attacks it violently in its values and fundamental requirements. Thus the family, which in God's plan is the basic cell of society and a subject of rights and duties before the state or any other community, finds itself the victim of society, of the delays and slowness with which it acts, and even of its blatant injustice.

For this reason the church openly and strongly defends the rights of the family against the intolerable usurpations of society and the state. In particular the synod fathers mentioned the following rights of the family:

—The right to exist and progress as a family, that is to say, the right of every human being, even if he or she is poor, to found a family and to have adequate means to support it;
—The right to exercise its responsibility regarding the transmission of life and to educate children;
—The right to the intimacy of conjugal and family life;
—The right to the stability of the bond and of the institution of marriage;
—The right to believe in and profess one's faith and to propagate it;
—The right to bring up children in accordance with the family's own traditions and religious and cultural values, with the necessary instruments, means and institutions;
—The right, especially of the poor and the sick, to obtain physical, social, political and economic security;
—The right to housing suitable for living family life in a proper way;
—The right to expression and to representation, either directly or through associations, before the economic, social and cultural public authorities and lower authorities;
—The right to form associations with other families and institutions in order to fulfill the family's role suitably and expeditiously;
—The right to protect minors by adequate institutions and legislation from harmful drugs, pornography, alcoholism, etc.;
—The right to wholesome recreation of a kind that also fosters family values;
—The right of the elderly to a worthy life and a worthy death;
—The right to emigrate as a family in search of a better life.[93]

Acceding to the synod's explicit request, the Holy See will give prompt attention to studying these suggestions in depth and to the preparation of a charter of rights of the family to be presented to the quarters and authorities concerned.

47. The Christian family's grace and responsibility

The social role that belongs to every family pertains by a new and original right to the Christian family, which is based on the sacrament of marriage. By taking up the human reality of the love between husband and wife in all its implications, the sacrament gives to Christian couples and parents a power and a commitment to live their vocation as lay people and therefore to "seek the kingdom of God by engaging in temporal affairs and by ordering them according to the plan of God."[94]

The social and political role is included in the kingly mission of service in which Christian couples share by virtue of the sacrament of marriage, and they receive both a command which they cannot ignore and a grace which sustains and stimulates them.

The Christian family is thus called upon to offer everyone a witness of generous and disinterested dedication to social matters through a "preferential option" for the poor and disadvantaged. Therefore, advancing in its following of the Lord by special love for all the poor, it must have special concern for the hungry, the poor, the old, the sick, drug victims and those who have no family.

48. For a new international order

In view of the worldwide dimension of various social questions nowadays, the family has seen its role with regard to the development of society extended in a completely new way: It now also involves cooperating for a new international order, since it is only in worldwide solidarity that the enormous and dramatic issues of world justice, the freedom of peoples and the peace of humanity can be dealt with and solved.

The spiritual communion between Christian families, rooted in a common faith and hope and given life by love, constitutes an inner energy that generates, spreads and develops justice, reconciliation, fraternity and peace among human beings. Insofar as it is a "small-scale church," the Christian family is called upon, like the "large-scale church," to be a sign of unity for the world and in this way to exercise its prophetic role by bearing witness to the kingdom and peace of Christ, toward which the whole world is journeying.

Christian families can do this through their educational activity—that is to say, by presenting to their children a model of life based on the values of truth, freedom, justice and love—both through active and responsible involvement in the authentically human growth of society and its institutions, and supporting in various ways the associations specifically devoted to international issues.

IV. Sharing in the Life and Mission of the Church

49. The family within the mystery of the church

Among the fundamental tasks of the Christian family is its ecclesial task: The family is placed at the service of the building up of the kingdom of God in history by participating in the life and mission of the church.

In order to understand better the foundations, the contents and the characteristics of this participation, we must examine the many profound bonds linking the church and the Christian family and establishing the family as a "church in miniature" (*ecclesia domestica*),[95] in such a way that in its own way the family is a living image and historical representation of the mystery of the church.

It is, above all, the church as mother that gives birth to, educates and builds up the Christian family by putting into effect in its regard the saving mission which she has received from her Lord. By proclaiming the word of God the church reveals to the Christian family its true identity, what it is and should be according to the Lord's plan; by celebrating the sacraments the church enriches and strengthens the Christian family with the grace of Christ for its sanctification to the glory of the Father; by the continuous proclamation of the new commandment of love the church encourages and guides the Christian family to the service of love so that it may imitate and relive the same self-giving and sacrificial love that the Lord Jesus has for the entire human race.

In turn, the Christian family is grafted into the mystery of the church to such a degree as to become a sharer, in its own way, in the saving mission proper to the church: By virtue of the sacrament Christian married couples and parents "in their state and way of life have their own special gift among the people of God."[96] For this reason they not only receive the love of Christ and become a saved community, but they are also called upon to communicate Christ's love to their brethren thus becoming a saving community. In this way, while the Christian family is a fruit and sign of the supernatural fecundity of the church, it stands also as a symbol, witness and participant of the church's motherhood.[97]

50. A specific and original ecclesial role
The Christian family is called upon to take part actively and responsibly in the mission of the church in a way that is original and specific by placing itself in what it is and what it does as an "intimate community of life and love" at the service of the church and of society.

Since the Christian family is a community in which the relationships are renewed by Christ through faith and the sacraments, the family's sharing in the church's mission should follow a community pattern: The spouses together as a couple, the parents and children as a family, must live their service to the church and to the world. They must be "of one heart and soul"[98] in faith, through the shared apostolic zeal that animates them and through their shared commitment to works of service in the ecclesial and civil communities.

The Christian family also builds up the kingdom of God in history through the everyday realities that concern and distinguish its state of life. It is thus in the love between husband and wife and between the members of the family—a love lived out in all its extraordinary richness of values and demands: totality, oneness, fidelity and fruitfulness[99]—that the Christian family's participation in the prophetic, priestly and kingly mission of Jesus Christ and of his church finds expression and realization. Therefore, love and life constitute the nucleus of the saving mission of the Christian family in the church and for the church.

The Second Vatican Council recalls this fact when it writes: "Families will share their spiritual riches generously with other families too. Thus the Christian family, which springs from marriage as a reflection of the loving covenant uniting Christ with the church, and as a participation in that covenant will manifest to all people the savior's living presence in the world, and the genuine nature of the church. This the family will do by the mutual love of the spouses, by their generous fruitfulness, their solidarity and faithfulness, and by the loving way in which all the members of the family work together."[100]

Having laid the foundation of the participation of the christian family in the church's mission, it is now time to illustrate its substance in reference to Jesus Christ as prophet, priest and king—three aspects of a single reality—by presenting the Christian family as 1) a believing and evangelizing community, 2) a community in dialogue with God, and 3) a community at the service of man.

A. The Christian family as a believing and evangelizing community

51. Faith as the discovery and admiring awareness of God's plan for the family
As a sharer in the life and mission of the church, which listens to the word of God with reverence and proclaims it confidently,[101] the Christian family fulfills its prophetic role by welcoming and announcing the word of God: It thus becomes more and more each day a believing and evangelizing community.

Christian spouses and parents are required to offer "the obedience of faith."[102] They are called upon to welcome the word of the Lord, which reveals to them the marvelous news—the good news—of their conjugal and family life sanctified and made a source of sanctity by Christ himself. Only in faith can they discover and admire with joyful gratitude the dignity to which God has deigned to raise marriage and the family, making them a sign and meeting place of the loving covenant between God and man, between Jesus Christ and his bride, the church.

The very preparation for Christian marriage is itself a journey of faith. It is a special opportunity for the engaged to rediscover and deepen the faith received in baptism and nourished by their Christian upbringing. In this way they come to recognize and freely accept their vocation to follow Christ and to serve the kingdom of God in the married state.

The celebration of the sacrament of marriage is the basic moment of the faith of the couple. This sacrament, in essence, is the proclamation in the church of the good news concerning married love. It is the word of God that "reveals" and "fulfills" the wise and loving plan of God for the married couple, giving them a mysterious and real share in the very love with which God himself loves humanity. Since the sacramental celebration of marriage is itself a proclamation of the word of God, it must also be a "profession of faith" within and with the church, as a community of believers, on the part of all those who in different ways participate in its celebration.

This profession of faith demands that it be prolonged in the life of the married couple and of the family. God, who called the couple to marriage, continues to call them in marriage.[103] In and through the events, problems, difficulties and circumstances of everyday life, God comes to them, revealing and presenting the concrete "demands" of their sharing in the love of Christ for his church in the particular family, social and ecclesial situation in which they find themselves.

The discovery of and obedience to the plan of God on the part of the conjugal and family community must take place in "togetherness," through the human experience of love between husband and wife, between parents and children, lived in the spirit of Christ.

Thus the little domestic church, like the greater church, needs to be constantly and intensely evangelized: hence its duty regarding permanent education in the faith.

52. The Christian family's ministry of evangelization

To the extent in which the Christian family accepts the Gospel and matures in faith, it becomes an evangelizing community. Let us listen again to Paul VI: "The family, like the church, ought to be a place where the Gospel is transmitted and from which the Gospel radiates. In a family which is conscious of this mission, all the members evangelize and are evangelized. The parents not only communicate the Gospel to their children, but from their children they can themselves receive the same Gospel as deeply lived by them. And such a family becomes the evangelizer of many other families and of the neighborhood of which it forms part."[104]

As the synod repeated, taking up the appeal which I launched at Puebla, the future of evangelization depends in great part on the church of the home.[105] This apostolic mission of the family is rooted in baptism and receives from the grace of the sacrament of marriage new strength to transmit the faith, to sanctify and transform our present society according to God's plan.

Particularly today the Christian family has a special vocation to witness to the paschal covenant of Christ by constantly radiating the joy of love and the certainty of the hope for which it must give account: "The Christian family loudly proclaims both the present virtues of the kingdom of God and the hope of a blessed life to come."[106]

The absolute need for family catechesis emerges with particular force in certain situations that the church unfortunately experiences in some places: "In places where anti-religious legislation endeavors even to prevent education in the faith, and in places where widespread unbelief or invasive secularism makes real religious growth practically impossible, 'the church of the home' remains the one place where children and young people can receive an authentic catechesis."[107]

53. Ecclesial service

The ministry of evangelization carried out by Christian parents is original and irreplaceable. It assumes the characteristics typical of family life itself, which should be interwoven with love, simplicity, practicality and daily witness.[108]

The family must educate the children for life in such a way that each one may fully perform his or her role according to the vocation received from God. Indeed the family that is open to transcendent values, that serves its brothers and sisters with joy, that fulfills its duties with generous fidelity and is aware of its daily sharing in the mystery of the glorious cross of Christ, becomes the primary and most excellent seed-bed of vocations to a life of consecration to the kingdom of God.

The parents' ministry of evangelization and catechesis ought to play a part in their children's lives also during adolescence and youth, when the children, as often happens, challenge or even reject the Christian faith received in earlier years. Just as in the church the work of evangelization can never be separated from the sufferings of the apostle, so in the Christian family parents must face with courage and great interior serenity the difficulties that their ministry of evangelization sometimes encounters in their own children.

It should not be forgotten that the service rendered by Christian spouses and parents to the Gospel is essentially an ecclesial service. It has its place within the context of the whole church as an evangelized and evangelizing community. Insofar as the ministry of evangelization and catechesis of the church of the home is rooted in and derives from the one mission of the church and is ordained to the upbuilding of the one body of Christ,[109] it must remain in intimate communion and collaborate responsibly with all the other evangelizing and catechetical activities present and at work in the ecclesial community at the diocesan and parochial levels.

54. To preach the Gospel to the whole creation

Evangelization, urged on within by irrepressible missionary zeal, is characterized by a universality without boundaries. It is the response to Christ's explicit and unequivocal command: "Go into all the world and preach the Gospel to the whole creation."[110]

The Christian family's faith and evangelizing mission also possesses this Catholic missionary inspiration. The sacrament of marriage takes up and reproposes the task of defending and spreading the faith, a task that has its roots in baptism and confirmation,[111] and makes Christian married couples and parents witnesses of Christ "to the end of the earth,"[112] missionaries, in the true and proper sense, of love and life.

A form of missionary activity can be exercised even within the family. This happens when some member of the family does not have the faith or does not practice it with consistency. In such a case the other members must give him or her a living witness of their own faith in order to encourage and support him or her along the path toward full acceptance of Christ the savior.[113]

Animated in its own inner life by missionary zeal, the church of the home is also called to be a luminous sign of the presence of Christ and of his love for those who are "far away," for families who do not yet believe and for those Christian families who no longer live in accordance with the faith that they once received. The Christian family is called to enlighten "by its example and its witness those who seek the truth."[114]

Just as at the dawn of Christianity Aquila and Priscilla were presented as a missionary couple,[115] so today the church shows forth her perennial newness and fruitfulness by the presence of Christian couples and families who dedicate at least a part of their lives to working in missionary territories, proclaiming the Gospel and doing service to their fellow man in the love of Jesus Christ.

Christian families offer a special contribution to the missionary cause of the church by fostering missionary vocations among their sons and daughters[116] and, more generally, "by training their children from childhood to recognize God's love for all people."[117]

B. The Christian family as a community in dialogue with God

55. The church's sanctuary in the home

The proclamation of the Gospel and its acceptance in faith reach their fullness in the celebration of the sacraments. The church which is a believing and evangelizing community is also a priestly people invested with the dignity and sharing in the power of Christ the high priest of the new and eternal covenant.[118]

The Christian family too is part of this priestly people which is the church. By means of the sacrament of marriage, in which it is rooted and from which it draws its nourishment, the Christian family is continuously vivified by the Lord Jesus and called and engaged by him in a dialogue with God through the sacraments, through the offering of one's life and through prayer.

This is the priestly role which the Christian family can and ought to exercise in intimate communion with the whole church through the daily realities of married and family life. In this way the Christian family is called to be sanctified and to sanctify the ecclesial community and the world.

56. Marriage as a sacrament of mutual sanctification and an act of worship

The sacrament of marriage is the specific source and original means of sanctification for Christian married couples and families. It takes up again and makes specific the sanctifying grace of baptism. By virtue of the mystery of the death and resurrection of Christ, of which the spouses are made part in a new way by marriage, conjugal love is purified and made holy: "This love the Lord has judged worthy of special gifts, healing, perfecting and exalting gifts of grace and of charity."[119]

The gift of Jesus Christ is not exhausted in the actual celebration of the sacrament of marriage, but rather accompanies the married couple throughout their lives. This fact is explicitly recalled by the Second Vatican Council when it says that Jesus Christ "abides with them so that just as he loved the church and handed himself over on her behalf, the spouses may love each other with perpetual fidelity through mutual self-bestowal... For this reason, Christian spouses have a special sacrament by which they are fortified and receive a kind of consecration in the duties and dignity of their state. By virtue of this sacrament, as spouses fulfill their conjugal and family obligations they are penetrated with the spirit of Christ, who fills their whole lives with faith, hope and charity. Thus they increasingly advance toward their own perfection as well as their mutual sanctification, and hence contribute jointly to the glory of God."[120]

Christian spouses and parents are included in the universal call to sanctity. For them this call is specified by the sacrament they have celebrated and is carried out concretely in the realities proper to their conjugal and family life.[121] This gives rise to the grace and requirement of an authentic and profound conjugal and family spirituality that draws its inspiration from the themes of creation, covenant, cross, resurrection and sign, which were stressed more then once by the synod.

Christian marriage, like the other sacraments, "whose purpose is to sanctify people, to build up the body of Christ, and finally, to give worship to God,"[122] is in itself a liturgical action glorifying God in Jesus Christ and in the Church. By celebrating it, Christian spouses profess their gratitude to God for the sublime gift bestowed on them of being able to live in their married and family lives the very love of God for people and that of the Lord Jesus for the church, his bride.

Just as husbands and wives receive from the sacrament the gift and responsibility of translating into daily living the sanctification bestowed on them, so the same sacrament confers on them the grace and moral obligation of transforming their whole lives into a "spiritual sacrifice."[123] What the council says of the laity applies also to Christian spouses and parents, especially with regard to the earthly and temporal realities that characterize their lives: "As worshippers leading holy lives in every place, the laity consecrate the world itself to God."[124]

57. Marriage and the eucharist

The Christian family's sanctifying role is grounded in baptism and has its highest expression in the eucharist, to which Christian marriage is intimately connected. The Second Vatican Council drew attention to the unique relationship between the eucharist and marriage by requesting that "marriage normally be celebrated within the Mass."[125] To understand better and live more intensely the graces and responsibilities of Christian marriage and family life, it is altogether necessary to rediscover and strengthen this relationship.

The eucharist is the very source of Christian marriage. The eucharistic sacrifice in fact represents Christ's covenant of love with the church, sealed with his blood on the cross.[126] In this sacrifice of the new and eternal covenant, Christian spouses encounter the source from which their own marriage covenant flows, is interiorly structured and continuously renewed. As a representation of Christ's sacrifice of love for the church, the eucharist is a fountain of charity. In the eucharistic gift of charity the Christian family finds the foundation and soul of its "communion" and its "mission": By partaking in the eucharistic bread, the different members of the Christian family become one body, which reveals and shares in the wider unity of the church. Their sharing in the body of Christ that is "given up" and in his blood that is "shed" becomes a never-ending source of missionary and apostolic dynamism for the Christian family.

58. The sacrament of conversion and reconciliation

An essential and permanent part of the Christian family's sanctifying role consists in accepting the call to conversion that the Gospel addresses to all Christians, who do not always remain faithful to the "newness" of the baptism that constitutes them "saints." The Christian family too is sometimes unfaithful to the law of baptismal grace and holiness proclaimed anew in the sacrament of marriage.

Repentance and mutual pardon within the bosom of the Christian family, so much a part of daily life, receive their specific sacramental expression in Christian penance. In the encyclical *Humanae Vitae,* Paul VI wrote of married couples: "And if sin should still keep its hold over them, let them not be discouraged, but rather have recourse with humble perseverance to the mercy of God, which is abundantly poured forth in the sacrament of penance."[127]

The celebration of this sacrament acquires special significance for family life. While they discover in faith that sin contradicts not only the covenant with God, but also the covenant between husband and wife and the communion of the family, the married couple and the other members of the family are led to an encounter with God, who is "rich in mercy,"[128] who bestows on them his love which is more powerful than sin,[129] and who reconstructs and brings to perfection the marriage covenant and the family communion.

59. *Family prayer*

The church prays for the Christian family and educates the family to live in generous accord with the priestly gift and role received from Christ the high priest. In effect, the baptismal priesthood of the faithful exercised in the sacrament of marriage constitutes the basis of a priestly vocation and mission for the spouses and family by which their daily lives are transformed into "spiritual sacrifices acceptable to God through Jesus Christ."[130] This transformation is achieved not only by celebrating the eucharist and the other sacraments and through offering themselves to the glory of God, but also through a life of prayer, through prayerful dialogue with the Father, through Jesus Christ, in the Holy Spirit.

Family prayer has its own characteristic qualities. It is prayer offered in common, husband and wife together, parents and children together. Communion in prayer is both a consequence of and a requirement for the communion bestowed by the sacraments of baptism and matrimony. The words with which the Lord Jesus promises his presence can be applied to the members of the Christian family in a special way: "Again I say to you, if two of you agree on earth about anything they ask it will be done for them by my Father in heaven. For where two or three are gathered in my name, there am I in the midst of them."[131]

Family prayer has for its very own object family life itself, which in all its varying circumstances is seen as a call from God and lived as a filial response to his call. Joys and sorrows, hopes and disappointments, births and birthday celebrations, wedding anniversaries of the parents, departures, separations and homecomings, important and far-reaching decisions, the death of those who are dear, etc.—all of these mark God's loving intervention in the family's history. They should be seen as suitable moments for thanksgiving, for petition, for trusting abandonment of the family into the hands of their common Father in heaven. The dignity and responsibility of the Christian family as the domestic church can be achieved only with God's unceasing aid, which will surely be granted if it is humbly and trustingly petitioned in prayer.

60. *Educators in prayer*

By reason of their dignity and mission, Christian parents have the specific responsibility of educating their children in prayer, introducing them to gradual discovery of the mystery of God and to personal dialogue with him: "It is particularly in the Christian family, enriched by the grace and the office of the sacrament of matrimony, that from the earliest years children should be taught, according to the faith received in baptism, to have a knowledge of God, to worship him and to love their neighbor."[132]

The concrete example and living witness of parents is fundamental and irreplaceable in educating their children to pray. Only by praying together with their children can a father and mother—exercising their royal priesthood—penetrate the innermost depths of their children's hearts and leave an impression that the future events in their lives will not be able to efface.

Let us again listen to the appeal made by Paul VI to parents: "Mothers, do you teach your children the Christian prayers? Do you prepare them in conjunction with the priests, for the sacraments that they receive when they are young: confession, communion and confirmation? Do you encourage them when they are sick to think of Christ suffering, to invoke the aid of the Blessed Virgin and the saints? Do you say the family rosary together? And you, fathers, do you pray with your children, with the whole domestic community, at least sometimes? Your example of honesty in thought and action, joined to some common prayer, is a lesson for life, an act of worship of singular value. In this way you bring peace to your homes: *Pax huic domui*. Remember, it is thus that you build up the church."[133]

61. Liturgical prayer and private prayer

There exists a deep and vital bond between the prayer of the church and the prayer of the individual faithful as has been clearly reaffirmed by the Second Vatican Council.[134] An important purpose of the prayer of the domestic church is to serve as the natural introduction for the children to the liturgical prayer of the whole church, both in the sense of preparing for it and of extending it into personal, family and social life. Hence the need for gradual participation by all the members of the Christian family in the celebration of the eucharist, especially on Sundays and feast days, and of the other sacraments, particularly the sacraments of Christian initiation of the children. The directives of the council opened up a new possibility for the Christian family when it listed the family among those groups to whom it recommends the recitation of the Divine Office in common.[135] Likewise, the Christian family will strive to celebrate at home and in a way suited to the members the times and feasts of the liturgical year.

As preparation for the worship celebrated in church and as its prolongation in the home, the Christian family makes use of private prayer, which presents a great variety of forms. While this variety testifies to the extraordinary richness with which the spirit vivifies Christian prayer, it serves also to meet the various needs and life situations of those who turn to the Lord in prayer. Apart from morning and evening prayers, certain forms of prayer are to be expressly encouraged, following the indications of the synod fathers, such as reading and meditating on the word of God, preparation for the reception of the sacraments, devotion and consecration to the Sacred Heart of Jesus, the various forms of veneration of the Blessed Virgin Mary, grace before and after meals and observance of popular devotions.

While respecting the freedom of the children of God, the church has always proposed certain practices of piety to the faithful with particular solicitude and insistence. Among these should be mentioned the recitation of the rosary: "We now desire, as a continuation of the thought of our predecessors, to recommend strongly the recitation of the family rosary . . . There is no doubt that . . . the rosary should be considered as one of the best and most efficacious prayers in common that the Christian family is invited to recite. We like to think and sincerely hope that when the family gathering becomes a time of prayer the rosary is a frequent and favored manner of praying."[136] In this way authentic devotion to Mary, which finds expression in sincere love and generous imitation of the Blessed Virgin's interior spiritual attitude, constitutes a special instrument for nourishing loving communion in the family and for developing conjugal and family spirituality. For she who is the mother of Christ and of the church is in a special way the mother of Christian families, of domestic churches.

62. Prayer and life

It should never be forgotten that prayer constitutes an essential part of Christian life, understood in its fullness and centrality. Indeed, prayer is an important part of our very humanity: It is "the first expression of man's inner truth, the first condition for authentic freedom of spirit."[137]

Far from being a form of escapism from everyday commitments, prayer constitutes the strongest incentive for the Christian family to assume and comply fully with all its responsibilities as the primary and fundamental cell of human society. Thus the Christian family's actual participation in the church's life and mission is in direct proportion to the fidelity and intensity of the prayer with which it is united with the fruitful vine that is Christ the Lord.[138]

The fruitfulness of the Christian family in its specific service to human advancement, which of itself cannot but lead to the transformation of the world, derives from its living union with Christ, nourished by the liturgy, by self-oblation and by prayer.[139]

C. The Christian family as a community at the service of man

63. The new commandment of love

The church, a prophetic, priestly and kingly people, is endowed with the mission of bringing all human beings to accept the word of God in faith, to celebrate and profess it in the sacraments and in prayer, and to give expression to it in the concrete realities of life in accordance with the gift and new commandment of love.

The law of Christian life is to be found not in a written code, but in the personal action of the Holy Spirit who inspires and guides the Christian. It is the "law of the Spirit of life in Christ Jesus":[140] "God's love has been poured into our hearts through the Holy Spirit who has been given to us."[141]

This is true also for the Christian couple and family. Their guide and rule of life is the Spirit of Jesus poured into their hearts in the celebration of the sacrament of matrimony. In continuity with baptism in water and the Spirit, marriage sets forth anew the evangelical law of love, and with the gift of the Spirit engraves it more profoundly on the hearts of Christian husbands and wives. Their love, purified and saved, is a fruit of the Spirit acting in the hearts of believers and constituting, at the same time, the fundamental commandment of their moral life to be lived in responsible freedom.

Thus the Christian family is inspired and guided by the new law of the Spirit and, in intimate communion with the church, the kingly people, it is called to exercise its "service" of love toward God and toward its fellow human beings.

Just as Christ exercises his royal power by serving us,[142] so also the Christian finds the authentic meaning of his participation in the kingship of his Lord in sharing his spirit and practice of service to man. "Christ has communicated this power to his disciples that they might be established in royal freedom and that by self-denial and a holy life they might conquer the reign of sin in themselves (cf. Rom. 6:12). Further, he has shared this power so that by serving him in their fellow human beings they might through humility and patience lead their brothers and sisters to that King whom to serve is to reign. For the Lord wishes to spread his kingdom by means of the laity also, a kingdom of truth and life, a kingdom of holiness and grace, a kingdom of justice, love and peace. In this kingdom, creation itself will be delivered out of its slavery to corruption and into the freedom of the glory of the children of God (cf. Rom. 8:21)."[143]

64. To discover the image of God in each brother and sister

Inspired and sustained by the new commandment of love, the Christian family welcomes, respects and serves every human being, considering each one in his or her dignity as a person and as a child of God.

It should be so especially between husband and wife and within the family, through a daily effort to promote a truly personal community, initiated and fostered by an inner communion of love. This way of life should then be extended to the wider circle of the ecclesial community of which the Christian family is a part.

Thanks to love within the family, the church can and ought to take on a more homelike or family dimension, developing a more human and fraternal style of relationships.

Love, too, goes beyond our brothers and sisters of the same faith since "everybody is my brother or sister." In each individual, especially in the poor, the weak and those who suffer or are unjustly treated, love knows how to discover the face of Christ, and discover a fellow human being to be loved and served.

In order that the family may serve man in a truly evangelical way, the instructions of the Second Vatican Council must be carefully put into practice: "That the exercise of such charity may rise above any deficiencies in fact and even in appearance, certain fundamentals must be observed. Thus attention is to be paid to the image of God in which our neighbor has been created, and also to Christ the Lord to whom is really offered whatever is given to a needy person."[144]

While building up the church in love, the Christian family places itself at the service of the human person and the world, really bringing about the "human advancement" whose substance was given in summary form in the synod's message to families: "Another task for the family is to form persons in love and also to practice love in all its relationships, so that it does not live closed in on itself, but remains open to the community, moved by a sense of justice and concern for others, as well as by a consciousness of its responsibility toward the whole of society."[145]

Part Four: Pastoral Care of the Family

I. Stages of Pastoral Care of the Family

65. The church accompanies the Christian family on its journey through life
Like every other living reality, the family too is called upon to develop and grow. After the preparation of engagement and the sacramental celebration of marriage, the couple begin their daily journey toward the progressive actuation of the values and duties of marriage itself.

In the light of faith and by virtue of hope, the Christian family, too, shares in communion with the church and in the experience of the earthly pilgrimage toward the full revelation and manifestation of the kingdom of God.

Therefore, it must be emphasized once more that the pastoral intervention of the church in support of the family is a matter of urgency. Every effort should be made to strengthen and develop pastoral care for the family, which should be treated as a real matter of priority, in the certainty that future evangelization depends largely on the domestic church.[146]

The church's pastoral concern will not be limited only to the Christian families closest at hand; it will extend its horizons in harmony with the heart of Christ and will show itself to be even more lively for families in general and for those families in particular which are in difficult or irregular situations. For all of them the church will have a word of truth, goodness, understanding, hope and deep sympathy with their sometimes tragic difficulties. To all of them she will offer her disinterested help so that they can come closer to that model of a family which the creator intended from "the beginning" and which Christ has renewed with his redeeming grace.

The church's pastoral action must be progressive also in the sense that it must follow the family, accompanying it step by step in the different stages of its formation and development.

66. Preparation for marriage
More than ever necessary in our times is preparation of young people for marriage and family life. In some countries it is still the families themselves that, according to ancient customs, ensure the passing on to young people of the values concerning married and family life, and they do this through a gradual process of education or initiation. But the changes that have taken place within almost all modern societies demand that not only the family but also society and the church should be involved in the effort of properly preparing young people for their future responsibilities.

Many negative phenomena which are today noted with regret in family life derive from the fact that in the new situations young people not only lose sight of the correct hierarchy of values but, since they no longer have certain criteria of behavior, they do not know how to face and deal with the new difficulties. But experience teaches that young people who have been well prepared for family life generally succeed better than others.

This is even more applicable to Christian marriage, which influences the holiness of large numbers of men and women. The church must therefore promote better and more intensive programs of marriage preparation in order to eliminate as far as possible the difficulties that many married couples find themselves in, and even more in order to favor positively the establishing and maturing of successful marriages.

Marriage preparation has to be seen and put into practice as a gradual and continuous process. It includes three main stages: remote, proximate and immediate preparation.

Remote preparation begins in early childhood in that wise family training which leads children to discover themselves as beings endowed with a rich and complex psychology and with a particular personality with its own strengths and weaknesses. It is the period when esteem for the authentic human values is instilled, both in interpersonal and in social relationships, with all that this signifies for the formation of character, for the control and right use of one's inclinations, for the manner of regarding and meeting people of the opposite sex, and so on. Also necessary, especially for Christians, is solid spiritual and catechetical formation that will show that marriage is a true vocation and mission, without excluding the possibility of the total gift to self to God in the vocation to the priestly or religious life.

Upon this basis there will subsequently and gradually be built up the proximate preparation, which—from the suitable age and with adequate catechesis, as in a catechumenal process—involves a more specific preparation for the sacraments, as it were, a rediscovery of them. This renewed catechesis of young people and others preparing for Christian marriage is absolutely necessary in order that the sacrament may be celebrated and lived with the right moral and spiritual dispositions. The religious formation of young people should be integrated, at the right moment and in accordance with the various concrete requirements, with a preparation for life as a couple. This preparation will present marriage as an interpersonal relationship of a man and a woman that has to be continually developed, and it will encourage those concerned to study the nature of conjugal sexuality and responsible parenthood, with the essential medical and biological knowledge connected with it. It will also acquaint those concerned with correct methods for the education of children and will assist them in gaining the basic requisites for well-ordered family life, such as stable work, sufficient financial resources, sensible administration, notions of housekeeping.

Finally, one must not overlook preparation for the family apostolate, for fraternal solidarity and collaboration with other families, for active membership in groups, associations, movements and undertakings set up for the human and Christian benefit of the family.

The immediate preparation for the celebration of the sacrament of matrimony should take place in the months and weeks immediately preceding the wedding so as to give a new meaning, content and form to the so-called premarital inquiry required by canon law. This preparation is not only necessary in every case, but is also more urgently needed for engaged couples that still manifest shortcomings or difficulties in Christian doctrine and practice.

Among the elements to be instilled in this journey of faith, which is similar to the catechumenate, there must also be a deeper knowledge of the mystery of Christ and the church, of the meaning of grace and of the responsibility of Christian marriage, as well as preparation for taking an active and conscious part in the rites of the marriage liturgy.

The Christian family and the whole of the ecclesial community should feel involved in the different phases of the preparation for marriage which have been described only in their broad outlines. It is to be hoped that the episcopal conferences, just as they are concerned with appropriate initiatives to help engaged couples to be more aware of the seriousness of their choice and also to help pastors of souls to make sure of the couples' proper dispositions, so they will also take steps to see that there is issued a directory for the pastoral care of the family. In this they should lay down in the first place, the minimum content, duration and method of the "preparation courses," balancing the different aspects—doctrinal, pedagogical, legal and medical—concerning marriage and structuring them in such a way that those preparing for marriage will not only receive an intellectual training, but will also feel a desire to enter actively into the ecclesial community.

Although one must not underestimate the necessity and obligation of the immediate preparation for marriage—which would happen if dispensations from it were easily given—nevertheless such preparation must always be set forth and put into practice in such a way that omitting it is not an impediment to the celebration of marriage.

67. The celebration

Christian marriage normally requires a liturgical celebration expressing in social and community form the essentially ecclesial and sacramental nature of the conjugal covenant between baptized persons.

Inasmuch as it is a sacramental action of sanctification, the celebration of marriage—inserted into the liturgy, which is the summit of the church's action and the source of her sanctifying power[147]—must be *per se* valid, worthy and fruitful. This opens a wide field for pastoral solicitude, in order that the needs deriving from the nature of the conjugal covenant, elevated into a sacrament, may be fully met and also in order that the church's discipline regarding free consent, impediments, the canonical form and the actual rite of the celebration may be faithfully observed. The celebration should be simple and dignified, according to the norms of the competent authorities of the church. It is also for them—in accordance with concrete circumstances of time and place and in conformity with the norms issued by the Apostolic See[148]—to include in the liturgical celebration such elements proper to each culture which serve to express more clearly the profound human and religious significance of the marriage contract, provided that such elements contain nothing that is not in harmony with Christian faith and morality.

Inasmuch as it is a sign, the liturgical celebration should be conducted in such a way as to constitute, also in its external reality, a proclamation of the word of God and a profession of faith on the part of the community of believers, Pastoral commitment will be expressed here through the intelligent and careful preparation of the liturgy of the word and through the education to faith of those participating in the celebration and in the first place the couple being married.

Inasmuch as it is a sacramental action of the church, the liturgical celebration of marriage should involve the Christian community, with the full, active and responsible participation of all those present, according to the place and task of each individual: the bride and bridegroom, the priest, the witnesses, the relatives, the friends, the other members of the faithful, all of them members of an assembly that manifests and lives the mystery of Christ and His church. For the celebration of Christian marriage in the sphere of ancestral cultures or traditions, the principles laid down above should be followed.

68. Celebration of marriage and evangelization of non-believing baptized persons

Precisely because in the celebration of the sacrament very special attention must be devoted to the moral and spiritual dispositions of those being married, in particular to their faith, we must here deal with a not infrequent difficulty in which the pastors of the church can find themselves in the context of our secularized society.

In fact, the faith of the person asking the church for marriage can exist in different degrees, and it is the primary duty of pastors to bring about a rediscovery of this faith and to nourish it and bring it to maturity. But pastors must also understand the reasons that lead the church also to admit to the celebration of marriage those who are imperfectly disposed.

The sacrament of matrimony has this specific element that distinguishes it from all the other sacraments: It is the sacrament of something that was part of the very economy of creation; it is the very conjugal covenant instituted by the Creator "in the beginning." Therefore the decision of a man and a woman to marry in accordance with this divine plan, that is to say, the decision to commit by their irrevocable conjugal consent their whole lives in indissoluble love and unconditional fidelity, really involves, even if not in a fully conscious way, an attitude of profound obedience to the will of God, an attitude which cannot exist without God's grace. They have thus already begun what is in a true and proper sense a journey toward salvation, a journey which the celebration of the sacrament and the immediate preparation for it can complement and bring to completion, given the uprightness of their intention.

On the other hand it is true that in some places engaged couples ask to be married in church for motives which are social rather than genuinely religious. This is not surprising. Marriage, in fact, is not an event that concerns only the persons actually getting married. By its very nature it is also a social matter, committing the couple being married in the eyes of society. And its celebration has always been an occasion of rejoicing that brings together families and friends. It therefore goes without saying that social as well as personal motives enter into the request to be married in church.

Nevertheless, it must not be forgotten that these engaged couples by virtue of their baptism are already really sharers in Christ's marriage covenant with the church, and that, by their right intention, they have accepted God's plan regarding marriage and therefore, at least implicitly, consent to what the church intends to do when she celebrates marriage. Thus the fact that motives of a social nature also enter into the request is not enough to justify refusal on the part of pastors. Moreover, as the Second Vatican Council teaches, the sacraments by words and ritual elements nourish and strengthen faith:[149] that faith toward which the married couple are already journeying by reason of the uprightness of their intention, which Christ's grace certainly does not fail to favor and support.

As for wishing to lay down further criteria for admission to the ecclesial celebration of marriage, criteria that would concern the level of faith of those to be married, this would above all involve grave risks. In the first place, the risk of making unfounded and discriminatory judgments; second, the risk of causing doubts about the validity of marriages already celebrated, with grave harm to Christian communities and new and unjustified anxieties to the consciences of married couples; one would also fall into the danger of calling into question the sacramental nature of many marriages of brethren separated from full communion with the Catholic Church, thus contradicting ecclesial tradition.

However, when in spite of all efforts engaged couples show that they reject explicitly and formally what the church intends to do when the marriage of baptized persons is celebrated, the pastor of souls cannot admit them to the celebration of marriage. In spite of his reluctance to do so, he has the duty to take note of the situation and to make it clear to those concerned that in these circumstances it is not the church that is placing an obstacle in the way of the celebration that they are asking for, but themselves.

Once more there appears in all its urgency the need for evangelization and catechesis before and after marriage, effected by the whole Christian community, so that every man and woman that gets married celebrates the sacrament of matrimony not only validly but also fruitfully.

69. Pastoral care after marriage

The pastoral care of the regularly established family signifies, in practice, the commitment of all the members of the local ecclesial community to helping the couple to discover and live their new vocation and mission. In order that the family may be ever more a true community of love, it is necessary that all its members should be helped and trained in their responsibilities as they face the new problems that arise, in mutual service and in active sharing in family life.

This holds true especially for young families, which, finding themselves in a context of new values and responsibilities, are more vulnerable, especially in the first years of marriage, to possible difficulties such as those created by adaptation to life together or by the birth of children. Young married couples should learn to accept willingly and make good use of the discreet, tactful and generous help offered by other couples that already have more experience of married and family life. Thus within the ecclesial community—the great family made up of Christian families—there will take place a mutual exchange of presence and help among all families, each one putting at the service of the others its own experience of life, as well as the gifts of faith and grace. Animated by a true apostolic spirit, this assistance from family to family will constitute one of the simplest, most effective and most accessible means for transmitting from one to another those Christian values which are both the starting point and goal of all pastoral care. Thus young families will not limit themselves merely to receiving, but in their turn, having been helped in this way, will become a source of enrichment for other longer established families through their witness of life and practical contribution.

In her pastoral care of young families the church must also pay special attention to helping them to live married love responsibly in relationship with its demands of communion and service to life. She must likewise help them to harmonize the intimacy of home life with the generous shared work of building up the church and society. When children are born and the married couple becomes a family in the full and specific sense, the church will still remain close to the parents in order that they may accept their children and love them as a gift received from the Lord of life and joyfully accept the task of serving them in their human and Christian growth.

II. Structures of Family Pastoral Care

Pastoral activity is always the dynamic expression of the reality of the church, committed to her mission of salvation. Family pastoral care too—which is a particular and specific form of pastoral activity—has as its operative principle and responsible agent the church herself, through her structures and workers.

70. The ecclesial community and in particular the parish

The church, which is at the same time a saved and a saving community, has to be considered here under two aspects: as universal and particular. The second aspect is expressed and actuated in the diocesan community, which is pastorally divided up into lesser communities of which the parish is of special importance.

Communion with the universal church does not hinder, but rather guarantees and promotes the substance and originality of the various particular churches. These latter remain the more immediate and more effective subjects of operation for putting the pastoral care of the family into practice. In this sense every local church and, in more particular terms, every parochial community must become more vividly aware of the grace and responsibility that it receives from the Lord in order that it may promote the pastoral care of the family. No plan for organized pastoral work at any level must ever fail to take into consideration the pastoral area of the family.

Also to be seen in the light of this responsibility is the importance of the proper preparation of all those who will be more specifically engaged in this kind of apostolate. Priests and men and women religious from the time of their formation should be oriented and trained progressively and thoroughly for the various tasks. Among the various initiatives I am pleased to emphasize the recent establishment in Rome, at the Pontifical Lateran University, of a higher institute for the study of the problems of the family. Institutes of this kind have also been set up in some dioceses. Bishops should see to it that as many priests as possible attend specialized courses there before taking on parish responsibilities. Elsewhere, formation courses are periodically held at higher institutes of theological and pastoral studies. Such initiatives should be encouraged, sustained, increased in number, and of course are also open to lay people who intend to use their professional skills (medical, legal, psychological, social or educational) to help the family.

71. *The family*

But it is especially necessary to recognize the unique place that in this field belongs to the mission of married couples and Christian families by virtue of the grace received in the sacrament. This mission must be placed at the service of the building up of the church, the establishing of the kingdom of God in history. This is demanded as an act of docile obedience to Christ the Lord. For it is he who, by virtue of the fact that marriage of baptized persons has been raised to a sacrament, confers upon Christian married couples a special mission as apostles, sending them as workers into his vineyard and in a very special way into this field of the family.

In this activity married couples act in communion and collaboration with the other members of the church, who also work for the family, contributing their own gifts and ministries. This apostolate will be exercised in the first place within the families of those concerned, through the witness of a life lived in conformity with the divine law in all its aspects, through the Christian formation of the children, through helping them to mature in faith, through education to chastity, through preparation for life, through vigilance in protecting them from the ideological and moral dangers with which they are often threatened, through their gradual and responsible inclusion in the ecclesial community and the civil community, through help and advice in choosing a vocation, through mutual help among family members for human and Christian growth together, and so on. The apostolate of the family will also became wider through works of spiritual and material charity toward other families, especially those most in need of help and support, toward the poor, the sick, the old, the handicapped, orphans, widows, spouses that have been abandoned, unmarried mothers and mothers-to-be in difficult situations who are tempted to have recourse to abortion, and so on.

72. *Associations of families for families*

Still within the church, which is the subject responsible for the pastoral care of the family, mention should be made of the various groupings of members of the faithful in which the mystery of Christ's church is in some measure manifested and lived. One should therefore recognize and make good use of—each one in relationship to its own characteristics, purposes, effectiveness and methods—the different ecclesial communities, the various groups and the numerous movements engaged in various ways, for different reasons and at different levels, in the pastoral care of the family.

For this reason the synod expressly recognized the useful contribution made by such associations of spirituality, formation and apostolate. It will be their task to foster among the faithful a lively sense of solidarity, to favor a manner of living inspired by the Gospel and by the faith of the church, to form consciences according to Christian values and not according to the standards of public opinion; to stimulate people to perform works of charity for one another and for others with a spirit of openness which will make Christian families into a true source of light and a wholesome leaven for other families.

It is similarly desirable that, with a lively sense of the common good, Christian families should become actively engaged at every level in other non-ecclesial associations as well. Some of these associations work for the preservation, transmission and protection of the wholesome ethical and cultural values of each people, the development of the human person, the medical, juridical and social protection of mothers and young children, the just advancement of women and the struggle against all that is detrimental to their dignity, the increase of mutual solidarity, knowledge of the problems connected with the responsible regulation of fertility in accordance with natural methods that are in conformity with human dignity and the teaching of the church.

Other associations work for the building of a more just and human world; for the promotion of just laws favoring the right social order with full respect for the dignity and every legitimate freedom of the individual and the family on both the national and the international level; for collaboration with the school and with the other institutions that complete the education of children, and so forth.

Notes

1. Cf. Gn. 1:26–27.
2. 1 Jn. 4:8.
3. Cf. Second Vatican Council, GS, 12.
4. Cf. Ibid., 48.
5. Cf. e.g., Hos. 2:21; Jer. 3:6–13; Is. 54.
6. Ez. 16:25.
7. Cf. Hos. 3.
8. Cf. Gn. 2:24; Mt. 19:5.
9. Cf. Eph. 5:32–33.
10. Tertullian, *Ad Uxorem*, II, VIII, 6–8: CCL, I, 393.
11. Cf. Council of Trent, Session XXIV, Canon 1: I.D. Mansi, *Sacrorum Conciliorum Nova et Amplissima Collectio*, 33, 149–150.
12. Cf. Second Vatican Council, GS, 48.
13. John Paul II, Address to the delegates of the *Centre de Liaison des Equipes de Recherche* (Nov. 3, 1979), 3: *Insegnamenti* II, 2 (1979), 1038.
14. Ibid., 4; loc. cit., 1032.
15. Cf. Second Vatican Council, GS, 50.
16. Cf. Gn. 2:24.
17. Eph. 3:15.
18. Cf. Second Vatican Council, GS, 78.
19. St. John Chrysostom, *Virginity*, X: PG 48:540.
20. Cf. Mt. 22:30.
21. Cf. 1 Cor. 7:32–35.
22. Second Vatican Council, *Perfectae Caritatis*, 12.
23. Cf. Pius XII, Encyclical *Sacra Virginitas*, II: AAS 46 (1954), 174ff.
24. Cf. John Paul II, Letter *Novo Incipiente* (April 8, 1979), 9: AAS 71 (1979), 410–411.
25. Second Vatican Council, GS, 48.
26. Encyclical *Redemptor Hominis*, 10: AAS 71 (1979), 274.

27. Mt. 19:6; cf. Gn. 2:24.
28. Cf. John Paul II, Address to Married People at Kinshasa (May 3, 1980) 4: AAS 72 (1980), 426–427.
29. GS, 49; cf. John Paul II, Address at Kinshasa 4: loc. cit.
30. Second Vatican Council, GS, 48.
31. Cf. Eph. 5:25.
32. Mt. 19:8.
33. Rv. 3:14.
34. Cf. 2 Cor. 1:20.
35. Cf. Jn. 13:1.
36. Mt. 19:6.
37. Rom. 8:29.
38. St. Thomas Aquinas, *Summa Theologiae*, II-II, q. 14, art. 2, ad 4.
39. Second Vatican Council, LG, II; cf. *Apostolicam Actuositatem*, 11.
40. Second Vatican Council, GS, 52.
41. Cf. Eph. 6:1–4; Col. 3:20–21.
42. Cf. Second Vatican Council, GS, 48.
43. Jn. 17:21.
44. Cf. Second Vatican Council, GS, 24.
45. Gn. 1:27.
46. Gal. 3:26, 28.
47. Cf. John Paul II, Encyclical *Laborem Exercens*, 19: AAS 73 (1981), 625.
48. Gn. 2:18.
49. Gn. 2:23.
50. St. Ambrose, *Exameron*, V 7, 19: CSEL 32, I, 154.
51. Paul VI, Encyclical *Humanae Vitae*, 9: AAS 60 (1968), 486.
52. Cf. Eph. 5:25.
53. Cf. John Paul II, Homily to the Faithful of Terni (March 19, 1981), 3–5: AAS 73 (1981), 268–271.
54. Cf. Eph. 3:15.
55. Cf. Second Vatican Council, GS, 52.
56. Lk. 18:16; cf. Mt. 19:14; Mk. 18:16.
57. John Paul II, Address to the General Assembly of the United Nations (Oct. 2, 1979), 21: AAS 71 (1979), 1159.
58. Lk. 2:52.
59. Cf. Second Vatican Council, GS, 48.
60. John Paul II, Address to the Participants in the International Forum on Active Aging (Sept. 5, 1980), 5: *Insegnamenti*, III, 2 (1980), 539.
61. Gn. 1:28.
62. Cf. Gn. 5:1–3.
63. Second Vatican Council, GS, 50.
64. *Propositio* 21. Section 11 of the encyclical *Humanae Vitae* ends with the statement: "The church, calling people back to the observance of the norms of the natural law, as interpreted by her constant doctrine, teaches that each and every marriage act must remain open to the transmission of life (*ut quilibet matrimonii usus ad vitam humanam procreandam per se destinatus permaneat*)": AAS 60 (1968), 488.
65. Cf. 2 Cor. 1:19; Rv. 3:14.
66. Cf. The sixth Synod of Bishops' Message to Christian Families in the Modern World (Oct. 24, 1980), 5.
67. GS, 51.
68. Encyclical *Humanae Vitae*, 7: AAS 60 (1968), 485.
69. Ibid., 12: loc. cit., 488–489.
70. Ibid., 14: loc. cit., 490.
71. Ibid., 13: loc. cit., *m* 489.
72. Cf. Second Vatican Council, GS, 51.

73. Encyclical *Humanae Vitae*, 29: AAS 60 (1968), 501.
74. Cf. Ibid., 25: loc. cit., 498–499.
75. Ibid., 21: loc. cit., 496.
76. John Paul II, Homily at the Close of the Sixth Synod of Bishops (Oct. 25, 1980), 8: AAS 72 (1980), 1083.
77. Cf. Paul VI, Encyclical *Humanae Vitae*, 28: AAS 60 (1968), 501.
78. Cf. John Paul II, Address to the Delegates of the *Centre de Liaison des Equipes de Recherche* (Nov. 3, 1979), 9: *Insegnamenti*, II, 2 (1979), 1035; and cf. Address to the Participants in the First Congress for the Family of Africa and Europe (Jan. 15, 1981): L'Osservatore Romano, Jan. 16, 1981.
79. Encyclical *Humanae Vitae*, 25: AAS 60 (1968), 499.
80. *Gravissimum Educationis*, 3.
81. Second Vatican Council, GS, 35.
82. St. Thomas Aquinas, *Summa Contra Gentiles*, IV, 58.
83. GE, 2.
84. Apostolic exhortation *Evangelii Nuntiandi*, 71: AAS 68 (1976), 60–61.
85. Cf. Second Vatican Council, GE, 3.
86. Second Vatican Council, AA, 11.
87. GS, 52.
88. Cf. Second Vatican Council, AA, 11.
89. Rom. 12:13.
90. Mt. 10:42.
91. Cf. GS, 30.
92. Second Vatican Council, *Dignitatis Humanae*, 5.
93. Cf. *Propositio* 42.
94. Second Vatican Council, LG, 31.
95. Cf. Second Vatican Council, LG, 11; AA, II; Pope John Paul II, Homily for the Opening of the Sixth Synod of Bishops (Sept. 26, 1980), 3: AAS 72 (1980) 1008.
96. Second Vatican Council, LG, 11.
97. Cf. Ibid., 41.
98. Acts 4:32.
99. Cf. Paul VI, *Humanae Vitae*, 9.
100. GS, 48.
101. Cf. Second Vatican Council, DV, 1.
102. Rom. 16:26.
103. Cf. Paul VI, *Humanae Vitae*, 25.
104. *Evangelii Nuntiandi*, 71.
105. Cf. Address to the Third General Assembly of the Bishops of Latin America (Jan. 28, 1979), IV A: AAS 71 (1979), 204.
106. Second Vatican Council, LG, 35.
107. John Paul II, Apostolic Exhortation *Catechesi Tradendae*, 68: AAS 71 (1979), 1334.
108. Cf. Ibid., 36: loc. cit., 1308.
109. Cf. 1 Cor. 12:4–6; Eph. 4:12–13.
110. Mk. 16:15.
111. Cf. Second Vatican Council, LG, 11.
112. Acts 1:8.
113. Cf. 1 Pt. 3:1–2.
114. Second Vatican Council, LG, 35; cf. AA, 11.
115. Cf. Acts 18; Rom. 16:3–4.
116. Cf. Second Vatican Council, AG, 39.
117. Second Vatican Council, AA, 30.
118. Cf. Second Vatican Council, LG, 10.
119. Second Vatican Council, GS, 49.

120. Ibid., 48.
121. Cf. Second Vatican Council, LG, 41.
122. Second Vatican Council, *Sacrosanctum Concilium*, 59.
123. Cf. 1 Pt. 2:5; Second Vatican Council, LG, 34.
124. Second Vatican Council, LG, 34.
125. SC, 78.
126. Cf. Jn. 19:34.
127. Section 25: AAS 60 (1968), 499.
128. Eph. 2:4.
129. Cf. John Paul II, Encyclical *Dives in Misericordia*, 13: AAS 72 (1980) 1218–1219.
130. 1 Pt. 2:5.
131. Mt. 18:19–20.
132. Second Vatican Council, GE, 3; cf. Pope John Paul II, *Catechesi Tradendae*, 36: AAS 71 (1979), 1308.
133. General Audience Address, Aug. 11, 1976: *Insegnamenti di Paolo VI*, XIV (1976), 640.
134. Cf. SC, 12.
135. Cf. *Institutio Generalis de Liturgia Horarum*, 27.
136. Paul VI, Apostolic Exhortation *Marialis Cultus*, 52, 54: AAS 66 (1974), 160–161.
137. John Paul II, Address at the Mentorella Shrine (Oct. 29, 1978): *Insegnamenti*, I (1978), 78–79.
138. Cf. Second Vatican Council, AA, 4.
139. Cf. John Paul I, Address to the Bishops of the 12th Pastoral Region of the United States (Sept. 21, 1978): AAS, 70 (1978), 767.
140. Rom. 8:2.
141. Rom. 5:5.
142. Cf. Mk. 10:45.
143. Second Vatican Council, LG, 36.
144. AA, 8.
145. Cf. Synod of Bishops' Message to Christian Families (Oct. 24, 1980), 12.
146. Cf. John Paul II, Address to the Third General Assembly of the Bishops of Latin America (Jan. 28, 1979), IV A: AAS 71 (1979), 204.
147. Cf. Second Vatican Council, SC, 10.
148. Cf. *Ordo Celebrandi Matrimonium*, 17.
149. Cf. Second Vatican Council, SC, 59.

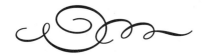

Marriage in Current Theology

14

Marriage

Francis Schüssler Fiorenza

Today marriage is a fragile institution. Societal changes have led to an increased rate of divorce. A growing number of couples decide to live together prior to or without a civil or church wedding. The number of families with a single parent as head of the household continues to grow. Violence within marriage, both the battering of wives and children and the sexual abuse of children, lead many to criticize the traditional patriarchal structure of marriage. Some persons see the very institution of marriage as challenged. "Is Marriage Obsolete?" was the provocative title of an article in *The Boston Globe*. The article described our society as "postmarital." It argued that the dominance of the single-parent family, the high rate of divorce, and the legal acknowledgment of survivorship and rights between unmarried persons are signs of the demise of marriage. Its author concluded: "By the third millennium marriage will be regarded as déclassé, a tacky arrangement practiced only by benighted and idolatrous monogamy freaks, an obscure and despised sect of something or other."[1] If this were to come to pass, people in the third millennium would obviously have no use for a theology of marriage as a sacrament and no sense for the religious significance of marriage.

Within the Roman Catholic church, exegetical and historical research has led Cardinal Joseph Ratzinger to offer a clear challenge to familiar ideas of marriage as a sacrament. Commenting on these traditional ideas, Ratzinger has asserted: "If one remains with the classic catechism, whereby a sacrament is an external sign, instituted by Christ, that signifies and effects inner grace, then these phrases say little; indeed they are in every respect questionable: neither has Jesus instituted marriage nor given it a specific external sign."[2] Moreover, Ratzinger continues, if the sacrament of marriage is understood as mechanically providing a couple with a grace that both makes their relation similar to the Christ-church relation and enables them to fulfill their tasks in the face of the reality of marriage, then the traditional teaching can "no longer be understood as a convincing, meaningful understanding of the notion of the sacrament."[3] In such cases, "the representative of systematic theology must appear, in more than one respect, as a hopeless dilettante."[4]

Such diverse challenges should impel us to examine carefully and critically the Roman Catholic tradition about marriage as a sacrament. A study of this tradition should take into account not only historical evidence about the long and diverse development of the Christian understanding of marriage. It should also examine philosophical and social background theories that have been the underlying assumptions of this tradition. Moreover, it would need to explore our contemporary experience and social constructs as articulated within diverse religious and social groups. This task can be approached here only in a very limited fashion. In this brief treatment, I shall first examine biblical teaching, then Roman Catholic theological and church traditions, and finally contemporary systematic expositions.

Biblical Teaching on Marriage

The canonical Hebrew and Christian Scriptures contain many chapters and verses touching on marriage and issues related to married life. Nevertheless, it would be highly inappropriate to look to the Bible for a theology of marriage, as if the Bible contained a "theology *of* marriage." Too often the Bible is looked upon as a source book for various "theologies of," be it a theology of work, a theology of nature, or a theology of sex. The Bible does not offer such a comprehensive systematic or conceptual analysis of marriage. On the other hand, it would be equally inappropriate if we did not attend to some of the diverse views and images of marriage that are reflected in biblical texts, for they have decisively influenced Christian theology.

Hebrew Scriptures

The Genesis accounts of the creation of the first human couple have influenced the interpretation of marriage in the West as much as the horizon of subsequent experience has influenced the interpretation of these verses. Historical-critical scholarship has shown, moreover, that the first chapters of Genesis contain two distinct accounts of the creation of the first couple: the Priestly account in Genesis 1 and the Yahwist account in Genesis 2 and 3.

The central verses of the Priestly tradition on the creation of humanity are Genesis 1:26–28: "Then God said, 'Let us make man ['*adam*] in our image, after our likeness. . . .' So God created ['*adam*] in his own image, in the image of God he created him; male and female he created them. And God blessed them, and God said to them, 'Be fruitful and multiply.'" This text describes the creation of human persons in the image of God as a creation of "the human" as male and female. The creation of the first couple takes place simultaneously. It is the human as both male and female that is created in the image of God and that represents God. This text is rather limited. "It says nothing about the image which relates '*adam* to God nor about God as the referent. . . . It is not concerned with sexual roles, the status or relationship of the sexes to one another or marriage. It describes the biological pair, not a social partnership; male and female, not man and wife."[5]

The Yahwist account in chapters 2 and 3 of Genesis contains the story of Adam and Eve in the Garden of Eden. In this narrative account Adam is created first and Eve is created afterward, formed from Adam's side in order to be his helpmate (Gen. 2:18–25). These verses have puzzled scholars. Traditional rabbinic literature interpreted these verses to mean that God originally created an "androgynous person," and those who translated the passage into Greek expressed this meaning by writing "a male with female parts." A more recent interpretation, however, suggests that '*adam* literally means "the earth creature." Consequently, the intent of the story is not so much to stress that God created a male being first as to emphasize that God created humankind.[6]

Throughout the history of Jewish and Christian literature, both biblical accounts have been diversely interpreted and the source of much philosophical and religious speculation.[7] Yet one must exercise a certain reserve in the appropriation and use of this material. The Genesis accounts do not contain an implicit theology of marriage that seeks to legislate for all time the meaning of male and female and their division into their proper roles. Rather the Genesis accounts function as mythic accounts of the origin of the world and of its inhabitants.

The Scriptures contain many verses and images about marriage. These have been the source of much poetic inspiration and theological reflection. Images of marriage and marital love can be found in the prophetic traditions, the Song of Songs, the story of Tobit, the Book of Proverbs, the Wisdom of the Son of Sirach, and Qoheleth. This literature is quite diverse in its conceptions and views. For example, the erotic imagery of the Song of Songs that so passionately exults in the beloved contrasts sharply with the skeptical advice of the Son of Sirach that there is no wickedness or wrath on the earth greater than that of a woman (c. 25:13).

The diverse literary genres and the contrasting social attitudes in these texts alert us to what can still serve as a source of inspiration and what needs to be assessed within its limited historical context. The negative attitudes toward women are pervasive, from the prophetic use of the harlot imagery[8] to Sirach's attribution of the origin of sin to women (25:24). At the same time, the ideals of fidelity and love are present in these texts. The negative texts must be acknowledged for what they are. They reflect not God's views, but the views of God's people—a sinful and wandering people like other peoples. The negative texts should be compared with more positive texts, and they should not be elevated above their socially and historically conditioned status to an eternal divine teaching about the sacrament of marriage.

Early Christian Scriptures

The early Christian Scriptures, like the Hebrew Scriptures, contain a variety of statements about marriage in diverse contexts. Quite often certain of these statements—e.g., Jesus' statements about divorce, the adultery exception of Matthew, or the Pauline exception—are highlighted from a particular systematic perspective. These verses, however, should not be isolated, but should be understood and interpreted within the context of diverse biblical traditions.

Relativization of Marriage for the Sake of Discipleship

The earliest texts in the New Testament that refer to marriage stem from the early Christian missionary movements. These texts indicate a disruption and disturbance of traditional family structures: "Jesus said, 'Truly, I say to you, there is no one who has left house or brothers or sisters or mother or father or children or lands, for my sake and for the gospel, who will not receive a hundredfold'" (Mark 10:29). Likewise: "Truly, I say to you, there is no man who has left house or wife or brothers or parents or children, for the sake of the kingdom of God, who will not receive manifold more in this time, and in the age to come, eternal life" (Luke 18:29).

The early Christian missionary movement, often referred to as the "Jesus movement," provides the context of these verses.[9] The earliest disciples of Jesus did not at first establish local communities. Instead they became wandering charismatics—traveling apostles, prophets, and disciples who moved from place to place and who left everything behind. As wandering preachers, they were homeless; they lacked possessions; and they lacked a family. The disciples left these behind for the sake of their preaching and missionary activity. For the sake of preaching God's kingdom, they chose a life with neither family nor possessions.

Eschatological Vision and the Command against Divorce

Another tradition of texts about marriage concerns divorce and remarriage.[10] These texts are Mark 10:11–12, Matthew 5: 31–32 and 19:3–9, Luke 16:18, and 1 Corinthians 7:10–11. These sayings against divorce belong to the oldest traditions in the New Testament. They are a part of the Jesus tradition. If any sayings can with some degree of historical certainty be attributed to the historical Jesus, then these statements would be among the prime candidates.[11]

Scholars offer diverse interpretations of these sayings. Some scripture scholars attempt to explain them away as allegorical. For example, Bruce Malina argues that when taken literally the statements make "as little sense as 'you are the salt of the earth.'"[12] Such an interpretation patently waters down the verses and substitutes personal conjecture for historical interpretation. Nothing in the text indicates metaphorical or allegorical language. In fact a literal interpretation of the texts conforms well to the historical situation within first-century Judaism.[13] During this period, Judaism permitted divorce but limited its conditions. Sectarian groups such as the Essenes, however, rejected divorce outright. They had a distinct eschatological perspective on which they based their rejection of divorce.

Instead of explaining away these verses, some scholars point to their context and trajectory, especially to the debate in Palestine between the Hillel school, with its more lenient interpretation allowing divorce for the husband, and the Schammai school, which permitted divorce only for the most extreme cases. This perspective suggests that Jesus sides with the stricter interpretation and goes beyond it. Some exegetes suggest that Jesus' interpretation offers a protection for women, as Matthew 5:28 implies.[14]

Other scholars suggest that these Matthean verses should not be interpreted as a debate between two schools, but as a part of Jesus' radical eschatological vision. It is pointed out that in the Jesus traditions that predate the Gospels (these traditions being reflected in Mark 10:2–9 and 12:18–27), Jesus' eschatological vision critically challenges traditional patriarchal marriage. It interprets marriage structures not in relation to an order of creation, but in relation to an apocalyptic theology of the restoration of original creation. The eschatological being of men and women is not based on sexual difference, but on freedom from sexual differentiation.[15] Jesus' imperatives do not provide valid norms for the historically conditioned circumstances of his time, but show that God's coming kingdom has an eschatological character that transcends the limits of traditional moral interpretations.[16]

Some exegetes have observed that in view of its liteary genre, argumentation, and textual quotations from the Greek version of Genesis, the controversial dialogue constituting the pericope Matthew 5:31–32 expresses not a Palestinian dispute, but a debate within a Jewish-Christian Hellenistic community.[17] Some argue, however, that this debate in the Hellenistic community presupposes as known a decision or statement going back to the historical Jesus.[18]

Since the "except for" (Matt. 5:31) clause has significantly influenced the systematic position concerning divorce, its interpretation has been controverted. Among contemporary Roman Catholic exegetes two divergent interpretations have emerged about the meaning of *porneia* in the text. One suggests that *porneia* refers to illegitimate marriages between relatives that were impermissible for Jewish Christians and that pagan Christians were also to avoid (Acts 15:20, 29). According to this interpretation, the exception adds not so much an exception as a further restriction. Divorce is not allowed except for marriages that are really impermissible.[19] The other solution points out that *porneia* can also mean "adultery." This interpretation suggests that divorce is allowed when the marriage is already broken.[20]

In 1 Corinthians 7 (one of the most difficult chapters to interpret), Paul touches on several themes of marriage. In the first instance, he affirms the early Christian missionary ideal of the excellence of ascetic celibacy. Such a priority of asceticism over marriage was significant in the early Christian movement, so much so that, as recent exegetical research has shown, many in early Christianity viewed baptism and marriage as incompatible.[21] Though Paul acknowledges a priority of the unmarried state and recommends that the unmarried remain such, he does display a realism that acknowledges marriage. Paul does not so much develop a theology of marriage as concede the possibility of marriage as a practical necessity. Despite the examples of married couples as missionary apostles in the early Christian movement, such as his co-workers Prisca and Aquila, Paul argues that commitment to the work of mission favors asceticism over Christian marriage.[22]

In charging that neither husband nor wife should divorce one another Paul refers to a word from the Lord. Such reference to a word from Jesus is a rare instance in Paul's writings. Nevertheless, in spite of the authority of this word, Paul argues from experience for an exception. In the history of Christianity Paul's action has led to a broadening of the exception, and it has raised the issue of the power and responsibility of the community.

Household Codes and Christian Marriage

The deutero-Pauline and the pastoral epistles contain a third tradition, the household codes, which were given that name because they were meant to regulate the behavior of the household. In contrast to the early Christian affirmation of asceticism and to the Pauline commendation of the unmarried state, these epistles affirm the importance of marriage and of family. Indeed, the pastoral epistles stipulate that bishops must be successful in marital and family life before their election to office; they must be married only once and have raised a solid family: "Now a bishop must be above reproach, the husband of one wife. . . . He must manage his own household well, keeping his children submissive and respectful in every way; for if a man does not know how to manage his own household, how can he care for God's church?" (1 Tim. 3:3–5).

Ephesians 5:21–33 contains a much more explicitly theological analysis of marriage. These verses have become the classic biblical reference for much theological reflection on marriage. The household codes in Ephesians deal not only with the relations between husbands and wives, but also with the proper relations in regard to children and slaves (6:1–9). The household codes provide three parallel orders of relation: husband and wife, parents and children, masters and slaves. The first member of each pair has the role of leadership and responsibility, whereas the second has the role of obedience. With regard to marriage, the husband as the head of the wife parallels Christ as the head of the church.

These household codes have been diversely interpreted. Some have viewed them as expressing a divinely ordered sphere of subordination.[23] Others underscore the element of Christ's love for the church with the concomitant demands of the husband's love for the wife. Recent scholarship on the New Testament has illumined the specific content and meaning of these texts. In the Greco-Roman world, the early Christians were considered disruptive of the socio-cultural order. The earliest Christians were in fact called atheists because they did not participate in emperor worship. Moreover, insofar as Christian communities allowed a wife, child, or slave to convert and to join the community without the permission of the male head of the household, they were looked upon as disruptive of the patriarchal family order of the time.

The early Christian communities with their emphasis on equality of discipleship and their admittance of individual women or individual slaves to the community seemed to bear out this charge. Consequently, the household codes, which are in the later books of the Christian Scriptures, represent in part an apologetic attempt to show that Christianity was not opposed to the Roman socio-cultural order. The texts, therefore, borrow from the Aristotelian philosophy current at that time, which was embodied in a set of codes that reinforced the patriarchal order. It is this apologetic context of the texts that should deter today's Christians from accepting the Roman social order of patriarchy in regard to wives, children, and slaves as a divinely ordained order.[24] Theological reflection and pastoral preaching, therefore, have to be alert to the socially conditioned background theories or assumptions in elaborating a theology of marriage for and in modern societies not based upon the Roman patriarchal order.

In assessing the theological appropriation of these verses from Ephesians, it is important to note that a specific translation has greatly influenced the understanding of these verses. Because the Greek word *mysterion* was translated in the Vulgate as *sacramentum*, Ephesians 5:32 has often been used as the basis for justifying the Scholastic doctrine of marriage as a sacrament. Some medieval theologians (for example, Peter Lombard) were aware of this translation problem. Moreover, Luther's polemic against the Roman Catholic teaching on marriage as a sacrament included this charge of mistranslation. As Walter Kasper has observed: "Most scholars are agreed now . . . that the later idea of sacrament should not be presupposed"[25] when one reads this passage from Ephesians. A theological justification of marriage as a sacrament should not be based exclusively on this passage.

Not Really a Harmony

One cannot bring these diverse traditions into harmony with one another as theologians of previous generations did when they attempted to synthesize ideas from various early Christian Scriptures into unified systematic concepts within a biblical theology or a theology of the New Testament. There is not a biblical theology of marriage as a unified set of ideas and concepts. Instead one has to view the richness and diversity of the various early Christian traditions.

The traditions that I have highlighted are central to the early Christian Scriptures. These traditions have impacted Christian thought throughout the centuries and can serve to criticize a one-sided appropriation of any particular tradition. The eschatological horizon of the Jesus movement with its emphasis on asceticism relativizes marriage and family for the sake of radical discipleship. Its emphasis sharply contrasts with the deutero-Pauline praise of the standard of a respectable family. The commitment to Jesus in a radical discipleship of equals relativizes the emphasis on the Roman patriarchal order in the household codes. Yet there is also the eschatological ideal of marriage in relation to the original human creation that represents a hope and a vision beyond the frailty in marriages. The insight that relations among humans are meant to mirror the divine-human relation provides a challenge for theological reflection that Christian theology has taken up in various ways throughout the centuries.

MARRIAGE IN THE HISTORY OF ROMAN CATHOLIC THEOLOGY

The history of Christian theological views toward marriage displays diverse attitudes, and the development of the Roman Catholic understanding of marriage as a sacrament is a complex topic. Rather than present a historical survey, I shall merely highlight a few salient points from the history of theology: first, Augustine's understanding of the sacrament in marriage within the context of his influential treatment of the goods of marriage; second, the development of medieval conceptions of marriage; third, the affirmations of the Council of Trent; and fourth, recent official teachings of the Roman Catholic church regarding marriage.

Augustine: The Sacrament in Marriage

Although many of the early Christian writers dealt with marriage, Augustine's views have most strongly influenced Western theology.[26] Augustine did not so much affirm marriage as one of the sacraments of the New Law; rather he affirmed that there is in all marriages, and not just Christian marriages, a sacrament. Augustine used the term *sacrament* in a general and a narrow sense.[27] In a very general sense, sacrament refers to visible words, things, and actions that are signs of what is invisible and transcendent. In a more narrow sense, sacrament refers specifically to the sacraments of the Catholic church, among which baptism and eucharist have a predominant role.

Augustine understands the sacrament in marriage in the broad rather than narrow sense, as is evident in his treatment of the goods of marriage—a specific teaching that has greatly influenced traditional Roman Catholic teaching about marriage. Though the words *goods* and to a lesser extent *blessings* or *benefits* are often used in the English translation of Augustine, the word *values* probably expresses more adequately Augustine's thought. In *The Good of Marriage*, Augustine taught that marriage has three values: fidelity, offspring, and sacrament.[28] Fidelity (*fides*) is the faithfulness in the mutual love that each spouse has for the other. Augustine interprets fidelity in relation to the sexual love and intercourse of the married couple. Yet he does so in a way that disallows the denigration of one partner or the other to a mere sexual object. In his view, even sexual relations open to procreation can be sinful if the partner is reduced to a mere object of libido. Fidelity relates to sexual love, but it entails more than a sexual commitment. Rather, it is a commitment of love and trust. Fidelity is the virtue that also supports the second value of marriage, offspring. This second value entails the acceptance of children in love, their nurturance in affection, and their upbringing in the Christian religion.

The third value of marriage is the sacrament of marriage. In chapter 18 of *The Good Marriage* Augustine explains that the sacrament is found in first marriages. It primarily refers to the union of the spouses as an indissoluble bond. For these marriages are a visible sign, that is, they signify the image of the one society of the blessed in eternity. A Christian marriage signifies visibly on earth the future unity of the people of God in eternity. The union of the spouses, their visible covenant with one another, is a tangible sign of the unity of all people in eternity.

These three values show that Augustine does not view marriage simply as a bond between two individuals. Instead he understands marriage as a sign and sacrament. He describes its sacramentality within the framework of the distinction between the old and new covenant. The marriages of the Hebrew patriarchs symbolized the future church that consisted of many nations and people, and this was signified by their polygamous marriage (*sacramentum pluralium nuptiarum*). The marriage of a bishop, as a marriage with one wife, differs from the marriage of the patriarchs. The one church from many nations already exists as a reality, even though it is not yet perfect. Therefore, the marriage of a bishop constitutes a sign of the radical unity and peace of the eschatological city (*sacramentum nuptiarum singularum*).[29] This vision of marriage as a sacrament underscores that marriage is a sign of societal peace and unity. It is not simply that the fidelity of two spouses aids in the continued nurturing of children, but also that the visible union of the couple signifies the eschatological unity of all people and nations.

Too often, contemporary theologians tend to neglect these positive elements within Augustine's theology and mention only what they perceive as the negative elements: for instance, his view of marriage as a remedy for concupiscence and his negative assessment of sexuality.[30] Augustine also taught that marriage "does not seem to be good only because of the procreation of children, but also because of the natural companionship between the sexes."[31] Moreover, as Augustine matured as a Christian, his belief in the incarnation led him to move further away from his early Manichean attitudes to a more positive assessment of human corporeality.[32]

Medieval Theology: Marriage as a Sacrament

A considerable development took place from Augustine's view of the sacrament of marriage as a visible sign of a transcendent unity of the people of God to the view of marriage as one of the seven sacraments. The incorporation of marriage into the rank of sacraments occurred during the medieval period between the eleventh and twelfth centuries. The context for this development was both doctrinal and liturgical. The doctrinal occasion was the spread of the Cathari or Albigenses, who were ascetics who viewed marriage as an evil. Their views prompted a theological response that affirmed the goodness of marriage and spurred the development of a theology of marriage as a sacrament. In fact, the first offical explicit affirmations of marriage as a sacrament occur in statements condemning the Cathari. In 1184 the Council of Verona under Pope Lucius III anathematized the Cathari for their opinions about marriage. In 1208 Pope Innocent III required as a condition for return to Catholicism that the Waldenses subscribe to a profession of faith that accepted all the church's sacraments, including marriage. In 1274 the Second Council of Lyons proposed a similar requirement as a condition for reunion for the Byzantine emperor Michael Palaeologus.

Liturgical celebrations also influenced the development of the notion of marriage as a sacrament.[33] The church's liturgical practice of the wedding ceremony appropriated Roman and Teutonic traditions. Germanic, Frankish, and Lombardic laws emphasized the handing over of the bride, different from though not unlike the Roman custom of the handing over of the bride to the husband as the paterfamilias. As a result, people came to equate the blessing of marriage with the "handing over of the bride." A parallel was seen between the veiling and handing over of the bride and the veiling and handing over of the consecrated virgin, as a "bride of Christ," to the church. This analogy between the bride and the consecrated virgin was significant for the developing understanding of marriage as a sacrament. Whereas the virgin was consecrated directly to Christ, the bride was consecrated through the human relationship with her husband, the figure of Christ. The bride's visible relationship to the husband was a sign of her invisible relation to Christ. The text of Ephesians 5:21–32 influenced this development. Since the virgin was consecrated directly to Christ, this consecration was not viewed as a sacrament. Since the consecration to the husband was a visible sign of a more profound relation to Christ, marriage was a sacrament. Such a development and view went beyond Augustine's view of the mutual fidelity in marriage as a sign of the unity of the people of God.

The doctrine of marriage as a sacrament developed gradually within the medieval period. Moreover, theological speculation about marriage during the medieval period was quite diverse. Three distinct theories existed about what constituted the nature of marriage. Does the marriage bond derive primarily from the consent of the two partners, from the consummation through sexual intercourse, or from marriage's social function? The consent theory, also known as the French theory, was advocated by theologians in Paris. They argued that the essence of marriage was the free consent of the individual couple. A marriage continued to be a full marriage even when sexual intercourse played no role, as in the example of Mary and Joseph. Procreation belonged to the task (*officium*) of marriage, but not its constitution. The second view, known as the *copula* theory, was advocated by canonists, especially in Italy. They argued that marriage was constituted by sexual intercourse and believed marital consent to sexual intercourse was the essential element of the marital relation. A third view argued that marriage was an institution that provided the social and human foundation for the bringing up of children.

Between proponents of the first two views there was a significant debate concerning the relation between mutual consent and the community of marriage.[34] Both agreed that mutual consent formed the basis of marriage, but they made a distinction between the contracted marriage (based on consent) and the ratified marriage (sealed through sexual consummation). Theologians such as Peter Lombard argued that the marriage bond was established by the mutual consent. It was this mutual consent that was the sacrament of the unity of Christ and the church. The canonists argued that a marriage, though valid due to mutual consent, could be dissolved if it was not consummated.

The influence of this debate, especially the Parisian emphasis on spousal consent, can be seen in Hugh of Saint Victor's theological treatment of marriage.[35] Hugh posited two sacraments of Christian marriage. The *sacramentum conjugi* consists of the love union between man and woman that signifies and images God's love for humans and the human love for God. The *sacramentum officii* is expressed in sexual intercourse that images the love of Christ and the church—a love in the flesh. The theological position that marriage requires consent led to an emphasis on love within marriage.[36] Richard of Saint Victor (d. 1173) gives a lyrical description of marital love in *Of the Four Degrees of Passionate Love*. His treatment gives a priority to human affection. "We know that among human affections conjugal love must take the first place, and therefore in wedded life that degree of love which generally dominates all other affections seems to be good. For the mutual affection of intimate love draws closer the bonds of peace between those who are pledged to each other, and make that indissoluble, life-long association pleasant and happy."[37]

The institution of the sacrament of marriage was viewed somewhat differently from that of the other sacraments. One could not simply affirm that Christ instituted the sacrament of marriage, since marriage existed before Christ, indeed was present even in paradise. Therefore, Scholastic theologians refer to stages in the institution of this sacrament. Anselm of Laon argued that marriage, in contrast to other sacraments, was instituted before the fall. Christ did not institute it, but confirmed it at the marriage in Cana. Three stages of institution are outlined in Thomas's *Summa Theologiae*. (Since Thomas died before completing the *Summa*, Reynaldo of Piperno completed the treatise on the sacraments by drawing on Thomas's earlier commentary on Peter Lombard's *Sentences*, where Thomas had basically followed Albert the Great.) These three moments of the institution of marriage are: the natural orientation prior to the fall, the healing institution of the Law of Moses after the fall, and finally, the institution of the New Law as a sign of union between Christ and the church.

Although it has been often noted that Thomas was much more negative in his assessment of women than Augustine due to the influence of Aristotle's biology,[38] he actually had a more positive view of human sexuality, as the debate about marriage in paradise showed. Some argued that in the Garden of Paradise prior to the fall, human procreation would have occurred without sexual intercourse. Against such a view Aquinas argued on the basis of the naturalness of human sexuality for procreation. It was not human sexuality, but "excessive concupiscence" that was absent.[39] Moreover, with a healthy realism, Thomas stressed the importance of friendship for marriage. "The greater that friendship, the more solid and long-lasting it be. Now, there seems to be the greatest friendship between husband and wife, for they are united not only in the act of fleshly union, which produces a certain gentle association even among beasts, but also in the partnership of the whole range of domestic activity."[40]

Bonaventure distinguished among three types of sacraments. The common sacraments of the old and new covenant are marriage and penance. They exist from the wisdom of nature and are merely confirmed by Christ.[41] Baptism, eucharist, and ordination are partially prefigured in the Old Testament, but they flourish in the New Testament. Only these three are established in a proper sense by Christ. Beyond these, there are sacraments distinctive to the New Testament, confirmation and the anointing of the sick. They were established in the church by the Holy Spirit.

The Council of Trent on Marriage

Prior to modern papal and conciliar teaching, two major councils were significant for the Roman Catholic church's teaching on marriage: the "Union" Council of Florence (1439–45) and the Council of Trent (1545–63). Whereas Florence was concerned with Eastern traditions, Trent affirmed both the sacramentality and the indissolubility of marriage in the context of Martin Luther's criticism of Roman Catholic teaching and practice.[42] The notion that marriage is indissoluble is evident in canon 7 (November 11, 1563): "Whoever says that the Church errs when it has taught and still teaches that, according to the evangelical and apostolic doctrine, because of the adultery of one spouse, the bond of marriage cannot be dissolved and that both, even the innocent party, who has not given cause for adultery cannot contract another marriage while the other spouse is still alive . . . may he be excluded."[43]

The Council of Trent made two basic affirmations about marriage. The first states that marriage is a sacrament and within the provenance of the church. Marriage is not simply a matter of private, personal, or individual decision, but concerns the community. Therefore, Trent required that Catholic marriages should take place in the presence of a priest. It, thereby, sought to curb the widespread practice of clandestine marriages. In addition Trent reaffirmed the church's teaching and practice, especially as it developed in the Western church, that prohibited divorce and remarriage for cases of adultery. The council maintained that this teaching and practice are "in accordance with" evangelical and apostolic doctrine. Scholars have maintained that the language used by the council pointed to obligatory teaching and practice, "not an ultimately obligatory dogma in the modern sense of the word."[44] It sought to underscore that the church's practice and teaching were in accordance with the New Testament. This affirmation was deliberately very nuanced. "In accordance with" is not the same as "identical with." In other words, "it is not simply the teaching of the Gospel."[45]

The decision of Trent, as Walter Kasper summarizes it, was limited. "The only intention was to come to a decision in the controversy that had been raging at the time between the Catholic Church and the Lutherans. Controversies within the Catholic Church itself were, however, left open. No previous decision of any kind was therefore made by the Council of Trent with regard to the pastoral problems of the twentieth century."[46]

Recent Official Roman Catholic Teaching

Within modern times, several statements on marriage provide the content of the Roman Catholic church's official teaching on the subject.[47] In *Arcanum Divinae Sapientiae,* published in 1880, Pope Leo XIII took issue with the trend toward seeing marriage as a purely secular event and as subject only to civil law. In contrast he argued for the sacramentality of marriage and the marital contract as a sign that imaged the relation between Christ and the church. Fifty years later in *Casti Connubii,* Pius XI took up many of the themes of Pope Leo's encyclical. He especially deplored the many abuses surrounding marriage. At the same time, he sought to further elaborate the religious meaning of marriage. In his view, "this mutual inward molding of husband and wife, this determined effort to perfect each other, can in a very real sense, as the Roman Catechism teaches us, be said to be the chief reason and purpose of marriage, provided marriage be looked at not in the restricted sense as instituted for the proper conception and education of the child, but more widely as the sharing of life as a whole and the mutual interchange and partnership thereof" (no. 24).[48] Pope Pius XII continued the basic teaching of his predecessor. In diverse talks to various groups, most notably his addresses to "Italian Catholic Obstetricians" and to "Italian Catholic Midwives," Pius XII sought to reaffirm the traditional papal teaching.[49] At the same time, he introduced some elements of the personalist philosophical approaches to marriage current at the time. These papal discourses provided the basic contours of Roman Catholic teaching prior to the Second Vatican Council.

The Second Vatican Council's constitution *Gaudium et Spes* (GS) made a decisive attempt to reflect theologically on marriage in the modern world. Though primarily concerned with the church in the modern world, this constitution deals also with marriage. It refers to marriage as an intimate community of love, a Christian vocation, a sacred bond and covenant, and mutual gift of two persons. It is noticeable that the traditional language describing marriage as a contract is missing. Its main theological point was to rethink the question of whether procreation constitutes the primary, natural end and purpose of marriage. Its formulation was very careful: Though it speaks of children as the gift of marriage and of the orientation of marriage toward the procreation and nurture of children, it affirmed that "while not making the other ends of marriage of less value, the true conduct of marital love and the entire meaning of family life that comes from it have this goal, that the spouses be willing to co-work courageously with the love of the Creator and Savior" (GS 50).[50]

Within Roman Catholic theology, contemporary reflections on many issues take as their starting point the documents of the Second Vatican Council. However, the situation differs in regard to marriage, and especially the issue of human sexuality. On June 23, 1964, Pope Paul VI removed the issue of the control of human fertility from the agenda of the Second Vatican Council. He expanded the Pontifical Study Commission, which Pope John XXIII had established, and instructed it to report directly to himself. The commission recommended a change in traditional teaching. Pope Paul VI rejected their concrete recommendation. His encyclical *Humanae Vitae* (1968) further developed the Roman Catholic understanding of marriage. In previous papal documents, the arguments against the limitation of birth were drawn from the end or purpose of marriage, namely, the procreation of children. Since the Second Vatican Council's statements broadened the understanding of the primary purpose of marriage, Pope Paul VI had to nuance the argumentation and gave it a more anthropological and personalist basis.

This argumentation has been echoed and further developed by Pope John Paul II's Apostolic Exhortation on the Family (*Consortium Socialis*) and in his Wednesday general audience talks on the "Theology of the Body."[51] To develop his understanding of sex and marriage John Paul II draws on phenomenology and personalist philosophy in order to explicate the importance of intersubjective bodily relations between the spouses. The human person is embodied as a sexual being with the task of integrating physical and spiritual acts. In the pope's view this integration requires that loving sexual unions be procreative.[52] In recent decades the issue of marriage has also been treated within the broader context of the nature and role of the family within modern society, as the documents of the bishops' synod and the International Theological Commission indicate.[53]

Marriage as a Sacrament in Current Systematic Theology

Within contemporary theology, the sacrament of marriage has been the subject of many studies. Much of the writing on marriage within theological literature concerns moral, pastoral, and canonical issues. Nevertheless, several important directions for a clearer understanding of marriage have been elaborated within contemporary systematic theology. In the following, I shall briefly sketch some contemporary directions, then offer some of my own systematic reflections on the sacrament of marriage, and finally summarize some of the discussion surrounding two practical pastoral issues that result from the Catholic theological view of marriage.

Three Contemporary Directions

Approaches to a theology of marriage as a sacrament reflect the general theological emphases of their historical contexts. During the last decades, three distinct trends within Roman Catholic theology have affected these approaches to marriage: christocentrism, the salvation-historical view, and the anthropological-ecclesial view. Due to the influence of Karl Barth, a christocentric focus entered not only Protestant neo-orthodox theology, but also Roman Catholic theology. Roman Catholic "christocentrism," however, displays its own distinctive forms with an emphasis on the sacramental notion of the body of Christ. Likewise the salvation-historical approach, exemplified by Oscar Cullmann and influential in French theology, made an impact upon Roman Catholic theology in the 1950s and 1960s and has affected the analysis of the sacrament of marriage. In addition, Karl Rahner's development of the anthropological-ecclesial foundation of marriage as a sacrament has deeply influenced Roman Catholic thought on the subject.

Christocentric View of Marriage

The christocentric focus that flourished within Roman Catholic theology in the 1950s has its roots in the nineteenth century. It was especially applied by Matthias Scheeben (1835–88) to marriage.[54] Within French Roman Catholic theology, the notion of the body of Christ or the mystical body of Christ, as it was then understood, became the key metaphor used to interpret marriage as a sacrament.[55] Whereas the sacrament of baptism signals an incorporation of a person into the body of Christ, the sacrament of marriage entails a further incorporation within the body of Christ. As a result the Christian couple participates in a distinctive and special vocation.

Salvation-historical View of Marriage

Roman Catholic theology has always been aware that the understanding of marriage as a sacrament has changed and developed throughout the ages. Many theologians interpret these changes not just as changes in the theological understanding of marriage. Instead they argue that the nature and meaning of marriage itself have changed within the history of salvation. Such a view is present within medieval theology, as exemplified by Bonaventure's understanding of marriage. Within recent decades, theologians have sought to relate marriage to salvation history in the same way that they have related it to the evolving history of the world and to the history of religious experience.[56]

Edward Schillebeeckx has elaborated a theological interpretation of marriage as a sacrament with this basic thesis: "Marriage is a secular reality which has entered salvation."[57] The relation between secular reality and religious reality is not a static relation but has a history. Human thought changes and develops in the process of continually reflecting on historical experience. Marriage has significance as a reality of created life. However, the historical experience by God's people of God's covenant and the Christian experience of Jesus as paschal event also contribute to the understanding of the significance of marriage. Marriage is then no longer understood simply as a secular reality within creation, but it is understood also as a promise in the light of the experience of God's covenantal promise. Created reality is both affirmed and relativized in the light of the eschatological hope. Love within marriage is understood not only in relation to natural attraction, but also in relation to the historical experience of Jesus' death and resurrection and the understanding of God and of love proclaimed by the gospel.

Anthropological-ecclesial View of Marriage

Karl Rahner contributes to the understanding of marriage as a sacrament by bringing together several key ideas of his theology: God's universal will for salvation, the fundamental unity of creation and salvation, the idea of a real symbol, and his understanding of the church as the basic sacrament.[58] For Rahner, God's love and gracious self-bestowal constitute the innermost dynamism of the world and of the history of humankind. It is God's gracious love that empowers us to love God and to love each other. Consequently, genuine love as a theological virtue is an event both of God's love for us and of our love for God.

The radical and real symbol of the unity of God's love for us and the human response of love is in the incarnate Christ. The church as a basic sacrament is real sign and symbol of God's love for humanity and the human love of God. In this context, marriage "is the sign of *that* love which is designed in God's sight to be the event of grace and a love that is open to all."[59] Moreover, marriage is a sacrament that concretizes and actualizes the church. For as Rahner expresses it: "The love that unites married spouses contributes to the unity of the Church herself because it is one of the ways in which the unifying love of the Church is made actual. It is just as much formative of the Church as sustained by the Church."[60]

Toward a Theology of Marriage as a Sacrament

These three directions have greatly enriched our understanding of marriage as a sacrament. Nevertheless, recent advances in fundamental theology, christology, and ecclesiology lead beyond these contributions. Recent shifts within fundamental theology regarding the foundation of the church and within ecclesiology concerning the nature of the church have suggested a new understanding of the church as a sacrament. It has thus become necessary to bring the conception of the sacramentality of marriage into accord with these changes. In addition, traditional theological expositions of marriage as a sacrament have, in some aspects, been based on patriarchal assumptions of marriage and family or have been shaped by outmoded social and anthropological assumptions about gender roles. It has become necessary to elaborate the meaning of the Roman Catholic vision and ideal of marriage in view of equalitarian assumptions about gender and marriage.

Marriage as Sacrament: The Community of the Spirit

Much of traditional theology focused on the text from Ephesians as the symbolic basis of the sacrament of marriage. Unfortunately, use of the image of the Christ-church relation as a model for the marital relation between husband and wife has certain shortcomings. In the image of the relation between Christ and the church, Christ is the one who rules, who saves, and who heals. The church is the one who is obedient and who needs healing and salvation. The application of such symbolism to the marriage relation between husband and wife places the husband in the role of ruler and savior and the wife in the role of sinner and subordinate.[61]

Even though the biblical verses emphasize that Christ's self-sacrificing love for the church should be paradigmatic for the husband's attitude and behavior, the symbolism still implies a superiority of the husband as the suffering redeemer in the marriage relation. Such imagery has as its background the prophetic tradition's description of the relation between God and Israel, with the images of a faithful God versus an unfaithful harlot. The image of the covenant relation between Christ and the church as the basic symbol of the marriage relation may stress God's fidelity, but may also unintentionally associate the husband with a faithful God and the wife with a fickle harlot. It also makes the husband superior to the wife and places her along with children and slaves in a subordinate obediential position.

In addition, the household codes' imagery as well as imperative of the superiority of the husband to the wife have had negative consequences within the history and practice of marriage. We have become increasingly sensitive to the prevalence of the problem of physical abuse of wives by husbands. But within the Christian tradition, such abuse was explicitly condoned and recommended in legislation with appeal to the household codes. Under the doctrine of "moderate correction," a husband was enjoined to beat or physically chastise his wife "moderately," as distinct from "excessively," as a loving correction for the good of her soul.[62]

For these reasons, which serve as retroductive warrants, I would like to suggest a fundamental shift in the underlying imagery of the relation between husband and wife in their relationship to God, Christ, and the church. As a part of my argument I would like to draw attention to an important shift in Roman Catholic systematic theology in the understanding of the church as a sacrament. Walter Kasper has argued for several good reasons that the church should be understood as the sacrament of the Spirit.[63] First, his proposal seeks to take into account the post-Easter emergence of the Christian community with its faith in the death and resurrection of Jesus. Kasper is following the Roman Catholic position elaborated by Eric Peterson, Heinrich Schlier, and Joseph Ratzinger concerning the origin and foundation of the church. In addition, the notion of the church as a sacrament of the Spirit takes into account the distinction between Christ and the church. If the church is viewed exclusively as the sacrament of Christ or as the continuation of the incarnate Christ, then the danger exists that the distinction between Christ and the church is neglected and the church is reduced to a "quasi-mythological hypostasis."[64] The metaphor of the church as the sacrament of the Spirit of Christ relates the church to Christ in a way that does not divinize the church. This metaphor allows one to understand the church as emerging in the post-Easter disciples. The church is the community of disciples that emerges under the impact of God's Spirit.

I suggest that an adequate theological understanding of the sacrament of marriage needs to take into account these developments in Roman Catholic theology concerning the foundation of the church and the sacramental nature of the church. If the church is understood primarily as the community of God's Spirit and as the sacrament of the Spirit, then marriage should be understood as a sign and symbol of the church precisely insofar as it is a sign of the community brought about by the Spirit of God and Christ. A marriage between two individuals is the beginning of a new community, a community of equal disciples and partners under the impact and power of the Spirit. The community of Christians arose after Jesus' death, in discipleship of Jesus, and in the proclamation of God's power in the face of death.[65]

To view marriage as both a symbol and an actual beginning of new community concurs with the insights of the recent salvation-historical approach that argues for a specific meaning of marriage within the Christian dispensation. Christians who view marriage in the light of faith see the meaning of marriage in relation to their experience, their Christian belief in Jesus, and their act of Christian discipleship. For Christians marriage has a specially Christian meaning. Marriage is not simply the new image of God's creative activity symbolized by the Adam and Eve narrative. Nor is marriage an image of the covenantal relation between God and Israel, as symbolized in the prophetic literature. Instead marriage is the symbol of a new community of life, one that images the origin of post-Easter, early Christian communities and one that anticipates the Christian eschatological hope of community. By stressing that the sacramental and symbolic function of marriage relates primarily to the church as the emergent post-Easter community of disciples rather than to the covenantal relation between Christ and the church, I seek to emphasize the fundamental equality of husband and wife in the role of forming a new community. Their equality in discipleship and in the formation of a new community of marriage and their hope for that community can symbolize the equality and hope of discipleship in the post-Easter Christian community.

Sacramental Vision and Roman Catholic Identity

When Roman Catholic theology affirms that marriage is a sacrament, it is not simply making a statement about the number of sacraments. Much more fundamentally it is bringing to expression the Roman Catholic vision of reality. We can distinguish two different cognitive and practical attitudes, in practice intermingled, in the way we relate to our world and society. One is instrumental or functional, the other symbolic or communicative. An instrumental attitude asks about how things function as instruments for some useful purpose. It asks: What utility or function does a particular institution have? A symbolic or communicative attitude is quite different. Its primary question focuses not on utility or function, but on meaning and value. What meaning does an action have? What ideal does an object symbolize? What do we want to communicate?

A similar distinction can be made with reference to C. S. Peirce's semiotic categories that enable us to place signs on a continuum according to their representational and communicative aspects. Some signs or complexes of signs are used referentially to convey information; others are used to communicate in a way that evokes participation. An engineer's model of the Brooklyn Bridge is referential and iconic, whereas a painter's picture is presentational and sensory.[66]

For Roman Catholic theology, then, the affirmation that marriage is a sacrament is an affirmation that marriage is not only instrumental or functional, but is also symbolic and communicative. Marriage is not merely an instrument by which various societies perpetuate themselves; nor is it simply a useful social arrangement by which the human race propagates itself. Instead marriage is also a symbol that communicates meaning, a meaning articulated in relation to a historical memory and a future hope. When Roman Catholic theology describes marriage as a sacrament, it is not so much giving a referential or iconic characterization of marriage, as it is seeking a presentational vision that should evoke one's participation in marriage in a specifically meaningful way.

Louis-Marie Chauvet, a French sacramental theologian, has applied the distinction between sign and symbol to the sacraments in general.[67] Arguing that the traditional doctrine of the sacraments has been based on the classical binary notion of sign, he suggests the appropriateness of the notion of symbol. Classically a sign refers to something else. For example, smoke is a sign of fire and grey hair is a sign of advanced age. The sign leads us to a new knowledge of something else. A symbol, however, introduces us to the cultural order to which it belongs. The sign of the cross, a religious habit, and a Bible are symbols of Christian identity. They do not primarily present new information or lead to new knowledge, as smoke leads us to suspect a fire. Instead they are visible ways in which we mediate our identity. The sign of the cross is more than a sign of something else; it is also a symbol of Christian identity.

It seems helpful in discussions about marriage to take up the distinction between sign and symbol and to ask how marriage is both a sign and a symbol. The liturgical celebration of the sacrament of marriage within the Christian community symbolizes the meaning that marriage has for Christians within the context of Christianity. Marriage takes place before a representative of the Christian community, the communities of two families and sets of friends come together, and the couple starts out beginning a new community. In many cases, and most appropriately, the celebration of marriage is linked with a eucharistic celebration by which the Christian community assembles and actualizes itself.

In my opinion, some theological treatments of marriage make romantic love the central notion of their thematizations. Such treatments can have several weaknesses. First, they overlook that for many centuries and in many areas, the romantic love of the partners for each other was not the personal and social condition of marriage.[68] Second, they sometimes apply an abstract ideal of love as self-gift to marriage without attending to the specific characteristics of love in marriage. Third, such an approach often leads to an intensification of expectations about marriage and the endurance of passion and romance that heightens the possibility for disappointment.[69]

If the meaning of marriage is seen primarily in relation to community rather than in relation to a romantic and individualistic ideal of love, then one is in a better position to understand the specific characteristics of both the marital community and the love that emerges in marriage, both the love of spouses for each other and the love of parents for their children and vice versa.

In a marriage commitment is primarily to a community. Obviously such a community has been differently understood. Traditionally marriage was viewed primarily as the continuation of the community of a particular family, whereas since the eighteenth century, marriage has been viewed as the beginning of a new community. What is important, however, in the stress on community and not simply on partnership or love, is that marriage entails a combination of personal and impersonal relations. It is not simply that the outside world is the world of the impersonal, whereas the family is the realm of the personal. (Often, one-sidedly understood, the public, outside world has been designated as the realm of the male, and the private, personal world has been designated as the domain of the female and family.) In my view, the commitment in marriage to community implies that the impersonal as well as the personal, the objective as well as the subjective, become the object of discourse and of life's energy. One develops a relationship not simply as an intimate relation to a private other, but rather as a community of intersecting relationships and interests.[70]

Love within marriage is often associated and equated with sexual attraction. Yet marital love entails not only desire, but also generosity and an ability to relate on diverse levels. As an eros, marital love includes passion and attraction. It grows from an initial attraction, pleasure, and happiness with one another to a full sexual passion and desire for one another. This passion and desire expand not only into a deeper passion but also into solidarity and commitment. Each spouse learns to respect the other as other and to encourage the other in his or her personal autonomy and hopes. The friendship that may bring the two together as an individual couple has to grow and develop to include others, has to broaden out to other tasks and to other communities. The more this broadening takes place, the more multiple the relationships, the more solid the foundation for the marriage. In the love of spouses for one another, all these elements are intermingled: friendship and passion, desire and generosity, communality and individuality, personal and communal interests. One does not pass from one to the other as if a stage of eros leads to a stage of agape, as if desire leads to solidarity, or friendship leads to love. Instead love, friendship, inclusion of others, and the intersecting of diverse and common interests coexist, each strengthening one another.

Just as the love between two spouses involves an intermingling of love and sexual attraction that is both powerful and multifaceted, so too does there also emerge in marriage the ambiguity of the love of parents for children. It is a love that begins as love for children as one's very own offspring and yet as such must give way and become transformed to give birth to a love and support that encourage freedom, independence, and autonomy, especially from the parents. The love of children for parents, to whom they owe their very existence, is at first a very dependent love that must eventually grow into a form of independence.

All of this suggests a dialectic of commitment and love in marriage that expresses a continued transformation parallel to the experience of the beginning of the Christian community. The Christian experience of Jesus' life-praxis solidarity, his suffering and death, is combined with an experience of new life after Easter and an experience of new life and hope. Yet this hope is based also upon the previous experience and community with Jesus. The new community of the church understands itself at first also as part of the community of Israel. Similarly, the experience of a new community and love in marriage continually gives birth to a transformed love, desire, hope, friendship, and responsibility.

If we take marriage as a sign or symbol of the new community of Christians under the impact of the Spirit, then we can better understand ourselves as Christians in relation to historical remembrance and history. We can understand marriage not simply as a self-giving love, but as a sign or symbol of a community that understands itself in relation to time and history and that is committed to a faith that trusts in a reality of love, hope, and transcendence. This faith is not above history, but is intermingled with disappointment, death, and weakness. For the Christian faith, reality is ultimately grounded in a gracious God, and this God is both manifest and present in Jesus. A couple's public promises of love and commitment within the context of a Christian assembly both signify and symbolize the Christian hope and faith. Their promises signify and symbolize a trust and hope in the face of the common experience of the fragility of marriage.

Meaning and Purpose of Marriage

Roman Catholic theological treatments of the meaning and purpose of marriage have discussed the question of procreation versus mutual fulfillment as the end of marriage and the question of individual gender roles within marriage. Whereas traditionally the procreation of children was considered the primary purpose of marriage, more recently a more personalistic view has gained favor. In my opinion, some reactions against traditional conceptions of the purpose of marriage have either caricatured the traditional position or have themselves offered an overly narrow understanding of the goal and purpose of marriage.

Contemporary treatments of marriage often announce an important shift between traditional and modern Catholic views on the goal and purpose of marriage. They often describe this shift as a shift from procreation to life partnership as the goal of marriage. They increasingly emphasize that the goal and purpose of marriage consist of this life partnership. They often present the Roman Catholic tradition as having asserted that the primary and exclusive end of marriage is the reproduction of children. It is important, however, not to caricature the tradition. Indeed throughout the tradition many theologians affirmed procreation as the purpose of marriage and often took Genesis 1:28 ("Be fertile and multiply") as a key code and biblical foundation for the meaning of marriage. Nevertheless, such affirmations were never exclusive. The Roman Cathechism (*Catechismus Romanus*) of the Council of Trent (1566) affirms that "nature itself by an instinct implanted in both sexes impels them to such companionship, and this is further encouraged by the hope of mutual assistance" (II, 8:13). Pius XI in the encyclical *Casti Connubii* distinguished between a narrow and broad sense of marriage. The former referred to the conception and education of the children, whereas the latter referred to "the mutual inward molding of husband and wife" and the "determined effort to perfect one another" as "chief reason and purpose" (no. 24).[71]

Many contemporary Catholic books on marriage view it primarily in the categories of interpersonal fulfillment, and the subject of marriage is seen as the individual couple. They argue against the traditional emphasis on procreation and children and they stress the interpersonal love, intimate sexual encounter, and mutual fulfillment of the couple as the meaning and purpose of marriage. Marriage is essentially a profound I-Thou relation between two individuals.[72]

Although this literature contains much of value, it may also risk replicating the individualism of much modern culture.[73] The very experience and phenomenon of marriage go counter, in my opinion, to this view of the married pair as an isolated individual couple. Moreover, insofar as such theologies of marriage make interpersonal affection and love the central component of marriage, they not only mirror the individualism of modern culture, but also, contrary to their very intention, contribute to the breakdown of marriages. For as one historian of divorce has noted, "The logical progress of this trend in modern Western society, where love is conceived as being the single most important consideration in the choice of spouse and in the relationship between husband and wife, is that the loss of sentiments of love on the part of one spouse toward the other (or mutually) is the more likely than ever to be perceived by them as indicative of the breakdown of their marriage."[74]

Rather, along with school and work, marriage socializes individuals beyond their intimate family into a new network of families and friends. Marriage is not just a life partnership, but the bringing together of families, groups of friends, and co-workers. Through children parents often come into greater contact with other families and with the community. Along with offspring comes the heightened responsibility that individuals bear not just for the next generation, but also for society as a whole, and for the earth on which the next generations are to live. Marriage as an encounter with another leads to the acceptance of responsibility for others. To define marriage primarily in terms of an interpersonal relation of two without recognizing the social and communal responsibilities that marriage entails is to offer a reductionistic view of marriage. The communal and social meaning of marriage needs to be explicated, especially in the face of an individualistic overemphasis on personal fulfillment.

The inclusion of this social and communal dimension helps insure an adequate understanding of the purpose of marriage. A theology of marriage must also steer the middle course between a romanticism of identity and a romanticism of difference. The romanticism of identity is present in writings that imagine some sort of mystical union takes place between two persons so that they become one. One popular Roman Catholic book on marriage divides the human person into three levels of being and action: the physical and biological (the animal level), the psychological (the level of human senses and emotions), and the spiritual (the religious level). The author concludes: "To become one biblical body, one whole person, a man and a woman must become one on all three levels."[75] The author does not critically reflect on the connection between his advocacy of the imagery of the couple becoming one body and the mythic belief that at first an androgynous being was created and that marriage brings split sexes back into one body. Fortunately, the author concedes that a husband and wife need not agree about everything on all three levels. One should affirm instead that the goal of mutual perfection should encourage each partner not only to develop self-respect and individuality, but also to achieve autonomy and self-possession. Ideals such as partnership or common good are indeed fine ideals, yet they can become oppressive to individuals. One of the merits of feminist theology and theory has been to demonstrate that too often such ideals as partnership or the common good lead to a sacrifice of the woman's own personal development—a sacrifice often with negative consequence for the wife, but also for the personal maturity of each spouse as well as the marriage itself.

The other romanticism is the glorification of sexual difference. This type of thinking became fully developed first in the Romantic period when the differences between male and female were considered essential differences. The novelty of this development is often overlooked. It has been observed that two basic views of gender or the sexes dominate the last two millennia of Western thought: the one-sex and the two-sex theories.[76] According to the one-sex theory, which dominates classical learning up until the modern Enlightenment, woman is an imperfect version of man. Her anatomy, physiology, and psychic makeup reflect this inferiority. The two-sex theory, which became dominant in nineteenth-century Romanticism, argues that the body determines gender differences and that woman is the opposite of man. She has incommensurably different organs, functions, and feelings. If the one-sex theories were once accepted as reflecting the divine order of creation and were used in order to justify a subordinate position of women within marriage and the exclusion of women from ordination, today two-sex theories are often used in theological analyses of marriage and in the interpretation of the order of creation. Such views of male and female as complementary poles have found popularity in pop-psychology and in a more nuanced fashion in Jungian psychoanalysis.

Within a theological analysis one must acknowledge the degree to which gender roles are social and historical constructions. The inadequacies of the one-sex theory have been widely discussed, but it is important to point out that the two-sex theory is also historically limited and appears increasingly inadequate to deal with gender roles in marriage and in the church. Theoretically, the two-sex theory has been criticized by feminist theologians.[77] Socially, it is inadequate for understanding the roles of male and female in the marriage of a dual-career couple, where both spouses bear mutual responsibility and equal time for the diverse tasks of parenting.

Pastoral-Practical Issues

Two of the most controversial issues within contemporary Roman Catholic teaching on marriage are birth control and divorce. Papal teaching on the nature and purpose of marriage has consistently excluded "artificial means" of birth control. The Council of Trent unambiguously affirmed the indissolubility of sacramental marriage. These issues are usually treated within pastoral and moral theology. Since, however, these issues pertain to the nature and meaning of marriage, it is appropriate here to include a brief sketch of the *status quaestionis* within Roman Catholic theology concerning these issues today.

A sharply controversial topic in contemporary Roman Catholic teaching in regard to marriage is the ethical issue of birth control—an issue related to the meaning and purpose of marriage. Its full treatment can be adequately developed only within a theological discussion of moral and ethical norms. From a systematic theological point of view, a shift has occurred within recent official church teaching. The importance of responsible parenthood together with the significance of mutual love as a primary purpose of marriage have received increasing affirmation within official church teachings. In turn, many Roman Catholic theologians and many married Roman Catholics infer from the shift that responsible parenthood and mutual love would allow various methods of birth control. Many theologians concur with what Cardinal Ratzinger wrote some years ago: "It is clear that the orientation of marriage to 'the procreation of offspring' and the model of 'in accordance with nature' that is closely connected with that view can no longer in its traditional form be the standard for the ethics [of marriage]."[78] At the same time, Ratzinger notes that the ideals of partnership and mutual fulfillment do not suffice as ethical standards. He concludes his analysis of the ethics of marriage in the following way: "We stand firm: One certainly no longer has an easily managed norm that is established from physiology."[79] Instead he argues that there is the responsibility before the totality of love, humanity, the future, the command of God, and the double mystery of death and hope. All of this means that there is "no unambiguity. These responsibilities can require the limitation of offspring, so that this limitation is what is ethically demanded and the opposite is immoral."[80]

Reflections similar to those of Ratzinger have led innumerable theologians to argue that the Catholic church should change its traditional opposition to "artificial means of birth control."[81] At the same time both Pope Paul VI and Pope John Paul II have consistently and unambiguously rejected that implication. When Pope Paul VI issued *Humanae Vitae,* more than 450 North American Roman Catholic theologians protested against this encyclical. Several episcopal conferences responded by recommending that the faithful should indeed attend to papal teaching, but they also suggested that the faithful should form their own conscience; such suggestions seemed to intimate cautiously the possibility of dissenting decision. Many theologians, such as Bernard Lonergan and Karl Rahner, elaborated the foundations for dissent, whereas many ethicists, such as Bernard Häring and Charles Curran, explicitly took dissenting views.[82] At present a crisis exists in the Roman Catholic church. There continues to be an enormous gap between the opinions of the majority of professional theologians and the principled practice of a majority of Roman Catholic married laity within the modern industrialized West, on the one hand, and the unambiguous and legitimate official teaching of recent popes, on the other.[83]

Despite this split and the controversy about the means of birth control, a fundamental unity of vision exists within the Roman Catholic church about the meaning and purpose of marriage. Its vision of marriage as sacrament entails the responsibility of the individual couple not only for themselves, but also for the community and society at large. This responsibility is an essential element of sexuality. It extends from the sphere of the individual family to encompass the future of the community and society. This responsible love, as a sign and a promise, gives marriage a mission to be a sacrament of the presence and power of God's creative love on earth.

The other difficult question is divorce and remarriage. The indissolubility of marriage has remained the ideal of Roman Catholicism from its very beginning. Nevertheless the fact remains that marriages do fail and remarried couples wish to participate actively as Roman Catholics in the church's sacramental life. Thus a pastoral problem of some weight arises out of the tension between the ideal and the actual practice. Despite all good intentions and all good will marriages do break down.[84] Sometimes, the breakdown results from a failure of commitment and trust. At other times, the breakdown results from a set of conditions and events beyond individual responsibility. In some situations, the two should quite clearly never have gotten married and the eventual collapse of the marital relation was obvious. In some circumstances a physical separation is the best for the individuals concerned as well as for the children—though no cases exist where there is not hurt that affects all involved. Proclamation of the ideal of marriage as indissoluble remains an important reminder not only of one's commitments and what one hopes for, but also of the suffering and hurt one seeks to avoid.[85]

In the face of the conflict between the religious ideal and the concrete practice, two pastoral solutions seem to have emerged in practice. One approach is canonical insofar as it involves the expanding of the canonical acknowledgment of the annulment of marriages. This has resulted in a de facto increase in annulments. The new Code of Canon Law expands the traditional grounds for nullity to include lack of understanding, lack of partnership and conjugal love, psychological immaturity, psychopathic and schizophrenic personality, and several other reasons.[86] In addition, an increased leniency in granting annulments has sought to deal in a practical and pastoral way with the breakdown of marriages. Yet in practical terms, this solution de facto renders children into bastards by declaring that a marriage was from the start null and void. Such an approach appears, in my opinion, to go against the spirit, if not the letter, of what was defined at the Council of Trent and affirmed in traditional Roman Catholic teaching. It is with considerable justification that unofficial Vatican statements have criticized the widespread use of this practice.

Another approach within contemporary Roman Catholic theology deals with the problem as a pastoral, practical issue. This approach is pastoral insofar as it highlights overlooked practices in the tradition of the church concerning second marriages. Three theologians now occupying episcopal offices, Walter Kasper, Karl Lehmann, and Cardinal Joseph Ratzinger, have defended this pastoral solution, though in different degrees. This approach points to more lenient practices in the first millennium of Christianity.[87] Origen and Basil mention that in cases where persons had become divorced because of adultery and then remarried, church leaders had allowed them to participate in the eucharist. Ambrosiaster and Augustine also made reference to this practice. In the beginning of the medieval period, several church synods and various penitential books permitted a second marriage even when the first partner was still alive. The Eastern church tolerated the possibility of second marriage, whereas the Western church as a result of Gratian's Decree established a stricter practice.

Diverse proposals have emerged from this historical data. Whereas some advocate that the Roman Catholic church should change its position and others advocate no change, the middle position takes a pastoral approach that still affirms the Council of Trent's teaching on marriage and yet suggests a change in pastoral practice.[88] Kasper writes:

> The Church should act in accordance with God's way of acting and for this reason, it should be possible to admit divorced persons who have remarried to the sacraments on three conditions: 1) when they are sorry for their guilt and have made amends for it as well as they can; 2) when everything humanly possible has been done to achieve reconciliation with the first partner; and 3) when the second marriage has become a morally binding union that cannot be dissolved without causing fresh injustice.[89]

Kasper's solution seeks to be faithful to traditional teaching as well as to pastoral practice. Personally, I would modify his formulation of the first condition. Obviously, there should be sorrow over a failed marriage and one should never consider oneself totally guiltless. Nevertheless, there are many situations where the failure of the first marriage results from situations and conditions for which an individual may not be primarily responsible. To admit this situation and to deal honestly with the issue of second marriages is not to reject what marriage is. To quote Karl Lehmann, "The toleration of a second marriage and the associated admission to the sacraments should in no way place in question the obligatory basic form of indissoluble marriage."[90]

One might even state that in face of the fragility of marriage, the celebration of the sacrament of marriage gives visible manifestation to the unconditionality of love as present in the conditions of human existence. The Roman Catholic church's affirmation of the indissolubility of marriage expresses the unconditionality of the commitment to a new community. It is the nature of solidarity, love, and commitment to be resolute, steadfast, and unreserved. To say that I am committed to you in solidarity on the condition that you stay healthy, wealthy, beautiful, and wise is absurd. Human commitment and solidarity have an unconditional, unreserved, transcending dimension. This dimension, which is symbolized in the sacrament of marriage, expresses the Christian faith in a transcendent hope and trust.

Such an ideal is often frightening, for we know too often of our own fragility and weaknesses. We know that marriages too often break down. We know that love and commitment are not certainties upon which we can rely. The mutual commitment in marriage is as much a hope as a faith or trust. It parallels in many ways our faith in God—an experience not of certainty, but of hope. It is this hope that the Catholic church expresses through its teaching and through its celebration of marriage as a sacrament.

For Further Reading

Barth, Karl. *The Doctrine of Creation.* Vol. 3, pt. 4 of *Church Dogmatics.* Edinburgh: T and T Clark, 1961, 116–323.
An influential presentation by a major Protestant theologian. Barth develops the nature of marriage as a life partnership. See the reprint of part of this text in *On Marriage* (Philadelphia: Fortress Press, 1968).

Brundage, James A. *Law, Sex, and Christian Society in Medieval Europe.* Chicago: University of Chicago Press, 1987.
Detailed historical research on neglected aspects of medieval law and practice.

Cahill, Lisa. *Between the Sexes: Foundations for a Christian Ethics of Sexuality.* Philadelphia: Fortress Press, 1985.
   An exposition of marriage that takes into account recent developments in biblical studies, gender studies, and anthropology. The work was written by a leading Roman Catholic ethicist.

Häring, Bernard. *Marriage in the Modern World.* Westminster, Md.: Newman Press, 1965.
   Somewhat dated but still provides an invaluable treatment of marriage with an emphasis on moral, pastoral, and social issues. Häring is a leading Roman Catholic moral theologian.

Kasper, Walter. *Theology of Christian Marriage.* New York: Crossroad, 1983.
   Offers a brief theology of marriage with special consideration to biblical and pastoral themes.

Kosnick, Anthony, et al. *Human Sexuality: New Directions in American Catholic Thought.* New York: Paulist, 1977.
   A controversial study commissioned and "received" (that is accepted but not approved) by the Catholic Theological Society of America.

Lawler, Michael G. *Secular Marriage, Christian Sacrament.* Mystic, Conn.: Twenty-Third Publications, 1985.
   Popular introduction to marriage with a strong personalist emphasis.

Mackin, Theodore. *The Marital Sacrament.* New York: Paulist, 1989.
   A comprehensive historical survey of the theological understanding of marriage from biblical to contemporary writings. Excellent bibliographies. This volume updates and completes a trilogy of volumes on marriage, the others being *What is Marriage?* (1982) and *Divorce and Remarriage* (1984).

Phillips, Roderick. *Putting Asunder: A History of Divorce in Western Society.* New York: Cambridge University Press, 1988.
   A comprehensive historical and sociological survey of divorce in the West that covers religious beliefs, legal regulations, and social practice.

Rahner, Karl. "Marriage as a Sacrament." In *Theological Investigations.* New York: Crossroad, 1973, 10:199–221.
   Develops Rahner's fundamental notions of marriage as a sacrament with reference to his ecclesial understanding of the sacraments.

Roberts, William P., ed. *Commitment to Partnership: Explorations of the Theology of Marriage.* New York: Paulist Press, 1987.
   A collection of essays by diverse authors. Offers distinct contemporary perspectives (exegetical, ethical, theological, and pastoral) on the nature of marriage.

Schillebeeckx, Edward. *Marriage: Secular Reality and Saving Mystery.* New York: Sheed and Ward, 1965.
   Two volumes have been printed together in the American edition. The first volume deals with the biblical writings; the second with marriage in the history of theology. Although a promised third volume has not appeared, Schillebeeckx's systematic theology of the sacraments is applied here in a theology of marriage.

Whitehead, James, and Evelyn Whitehead. *Marrying Well: Stages on the Journey of Christian Marriage.* New York: Doubleday, 1984.
   An important treatment of marriage that is highly recommended for counselors. Reflects on the relation between marriage and maturation.

Whitehead, James, and Evelyn Whitehead. *A Sense of Sexuality: Christian Love and Intimacy.* New York: Doubleday, 1989.
   Well-written with a thorough development of the pastoral and psychological dimensions of sexuality. Deals with important topics that are often neglected in theological treatments, such as intimacy, pleasure, and sexual experience.

NOTES

1. David B. Wilson, "Is Marriage Obsolete?" *The Boston Globe*, Sunday, August 6, 1989, sec. A.
2. Joseph Ratzinger, "Zur Theologie der Ehe," *Theologische Quartalschrift* 149 (1969) 53–74, here 54. See also Ratzinger's expositions of sacraments in general, *Die sakramentale Begründung christlicher Existenz* (Friesing: Kyrios Verlag, 1973), and *Zum Begriff des Sakraments*, Eichstätter Hochschulreden, vol. 13 (Munich: Minerva, 1979).
3. Ratzinger, "Zur Theologie der Ehe," 54.
4. Ibid., 53.
5. Phyllis Bird, "'Male and Female He Created Them': Gen. 1:27b in the Context of the Priestly Account of Creation," *Harvard Theological Review* 74 (1981) 129–59, here 155. Bird's analysis counters Karl Barth's influential analysis of the *imago* passage; see Karl Barth, *Church Dogmatics* (Edinburgh: T and T Clark, 1958), 3/1:183–206.
6. Phyllis Trible, *God and the Rhetoric of Sexuality* (Philadelphia: Fortress Press, 1978).
7. See Elaine Pagels, *Adam, Eve, and the Serpent* (New York: Random House, 1988).
8. See the critical analysis by T. Deborah Setel, "Prophets and Pornography: Female Sexual Imagery," in Letty M. Russell, ed., *Feminist Interpretation of the Bible* (Philadelphia: Westminster Press, 1985).
9. For a social analysis of the Jesus movement, see Gerd Theissen, *Sociology of Early Christianity* (Philadelphia: Fortress Press, 1978).
10. For general Roman Catholic exegetical treatments, see Rudolf Pesch, *Freie Treue: Die Christen und die Ehescheidung* (Freiburg: Herder, 1971); Rudolf Schnackenburg. "Die Ehe nach der Weisungen Jesus und dem Verständnis der Urkirche," in Franz Henrich and Volker Eid, eds., *Ehe und Ehescheidung*, Münchener Akademie Schriften, vol. 59 (Munich: Kösel, 1972), 11–34.
11. Paul Hoffmann, "Jesus' Saying about Divorce and Its Interpretation in the New Testament Tradition," in Franz Böckle, ed., *The Future of Marriage as an Institution* (entire issue of *Concilium* 55 [New York: Herder and Herder, 1970]: 51–66).
12. Bruce Malina, *The New Testament World: Insights from Cultural Anthropology* (Atlanta: John Knox Press, 1981), 118–21.
13. Joseph Fitzmyer, "The Matthean Divorce Texts and Some New Palestinian Evidence," *Theological Studies* 37 (1976) 197–226; reprinted in *To Advance the Gospel* (New York: Crossroad, 1981) 79–111.
14. See Dieter Luhrmann, "Eheverständnis und Eheseelsorge im Neuen Testament," in Günther Gassmann, ed., *Ehe, Institution im Wandel* (Hamburg: Lutherische Verlagshaus, 1979) 67–81.
15. See Elisabeth Schüssler Fiorenza, *In Memory of Her* (New York: Crossroad, 1983) 140–45.
16. Kurt Niederwimmer, *Askese und Mysterium: Über Ehe, Ehescheidung und Eheverzicht in den Anfängen des christlichen Glaubens*, Forschungen zur Religion und Literatur des Alten und Neuen Testaments, no. 113 (Göttingen: Vandenhoeck, 1975) 12–41.
17. See Pesch, *Freie Treue*, 10–60.
18. Rudolf Schnackenburg, *Die sittliche Botschaft des Neuen Testaments* (Freiburg: Herder, 1986), 1: 148–53.
19. Jean Bonsirven, *Le Divorce dans le Nouveau Testament* (Paris: Desclée, 1948), and Joseph Fitzmyer, *To Advance*, 79–111.
20. Carlo Marruci, *Parole di Gesù sul divorzio* (Brescia: Morcelliana, 1982); Gerhard Schneider, "Jesu Wort über die Ehescheidung in der Überlieferung des Neuen Testaments," *Trierer theologische Zeitschrift* 80 (1971) 65–87. See also the works of Paul Hoffmann, Rudolf Pesch, and Rudolf Schnackenburg quoted above. In *Die sittliche Botschaft*, Schnackenburg retracts his earlier advocacy of the first interpretation.
21. Niederwimmer, *Askese und Mysterium*, 42–124. Niederwimmer shows the ascetic, christological, and eschatological basis for such a priority in early Christianity.
22. See Schüssler Fiorenza, *In Memory of Her*, 160–204.
23. Most recently, Hans Urs von Balthasar, *Theologik* (Einsiedeln: Johannes Verlag, 1987), 3:317–18.
24. Elisabeth Schüssler Fiorenza, *Bread Not Stone* (Boston: Beacon Press, 1984). For a more popularly written version, see her "Marriage and Discipleship," *The Bible Today* 102 (April 1979) 2027–33.

25. Walter Kasper, *Theology of Christian Marriage* (New York: Crossroad, 1983) 30.

26. For a survey of the views on marriage in the ancient church, see Alfred Niebergall, *Ehe und Eheschliessung in der Bibel und in der Geschichte der alten Kirche* (Marburg: N. G. Elwert, 1985) 101–253.

27. Charles Couturier,"'Sacramentum' et 'Mysterium' dans l'ouvre de Saint Augustin," in *Études Augustiniennes,* Théologie, vol. 28 (Paris: Aubier, 1953) 161–332.

28. Augustine, *The Good of Marriage,* in Saint Augustine, *Treatises on Marriage and Other Subjects,* Fathers of the Church, vol. 15 (New York: Fathers of the Church, 1955) 9–51.

29. Ibid., chap. 18: "Just as the many wives of the ancient fathers signified our future churches of all races subject to one man-Christ, so our bishop, a man of one wife, signifies the unity of all nations subject to the one man-Christ."

30. Augustine often argues against several fronts. It is in his writings against the Manicheans that his most positive evaluations of marriage are made.

31. Augustine, *The Good of Marriage* chap. 3.

32. See Margaret Miles, *Augustine on the Body* (Missoula, Mont.: Scholars Press, 1979).

33. For a discussion of this development, see Edward Schillebeeckx, *Marriage: Secular Reality and Saving Mystery* (New York: Sheed and Ward, 1965) 302–43.

34. For a description of the medieval controversies, see James A. Brundage, *Law, Sex, and Christian Society in Medieval Europe* (Chicago: University of Chicago Press, 1987).

35. See Hugh of Saint Victor *De Beatae Mariae Virginis Virginitate,* written between 1131 and 1141. His *De Institutione Sacramentorum* treats of marriage in book 2, 11: *De Sacramento Conjugii.* See Roy J. Defarrari, ed., *Hugh of St. Victor: On the Sacraments of the Christian Faith* (Cambridge: Medieval Academy of America, 1951). For a general treatment of diverse monastic views of marriage, see Jean Leclercq, *Monks on Marriage: A Twelfth-Century View* (New York: Seabury Press, 1982); for a broader historical survey see Georges Duby, *Medieval Marriage: Two Models from Twelfth-Century France* (Baltimore: John Hopkins Press, 1978).

36. Although medieval marriages were first of all social and economic relationships, one should not underestimate the importance of affective criteria in the choice of partners. See David Herlihy, "The Making of the Medieval Family: Symmetry, Structure and Sentiment," *Journal of Family History* 8 (1983) 116–30.

37. Richard of Saint Victor, *Selected Writings on Contemplation* (New York: Harper and Brothers, n.d.) 215.

38. See Kari Elisabeth Borresen, *Subordination and Equivalence: The Nature and Role of Woman in Augustine and Thomas Aquinas,* rev. ed., (Washington, D.C.: University Press of America, 1981).

39. Thomas Aquinas, *Summa Theologiae* 1, q. 98. For a defense of Thomas's view of human sexuality, see Otto Hermann Pesch, *Thomas von Aquin: Grenze und Grösse mittelalterlicher Theologie* (Mainz: Matthias-Grünewald, 1988) 254–56, and in regard to women, 20–227. See also Lisa Sowle Cahill, *Between the Sexes: Foundations for a Christian Ethics of Sexuality* (Philadelphia: Fortress Press, 1985), 105–22.

40. Thomas Aquinas, *Summa Contra Gentiles* 3.123.6 (trans. Vernon J. Bourke [New York: Image Books, 1956]).

41. Ratzinger, "Zur Theologie der Ehe," 59.

42. Martin Luther, "The Babylonian Captivity of the Church," in Theodore G. Tappert, ed., *Selected Writings of Martin Luther, 1517–1520,* vol. 1 (Philadelphia: Fortress Press, 1967); for the section on marriage, see 444–58. See also "A Sermon on the Estate of Marriage," in Timothy F. Lull, ed., *Martin Luther's Basic Theological Writings* (Minneapolis: Augsburg Fortress Press, 1989), 630–37, where Luther develops a complementary idea of marriage as an estate.

43. Denzinger-Schönmetzer, *Enchiridion Symbolorum* (hereafter DS), 1807; for literature on the Council of Trent, see Hubert Jedin, "Die Unauflöslichkeit der Ehe nach dem Konzil von Trient," in Klaus Reinhardt and Hubert Jedin, *Ehe-Sakrament in der Kirche des Herrn,* Ehe in Geschichte und Gegenwart, vol. 2 (Berlin: Morus, 1971) 61–135; Piet Fransen, "Divorce on the Ground of Adultery—The Council of Trent (1563)," in Böckle, ed., *The Future of Marriage as an Institution,* 89–100; Peter J. Huizing, "La dissolution du mariage depuis le Concile de Trent," *Revue de Droit Canonique* 21 (1971) 127–45.

44. Kasper, *Theology,* 61

45. See Karl Lehmann, *Gegenwart des Glaubens* (Mainz: Matthias-Grünewald, 1974) 274–308, here 285. Lehmann relies on the interpretations of Piet Fransen (in Böckle, ed., *The Future of Marriage as an Institution*, 89–100) and Joseph Ratzinger, "Zur Frage nach der Unauflöslichkeit der Ehe," in Henrich and Eid, eds., *Ehe und Ehescheidung*, 35–56, esp. 49ff.

46. Kasper, *Theology*, 62.

47. See Benedictine Monks of Solesmes, eds., *Papal Teaching: Matrimony*, trans. Michael J. Byrnes (Boston: St. Paul's Editions, 1963).

48. The English translation of the encyclical is in Benedictine Monks of Solesmes, eds., *Papal Teaching*, 219–21.

49. For a collection of Pius XII's discourses, see ibid., 301–506.

50. For an exposition of the teaching of *Gaudium et Spes* on marriage, see Joseph A. Selling, "A Closer Look at the Doctrine of Gaudium et Spes on Marriage and the Family," *Bijdragen* 43 (1982) 30–48, and idem, "Twenty Significant Points in the Theology of Marriage and Family Present in the Teaching of Gaudium et Spes," *Bijdragen* 43 (1982) 412–41.

51. John Paul II's Apostolic Exhortation on the Family is published with commentaries in Michael J. Wrenn, ed., *Pope John Paul II and Family* (Chicago: Franciscan Herald Press, 1983). For the "Theology of the Body" series, see vol. 3 of *Reflections on Humanae Vitae: Conjugal Morality and Spirituality* (Boston: Daughters of St. Paul, 1983).

52. For a critical analysis and interpretation, see Lisa Sowle Cahill, "Community and Couple: Parameters of Marital Commitment in Catholic Tradition," in William P. Roberts, ed., *Commitment to Partnership: Explorations of the Theology of Marriage* (New York: Paulist Press, 1987), 81–101. For a different perspective that defends papal teaching, see Richard M. Hogan and John M. LeVoir, *Covenant of Love: Pope John Paul II on Sexuality, Marriage, and Family in the Modern World* (Garden City, N.Y.: Doubleday and Co., 1985).

53. Jan Grootaers and Joseph Selling, eds., *The 1980 Synod of Bishops "On the Role of the Family": An Exposition of the Event and an Analysis of Its Texts*, Bibliotheca Ephemeridum theologicarum Lovaniensum, 64 (Louvain: University of Louvain Press, 1983); and International Theological Commission, "Propositions on the Doctrine of Christian Marriage," *Origins* (September 28, 1978) 235–39.

54. Matthias Scheeben, *The Mysteries of Christianity* (St. Louis: B. Herder, 1946), chap. 21.

55. Gustav Martelet, "Mariage, amour et sacrement," *Nouvelle Revue Théologique* 85 (1953) 577–97; Henri Rondet, *Introduction à l'étude de la théologie du mariage* (Paris: Lethielleux, 1960).

56. Piet Schoonenberg, "Marriage in the Perspective of the History of Salvation," in his *God's World in the Making* (Techny, Ill.: Divine Word Publications, 1964) 106–34.

57. Schillebeeckx, *Marriage*, 384.

58. Karl Rahner, "Marriage as a Sacrament," in *Theological Investigations* (New York: Crossroad, 1973), 10:191–221. For his basic understanding of sacraments, see *The Church and the Sacraments* (New York: Herder and Herder, 1963).

59. Rahner, "Marriage as a Sacrament," 209.

60. Ibid., 212.

61. Whereas Rahner argues that the subordination of wife to husband depicted in Ephesians is time-conditioned in that it "belonged to *that period alone*" (ibid., 221), von Balthasar argues for its relevance (*Theologik*, 3:318).

62. For example, Friar Cherubino of Ciena (ca. 1450–81) writes that if pleasant words do not work, "scold her sharply, bully, and terrify her. And if this still does not work . . . take up a stick and beat her soundly, for it is better to punish the body and correct the soul than to damage the soul and correct the body. . . ." Quoted in William J. Hawser, *Differences in Relative Resources: Familial Power and Abuse* (Palo Alto, Calif.: Mayfield, 1982) 8. A customary law in thirteenth-century France stated: "It is licit for the man to beat his wife, without bringing about the death or disablement, when she refuses her husband anything." Quoted in Jean-Louis Flandrin, *Families in Former Times: Kinship, Household, and Sexuality* (New York: Cambridge University Press, 1979), 123. See also Edward Shorter, *A History of Women's Bodies* (New York: Basic Books, 1982).

63. Walter Kasper and Gerhard Sauter, *Kirche—Ort des Geistes* (Freiburg: Herder, 1976).

64. Walter Kasper, *Glaube und Geschichte* (Mainz: Matthias-Grünewald, 1970) 294.

65. For an interpretation of the post-Easter emergence of the church in relation to the life-praxis of Jesus and of the earliest Christian proclamation of God's power in relation to Jesus, see Francis Schüssler Fiorenza, *Foundational Theology: Jesus and the Church* (New York: Crossroad, 1984) 3–192.

66. See Stanley Jeyariaja Tambiah, *Magic, Science and Religion and the Scope of Rationality* (New York: Cambridge University Press, 1990) 84–110.

67. Louis-Marie Chauvet, *Symbole et sacrement: Une relecture sacramentelle de l'existence chrétienne*, Cogitatio Fidei, vol. 144 (Paris: Éditions du Cerf, 1988). See also his earlier work, *Du symbolique au symbole: Essai sur les sacrements* (Paris: Éditions du Cerf, 1979).

68. Edward Shorter and Lawrence Stone argue that it was in the eighteenth century that a shift took place from marriages based on interest to those based on affection and romantic love. See Lawrence Stone, *Family, Sex, and Marriage in England: 1500–1800* (New York: Harper, 1977), and Edward Shorter, *The Making of the Modern Family* (New York: Basic Books, 1975). A nuanced correction of this view is offered by Herman R. Lantz, "Romantic Love in the Pre-modern Period: A Sociological Commentary," *Journal of Social History* 15 (1982) 349–70. Lantz points to the existence of romantic love further back in Western history, but sees its spread as a part of the process of modernization.

69. Compare Ernest W. Burgess, et al., *The Family: From Traditional to Companionship* (New York: Van Nostrand, 1971); Niklas Luhmann, *Love as Passion: The Codification of Intimacy* (London: Polity Press, 1986); George Levinger and Harold L. Raush, *Close Relationships: Perspectives on the Meaning of Intimacy* (Amherst: University of Massachusetts Press, 1977).

70. For some recent literature, see Mark Cook and Glenn Wilson, eds., *Love and Attraction: An International Conference* (Oxford: Clarendon, 1979).

71. See Benedictine Monks of Solesmes, eds., *Papal Teaching*; DS 2232.

72. Examples of the personalist direction are: Dietrich von Hildebrand, *Marriage* (London: Longman, Green and Co., 1942), and Herbert Doms, *The Meaning of Marriage* (London: Sheed and Ward, 1939). More recently, Theodore Mackin, *The Marital Sacrament* (New York: Paulist, 1989). Mackin polemicizes against the traditional understanding of marriage as a contract at a time when feminist theory is pointing to the importance of contracts within marriage to underscore the mutual responsibilities and obligations in regard to the common tasks that a couple face. See also Michael G. Lawler, *Secular Marriage, Christian Sacrament* (Mystic, Conn.: Twenty-Third Publications, 1985); Lenore J. Weitzman, *The Marriage Contract: Spouses, Lovers, and the Law* (New York: Free Press, 1981).

73. For criticism of this individualism in relation to marriage, see Robert N. Bellah, et al., *Habits of the Heart: Individualism and Commitment in American Life* (New York: Harper and Row, 1985) 85–112.

74. Roderick Phillips, *Putting Asunder: A History of Divorce in Western Society* (New York: Cambridge University Press, 1988), 359.

75. Lawler, *Secular Marriage*, 71.

76. Thomas Laqeur, *Making Sex: Body and Gender from the Greeks to Freud* (Cambridge: Harvard University Press, 1990).

77. I have been especially influenced by Elisabeth Schüssler's critique of Gertrude LeFort's advocacy of duality; see Elisabeth Schüssler, *Der Vergessene Partner* (Düsseldorf: Patmos, 1964).

78. Ratzinger, "Zur Theologie der Ehe," 70; my translation here and following.

79. Ibid., 71.

80. Ibid.

81. For an invaluable historical survey, see John Noonan, *Contraception*, 2d ed. (Cambridge: Harvard University Press, 1988).

82. Karl Rahner, "On the Encyclical '*Humanae Vitae*,'" in *Theological Investigations* (New York: Crossroad, 1974), 11:263–87. See also his "Magisterium and Theology," in *Theological Investigations* (New York: Crossroad, 1983), 18:54–73. An important early article on the philosophical presuppositions of the debate was Bernard Lonergan's "Finality, Love, Marriage," in his *Collection* (New York: Herder and Herder, 1967), 16–53. See essays by diverse theologians in Charles E. Curran, ed., *Contraception: Authority and Dissent* (New York: Herder and Herder, 1969).

83. For a discussion of the reception of *Humanae Vitae*, see Joseph Komonchak, "*Humanae Vitae* and Its Reception: Ecclesiological Reflections," *Theological Studies* 39 (1978) 221–57.

84. For the causes of the breakdown of marriages as well as of divorce (two distinct issues), there is much recent literature. For a survey of recent research, see Gay C. Kitson and Helen J. Raschke, "Divorce Research: What We Know; What We Need to Know," *Journal of Divorce* 4 (1981): 1–37; George Levinger and Oliver C. Moles, eds., *Divorce and Separation: Contexts, Causes and Consequences* (New York: Basic Books, 1979); Stan L. Albrecht, et al., *Divorce and Remarriage: Problems, Adaptations and Adjustments* (Westport, Conn.: Greenwood Press, 1983); and Barbara Thornes and Jean Collard, *Who Divorces* (London: Routledge and Kegan Paul, 1979).

85. It should still be noted that despite the increase in the number of divorces in the West in the twentieth century, the majority of marriages do not end in divorce. Moreover, Robert H. Lauer and Jeanette C. Lauer ("Factors in Long-Term Marriages," *Journal of Family Issues* 7 [1986]: 382–90) have noted that in marriages lasting more than fifteen years, 83 percent of both partners consider themselves happily married.

86. As an example of such practical recommendations, see Joseph P. Zwack, *Annulment* (New York: Harper, 1983). For a study of marriage and the new code, see Ladislaus Orsy, *Marriage in Canon Law* (Wilmington, Del.: Glazier, 1986).

87. Henri Crouzel, *L'Église primitive face au divorce, du premier au cinquième siècle*, Théologie historique, vol. 13 (Paris: Beauchesne, 1971). For corrections and modifications of Crouzel's arguments, see Peter Stockmeier, "Scheidung und Wiederverheiratung im Neuen Testament," *Theologische Quartalschrift* 151 (1971): 28–38.

88. See Joseph Ratzinger, "Zur Frage nach der Unauflöslichkeit der Ehe," 35–56.

89. Kasper, *Theology*, 70.

90. Lehmann, *Gegenwart des Glaubens*, 292 (my translation).

15

The Sacramental Dignity of Marriage

Walter Kasper

1. Its Foundation in the History of Salvation: The Unity of Creation and Redemption

(i) Its Basis in Creation

The attitude of the Old Testament authors towards human sexuality, love between man and woman, and marriage and the begetting of children, is extremely open, frank, and positive. The Song of Solomon, for example, is a celebration of human love, which is presented as an experience of great happiness and fulfillment. The experience is certainly not seen in terms of naive sexual euphoria. The biblical authors were certainly also aware of the other aspects of human sexuality—its temptations and brokenness, the pain of giving birth, the oppression of woman by man, unfaithfulness and guilt. But sexuality is never fundamentally devalued or defamed in the Old Testament. The sexual difference between man and woman and their sexual encounter with each other are presented as belonging to the order of creation and as part of God's plan. Of God's creation it is said that "it was very good" (Gen. 1:31), and this also applies to the relationship between man and woman.

This relationship is so fundamental in the Bible that it forms part of the theological definition of humanity's being that is provided in Genesis, when people are described as having been made in God's image: "So God created man in his own image . . . male and female he created them" (Gen. 1:27)[1] The sexual difference clearly forms an essential part of humanity's created being. Humanity as such does not exist. It exists only as man and woman. It is only in togetherness that human existence can be fulfilled in the fully human sense. This mystery between man and woman is so deep that the covenant between man and woman is, in the Bible, the image and likeness of God's covenant with man and the reproduction of his love, faithfulness and creative power. In this way, an almost inestimable value is given to marriage, and hostility between the sexes is excluded from the relationship.

Despite the fact that the Bible raises human sexuality and the relationship between man and woman to such a high level, it never deifies sex or erotic love in the way that it was deified in the other religions of the ancient Near East. On the contrary, this sacralization and deification of sexuality was regarded by the biblical authors as typically pagan and was therefore rejected by them. This desacralization is based on the Old Testament faith in creation and the consequent distinction made between the creator and the creature. It is only if people have this natural or rather creaturely view of sexuality that they can be inwardly free and responsible for themselves in this sphere as in others. As factors in human creation, sexuality and marriage never have an ultimate value. They can only have a penultimate value because, in their created goodness and beauty, they point to something beyond themselves. Like other aspects of creation, they do not have their basis or their aim in themselves. For this reason, people cannot find ultimate fulfillment in a purely horizontal love relationship. The finite and limited love between man and woman is rather the image of an unconditioned and definitive acceptance of man that can only come from God. Both in its greatness and in its limitations, then, marriage is an actual form of human hope of salvation. It is therefore possible to speak, in this sense, of a natural sacrament of marriage, as indeed the Church's tradition does.

(ii) Instituted by Jesus Christ?

In the Old Testament, the covenant between man and woman becomes the "image and likeness" of the covenant between God and man (see, for example, Hos. 1, 3; Jer. 2, 3, 31; Ezek. 16, 23; Isa. 54, 62). Marriage, then, is the grammar that God uses to express his love and faithfulness. This covenant between God and humanity is realized in a definitive and unsurpassable way in Jesus Christ, who is in person God's covenant with human beings. He is the bridegroom of God's people of the new covenant (see Mark 2:19). It is through him that we are definitively invited to share the wedding feast in the kingdom of God (see Matt. 22:2ff). Our understanding of marriage as a sacrament is based above all on this understanding of marriage as a sign of God's covenant.[2] The sacramental nature of marriage cannot be proved by using individual words of institution. It is more important to show that marriage is sacramental because it is fundamentally related to the saving work of Jesus Christ.

Jesus' attitude towards marriage[3] is expressed most clearly in Mark 10:2–9. In a controversy with the pharisees, Jesus is here confronted with the question as to whether it is lawful for a man to release his wife. The controversy as a whole is about the interpretation of Deuteronomy 24:1, which is disputed by the Jews. Jesus does not become involved in the casuistry of the controversy, but raises the whole matter to a higher level and points to the original order of God's creation. His conclusion is that "what God has joined together, let no man put asunder."

If this statement is viewed simply from the outside, it points to a strengthening on Jesus' part of the law. If, however, we consider it within the whole context of Jesus' preaching and teaching, it is clear that the level of the law as such is completely transcended. Like the prophets, Jesus was aware of human hardness of heart. It is only when God gives people a "new heart" (see Jer. 31:33) that they are capable of living in accordance with God's will. This messianic expectation was fulfilled in Jesus' proclamation of the closeness of the eschatological kingdom of God. It would therefore be wrong to understand his pronouncement about marriage as a legal statement. It is above all a prophetic and messianic statement, an affirmation of salvation and grace. In Jesus' proclamation, then, marriage is seen both as part of the original order of creation and as an aspect of the order of salvation of God in his kingdom of love and faithfulness.

The coming of the kingdom of God is closely linked to the coming of Jesus. He is the new Moses who, with his full authority, goes back beyond the words of Moses and surpasses them eschatologically. He is the coming of the kingdom of God in person. This aspect of his appearance was developed in the early communities of the Church after the Easter event, and the Christological link with marriage was also expressed at a relatively early period in the history of Christianity. There is a reference to this in the first letter to the Corinthians, where Paul says that Christians should marry "in the Lord" (1 Cor. 7:39). It is clear from this and other references that marriage is included in humanity's new being in Christ that is based on baptism. This is why marriage and family life feature again and again in the household codes of the New Testament as a place where Christian faith proves its value in a very special way. In practice, the partners in Christian marriage behave in such a way towards each other that their conduct is always oriented towards the obedience, love, faithfulness and self-giving of Christ for his church. In this sense, marriage is a Christian emergency because it is in it that "being of the mind of Christ" (Phil. 2:5) in obedience, love and faithfulness is made a reality here and now in a very special way (see, for example, Col. 3:18ff; 1 Pet. 3:1–7; 1 Tim. 2:8–15; Titus 2:1–6).

The most important of these household codes for our purpose is found in Ephesians 5:21–33.[4] In this text, the covenant between man and wife in marriage is seen as the image of the covenant between Christ and the Church. The passage closes with the words: "This is a great mystery (*mysterion*) and I take it to mean Christ and the Church." A sacramental interpretation of this passage was suggested in the later tradition of the Church by the translation in the Vulgate of the Greek concept of *mysterion* by the Latin word *sacramentum*. Most scholars are agreed now, however, that the later idea of sacrament should not be presupposed in this biblical periscope. Three different interpretations have been suggested in recent years and these can be summarized as follows. The word *mysterion* can be understood as the hidden meaning of the passage quoted (Gen. 2:24). It can be seen as referring to marriage itself. Thirdly, it can be regarded as pointing to the connection between Christ and his Church. It is certainly this last interpretation that is most fully in accordance with the linguistic usage of the Pauline and the Deutero-Pauline letters, since, in those writings, *mysterion* always points to God's eternal plan of salvation and his saving will that became a historical reality in Jesus Christ and a present reality in the Church. It is within this all-embracing reality of salvation that marriage is included.

Marriage, then, is in its own way a form by means of which God's eternal love and faithfulness, revealed in Jesus Christ, are made historically present. The love and faithfulness existing between Christ and his Church is therefore not simply an image or example of marriage, nor is the self-giving of man and wife in marriage an image and likeness of Christ's giving of himself to the Church. The love that exists between man and wife is rather a sign that makes the reality present, in other words, an epiphany of the love and faithfulness of God that was given once and for all time in Jesus Christ and is made present in the Church. In this sense, it is possible to see that the sacramental nature of marriage is indicated in Ephesians 5:32, as did the Council of Trent.[5]

It is, however, hardly possible to base the sacramentality of marriage exclusively on a few isolated passages in Scripture. It is only possible to do this by applying the argument of convergence. The sacramentality of marriage emerges from Ephesians 5:21ff above all on the basis of a number of suppositions. These are "that the total self-giving of the person that takes place in marriage implies a relationship with God as the ground and the aim of this self-giving; that Christ included marriage in the Christian order; that the relationship involved in marriage is different from other relationships between human beings; that, wherever fundamental signs that are intimately connected with the life of Christians and the Church exist and these point to the reality of grace, such signs cannot, within the new covenant, be empty and meaningless; that every community of Christians in Christ includes a making present of Christ and therefore of the Church (see Matt. 18:20), with the result that this can also be said especially of the smallest community in Christ, namely marriage. It is possible to understand the sacramental nature of marriage and its historical institution on the basis of these presuppositions. Christ instituted the sacrament by establishing the new covenant as an eternal sign of God's grace and by giving that sign a sacramental reality. This sacramental sign represents and expresses the unity of Christ and the Church."[6]

(iii) The Development of Marriage as a Sacrament in the Tradition of the Church

It was not until relatively late in the history of the Church that marriage was declared to be a sacrament. From that time, that is the twelfth century, onwards, explicit statements were made by the Church's teaching office.[7] We cannot, of course, enter into details here about this complicated historical process. It should, however, be clear that the fact that marriage was not until that time explicitly regarded as a sacrament did not mean that it was on the contrary seen, until about the twelfth century, simply as a secular reality and only later sacralized. The very opposite is true. The whole of reality, including marriage, was regarded almost without question as sacral, and it was only as a result of the long and difficult controversies that took place in the eleventh and twelfth centuries, following the Gregorian reform of the Church, that the latter became free from involvement in the dynastic structure and political order of the Carolingian and Ottonian empire and its overemphasis of the sacral nature of reality. It was at this time that the process of secularization first began, and it was only after this secular view of reality had become firmly established that individual signs and rites could be consciously presented as sacraments. The conscious appreciation of marriage as a sacrament, then, presupposes its desacralization and its recognition as a reality of creation. This also applies to marriage in a very special sense. In each sacrament, after all, an element of the world (water, bread, wine, for example) becomes an effective sign of salvation. Whereas birth, however, is not baptism, marriage as such is really a making present of God's love and faithfulness in Jesus Christ for a baptized Christian. Among baptized Christians, then, marriage as a reality of creation is at once and at the same time a sacrament of Christ.

This close connection between the order of creation and the order of redemption in Christian marriage is of importance in our assessment of the controversy between Catholicism and Protestantism about the sacramental nature of marriage.[8] Luther called marriage a "worldly affair"[9] and an "external and worldly thing."[10] He did not, however, mean by these statements that marriage was a purely profane reality, since, only a few lines further on, he called marriage "God's work and commandment," a holy state worthy of God's blessing.[11] He was only concerned to stress the fact that marriage was part, not of the order of salvation, but of the order of creation.[12] The controversy about the sacramentality of marriage, then, was not a dispute about an isolated statement about faith, but a far-reaching debate about the fundamental problem of the relationship between the order of creation and the order of redemption and the relationship between the Church and the world. The whole Catholic-Protestant controversy, which was fundamentally about human justification by God, was concentrated here in one concrete and individual question, that of the sacramentality of marriage. This question is of great contemporary importance because the increasing numbers of marriages between Catholics and Protestants today make it necessary for us to strive towards a greater degree of agreement about this central point of controversy and eventually to find a solution to the problem of the sacramentality of marriage. In the meantime, such marriages present us with a pressing pastoral need which can only be satisfied by reaching a common understanding.

Many people find it difficult to understand marriage as a sacrament and think of it as a mystification, a sacralization, a spiritualization or an idealization of marriage, of a kind that can hardly be expressed in the day-to-day experience of marriage. This giving of a higher, supernatural and even false value to marriage (which is often coupled with a shameful justification of the reality) is not without its dangers, because it can easily lead to giving a much lower value to the natural reality of marriage or even to isolating it altogether. It is really a question of including marriage as such, as a reality of creation, in the reality of Christ and regarding it as an effective sign of the salvation given by Christ.

2. The Essence of the Sacramentality of Marriage

(i) Marriage as the Sign of Christ

The bond or covenant of marriage has in itself an essential religious dimension. Even "natural" marriage is a religious symbol that points to God's faithfulness. This is why it was possible for the Old Testament authors to use marriage as the image and likeness of God's covenant with human beings. In Scripture, covenant is the reality of salvation as such. Salvation consists of God's definitive acceptance of man, his "yes" to humanity. It is God's communication of himself as love. God's "yes" really reaches people for the first time when they accept that "yes" in faith, hope and love and, in saying "yes" to God, respond to God in love. This unity in love existing between God and human beings is made present as a sign in marriage. It is realized in the highest and most unique way in Jesus Christ, in whom God said "yes" to human beings in a unique, definitive and unsurpassable way by communicating himself totally and making the humanity of Jesus the form of his existence in the world. On the other hand, Jesus opened himself completely to the reality of God even in his total obedience on the cross. In this way, he made himself, in his human self-surrender, the sign of the presence of God's love. Jesus Christ is therefore in person God's covenant with people. In him, God has once and for all time accepted everything human and has at the same time also affirmed it in its human dignity.

The marital love and faithfulness of those who are, through faith and baptism, "in Christ" are, in a very special way, included, borne up, purified and fulfilled by God's love and faithfulness in Jesus Christ. This situation is defined in the document on the Church of Vatican II in these words: "Authentic marital love is included in divine love and guided and enriched by the redeeming power of Christ and the Church's mediation of salvation."[13] The love and faithfulness that Christian husbands and wives have for each other, then, are not simply the sign and symbol of the love of God—they are the effective sign, the fulfilled symbol and the real epiphany of the love of God that has appeared in Jesus Christ.

If marriage represents a special form of being human in Christ that is based on baptism, it is also a special form of sharing in the death and resurrection of Christ. If marital love is seen as existing under the sign of Christ's cross, it must also be seen as being sustained by giving and being given, forgiving and being forgiven and a continuous process of new beginnings. Just as Christ loves the Church as a Church of sinners, purifies it and makes it holy, so too must married couples accept each other again and again with all their conflicts, in all their dissatisfactions and with all their guilt. This growth in love and this transformation are possible for married couples because they are able to have confidence that their human love and faithfulness are always surpassed and completed by the Easter victory of God over human lack of love and faithfulness.

It is possible to describe the participation of Christian marriage in the reality of Jesus Christ more precisely in both the negative and the positive sense.[14] The negative aspect was stressed above all by the theologians and canonists of the early Middle Ages, who defined marriage as a remedy against concupiscence. This definition strikes us as strange today, but it is possible to understand it when we remember the theological meaning of the term "concupiscence." It should not be thought of as synonymous with sensuality or sexual desire. It is, in the theological sense, the inner disintegration and fragmentation of human existence caused by sin—human sensuality insofar as it is opposed to the whole orientation of the person. It is as a remedy for this disintegration that the sacrament of marriage was defined by the early medieval theologians, who saw that marriage had a healing part to play in the integration of sex and eroticism into the whole human and religious structure of the individual and society. The beginning of a new creation is made by the sacrament of marriage.

This redemption from the "powers" of "flesh and blood" and their integration into the totality of human and Christian existence should make people free to serve God in his love (see 1 Cor. 6:20), that is, in their bodily and worldly relationships. This positive aspect can be described as the sanctification of those who are married. According to the New Testament, all those who are baptized are saints, that is, they have all been raised to the sphere of God's holiness (see 1 Cor. 1:2, 30; 6:11, etc.). The sacrament of marriage is in a special way a participation in the sanctifying service of Christ (see Eph. 5:26). This sanctification includes two elements: being taken into the service of God and his work in creation and redemption (*consecratio*) and being made inwardly capable of carrying out that service by sanctifying grace (*santificatio*).[15] Taken together, both of these aspects mean that married couples are, in their love for and faithfulness to each other, included in the love and faithfulness of God in Jesus Christ, with the result that their love for each other is an effective and fulfilled sign of the love of God. The life that man and wife share together in marriage therefore serves to glorify God. As M. J. Scheeben pointed out, sacramental marriage is not simply a symbol or an external example of the mystery of Christ and the Church, "but a copy of that mystery that has grown out of the union of Christ with the Church and is borne up by and penetrated with that union. Marriage does not merely symbolize that mystery. It really represents it in itself and represents it by showing itself to be active and effective in it."[16]

(ii) Marriage as the Sacrament of the Church

God's love and faithfulness in Jesus Christ applies to people in actuality. They are therefore present in human life in a visible and truly human way, that is, through the service of the Church as the community of believers. The love and faithfulness of God are made present by the love and faithfulness that Christians have for and towards each other. They are moreover, made present in this way in history. The Church is therefore the all-embracing sacrament of Christ, just as Christ himself is the sacrament of God.[17] What applies to the Church as a whole is concentrated in the sacraments and given its most complete form in them. What takes place in the sacraments, then, is not something that does not take place at all elsewhere in Christian life. The sacraments are, in other words, not an isolated and special sphere of activity. They are only capable of being fully understood and expressed as the supreme expression of what takes place in the rest of the life of the Church and its members.

Married and family life are in a very special sense the Church in miniature—Vatican II spoke of the family as the "domestic Church."[18] In this function, married and family life are not, however, simply a development of the essential being of the Church. They in fact make an active contribution to the building up of the Church. That is why married couples have a special charism, that is, a distinctive call, gift, and form of service, within the Church (see 1 Cor. 7:14). In a special way they contribute, by accepting and bringing up the children whom they are given, to both the internal and the external growth of the Church. They are also able to form living cells in the Church by the example of their life together as believers, and by the hospitality and openness of their "domestic Church."

The inner connection between marriage and the Church is most clearly expressed in the solemnization of marriage. It would be quite wrong to see this simply as an aspect of the Church's authority over marriage and as a formal duty that is justified by that authority. There has only been a formal duty of this kind in the Church since the appearance of the Tridentine decree on marriage *Tametsi* in 1563.[19] What is more important in this context is that marriage is, because of its inner and essential being, not simply a private matter, but also a public and ecclesial matter. This public and ecclesial aspect of marriage means that it is most important for the couple to enter into marriage in the presence and with the active participation of the Christian community gathered together within the framework of the liturgy. According to the Catholic understanding of this matter, the active collaboration of the Church's office is required for the full and official constitution of a community of believers. This is the theological basis of the Church's ruling that marriage must be solemnized in the presence of a priest. The latter's task is, moreover, not purely formally legal. The questioning procedure and the acceptance of the consensus by the priest should be understood as a clarification of the ecclesial dimension of the marriage itself. The priest also makes that dimension clear by his function as the Church's official witness to the marriage, his proclamation of the word of God and his prayer over and blessing of the bride and bridegroom. In this way, the Church is as it were answerable to God in an official sense for the success of the marriage that has just been solemnized.

Even though the Church collaborates in the solemnization of marriage because this participation is in accordance with the essential being of marriage itself, Christian marriage nonetheless remains independent within the Church. According to the most widely accepted theological opinion, it is not the priest who bestows the sacrament of marriage, but rather the bride and bridegroom who give the sacrament to each other. Sacramental marriage, then, is founded on the personal act "whereby spouses mutually bestow and accept each other"[20] and their mutual consent constitutes the marriage. There is a difference between the Western Church and the Orthodox Church with regard to this aspect of Christian marriage that has persisted up to the present day. In the Orthodox Church, which has not experienced the separation between the Church and the world that has marked the theology of the Western Catholic Church since the twelfth century, the priest is regarded as the one who bestows the sacrament of marriage.[21] The Reformed Churches have a different view from both the Orthodox and the Western Catholic Churches. They were, because of their presuppositions regarding the reality of marriage, obliged to hand over the solemnization of marriage to the secular authorities.[22] This has led, in recent centuries, to a far-reaching process of secularization in the institution of marriage on the one hand and, at the same time, a privatization and spiritualization of the Christian life of married couples.

It is clear from the concepts used in connection with marriage that the difficult balance in the Catholic doctrine between the personal and the ecclesial elements has not yet been fully resolved. Traditionally, both aspects are expressed in the term "marriage contract."[23] It is, however, obvious that the legal term "contract" can only be applied to marriage in an analogous sense. It is especially since the rise of the individualistic and liberal theories of law in the eighteenth and nineteenth centuries that the term "marriage contract" has been open to misunderstanding. Several Christian authors have therefore argued that the term "institution" rather than "contract" should be applied to marriage.[24] There is no doubt that this term expresses more clearly than the word "contract" the fact that marriage is a reality that is previously given, that both embraces and transcends the partners and that is not simply placed arbitrarily at their disposal. The Second Vatican Council followed this linguistic usage and preferred to speak of the institution rather than the contract of marriage.[25] On the other hand, however, it cannot be denied that the word "institution" can be interpreted in various ways and can only be applied to marriage partially and analogously. The most suitable word, then, would seem to be the biblical term "covenant," which was also used in the documents of the Second Vatican Council. "Covenant" expresses the personal character of the consensus better than "contract" or "institution." It is also able to express the legitimate intention of marriage, its public character, which is contained in the term "contract." A covenant is both private and public. The covenant of marriage is not simply a personal bond or covenant of love—it is also a public and legal matter concerning the whole community of believers. This is, of course, why the covenant is normally concluded *in facie ecclesiae*.

This unity, dynamic tension and mutually complementary nature of the personal and the ecclesial aspects of marriage must go further than the simple act of solemnization and be worked out in the whole continued history of the marriage relationship.[26] This tension forms the basis both of the obligation that the married couple have to collaborate in the Church and the community and of the coresponsibility that the Church and the community of believers have with regard to the human and Christian success of the marriage in its early period and its later stages. In addition to its material and spiritual diaconate or ministry in the widest sense, one expression of which is marriage counselling, the Church also has a supportive function. In the present situation, pastoral work with families and the formation and strengthening of family groups are of fundamental importance in the task of revivifying the Church and its communities of believers and therefore in enabling it to carry out its mission in the world. It is also possible that attempts of this kind may form at least one step towards leading the Church and society as a whole out of the impasse into which they have in recent decades been drawn by an understanding of marriage and family life that has been one-sidedly based on the model of the individual partnership. Why should vital Christian communities consisting of family groups not take over at least some of the functions of the earlier extended family?

(iii) Marriage as an Eschatological Sign

This dynamic relationship that exists between the Church and marriage also has a further dimension. Neither the Church nor marriage exist in themselves. The Church always continues to be a sacramental sign and instrument and a symbolic anticipation of the gathering together and reconciliation of mankind at the end of time and the establishment of peace among the nations. Marriage too is a sign of eschatological hope. The festive mood at a wedding is a symbol of the joy and the fulfillment of human hopes that will be present at the end of time (see Mark 2:19ff; Matt. 22:1–14; 25:1–13 etc.). It is therefore not simply necessary from the human point of view alone to celebrate the wedding as festively as possible, it is also important to mark the occasion in this way as a hopeful anticipation and celebration in advance of the feast at the end of time.

Marriage, then, has the value of an eschatological sign, but there is also an eschatological reservation in the New Testament with regard to marriage (see Mark 12:25; 1 Cor. 7:25–38). Marriage belongs to the form of this world which is transient. According to Christian teaching, it is not an ultimate, but a penultimate and to the extent a temporary value. This eschatological relativization of marriage is not a fundamental devaluation—on the contrary, marriage is given a new content and meaning by being given a relative value in the eschatological sense. By being classified as a penultimate rather than as an ultimate value, marriage is demythologized, demystified and desacralized, and in this way its immanent beauty and inner wealth are more perfectly expressed. If, on the other hand, exaggerated expectations are projected onto marriage and the partners in marriage, the inevitable result is almost always disappointment. No partner can give the other heaven on earth. A person's urge to make such penultimate values absolute and his tendency to do violence to them in this way can only cease when he recognizes God as the ultimate reality. A person can only be fully human when he or she sees God fully as God.

The eschatological glorification of God is the final humanization of humanity. The eschatological reservation regarding marriage is therefore the source of freedom in marriage. It binds both partners to God and prevents them from becoming enslaved to each other.

This eschatologically-based Christian freedom, however, presupposes that marriage is not the only possible call made by God to people or the only way in which people can be fulfilled.[27] The charism of the unmarried state is there precisely for the sake of this freedom in marriage (see 1 Cor. 7:7). A Christian who voluntarily remains unmarried for the sake of the kingdom of heaven (see Matt. 19:12) is not a better Christian than the one who marries. He or she does, however, express through the unmarried state an aspect that is essential for all Christians—he or she is there entirely for the Lord and his affairs (see 1 Cor. 7:32). He or she makes it clear, as a sign, through this eschatologically-based Christian freedom what the fundamental attitude of every Christian should be. According to the New Testament, then, this freely chosen unmarried state is an essential sign in the Church. The Church needs this sign at every period of its existence. It is also necessary for the success of Christian marriages.

Just as the Christian who remains unmarried for Christ's sake discloses the married Christian's freedom as a sign to the latter, so too does the eschatological character of marriage show the unmarried Christian that eschatological existence should not imply a flight from the world, but is in fact a special form of service in the world and for others. Both forms of Christian life have therefore to be understood in their mutual relationship. Each stands or falls with the other. A call to remain unmarried is a sign to the healthy Christian marriage, and a devaluation of the unmarried state is inevitably bound to lead to a distortion of Christian values in marriage. Both aspects of Christian life must therefore be borne in mind in any responsible pastoral policy for marriage.

Notes

1. Karl Barth elaborated—rather one-sidely—the connection between man's having been created in the image of God and creation as man and woman; see his *Kirchliche Dogmatik* (*Church Dogmatics*), III / 1, pp. 204–33; III / 2, pp. 344–91. See also C. Westermann, *Genesis* (*Bibl. Kommentar AT,* I / 1), (Neukirchen and Vluyn, 1974), pp. 208ff., 220ff, 306–22.

2. For the sacramentality of marriage, see H. Volk, *Das Sakrament der Ehe*, (Münster, ²1956); K. Rahner, "Die Ehe als Sakrament," *Schriften zur Theologie* VIII, (Einsiedeln, Zürich & Cologne, 1967), pp. 519–40; J. Ratzinger, "Zur Theologie der Ehe," *Theologische Quartalschrift* (1969), pp. 53–74 (*Theologie der Ehe*), (Regensburg and Göttingen, 1969), pp. 81–115); W. Kasper, "Die Verwirklichung der Kirche in Ehe und Familie," *Glaube und Geschichte* (Mainz, 1970), pp. 330–54; M. Schmaus, *Der Glaube der Kirche* II (Munich, 1970), pp. 491–531; D. O'Callaghan, "Marriage as Sacrament," *Concilium* 5 (1970), pp. 101–10; W. Beinert, "Die Ehe als Sakrament der Kirche," *Beiträge zur Theologie der Ehe*, (Kevelaer, 1971), pp. 11–36; K. Reinhardt, "Sakramentalität und Unauflöslichkeit der Ehe in dogmatischer Sicht," K. Reinhardt and H. Jedin, *Ehe—Sakrament in der Kirche des Herrn* (*Ehe in Geschichte und Gegenwart* 2) (Berlin, 1971), pp. 7–59; K. Lehmann, "Zur Sakramentalität der Ehe," *Ehe und Ehescheidung*, (Munich, 1972), pp. 57–72; E. Christen, *Ehe als Sakrament—neue Gesichtspunkte aus Exegese und Dogmatik* (*Theologische Berichte* 1) (Einsiedeln, 1972), pp. 11–68; L. Boff, "The Sacrament of Marriage," *Concilium* 7 (1973), pp. 22–33; L. Duss-von Werdt, "Theologie der Ehe. Das sakramentale Charakter der Ehe," *Mysterium Salutis* IV / 2, pp. 422–49; H. Volk, "Von der sakramentalen Gnade der Ehe," *Christus alles in allen* (Mainz, 1975), pp. 70–95. See also the works by P. Adnès and E. Schillebeeckx, op. cit., in note 9.

3. See H. Baltensweiler, *Die Ehe im Neuen Testament. Exegetische Untersuchungen über Ehe, Ehelosigkeit und Ehescheidung* (*Abhandlungen Theol. AT. und NT.* 52) (Zürich & Stuttgart, 1967), pp. 43–81; R. Schnackenburg, "Die Ehe nach dem Neuen Testament," *Theologie der Ehe*, ed. G. Krems and R. Mumm (Regensburn & Göttingen, 1969), pp. 40–55; H. Greven, "Ehe nach dem Neuen Testament," *Theologie der Ehe*.

op. cit., pp. 40–56; P. Hoffmann, "Jesus' Saying about Divorce and its Interpretation in the New Testament Tradition," *Concilium* 5 (1970), pp. 51–66; R. Pesch, *Freie Treue. Die Christen und die Ehescheidung* (Freiburg, Basle & Vienna, 1971), pp. 22–32. See also J. Ratzinger, "Zur Theologie der Ehe," op. cit., p. 54ff.

4. See H. Baltensweiler, *Die Ehe im Neuen Testament,* op. cit., pp. 218–35; R. Schnackenburg, *Die Ehe nach dem Neuen Testament,* op. cit., p. 25ff; H. Schlier, *Der Brief an die Epheser* (Düsseldorf, 1957), p. 262ff; J. Gnilka, *Der Epheserbrief* (*Herders Theologischer Kommentar zum Neuen Testament* X, 2) (Freiburg, Basle & Vienna, 1971), p. 274ff; G. Bornkamm, *"Mysterion," ThWNT* IV, p. 829ff.

5. See *DS* 1799; the Council of Trent does not argue on the basis of Scripture so much as on a suggestion (*innuit*) of Scripture.

6. H. Volk, "Ehe," *LThK* III (²1959), p. 681.

7. Second Lateran Council (1139): *DS* 718; Council of Verona (1184): *DS* 761; Innocent III (1198–1216): *DS* 769, 793; Second Council of Lyons (1274): *DS* 860; John XXII (1318): *DS* 916; Council of Florence (1439–1345): *DS* 1327; Council of Trent (1545–1563): *DS* 1801; Pius IX, *Syllabus* (1864): *DS* 2965–2974; Leo XIII, Encyclical *Arcanum divinae* (1880): *DS* 3142f; Pius X, Decree *Lamentabili* (1907): *DS* 3451; Pius XI, Encyclical *Casti Connubii* (1930): *DS* 3700, 3710ff; Second Vatican Council, Pastoral Constitution *Gaudium et Spes,* 48.

8. See Martin Luther, "De captivitate Babylonica ecclesiae" (1520): *WA* 6, p. 550ff; summarizing p. 553: *Sit ergo Matrimonium figura Christi et Ecclesiae, sacramentum autem non divinitus institutum, sed ab hominibus in Ecclesia inventum.* For the contemporary Protestant attitude towards marriage, see W. Lohff, "Die Ehe nach evangelischer Auffassung," *Ehe und Ehescheidung. Ein Symposium* (Stundenbücher, 30), (Hamburg, 1963), p. 53. It is not without significance that most Protestant theologians deal with the subject of marriage not within the framework of dogmatic theology, but as an ethical question. (See, for example, the writings of W. Elert, K. Barth, E. Brunner, H. Thielecke, P. Althaus, W. Trillhaas and others.) M. Thurian, in *Mariage et célibat* (*Foi vivante,* 135) (Neuchâtel, 1964), is exceptional among Protestants in his attitude towards marriage. See also, "Ehe," *Religion in Geschichte und Gegenwart* II (³1958), p. 322ff; *EKL* I (1956), pp. 1001–1003; *Lexikon für Theologie und Kirche* III (²1959), p. 698ff (bibliography). It is not possible for me to go into the many problems of mixed marriages in this context; the reader should consult R. Beaupère and others, *Die Mischehe in ökumenischer Sicht* (Freiburg, 1968); P. Lengsfeld, *Das Problem der Mischehe. Einer Lösung entgegen* (Freiburg, Basle & Vienna, 1970).

9. Martin Luther, "Ein Traubüchlein für die einfältigen Pfarrherrn" (1529): *WA* 30, III, 74.

10. Martin Luther, "Von Ehesachen" (1530): *WA* 30, III, p. 205.

11. Martin Luther, "Ein Traubüchlein" (1529): *WA* 30, III, p. 75ff.

12. Martin Luther, *Tischreden,* No. 233.

13. Dogmatic Constitution on the Church, *Lumen Gentium,* 11; see also *DS* 1799.

14. See the synthesis in Thomas Aquinas, Suppl. 42, 3.

15. For this distinction, see H. Volk, "Das Wirken des Heiligen Geistes in den Gläubigen," *Gott alles in allem. Gesammelte Aufsätze* I (Mainz, 1961), p. 90ff.

16. M. J. Scheeben, *Die Mysterien des Christentums,* ed. J. Höfer (*Gesammelte Schriften* II) (Freiburg, 1951), p. 496.

17. Vatican II defined the Church as a "sacrament of intimate union with God and of the unity of all mankind, a sign and an instrument of that union and unity" (Dogmatic Constitution on the Church, *Lumen Gentium,* 1). See also the works of O. Semmelroth, K. Rahner, and E. Schillebeeckx. A good summary will be found in L. Boff, *Die Kirche als Sakrament im Horizont der Welterfahrung. Versuch einer Legitimation und einer struktur-funktionalistischen Grundlegung der Kirche im Anschluß an das II. Vatikanische Konzil* (Paderborn, 1972).

18. Dogmatic Constitution on the Church, *Lumen Gentium,* 11.

19. See *DS* 1813–16. See also K. Mörsdorf, "Die Eheschließung nach dem Selbstverständnis der christlichen Bekenntnisse," *Münchener Theologische Zeitschrift* 9 (1958), pp. 241–56; R. Lettmann, *Die Diskussion über die klandestinen Ehen und die Einführung einer zur Gültigkeit verpflichtenden Eheschließungsform auf dem Konzil von Trient* (Münster, 1967); H. Dombois, *Kirche und Eherecht. Studien und Abhandlungen 1953–72* (Stuttgart, 1974), pp. 117–34.

20. Pastoral Constitution, *Gaudium et Spes,* 48.

21. See H. Dombois, *Kirche und Eherecht,* op. cit., pp. 197–213.

22. See Martin Luther, "Von Ehesachen" (1530): *WA* 30, III, p. 207.

23. See the *Codex Iuris Canonici,* canon 1012 § 2. See also U. Mosiek, *Kirchliches Eherecht unter Berücksichtigung der nachkonziliaren Rechtslage* (Freiburg, ²1972), pp. 35, 42.

24. J. Leclercq and J. David, *Die Familie,* op. cit., pp. 32–37; H. Dombois, *Kirche und Eherecht,* op. cit., pp. 84–95.

25. Pastoral Constitution, *Gaudium et Spes,* 47ff.

26. See F. Böckle, F. Betz and N. Greinacher, "Die Ehe als Vollzug der Kirche," *Handbuch der Pastoraltheologie* 4 (Freiburg, Basle & Vienna, 1969), pp. 17–94; *Ehe und Familie (Pastorale* 2), (Mainz, 1973).

27. See M. Thurian, *Mariage et célibat* (Neuchâtel, 1964); E. Gössmann, "Ehe und Ehelosigkeit. Eine Literaturübersicht," *Bibel und Leben* 9 (1968), pp. 230–36.

16

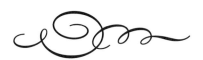

Marriage as a Sacrament

Karl Rahner, S.J.

In the current scene both within and without the Catholic Church marriage constitutes one of the most popular topics of discussion. Admittedly in this, even in the case of discussions within the Catholic Church, it is only rarely that the discussion centres upon marriage as a sacrament. Here, however, it is precisely this question of dogmatic theology, however 'theoretical' and out of touch with current thought it may seem to be, that is to be treated of. This question and no other besides. For in fact that which has been forgotten, neglected and thrust into the background is still very far indeed from being less important than that which fills the columns of the newspapers and the Church's periodical literature, or even which has been made the subject of a papal commission. Perhaps it is not altogether useless from the 'practical' point of view too to enquire into what is, *precisely on a Christian understanding,* the heart and centre of marriage. What does it mean to say that married love is sanctified by God's grace? How does that which every marriage is in any case and of its very nature acquire new and deeper roots in virtue precisely of what takes place at the *sacramental* level? What part does marriage as understood in this sense play in the life of the Church at the level of theology and faith? Is it not necessary to view the institution of marriage once more in its theological and spiritual origins, seeing that at the deepest level it is on this basis alone that the concrete problems of life can be endured and solved? In the article which follows an attempt will be made to take a first step in this direction.

A valid marriage between two baptized Christians is a sacrament, one of the seven sacraments of the Church of Christ. In what follows we shall be exploring, to some extent, this straightforward statement which has been defined as part of the faith of the Catholic Church.[1] For in fact it cannot be said that we have really understood this statement merely on the grounds that we 'know' about it in the sense that it strikes us as well-known and familiar, and to this extent is firmly rooted in the contents of our catechism, whether in its printed or unprinted form. The aim we have set ourselves is not directly or properly speaking to establish that this statement is contained in the 'sources' of revelation.[2] Nor shall we be defending it as a matter of theological controversy against the theology of the Reformation.[3] Here we shall only be attempting simply and straightforwardly to understand precisely *what* this statement really means and says. It is inevitable in the very nature of the case that in this we will have to concern ourselves with questions which are both extremely difficult and extremely obscure.

I

We must begin by enquiring briefly into the nature of the *sacrament in general*. In doing so we are conscious of the fact that we are embarking upon a way which is, from the aspect of the history of dogma, as also from that of the methodology employed in this field, a dangerous one. For the general concept of 'sacrament' is—historically speaking and from the point of view of the subject matter itself—a subsequent abstraction which has emerged at a relatively late stage from those seven sacred realities which take place in the life of the Church, but which, when we compare them with one another, turn out to be of very different kinds. An ill-thought out application of this concept which has subsequently been abstracted from them, therefore, in which it is taken as an overall model which is capable only of secondary variations, can make it extremely difficult for us to perceive the real nature of the individual sacrament. However our only purpose in beginning with a consideration of sacrament in general is thereby to acquire an initial orientation. The significance of it is that in a certain sense it makes sure that in our treatment of marriage as such certain definite aspects of it will not be able to escape our notice from the outset.[4]

The first point to be recognised about a sacrament is that it is essentially something that takes place in the *Church,* i.e. not merely something which the Church brings about, as it were, externally in the life of specific individuals, but an event in which the Church realizes her own nature and thereby 'actualizes' herself. A sacrament is something that takes place at that manifest level which belongs to the nature of the Church, not a 'private treatment' in which the Church merely collaborates in some way. This event has the force of a cultic manifestation, an objective symbol, a physical embodiment. It belongs palpably to the historical dimension of space and time, as well as to that of God's self-bestowal in grace upon man.[5] At the same time it also belongs to the nature of the Church which in Christ is the arch-sacrament, eschatologically victorious and indefectible, of precisely this same self-bestowal of God.[6] And finally it is also the free act by which this gracious self-bestowal of God is accepted by him who allows the sacrament to take effect in him, and by his act plays his own part in constituting it as such. In accordance with this we have to distinguish in the sacrament between the sign and that which is signified, between the manifestation and that which is manifested and which has a message to proclaim in hidden form in the manifestation. In the order of the physical person endowed with freedom as he exists in space and time, and in the order of the incarnation, both elements have a connatural relationship to one another, yet are not identical with one another.[7] The sacramental sign proceeds from the will of God truly to save men, and from the nature of the Church as the arch-sacrament of the grace of God, eschatologically victorious and indefectible. And as rooted in these this sign always has an 'exhibitive' force as the effective and unconditional offering of salvation by Christ and the Church. In this sense, then, the sacramental sign is *opus operatum*.[8] But since grace is only the event of salvation as brought about when it is accepted in freedom, and since this free acceptance can precisely be withheld by man, the sacramental manifestation of grace remains radically indeterminate *precisely from the human aspect*. It can remain an 'empty' manifestation. It can be an invalid or ineffective sacrament, or alternatively it can have the force of really being that 'exhibitive' word which carries what it expresses within itself, the word in which and through which that which it signifies takes place in very truth. Certainly this is far from being an exhaustive description of the nature of the sacrament in general.[9] But nevertheless certain aspects of it have been indicated to which we have to pay due heed in any consideration of marriage as a sacrament.

Marriage is a *sign*. It possesses this character prior to any theological consideration and prior to its bearing upon the relationship between Christ and the Church, because in itself it has a physical and social dimension of reality. Here we have the incarnation, as it were, the real symbol, the manifestation, the 'space-time' dimension, the expression of the most interior and most personal union in love of two individuals at the very roots of their being as orientated in freedom to God. Already here, then, we can perceive that difference and that unity in the elements which go to make up this sacrament inasmuch as this too is the sign at the physical and social level of a personal faith and love manifested in the appropriation of the grace of God as addressed to the individual in the sacrament. Considered purely in itself marriage already constitutes such a unity, in which the two elements remain distinct, of personal love, on the one hand, and its sign at the physical and social level on the other.[10] This sign, therefore, is both the 'other factor' in which and through which the personal love expresses itself, declares itself and makes itself manifest, and also, under certain circumstances, the *mere* sign which remains 'empty', deprived of its true basis, in which case it precisely does *not* carry with it what it signifies. Obviously this applies to marriage considered both as the sealing of a covenant and as the 'concluding of a contract' (as the canonists put it), and it also applies to married life as such. In both respects we can speak of the unity and the difference which exist between the sign and the reality signified.

II

For the present we shall still be remaining in this dimension of marriage in itself, without explicitly adverting to the precise *sacramental* significance of this sign. The question for us is, therefore, in view of what has been said, precisely *what* is made manifest in marriage in the dimension of the physical, of space and time, and of social living? Up to this point we have concluded that it is the most intimate and personal unity in love between two individuals (of different sexes). We must now see a little more deeply into what this statement signifies. Admittedly this could be achieved in various ways and at various levels. For instance that personal love which forges the most intimate possible unity between two human individuals would have to be considered in its own distinctive nature. Every word of this definition is capable of yielding the deepest insight into the meaning of marriage. Here three further specific aspects are particularly to be brought out: how this love relates to God, the process by which this personal love acquires fresh roots through that which we call grace, personal love as uniting us with the whole community of men.

1. We would have to begin by saying something about how this personal and unifying love relates to God. To do this we would have to give an account of the entire theological problem of the unity which exists between love of God and love of neighbour, of the relationship which we bear to God, and of our intercommunication among ourselves. And of course this is not possible here.[11] Love of God and love of neighbour *mutually* condition one another, even if at first we do not explicitly reflect upon the fresh roots which both acquire through grace. Love of neighbour is not merely a moral task and a duty which is demanded by love of God. More than this, it is the means without which love of God, a right knowledge of God and of our true and total commitment to him, is quite impossible. The transcendental reference which man bears to God can only be realised to the full, can only be experienced for what it truly is and as such freely entered into, in the experience which we have through love of our neighbour. For the 'world' in and through which, according to Christian philosophy and theology, God can be 'recognized' is precisely in its ultimate depths, not merely our material environment, but first and last the world of personal interrelationships. Only one who has encountered this world as a matter of concrete experience, has accepted it in love and freely committed himself to it, can make

real to himself and freely accept that transcendental orientation of the spirit in terms of knowledge and freedom, the ultimate basis and absolute goal of which is that Mystery upholding all and upheld by none which we call 'God'. It is this that makes it possible to realise what it is to be so orientated. In this context it is a question of secondary importance (in the light of what is ultimate) how far we succeed in arriving at a free and loving commitment to the world of personal interrelationships such that this involves, at least as something included in it, an experience of our own transcendence, and in this of God also. The question, in other words, of how we succeed in objectifying in conceptual and thematic terms, and setting out in propositional form, that orientation to God which we realise and accept as something that is included in our personal relationships. Even the atheist who truly loves makes experience in his love (provided only that it is what it must be) of God, whether or not he can express this to himself in his conscious thoughts or words.[12] Even in his case the absolute quality of personal love for the 'thou' of his fellow man utters a silent 'yes' to God. It has that quality of self-surrender which is achieved, and necessarily must be achieved, in love, and which can only take place provided that its basic origin and its ultimate goal consist in that which we call God. Or, to put the matter in another way, a love of this kind between human beings is based in its ultimate and connatural depths precisely upon this orientation to God. These ultimate and connatural depths of love consist in its power to attain to the other at the very deepest and most ultimate levels of his personhood and his uniqueness. Thus there is a hope of the two beings as they actually exist arriving at what is ultimate and definitive in the existence of them both, and in a love of this kind this hope is positively affirmed. This too has its basis in the ultimate orientation to God as also has the basic faithfulness which such love involves.

2. Now this personal love, which creates the state of marriage as the mode in which to manifest itself, is in fact[13] in the present order of salvation sustained by the grace of God which *always* imbues this love with its salvific power, exalts it and opens it to the immediacy of God himself. Now this can take place even before this love encounters the message of the gospel proclaimed and made known as such in explicit words.

We cannot here set out the special reasons for holding this. Instead we shall assume it as an application of a more general theological principle.[14] This can be formulated in the following terms: *in the present order of salvation a moral act that is truly positive ('actus honestus') is in fact also a salvific act ('actus salutaris') in the proper sense in virtue of the grace which always exalts it and which is offered always to every man by the universal salvific will of God.* This more general principle is, it is true, not universally accepted in Catholic theology. Nevertheless in different forms it has already been maintained in it for a long time, for instance by Vasquez and Ripalda,[15] and materially speaking should certainly be accorded recognition as a prolongation of what the Second Vatican Council teaches with regard to the possibility of salvation for the non-Christian and the inculpable atheist.[16] Doubts have been cast upon, or opposition offered to this principle hitherto by theologians only because they were incapable of rightly appreciating how it is possible, outside the sphere of the *explicit* preaching of the gospel, for that true faith to exist which is necessary for salvation, and also for a salvific act in the true sense to be posited. But if, for reasons which cannot be treated of here and now,[17] we accept the fact that revelation, and therefore faith too, can also be granted to him who has not been touched in any direct sense by the historical message of the Old or New Testaments, then neither the general principle already mentioned nor its particular application to the special question we are considering here continue to constitute any insuperable difficulty. In other words we can say: in the order of salvation as it *de facto* exists there are no merely 'natural' moral acts on man's part. These acts are *de facto,* when they are posited at all, also upheld by grace and supernaturally orientated to God in his direct act of self-bestowal, and indeed are already in themselves acts which have been made possible by this self-bestowal even though this has not become objectified or explicitated in terms of man's own conscious awareness.

The situation as set forth above applies primarily to the love between human beings where this is made real in the form of a personal and selfless union between two individuals. But this means: *genuine love is* de facto *always that theological virtue of* caritas *which is sustained by God himself through his grace.* In this virtue love is extended to both God and man both in a mutual interrelationship and according to their respective conditions *in such a way that in this relationship the lover achieves his salvation in the event of justification. In this salvation of his he wills salvation for the other also, and in both God is attained to immediately as this salvation in person.* The human love of which we are speaking here, therefore, 'intends' God not merely as a transcendental (not explicitly objectified) origin and goal in his infinite remoteness, but rather attains to God in that absolute proximity in which he imparts his own self—and not in the form of any merely creaturely gift—as the innermost mystery and life of man. In virtue of the fact that it is *caritas,* therefore, this love is also the event of the loving self-bestowal of God upon us which alone empowers us to love God and man. *Caritas,* therefore, is the event of the love of God for us and of our love for God taken as a unity. Unfortunately here we must forego the attempt to translate this statement, which has been made in very abstract terms and on the basis of theological data, as it were into phenomenological terms and to express it as an existential and ontological fact. In this way, and on the basis of the experience of this radical love in itself, we could show that these theological implications of the nature of love are actually present in it, or at least we could demonstrate the possibility of this.

3. But this love signifies at the same time a unity with mankind as a whole also. This needs to be shown from various aspects. We are accustomed to attribute to married love the character of a special intimacy and exclusiveness in relation to others outside the married partnership itself. We actually go so far as to regard these qualities as constituting what is special in married love as opposed to other forms of love such as love of neighbour in general, comradeship, friendship etc.

Now we do not for a moment intend to deny that married love has this character. Certainly it is consonant with the nature of married love. Nevertheless we ought to ask ourselves precisely *whence* the character of this somewhat startling exclusiveness derives. Is it based upon the ultimate nature of this personal love or are there *also* less basic reasons for it which have to do, rather, with the concrete physical forms and manifestations of this love as these are limited by space and time? Or can it even be that still further determining factors in this exclusiveness are the cultural, social and sociological factors of human living? In other words are some of the factors which go to determine this exclusiveness susceptible of alteration?[18]

But in any case it must be of service to point this out, if only because of the fact that it would be false if we sought to understand married love from the outset as an act of withdrawing behind closed doors where the two partners are isolated from the rest, for this would be, at basis, an egoistical state. Marriage is not the act in which two individuals come together to form a 'we', a relationship in which they set themselves apart from the 'all' and close themselves against this. Rather it is the act in which a 'we' is constituted which opens itself lovingly precisely to *all*. This aspect of the basic essence of such love 'appears' already in the very fact that those united by married love themselves already come from a community. In their love they do not abandon this—indeed they must not abandon it. And their love becomes fruitful in the child that they produce, which for its part in turn must not become enclosed within the 'we' relationship, but must be set free to enter into the wider community of the 'all'. Married love, therefore, is, even in respect of its concrete physical forms, a source of, and an initiation into a wider community, and must therefore itself also intend this right from the outset.

This idea needs to be still further deepened. Married love cannot be so intimate and exclusive that it ceases to be love at all. Now of its very nature it is love only when it does not exclude, but rather opens itself to and includes, when it really commits itself ever anew to that which is strange in the other even before it has explored and seen into it; when it trusts itself without condition to accept that which is really 'other' in the beloved as its own (which, in fact, must also constantly be taking place in the intimate partnership of the marriage itself). In the *specific* love for the *concrete* individual man must precisely *experience* what 'love' is in general. He must experience that this is possible really as love and not as flattery, behind which, contrary to all appearances, only egotism and self-assertion lie concealed, in order that he may be able to trust himself in his relationship with the other. But then when he has achieved this his love must not be smothered by both the married partners becoming egoistical to all others. They must not seek to use their mutual love so as to justify a position in which they precisely do *not* love others. They must maintain an openness to all, however much their finite powers and possibilities may in fact impose limitations upon them in this.

Married love too is a readiness, an exercise, a promise and a task, to *love* man *in himself*—something which is more than merely 'respecting' him, merely giving him 'his due' instead of being ready again and again to trust him with one's *self*, to commit one's self to him 'with one's whole heart and with all one's resources'. We are always in debt to all, often, perhaps to those most remote from us even more than to those who are closest. Marriage is the concrete state in which we begin to pay this endless debt, not a dispensation from this endless task which can only be fulfilled by God's help.

A further aspect must now be added to what has just been said. That grace which, as we have seen, sustains married love and renders it open to God in his radical immediacy is the grace of a covenant, which constitutes the innermost dynamism of the world and of the history of mankind in its unity. It is a grace which establishes the one dominion of God over all. So individual a grace, which, in its ultimate depths, is God himself, is directed to the individual in his uniqueness, and this is true however much it may also be the case that, while never ceasing to be this, it is at the same time an 'universal concrete', a unifying grace through which the individual is intended precisely as *belonging to* the *unity* of mankind, as having a place in the people of God.[19] This is not surprising. For the true uniqueness of the existence of each particular individual consists, if it is genuinely to be brought to its fulness and not to lead to an egoistical self-gratification of one's own 'personality', in the unique singleness with which one actually *loves* all. If grace is in this sense the event in which God becomes, for the particular individual, *his* God, it is also, and precisely in virtue of this, the event in which grace not only breaks out of the bonds of egoism in a 'moral' sense and, so to say, at the external level of man's life, but does so in such a way that thereby man is *set free* to transcend the possibilities of his own nature and to attain to *that* infinitude of the freedom of God in which *all* are comprehended in love from the very roots of their existence, and in God can actually be loved in this way even by the creature.

Married love, therefore, is—in spite of, and in its intimacy or exclusiveness—of its very nature and on the basis of the grace of God which sustains it, a state in which we achieve union with mankind, impelled as it is by the selfsame grace. It follows, then, that right from its very origins married love, if its true nature is really attained to, also constitutes a relationship with God, an event of grace, a loving concord with that basic movement in which, through grace, mankind considered as the people of God arrives at the unity of the kingdom of God.

Marriage, as we have said at the outset (1), is the physical manifestation, the sign, the real symbol and the embodiment of this married love, which achieves reality through this manifestation of itself. Marriage—this is what we now have to conclude—is the sign of *that* love which is designed in God's sight to be the event of grace and a love that is open to all. Yet even this insight is still only at the provisional stage in its development. The actual structure of 'sign' in itself has now to be examined more precisely, and that in its *sacramental* character. To accomplish this we shall first compare the sacramental structure of the Church and of marriage in general.

III

What has just been said about marriage considered as a 'real symbol' of the love which has thus been specified can now also be asserted of the *Church*. Of course in drawing this parallel we have to maintain the force of the distinction which exists between the individual (or a few individuals) and the community made up of all. But this distinction as applied to mankind is not *ipso facto* the same as that between a unity merely in the numerical sense and a numerical multitude. The mutual relationship which exists between the individual and mankind as a whole is different from this. In every individual man everything is present (*homo quodammodo omnia*), and the whole achieves a unique manifestation of itself in each particular individual. The community of mankind for its part is not the agglomeration of the many—all too many, but the unity in love of those, each of whom is unique in his own right, a love which sets each free for his own, which assembles all this and so once more unifies it. In the light of this it is not surprising that we can make the same assertion about the Church *and* about the individual, the more so seeing that even from the point of view of the individual it is genuine community that is in question.

Allowing, therefore, for the general differences in the relationship which the individual bears to the community and that which the community of all taken together bears to the individual, we shall put forward the following proposition: the same 'sign' function which is found in marriage is also present in the Church. For the Church is, in Christ, the arch-sacrament, the basic sacrament: in him the love of God for mankind in his act of self-bestowal achieves its historical manifestation through grace in the loving unity of mankind.[20] In this parallelism which exists between the 'sign' function in marriage and in the Church respectively, one further particularly noteworthy element, as well as a difference which will be of importance in our later considerations, must be brought out. The special aspect in this parallelism is the following one. We have said that in marriage a difference exists between the sign and that which is signified, between the marriage as it exists at the physical and social level and married love. This difference can be so far-reaching that in the individual case the two entities—even though this is against the mutual relationship which is connatural to them—can actually be torn apart. The same is also true of the Church. Here too the sign ('Church as basic sacrament') and the reality signified are not simply identical. For what the Church points to is not herself. Rather as sign, i.e. as a socially organised community constituted by a common creed, a common cult and common works of charity, she is precisely the sign of that humanity, consecrated and united by grace (in interior faith and justification), the grace-given unity of which extends far beyond the social organism of the Church.[21] On the other hand a further and more essential distinction is to be found within this common difference: the 'sign' function in the case of a particular marriage can sinfully be degraded into a lie when that which it is intended to manifest and to render present is not present in itself, namely the love that is grace-given and unifying. In the

Church as a whole the intrinsic connection between sign and reality signified can no longer radically be destroyed in virtue of the eschatological victory of grace in Christ. Nevertheless the basic parallelism between marriage and the Church continues to exist. The following proposition applies just as much to the Church as it does to marriage: she is the sign, at the palpable level of historical and social human life, of the fact that *that* love is being made effective and victorious throughout the whole of humanity which is the love of God for us and of us for God, the love which comprehends and unifies all so long as no-one sinfully denies it.

We cannot develop any further the doctrine of the Church as the basic sacrament of salvation (and therefore of that love which is salvation) at this point.[22] Here we must be satisfied with what has already been said, since what we are concerned with is the parallelism between marriage and the Church. When we compare the Church with marriage we are thinking of the Church simply as she is, the Church who is what she is simply in virtue of the mutual love between her and Christ. But while Christ is in this sense included, at the same time it is not *merely* a summary description when we say simply 'Church'. For she is also the basic sacrament of grace and of the love which unites us all precisely in virtue of the fact that in her a *social* unity of truth, hope and love is brought about among men in themselves. This aspect belongs just as much to her character as basic sacrament as her unity with Christ which she expresses in creed and cult, and which thereby constitutes the manifestations of her unity with Christ in the *pneuma*.

Indeed we can actually make bold to proceed a stage further: the unity of the Church which she presents as the model and basis for the unity of marriage—in the dimensions of the sign and of the reality signified alike—is, nevertheless, so far as that precise aspect is concerned which we are considering here, *de facto* constituted through the love of men in the Church and the manifestation of this at the level of social and communal life. But this love is not something that belongs to another dimension altogether, but rather precisely that same love which unites married spouses—including all that deeper theological dimension which belongs to it. But in that case we can also say: *the love that unites married spouses contributes to the unity of the Church herself because it is one of the ways in which the unifying love of the Church is made actual. It is just as much formative of the Church as sustained by the Church.* The term 'Church-house', signifying the sort of local Church which is constituted by a family unit, is more than a mere pious image.[23]

This correspondence and parallelism between Church and marriage, therefore, is not merely an external similarity between two entities each of which exists on its own and independently of the other. On the contrary the conformity between the two is due to the fact that both have a common root. For marriage as such is, taken as a whole, the manifestation which is creative of *that precise* love which, as the love of God and for God in the divine act of self-bestowal, is constitutive of the union of mankind with one another and with God, and constitutive too of the basic sacrament of this which is the Church. In this we must not overlook the fact that the Church and humanity as made manifest, sanctified and unified in her are in no sense mythical entities but precisely those concrete individuals in themselves who love God and love in God, and give their intrinsic unity a manifest expression in the dimension of history in the unifying society that is the Church.[24]

Now let us see what happens when, on the basis of this fundamental conformity marriage takes place precisely in the sphere of the Church. It becomes precisely that which we are seeking to express when we explain that it is a 'sacrament'. In the light of the principle we have laid down this statement acquires the force not merely of a principle which we already know and understand. Rather this principle only truly becomes intelligible to us in the truths which it itself is intended to express, so that it is no mere abstract concept of sacrament which is applied to the institution of marriage *ab externo*. We must now attempt to clarify this point.

IV

Two baptised individuals voluntarily bind themselves in marriage. In this something takes place in the Church too. Here we do not need to adopt the approach of canon law, or to ask what precise conditions are required by the divine or human law upheld by the Church and from the nature of the case in order that such a bond of marriage (let us not call it a 'contract'!) may take place precisely *in* the Church and in the context of her life as a 'visible society'. But at basis all this is already given in virtue of the fact that it is two baptised individuals that are involved, and a marriage between them, something which always has a social relevance. Because married love has the character of a pointer and a sign, marriage itself is never a mere 'worldly affair'. For this love itself is no worldly affair, but rather the event of grace and love which unites God and men. When a marriage of *this* kind, therefore, takes place in the Church, it is an element in the process by which the Church fulfils her own nature as such, one which is brought into being by two baptised Christians who, through their baptism, have been empowered to play an active part in this self-realisation.[25] As baptised, therefore, they act in a manner which is precisely proper to the Church herself. They make manifest the sign of love in which *that* love is visibly expressed which unites God and men.

Now when the Church achieves the fulness of her own nature in this way precisely at this *essential* level, making it effective in the concrete and decisive living situation of a human individual, there we have a sacrament.[26] In that case there is no need for this purpose of any *explicit* words of institution uttered by Jesus (we could never establish as a matter of historical fact that he ever uttered such words, nor is it even probable that he did so), such as for instance are to be found in the case of the Eucharist.[27] The 'word of institution' in this case consists in two factors: on the one hand in the fact that the religious relevance of marriage is acknowledged and that it is recognised that this too is something that is achieved through the word and the deed of Jesus himself.[28] It also consists in the fact that marriage has been instituted by the Church as an eschatological sign of salvation for the kingdom of God (considered as the absolute proximity of God to man) until the end of time.[29] On the other hand marriage itself and of itself carries with it its own profoundly significant theological dimension.

Those theologians who invoked the support of Eph 5 for the sacramental nature of marriage were unable to perceive this point clearly. And because of this there has always been a certain embarrassment about this theology which, ultimately speaking, proves to be utterly unnecessary. For the saying from Gen 2:24 which is quoted in Eph 5 appeared to raise marriage *in general*—not merely that between Christians—to a sign of the unity between Christ and the Church, and it was believed that this could not be conceded without difficulty. In reality this is perfectly possible if we think out exactly the full implications of what we have said with regard to the character of marriage as a sign referring to married love and the special theological dimensions belonging to this. In Christian theology, in fact, we certainly do not have to maintain that a sacramental marriage is related to a non-sacramental marriage as a sacrament to a purely secular human activity. On the contrary both are related to one another as the *opus operatum* to an *opus operantis*, and this latter too is wholly an event of grace.[30] The order in which the one stands to the other here is similar, for instance, to that relationship which a sacramental forgiveness of sins bears to a non-sacramental one achieved merely through repentance. For this too takes place as the outcome of grace and in grace.[31] Marriage does not become an *event of grace* only at that stage at which it acquires the status of a 'sacrament'. On the contrary the event of grace in marriage becomes a *sacramental* event of grace as *opus operatum* in those cases in which it takes place between two baptised individuals in the Church. The case here is exactly as with the faith which justifies of itself even *prior to* baptism, and which then becomes *opus operatum* in baptism.[32] Up to the present, if I am not mistaken, there has been a strange naiveté among theologians in their approach to marriage in that that distinction and that unity which is familiar to every theologian in the case of faith—baptism, penance—sacrament of penance has not consciously been worked out and applied here. In the two former cases the grace-given event of justification is initiated not merely at the moment when the sacrament as such is conferred, but already prior to this at the stage of faith and repentance. *On the other hand* in the dimension of historical manifestation as such this sign only acquires the character of an *unconditional* pledge of grace from God, in other words that of an *opus operatum* and so of a 'sacrament', when it takes place in the Church and takes its place in the concrete in the context in which such a pledge acquires its historical manifestation. This is the Church herself considered as basic sacrament. When a marriage takes place between baptised people in the Church it constitutes an element in the Church's role as basic sacrament, so that the parties actively share in and contribute to the Church's role as basic sacrament, for both give manifest expression to the unifying love of the grace of God, and a marriage of this kind between them achieves this precisely *as* an element in the social unity of the Church herself. Now because of this the marriage as an event of grace gives rise to a 'sacramental' event of grace in which this sign actively contributes to the irrevocable manifestation of God's pledge of grace to mankind, that pledge which is constantly in force and of which God himself never repents. And this manifestation is nothing else than the Church herself.

On the basis of this conception of the 'institution' of this sacrament we can now proceed more freely to evaluate the findings of dogmatic tradition with regard to the doctrine of marriage as a sacrament. We do not need to force the evidence here so as either to postulate or to construct for ourselves any explicit doctrine hypothetically supposed to have existed right from the outset, in which marriage would always have been considered as a 'sacrament' and as such subsumed under a general concept of sacrament. The less we make use of any such idea—so long as we still understand and experience the 'sacramental' nature of a sign of salvation in the Church—the better it will be. When, therefore, we find this also confirmed by the dogmatic tradition we should regard this as neither surprising nor shocking.[33]

V

What has been said, however, still needs clarification to some extent in terms of what is familiar to us from the catechism as a formal statement of what constitutes marriage as a sacrament. It is customarily said that marriage is an image of the unity of Christ and the Church, and that it is a sacrament in virtue of this. On an initial reading of Eph 5:22–33[34] we may, perhaps, receive the impression that the vital common basis for the similarity between the relationship which Christ bears to the Church on the one hand and that involved in marriage on the other consists in the fact that the husband represents Christ while the wife represents the Church. In that case the unity of marriage as such would itself be a relatively secondary reflection of the unity between Christ and the Church, which in turn would be based on a reflection in which the married partners were regarded as separate from one another precisely in respect of the different roles they play. But surely we would still have to say that even for Paul himself this way of viewing the matter is secondary, conditioned perhaps by the parenetic context and more or less conditioned too by the sociological factors prevailing at the time. On this showing, then, it would not simply be the text quoted as a whole which would constitute a statement of central theological importance, but rather the particular passage of 5:29–33 that would have primary importance in it, for these particular verses bear upon the unity of love as such, as constituted in *one* flesh and body. The relationship of leadership and subordination as expressed in the love of solicitude and help on the one hand, and in obedience, submissiveness and 'fear' on the other, is not the objective factor that is decisive in this parallel.[35] If for our present purposes we can take this as established, then all that needs to be clarified here is where, in more precise terms, Christ is to be fitted in in the basic conception put forward in this study. First in the case of Paul it is clear that he regards the order of creation depicted in Gen 2 as belonging to the order of grace and redemption,[36] so that right from the outset that order of creation, and so too of the marriage of Adam, had the significance of pointing forwards to this order of grace. In our terms this is implicitly asserted—albeit on quite different theological principles—when we emphasise that every moral attitude on man's part (and this includes also what is presupposed to such an attitude) is everywhere and in all cases sustained and subsumed by the bestowal of grace by God upon the creature. 'Covenant' is the more sublime and more ultimate factor which, by comparison with the creation considered as the positing of a creature still not determined in a specific direction, has in turn the character of unmerited grace.[37] But precisely because of this 'covenant' is the goal and the all-embracing factor which sustains and subsumes creation as the positing of the condition which makes covenant possible, since it provides the potential covenant partner. This means that objectively speaking everything that takes place in terms of human morality has a hidden relationship to Christ, in whose being and work precisely this imparting of grace finds its eschatological culmination and manifestation. Because he is the goal of it all he provides the basis for the whole dynamism of human history as imparted to it through grace, impelling it towards the immediacy of God.

We are speaking, then, of a unity in love between two human individuals. They are united in a love which consists not merely in the fact that both are aiming at a single common goal in this earthly dimension. This unity, rather, refers to the persons themselves in so far as their orientation to the last end has an eternal validity. And where the unity of love in this sense is achieved, there we have the operation and manifestation of that grace which constitutes the unity of men in the truest and most proper sense. But the converse is also true. Precisely this same grace, considered as establishing a unity between God and man, is manifested in the unity between Christ and the Church, and that too in a manifestation which has an absolute and eschatological force, and which as goal provides the basis for all other graces and their function as establishing unity in the world. For this reason there exists not merely an external similarity between the unity in love of two human individuals on the one hand and the unity between Christ and the Church on the other, but also a relationship between the two unities such that they condition one another: the former exists *precisely because* the latter exists. Their mutual relationship of similarity is not subsequent to the two but is a genuine relationship of participation due to the fact that the unity between Christ and the Church is the ultimate cause and origin of the unity of marriage.

In the light of this we can also understand that the more precise quality of the relationship between Christ as the *directing and controlling head* on the one hand, and the Church as the *obedient* and submissive *bride* on the other is not simply projected in precisely the selfsame sense into the unity of those united in love through marriage. The unity between Christ and the Church is the basis for the unity between husband and wife prior to the question of whether, and to what extent this unity which is brought about also carries with it all the special attributes of the unity which brings it about. To the extent that the unity of Christ and the Church itself has its source in God's gracious will to bestow himself, both *this* unity *and* the unity of marriage have their basis in the selfsame grace of God, which unites mankind to God and men among themselves. To the extent that the goals of this *one single* will to bestow grace are related to one another as 'cause' and 'effect', since precisely *in* the will by which God intended Christ and the Church everything else is willed, this one particular effect of this grace-giving will (namely married unity) is also brought about by the other effect (the unity of Christ and the Church).

By reason of this mutual interrelationship of the two unities, the unity of marriage achieves its *full* manifestation precisely in the unity of Christ and the Church. And because of this much that would otherwise perhaps have remained obscure and unrecognised in the unity of married love can be deduced from the unity of Christ and the Church. And this remains true in spite of the caution which is necessary in adopting this approach. Thus with regard to the relationship of leadership and subordination between husband and wife in marriage Paul had already, and rightly, perceived that the basis of this was the unity of Christ with the Church, even though it may be true that the relationship which he was seeking to justify in part belonged to *that period alone,* and to that extent cannot have been a *moral demand* in the same sense at all periods. But if we were to take the same principle as our starting-point we could recognise other and similar parallels too: the character of the Cross with which both are imprinted; the irrevocability of the covenant; the provisional nature of both measured by the final and eternal consummation for with the Church[38] and marriage[39] are still waiting. However we cannot delay any longer in this article in explaining and rounding off this point.

Marriage, therefore, reaches upwards into the mystery of God in a sense which is far more radical even than we could have guessed merely from the nature of human love as unconditioned. Certainly all still remains hidden under the veil of faith and hope, and all this may still not be lifted from the lowly circumstances of our everyday lives. There is no question that such a truth does not take place either at a level which is utterly beyond man, his freedom, and his interior assent. There is no doubt, therefore, that those united in married love experience this reality in the same measure as they open their hearts to it in faith and love. Surely it has become clear that such a theology of marriage cannot be understood in that sense in which we introvertedly make it our own 'private affair'. On the contrary genuine Christian marriage has at all times the force of a real representation of the unifying love of God in Christ for mankind. In marriage the Church is made present. It is really the smallest community, the smallest, but at the same time the true community of the redeemed and the sanctified, the unity among whom can still be built up on the same basis on which the unity of the Church is founded, in other words the smallest, but at the same time the genuine individual Church. If we were able to recognise[40] and to live out such a truth in its full significance then we could return somewhat more consoled and more bravely, in a spirit of truly Christian freedom, to our 'married problems', so urgent as they are, yet almost talked to death.

Notes

1. cf. D.S. 1001, 1801. For a more detailed treatment on this (with bibliography) P. Adnès, *Le Mariage = Le Mystère chrétien. Théologie sacramentaire* (Tournai 1963), pp. 100–104; H. Rondet, 'Introduction à l'Étude de la théologie du mariage' = *Théologie, Pastorale et Spiritualité. Recherches et Synthèses* 6 (Paris 1960), pp. 97 ff., 175 ff.; H. Volk, *Das Sakrament der Ehe* (Munster 1952); M. Schmaus, *Katholische Dogmatik* IV/I (Munich, 6th ed., 1964), pp. 767–828; E. Schillebeeckx, *Le Mariage* I (Paris 1967).

2. cf. also the manuals of dogmatic theology, e.g. in P. Adnès, *Le Mariage*, op. cit., pp. 135 ff.; M. Schmaus, op. cit., pp. 781 ff.; cf. also J. Michl and H. Volk, 'Ehe', *L.T.K.* III (Freiburg, 2nd ed., 1959), 677–684; W. Molinski, 'Marriage', *Sacramentum Mundi*.

3. This is set forth in P. Adnès, op. cit., pp. 95 ff. (with bibliography); cf. also P. Althaus, *Die Ethik Martin Luthers* (Gütersloh 1965), pp. 88 ff.; O. Lähteenmäki, *Sexus und Ehe bei Luther = Schriften der Luther–Agricola–Gesellschaft* (Turku, 1955).

4. For more precise details on the emergence of the general concept of 'sacrament' see G. van Roo, *De Sacramentis in Genere* (Rome 1957), pp. 1–61; J. Finkenzeller, 'Sakrament' III, *L.T.K.* IX (Freiburg, 2nd ed., 1964), 220–225 (with bibliography). On the problem of the sacramentality of marriage in particular cf. P. Adnès, op. cit., pp. 43 ff., 71 ff. (the Fathers), 89 ff. (the Middle Ages), 104 ff. (Post-Tridentine), 132 ff., 134 ff. (Systematic theology); H. Rondet, op. cit., pp. 79 ff. (Middle Ages), 97 ff. (Trent), 145 ff., 153 ff. (Systematic theology); H. Volk, op. cit., pp. 7–18; M. Schmaus, op. cit., pp. 787 ff.

5. On this cf. K. Rahner, 'The Word and the Eucharist', *Theological Investigations* IV (London and Baltimore 1966), pp. 253–286. My reason for referring to my own works in the course of this article is to give the reader the opportunity to achieve a better understanding of unusual and difficult lines of thought in the context of the general theological system which I have worked out.

6. On this K. Rahner, *Handbuch der Pastoraltheologie* I (Freiburg 1964), pp. 118 f., 121 ff., 132 ff. See also below, nn. 7, 20, 21, 22. Cf. in addition E. Schillebeeckx, *Christus Sakrament der Gottbegegnung* (Mainz 1960), pp. 17–95.

7. Apart from the treatments mentioned in nn. 5, 6 with references, cf. on this also K. Rahner, 'The Church and the Sacraments', *Studies in Modern Theology* (Freiburg/London 1965), pp. 206–215; idem, *Handbuch der Pastoraltheologie* I, pp. 323 ff.

8. cf. K. Rahner, 'Personal and Sacramental Piety', *Theological Investigations* II (London and Baltimore 1963), pp. 109–133; idem, *Kirche und Sakramente*, pp. 22 ff.

9. cf. G. van Roo, op. cit., pp. 62 ff., 82 ff., K. Rahner, 'Sakrament' IV, *L.T.K.* IX (Freiburg, 2nd ed., 1964), 225–230.

10. This is precisely what we mean when we use the term 'real symbol', cf. K. Rahner, 'The Theology of the Symbol,' *Theological Investigations* IV (London and Baltimore 1966) pp. 221–252.

11. cf. K. Rahner, 'Reflections on the Unity of the Love of Neighbour and the Love of God', *Theological Investigations* VI (London and Baltimore 1969), pp. 231–249; idem, *Der eine Mittler und die Vielfalt der Vermittlungen* = Institut für Europäische Geschichte, Mainz. Vorträge Nr. 47 (Wiesbaden 1967), also Vol. IX of this series, pp. 169–184.

12. For more exact details on this cf. the author's recent work, 'Atheismus und implizites Christentum', *Handbuch des Atheismus*, J. Girardi ed. (Munich 1967), also Vol. IX of this series, pp. 145–164.

13. The character of this grace as unmerited is not destroyed by the fact that this *de facto* situation is inescapable. Nor can this be presented as a 'demand' arising from human nature as such at the purely natural level. On this cf. the author's article, 'Concerning the Relationship between Nature and Grace', *Theological Investigations* I (London and Baltimore 2nd ed. 1965), pp. 297–317; 'Nature and Grace', *Theological Investigations* IV (London and Baltimore 1966), pp. 165–188, cf. also below, n. 37.

14. On this cf. K. Rahner, *Zur Theologie des Todes* = Quaestiones Disputatae 2 (Freiburg⁵ 1965), pp. 79 ff., 85 ff.

15. On this cf. Patres Societatis Jesu in Hispania professores, *Sacrae Theologiae Summa* III (Matriti, 3rd ed., 1956), pp. 516 ff. (bibliography).

16. More precise details are provided in the study referred to above in n. 12.

17. Apart from the article referred to above in n. 12, cf. K. Rahner (with J. Ratzinger), *Revelation and Tradition* = Quaestiones Disputatae (London 1965), pp. 9–25; idem, *Zur Theologie des Todes*, pp. 80 ff.

18. From this point of view we would have to concern ourselves with certain aspects of the 'crisis' in marriage as this is defined principally by sociologists. It is only by ridding our minds of certain specific patterns of marriage which have arisen in the course of social history that the true essence of Christian marriage can be established in its pristine force.

19. Attention has once more plainly been drawn to this aspect in the Constitution on the Church, *Lumen gentium* (Chap. I–II).

20. On this cf. J. Alfaro, 'Cristo, Sacramento de Dios Padre, La Iglesia, Sacramento de Christo Glorificado', *Gregorianum* 48 (1967), pp. 5–27; P. Smulders, 'Die Kirche als Sakrament des Heils', *De Ecclesia* I, G. Baraúna ed. (Freiburg 1966), pp. 289–312; idem, 'Sacramenten en Kerk', *Bijdragen* 17 (1956), pp. 391–418.

21. On this cf. K. Rahner, *Handbuch der Pastoral Theologie* I, pp. 121 ff., 132 ff.; idem, 'The New Image of the Church', pp. 3–43, esp. pp. 12–25 in this volume [the author's *Theological Investigations*, vol. 10].

22. On this cf. the studies quoted above, nn. 6, 7, 20, 21. In addition, K. Rahner, *The Church and the Sacraments*, pp. 193–201.

23. On this cf. the Constitution on the Church, *Lumen gentium*, No. 11. This passage deserves greater attention, and not merely in the context with which we are here concerned.

24. On the concrete problem thereby entailed cf. K. Rahner, *Theological Investigations* VI (London and Baltimore 1969), pp. 289 ff.

25. On this cf. K. Rahner, *Handbuch der Pastoraltheologie* I, pp. 146 ff., 151 ff.; idem, *The Church and the Sacraments*, pp. 269–272, 289–294.

26. cf. K. Rahner, *Handbuch der Pastoraltheologie* I, pp. 323–332; idem, *The Church and the Sacraments*, pp. 202 ff.

27. On these problems cf. K. Rahner, *The Church and the Sacraments*, pp. 258–264, and M. Schmaus, *Katholische Dogmatik* IV/I, pp. 75 ff.; E. Schillebeeckx, op. cit., pp. 117 ff.

28. On this cf. the brief survey by J. Michl, 'Ehe', *L.T.K.* III (Freiburg, 2nd ed., 1959), 677–680 (bibliography); P. Adnès, op. cit., pp. 7–42; M. Schmaus, op. cit., pp. 781 ff.; J. Dupont, *Mariage et divorce* (Bruges 1959); P. Grelot, *Le couple humain dans l'Ecriture* (Paris, 2nd ed., 1964); cf. also pp. 210, nn. 34 and 35.

29. On this cf. K. Rahner, 'The Church and the Parousia of Christ', *Theological Investigations* VI (London and Baltimore, 1969), pp. 295–312.

30. On this cf. K. Rahner, *Theological Investigations* II (London and Baltimore 1963), pp. 114–133; idem, *Handbuch der Pastoraltheologie* I, pp. 330 ff.; idem, *The Church and the Sacraments*, pp. 206–215 (supplement with A. Häussling); *Die vielen Messen und das eine Opfer = Quaestiones Disputatae* 31 (Freiburg² 1960), pp. 208–253.

31. On this cf. K. Rahner, 'The Meaning of Frequent Confession of Devotion', *Theological Investigations* III (London and Baltimore 1967), pp. 177–189; idem, 'Die Priesterbeichte', *Knechte Christi. Meditationen zum Priestertum* (Freiburg 1967), pp. 208–253.

32. Apart from the studies already mentioned in n. 30 cf. K. Rahner, 'The Word and the Eucharist', *Theological Investigations* IV (London and Baltimore 1966), pp. 253–286; idem, *The Church and the Sacraments*, pp. 269–272.

33. On the dogmatic tradition of the sacramentality of marriage cf. especially P. Adnès, *Le Mariage*, pp. 43 ff., 71 ff., 76–110; H. Rondet, 'Introduction à l'étude de la théologie du mariage', op. cit., pp. 11–135; E. Schillebeeckx, *Le Mariage* I (Paris 1967). The principle we are stating here could also be taken as the starting-point for a new oecumenical approach. Many Protestant theologians maintain that marriage is not indeed a 'sacrament' but is, nevertheless, a *sanctum*. (Thus, for instance E. Brunner.) In view of this, and setting aside all polemical attacks against an alleged Romish 'sacramentalism'—which, however is based upon a wrong interpretation—the question has still to be raised whether a serious discussion, or even a mutual enlightenment is not possible on this point, to the extent that from the Catholic side we understand how rightly to interpret the sacramentality of marriage. In any case we should not simply apply to it a general and abstract concept of 'sacrament'. This procedure is adopted, for instance, by M. Schmaus, *Katholische Dogmatik* IV/I, pp. 803 f., 806 f., and probably also by K. Mörsdorf, *Lehrbuch des Kirchenrechts* II (Paderborn, 10th ed., 1960), pp. 238–249; cf. also *Münchener Theologische Zeitschrift* 9 (1958), pp. 241–256, esp. 248 f. These authors believe that they have to evaluate the function of the presiding priest in dogmatic terms, and so to treat of marriage in a way which is exactly parallel to the treatment appropriate to the other sacraments. K. Mörsdorf enters quite explicitly into the question with which we are concerned in his article 'Der ritus sacer in der ordentlichen Rechtsform der Eheschliessung', *Liturgie. Gestalt und Folgzug. Festschrift für J. Pascher*, W. Dürig ed. (Munich 1963), pp. 252–266, esp. 265 f. Mörsdorf sees an intrinsic connection between the marriage liturgy and the juridical form of marriage, with the result that he posits the closest possible relationship between the solicitude to ensure the juridical validity of marriage, and the activity of the Church in her function as mediator of salvation. Mörsdorf regards the more recent history of the Church's practice in the case of mixed marriages (especially as a result of the decree *Ne temere* of 1907) as the expression of the Church more and more realising her own power with regard to the forms by which marriage is validly celebrated. In this, according to Mörsdorf's own interpretation, the fathers of the Tridentine Council were not yet able to attain to this realisation. The active assistance of the priest in the liturgical sense is raised to the function of the priest as an active contributor (*persona*

agens), so that the 'collaboration of the priest presiding over the marriage is an essential element in the performance of the sacramental sign' (op. cit., p. 266). Mörsdorf is followed in his views by his pupil, G. May, *Die kanonische Formpflicht beim Anschluss von Mischehen* (Panderborn 1963), p. 42. At this point we shall not undertake any investigation of the historical aspects of this problem, even though these continue to be of decisive importance (the function of the marriage customs and rituals in the early and main periods of the Middle Ages, the interpretation of the decree *Tametsi* etc.). Nor can we examine the ways in which Mörsdorf and May use the concepts of 'passive' and 'active' 'assistance'. Nor do we propose to challenge these authors on the question of whether, and to what extent, the Church has the right to decide (in part) the external signs or form of the sacraments. A more important point is the fact that there are phenomena or factors in the Church's theology and practice of marriage which it is hard to reconcile with this thesis: marriages of baptised non-Catholics are indeed not bound by the canonical form, but are rather valid and sacramental as *matrimonia rata* even without the priest playing any part in them. The marriages between persons of different confessions prior to 1918 in Germany were valid and sacramental even without any Catholic ceremony taking place. Finally reference may be made to canon 1098 (the possibility of concluding a marriage without any collaboration by the priest). When, therefore, Mörsdorf seeks to regard the active intervention of the priest as an '*essential*' element' in the sacramental act, then this term 'essential' cannot be taken in a strict sense. For with regard to a requirement that is essential in the *true* sense in the context of the sacraments, the Church has *no* power of dispensation. But if the priest has no constitutive function in the concluding of a sacramental marriage in the strict sense, then it is not immediately clear what is meant here by 'essential element', '*persona agens*', 'active contributor' etc., or whether this in fact demands any theological interpretation. In any case from the standpoint of a sacramental theology such an interpretation is quite unnecessary. With regard to those cases in which the priest plays no active part, or at any rate not an 'essential' one, it is not asserted that the Church has no mediating function at all, as is proved from the example of valid baptism by laymen. Even in historical terms it must be maintained that the introduction of the form made obligatory by the Council of Trent derives primarily from the Church's anxiety for the welfare of the Christian community (clandestine marriages), but in no sense has this anything directly to do with the progressive development of the Church's authority. On this cf. *C.T.* IX, 639 f., 682–685, 761–764, 668 f. Precisely with regard to the problems which are raised today on the subject of mixed marriages, the acceptance of this theological interpretation of the essence of marriage would in practice raise a fresh difficulty which, from the point of view of dogmatics, is quite unnecessary. On this problem cf. also L. Hofmann, 'Formpflicht oder Formfreiheit der Mischehenschliessung', *Catholica* 18 (1964), pp. 241–257, esp. 245 f.; F. Böckle, 'Das Problem der Mischehe', *Lutherische Monatshefte* 5 (1966), p. 342 with n. 6; P. J. Kessler, *Die Entwicklung der Formvorschriften für die kanonische Eheschliessung* (Diss. iur. Bonn, 1934, Borna-Leipzig 1934); H. Portmann, *Wesen und Unauflösigkeit der Ehe in der kirchlichen Wissenschaft und Gesetzgebung des 11. und 12. Jahrhunderts* (Emsdetten / Westfalen 1938); R. Lettmann, *Die Diskussion über die klandestinen Ehen und die Einführung einer zur Gültigkeit verpflichtenden Eheschliessungsform auf dem Konzil von Trient* = Münsterische Beiträge zur Theologie 31 (Munster 1967), pp. 166 ff. (Conclusion). Unfortunately even with regard to the historical aspects Lettmann does not adopt any position with regard to Mörsdorf's works (for his only remarks on this cf. p. 19, n. 21), and attaches himself without any discussion of other attempts at a theological interpretation to the theses of Wilhelm Bertram, which are primarily influenced by factors of social philosophy. In reply to the more recent hypothesis of K. Mörsdorf I can only offer the present outline of a theology of marriage in general and in numerous points of detail as an alternative suggestion. This could then constitute a starting-point for a further attempt to solve the dogmatic problems entailed in the question of mixed marriages. Even on the interpretation of the form made obligatory by the Council of Trent the last word has not yet been said from the point of view of the history of canon law, a fact which is brought out strikingly in the inaugural address of P. J. M. Huizing, the official canonist for the diocese of Nijmegen, *De Trentse Huwelijksvorm* (Hilversum / Antwerp 1966).

34. For the exegesis of this cf. especially H. Schlier, *Der Brief an die Epheser* (Düsseldorf, 2nd ed. 1958), pp. 252–280.

35. In view of the number of studies a detailed exegetical cannot be undertaken here. On this cf. N. A. Dahl et al., *Kurze Auslegung des Epheserbriefes* (Göttingen 1965), pp. 68–72; F. Foulkes, *The Epistle of Paul*

to the Ephesians (Michigan 1963), pp. 154–163; H. C. G. Moule, *Ephesian Studies* (Michigan, 2nd ed., 1955), pp. 281–296; F. F. Bruce, *The Epistle to the Ephesians* (London 1961), pp. 114–120; J. N. Sanders, 'The Theology of the Church', *Studies in Ephesians*, F. L. Cross ed. (London 1956), pp. 64–75, esp. pp. 71 ff.; H. Schlier and V. Warnach, *Die Kirche im Epheserbrief* (Munster 1949), pp. 25 ff.; H. Conzelmann, *Die kleineren Briefe des Apostels Paulus = N.T.D.* 8 (Göttingen, 9th ed., 1962), pp. 86–88; F. Mussner, *Christus, das All und die Kirche. Studien zur Theologie des Epheserbriefes = Trierer theolog. Studien* 5 (Trier 1955), pp. 147–153; E. Kähler, *Die Frau in den paulinischen Briefen* (Zürich 1960), pp. 88 ff.; J. J. von Allmen, *Maris et femmes d'après Saint Paul = Cahiers théologiques* (Nauchâtel / Paris 1951), pp. 28 ff.; P. Grelot, *Le couple humain dans l'Écriture* (Paris, 2nd ed., 1964); P. Adnès, *Le Mariage*, pp. 39 ff.; H. Greeven, 'Zu den Aussagen des N.T. über die Ehe', *Zeitschrift für evangelische Ethik* I (1957), pp. 109–125, esp. 121 ff.; P. Colli, *La pericopa paolina ad Eph. V 32 nella interpretazione dei SS Padri e del Concilio di Trento* (Parma 1951). cf. also n. 36.

36. On this cf. H. Schlier, *Der Brief an die Epheser*, pp. 262 f., 276 ff. Most recently, especially R. Batey, 'The υία σάρξ Union of Christ and the Church', *N.T.S.* 13 (1967), pp. 270–281; N. A. Dahl, 'Christ, Creation and the Church', *The Background of the New Testament and its Eschatology* (Festschrift for C. H. Dodd), W. D. Davies and D. Daube eds. (Cambridge 1965), pp. 422–443, esp. 437.

37. On this, in addition to the articles mentioned in n. 13, cf. esp. K. Rahner, 'Erlösungswirklichkeit in der Schöpfungswirklichkeit', *Sendung und Gnade* (Innsbruck, 4th ed., 1966), pp. 51–87, esp. 52–75 = *Handbuch der Pastoraltheologie* II/2 (Freiburg 1966), pp. 203–228.

38. cf. the Constitution on the Church *Lumen gentium*, No. 48.

39. cf. ibid., No. 35.

40. On this cf. K. Rahner, *Glaubend und liebend* (Munich 1957); idem, 'Vom Gottgeheimnis der Ehe', *Geist und Leben* 31 (1958), pp. 107–109 = K. Rahner, *Glaube der die Erde liebt* (Freiburg, 2nd ed. 1967), pp. 125–128.

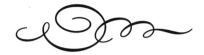

Divorce and Remarriage

17

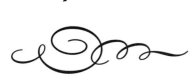

The Indissolubility of Completed Marriage: Theological, Historical, and Pastoral Reflections

E. Hamel, S.J.

1. Indissolubility in the Fathers of the Church

It has been recently maintained in various places that in the early centuries many Fathers of the Church and ecclesiastical authorities permitted remarriage or at least the remarriage of husbands betrayed by their wives. This statement is obviously heavy with serious implications. It calls for a new inquiry into the discipline of the Church and its historical development.[1]

We offer here a few reflections which touch upon the following questions: Did the ancient Church permit a separation that did not include remarriage? What conception of marriage did the Fathers advocate? How should we interpret instances of tolerance in their pastoral practice?

Was Simple Separation Unknown?

It has been said that separation without remarriage was unknown in Roman and Jewish law and was therefore unthinkable for converts to Christianity or for the Church Fathers. But is it historically certain that people would not think of this option or that they were not interested in thinking of it? Is this so novel and modern a notion that no generation prior to the Middle Ages could conceive it, at least as an hypothesis? After new converts heard Christ's and Paul's declarations on marriage, could they not think of this possibility, and would they not have to think of it, even if it seemed harsh to them? New exigencies call for new solutions. A reality which, historically, had never been thought of, but was thinkable as hypothesis, could begin to be envisaged *de facto* because something new had happened, namely, the commandment of Christ, a commandment which amounted to a radical novelty.

Paul's First Letter to the Corinthians was written in the spring of the year 57 A.D. It mirrors the oldest tradition of the Church and shows that Paul did not reject all separation. He alludes to the fact that it is possible for a wife to live apart from her husband: "If she does separate, she must either remain single or become reconciled with her husband again" (1 Cor 7:11). Are we dealing here with a permission which Paul gives or with a concession made to a *fait accompli*? The reason for the separation is not mentioned. The context suggests that the reason was not adultery or lewd conduct (Dt 24) but a disagreement spiritual in nature. To be sure, we cannot maintain on the basis of this text that Paul devised a final solution for the problem of the juridical status of separation. He does exclude remarriage in the name of Christian demands and values. He does lay the incontestable foundations of the institution which church law will later formalize, especially since he speaks in the name of the Lord.[2]

The question has been asked whether the Church Fathers did not make the fatal mistake of falling in line with civil law in this area, allowing for a repudiation followed by remarriage. To begin with, note that postclassical Roman law (that is, after Constantine) was already beginning to recognize the notion of a separation without remarriage. Remarriage was henceforth forbidden and punished by law whenever the repudiation was not motivated. Should a citizen choose to ignore this prohibition and contract another marriage, was the bond of the first marriage rescinded? Opinions differ, but in any case, a penalty was inflicted for remarriage, so that a divorced person who wanted to escape punishment had either to return to his first wife or live alone.

Besides, the notion of separation without remarriage had already appeared in the *Shepherd of Hermas* (100–150 A.D.). In his *Moralia,* St. Basil made a clear distinction between separation and remarriage. He first deals with separation and with the reasons why it may be permitted or must be imposed. In a second chapter, he speaks of the possibility of remarriage for spouses who have separated.

It is difficult, threfore, to take for granted that because remarriage was accepted by Roman law the Fathers of the Church meant more than the termination of conjugal life when they spoke of dissolution in relation to marriage. Unless the opposite is explicitly asserted—a given Father of the Church explicitly stating that separated spouses are free to remarry, or using words to that effect—we may conclude that, when the Fathers speak of repudiation or broken marriage, they are implicitly referring to the termination of conjugal life, not to the right to remarry. The notion of separation without remarriage was known, even though there was no technical vocabulary by which to refer to it. The creation of a specific language, institutionalization, and the legal-technical modalities of institutionalization came later. As we are frequently told nowadays, praxis often precedes legislation.

Thus the repudiation of which the Fathers speak would be a moral, not yet a juridical, institution. It effected separation but did not give the spouses the freedom to remarry. Since theologico-juridical reflection was still embryonic at this time, the prohibition to remarry retained no doubt the quality of a moral prohibition.[3]

Mandatory Separation in Case of Adultery

Many Fathers believed that adultery by itself brought about the termination of marriage (Origen, Chrysostom, Theodoret), at least in the sense that the innocent spouse was obliged to separate from the adulterous spouse in order not to be an accomplice in his or her sin. To maintain association with an adulterous spouse was looked upon as equivalent to condoning adultery, and so ignoring the precept of the Old Testament.

From the theological perspective that sees marriage as a holy institution and salvation as an important concern, separation without remarriage makes sense. The writers who require the innocent spouse to refrain from cohabitation in case of adultery do so in the name of the holiness of marriage. The adulterous spouse must be dismissed, lest the innocent one should share in his or her guilt. Origen: "Thus, a man who has only one eye shall be saved, namely the man who has gouged out the eye of his own household, the adulterous wife, lest having kept her he should march with two eyes into the eternal fire." Basil says that a husband has not only the right but the duty to dismiss his unfaithful wife. His reason is not so much that Roman law demands this separation, but rather a conflation of Matthew 19:9, Jeremiah 3:1 and Proverbs 12:22a: "The man who keeps an adulterous wife under his roof is a godless fool."

The position that separation is required to safeguard the holiness of marriage in case of adultery was advocated by the ante-Nicene and the post-Nicene Fathers. This explains the very strong language which, if taken in a strictly juridical sense, could lead to the conclusion that the innocent spouse is entitled to remarry. The adulterous spouse is no longer a spouse, and the husband is no longer a husband. The couple is a small community. If one of the spouses lapses into adultery, he separates himself from Christ. For the Fathers, adultery was truly the offense against the holiness of the conjugal bond. What we have here is a strictly moral conception of adultery. Adultery was in their eyes the only legitimate ground for separation. The dismissal of a spouse without sufficient reason goes counter the law of the Lord. It was forbidden because it leads to adultery (Mt 5:32).[4]

Conversion and Return of the Guilty Spouse

There is another consideration which justifies separation without remarriage. The Fathers had a moral, not a juridical, conception of adultery. Adultery is thus an obstacle to conjugal life, but one that can be removed by conversion, forgiveness, baptism, penance. The innocent spouse has grounds for hoping that the guilty spouse will repent and return, in which case charity and patience are required. Tertullian: "Patience does not make an adulterer out of the innocent spouse; it rather favors amendment." If the repentant wife returns home, may the husband receive her? Hermas answers categorically: the husband is under serious obligation to receive her.

Why? Because this is an opportunity for conversion, offered to God's servants. Remarriage is forbidden for the same reason. Marry again, and there is no longer any possibility for going back. For the sake of the repentance of the adulterous wife the husband should not remarry. In conclusion, persistent adultery is the only valid reason for separation. As noted, according to the mentality of the time and the way the scriptures were being read, this exception was meant to preserve the holiness of life together.

Ambiguity of the Term "Divorce"

How did the Fathers understand the term *divorce*? For them, this word did not have the strict and precise sense it has in contemporary usage. It could refer both to divorce as we understand it and to mere physical separation. When the Fathers used this word, they did not supply the necessary qualifications. Likewise, they used the synonymous expressions *to loose* and *to separate* (*solvere, dissolvere*) with no precise distinctions.

In Roman law, these expressions did indeed presuppose the possibility of remarriage. But are we to conclude that the Fathers used them in the sense which Roman law assigned to them? As a rule, the Fathers used the vocabulary current in their time with considerable freedom. They did not feel obligated to use words in keeping with their technical meaning. Therefore, one must consult the context to ascertain what they meant. Augustine, for example, had no doubt that remarriage is forbidden in case of adultery, and yet he spoke of the dissolution (*solutio*) of conjugal unions. If we are going to maintain that a particular Father of the Church permitted remarriage in case of adultery, it is not enough to point out that he says that the spouses can or should separate through divorce. He would have to say in addition that a divorced spouse may legitimately and in accordance with the Christian faith contract a new marriage while the other spouse lives. It turns out that Ambrosiaster is the only one who says this explicitly.

In this controversy, it has been too often overlooked that with the passing of time, the Church acquires a surer knowledge of the scriptures, and her awareness of what they mean grows more distinct. We should not be surprised, therefore, if we come upon ambiguous texts which seem to favor divorce and remarriage and which, taken in isolation, could be read to favor remarriage or the possibility of it. The ambiguity, if there be ambiguity, concerns only the way in which we should assess the consequences of adultery. Does adultery make another marriage possible, or only separation?

But let us suppose for a moment that what some people assert is true: namely, that some church fathers and councils did grant that marriage can be totally dissolved and that therefore remarriage after divorce is possible. Note, however, that the case with which they were dealing was very specific, that the ground was precise—adultery—and that they stressed an interpretation of the Matthean clause, *nisi fornicationis causa,* which has never gained currency because it is opposed to the texts of Mark, Luke, and Paul. We would have to conclude that we are dealing with a practice which, compared to what was permitted by civil law, was very limited.[5]

Moral, Nonjuridical Conception of Marriage

The Church has concerned herself with marriage since the beginning, at least by way of prohibiting remarriage. In spite of the absence of legal texts and precise canonical norms, a certain praxis existed. Athenagoras speaks of people who get married "in keeping with the laws current among us."[6]

However, there was as yet no in-depth reflection concerning the indissolubility of marriage. When the Fathers assert that separation dissolves, breaks, or loosens the bond of marriage, when they speak of a transgression that breaks the bond, we should not interpret these texts as meaning that they favored a juridical automatism and necessarily advocated a total severance with the right to remarry. When, on the basis of their interpretation of the clause *nisi fornicationis causa* (Mt 19:9), the Fathers allowed separation from an unfaithful spouse, the innocent spouse was indeed entitled to make use of the repudiation (*repudium*) allowed by civil law, but it did not necessarily follow that remarriage was permitted. Adultery did indeed rescind the obligation to live under the same roof, but solid proof would be needed before we could go on to say that, according to the Church Fathers, adultery made a total end of the conjugal bond and gave access to remarriage.

Remarriages Morally Null and Void

The early Church never issued pronouncements about marriage in terms of juridical validity or juridical nullity. Besides, if the ecclesiastical authorities had decreed the juridical nullity of a mariage which was not regarded as invalid by Roman law, they would have placed the faithful in a difficult predicament. However, granted that such terms as *nullity, validity, invalidity,* and the like, were never used, a certain notion of moral, nonjuridical nullity was already present in the thinking of the Church Fathers. When they speak of remarriage following repudiation, they never use the word *marriage* (*coniugium,* γάμος). Origen speaks of a liaison and says that the man does not really marry. Basil speaks of cohabitation. The Synod of Elvira uses the word *incest* for a union of a man with his daughter-in-law. The Fathers did, therefore, have some expressions by which to refer to a marriage that was null and void. Thanks to this notion of moral nullity, they were able to deny to certain unions the quality of a real marriage. Could we not perhaps speak here of an embryonic Christian legislation? When the Church decrees penalties against remarriages, should not this be taken to mean that she did not purely and simply canonize all the civil regulations relative to marriage?[7]

Toleration of Remarriages

The practice of divorce in case of adultery, sanctioned by civil law, was so deeply anchored in the ethos of the day that the Church Fathers felt constrained at times to tolerate the *fait accompli* in order to preclude even greater mischief. Origen says that those who, contrary to the teaching of the gospel, have allowed people to remarry have not done this entirely without reason or excuse. Basil speaks of remarriage as a custom which is contrary to scripture and for which justification is difficult to find, but he also says that the spouse who has been deserted and has remarried is "forgivable."

The large measure of tolerance exhibited toward men can be explained at least in part by pointing out that men and women did not enjoy equal rights at this time and that inequality was accepted even by ecclesiastical custom. The tolerance toward the wife is traceable to the fact that a deserted wife would find it almost impossible, both materially and morally, to live alone. The law would afford her no protection, and she had no means of subsistence.

Pastoral Silences

In the early Church, the pastors were often at a loss in dealing with divorced persons who had remarried. That was a time when the wedding was celebrated in the family, and the marriage contract was kept in the family archives, although very early a liturgical celebration was added to the wedding ceremony itself. The bishops were often unable to recognize the remarried divorced people as they mingled with the other faithful. In principle, of course, the culprits were supposed to request the penance prescribed by canon law. But if they failed to do so, was the bishop in a position to impose such a penance? In short, in many cases the bishops did not know which way to turn. This is why they elected at times to remain silent with regard to a union which had been contracted before the civil authority and which could not be dissolved because of the consequences that would ensue.

Unable to Christianize in one stroke an institution so alien to the faith of the gospel, the Church hesitated to impose a burden too heavy to carry. It patiently tolerated what it knew was an abuse. The law of the Church, too revolutionary for the people of that time, was difficult for them to accept. This explains the tolerance of a Church that chose not to alienate peoples whose social structures were not yet Christianized. Without explicitly conceding the legitimacy of a marriage contracted by innocent spouses, the Church merely passed over their situation in silence, which is an act of tolerance, not of approval. Is this not the classic doctrine of profitless admonition (*monitio non profutura*)? People were simply allowed to go on in good faith.

Pastoral Silence Today?

These scattered cases of practical tolerance on the part of the ancient Church may be interpreted as an example of how an unflawed strictness in matters of doctrine can be combined with a measure of pastoral flexibility. For we should not overlook the fact that, in the early centuries of Church history, an impressive consensus existed as to the fundamental principle of the indissolubility of Christian marriage.

Against this historical background, some pastors ask today whether one cannot still follow this example and somehow reconcile fidelity to the gospel with mercy, punctiliousness with 'economy.'

The answer is surely yes, if what is involved is a pastoral practice that emphasized benevolent attentiveness rather than rejection. But can we go even further? Specifically, can we allow divorced Catholics to participate in the Eucharist, as they so loudly demand? We think not.

Besides noting the doctrinal reasons developed by Martelet, we must realize that, in spite of surface similarities between situations, the life and tradition of the Church cannot be a cyclic duplication of the past.

It is one thing to bide one's time, to shut an eye in the presence of abuses in an effort to restructure moral conduct in accordance with the severity of the gospel, and another thing to abandon this severity theoretically and practically once it has been established. Would we be willing to accept regression in matters of social justice and social progress on the grounds that it took a long time for people to perceive the rightness of social demands?

In the ancient Church, tolerance was equivalent to a preparation for the gospel (*preparatio evangelica*); it was part of the task of getting people to understand still obscure requirements. But after theological research has reached clear positions and the teaching of the popes has driven the obscurity away, after an ecumenical council has defined its position in the matter, can we still revert to a practice which, casuistic subtleties apart, legitimizes remarriage after divorce, whether or not we have the courage to say so?

2. Indissolubility in the Teaching of the Popes 5th to 12th Century

In the early centuries, Christians lived in an environment in which divorce was admitted, and were exposed to the influence of that environment. Since the beginning of the fifth century, the popes have been consulted by bishops concerning cases in which the indissolubility of marriage was threatened. At times, the cases calling for resolution were unprecedented and difficult. Faced with the questions, the hesitations, and the excessively liberal interpretations of local churches, the popes, whose authority was unchallenged in the West, reasserted the principle of indissolubility and endeavored to contain and counteract abuses. Although the Church often adopted secular views when deciding which element was constitutive of the conjugal bond, she parted company with such views when it came to asserting the solidity of that bond. The demanding originality of the gospel in the matter of indissolubility was proclaimed and upheld.

Innocent I (401–17)

Letter to Exuperius, Bishop of Toulouse (PL 20, 500–501)
Was a husband entitled to remarry after divorcing his wife? Exuperius, Bishop of Toulouse, was uncertain on what course of action to take. In 405 he contacted Pope Innocent I in order to have the benefit of his opinion. This is how the Bishop of Rome replied: men who remarry while their spouses are still among the living, even if their marriage appears to be broken (*dissociari videatur*), cannot but be regarded as adulterers (*neque possunt adulteri non videri*). As for the women with whom they are now living, they too must be looked upon (*videantur*) as guilty of adultery. This accords with what we read in the gospel: "... whoever divorces his wife and married another commits adultery, and the man who marries a divorced woman commits adultery." Note that the pope omits the clause *nisi fornicationis causa* in quoting Matthew 19:9. Why? Is it because he thinks the clause does not entail an exception and that it fails to accord exactly

with Mark 10:12 and Luke 16:18? Or does he state here only a general principle, without considering the specific case of the deserted husband? The former hypothesis seems more plausible, since the gist of the answer is that the repudiation (*repudium*) to which the husband is entitled does not give him the right to a second marriage, and that because of Matthew 19:9.

In a letter to Victricius, Bishop of Rouen, written a year earlier, Innocent I had already declared that any woman who remarries during the lifetime of her husband must be looked upon as an adulteress (*adultera habeatur*). She will not be allowed to do penance (*nec si agendae poenitentiae licentia conceditur*). He declares that this is a common and unchallenged doctrine (*in omnibus haec ratio custoditur;* PL 20, 478–79).

Letter to the Magistrate Probus (PL 20, 602)

During the barbarian invasions, many were taken prisoner. The absence of a spouse was bound to exacerbate the indissolubility problem. Fortinius remarried because his wife Ursa, taken captive when Rome was besieged by Alaric in 409, had long been absent. But Ursa returned, went to Pope Innocent and announced that she was Fortinius's lawful wife.

Note first that according to Roman law, even under Constantine, captivity entails the immediate dissolution of the conjugal bond, both because life in common is no longer possible and because the spouse in captivity can no longer be juridically regarded as possessing the will required for the maintenance of the conjugal bond. Therefore, when Fortinius remarried, he did not violate any civil law. The pope, fully conscious of his authority and with the support of the Catholic faith (*fide catholica suffragante*), decided that the marriage which Fortinius has contracted with Ursa was the true one. A long absence is not sufficient grounds for dissolution and therefore, the second union was not legitimate (*nullo pacto posse esse legitimum*). The pope, then, did not admit the solution advocated by imperial law. Why? Because Ursa was alive, and she had not been dismissed by divorce (*nec divortio ejecta*). The first reason is clear; the second creates a problem. What is the point of the reasoning: Ursa has not been dismissed by divorce? At that time, captivity did cancel out marriage *ipso facto* but was not yet grounds for divorce. It became grounds only in the year 542, under Justinian. Therefore, Fortinius had no need to divorce Ursa, his captive wife. Did the pope suppose that Fortinius could have divorced Ursa on other grounds, but had not done so? Does the pope's reasoning imply that, had Ursa been dismissed through divorce, Fortinius's second marriage would have been valid? It does not seem so. The solution of a specific case is one thing; the argument supporting that solution is another. A specific response is not a doctrinal premise from which inferences not pertinent to the case may be drawn.

But why did the pope address his answer to the magistrate in the first place? In the year 399, Emperor Honorius had restricted the authority of bishops to religious matter. A bishop who rendered a decision on marital matters was not bound to apply the civil law, only the religious law. In accordance with this decree, Innocent declared: "Because of the captivities which had occurred, the marriage validly contracted by Fortinius and Ursa would have been dealt a demeaning blow had the holy decisions of religion not intervened." In the year 408, Honorius enjoined public officials to execute episcopal decrees whenever the parties involved agreed to submit their case to the bishop. This is why the Pope addressed his decision to the magistrate: he was responsible for executing it.

Leo the Great (440–61)

Letter to Nicetas, Bishop of Aquileia (DS 311–14)

During his expedition against Rome, Attila too took a large number of captives. The spouses of some of these captives remarried. But some captives were subsequently released and returned home. Nicetas wrote to the Pope and submitted the case of husbands reunited with their families.

In his response, the pope spoke especially of the wives who had remarried and exhibited great severity with respect to them. He decreed that they were to return to their first husbands in keeping with the precept of the gospel: "Let no man separate what God has joined" (Mt 19:6). By way of corroboration, the pope uses a comparison which is none too complimentary to the wife. He compares her to goods abandoned in time of war (*bona tempore belli derelicta*) which must be returned to their rightful owner at war's end (*Omnique studio procurandum est, ut recipiat unusquisque quod proprium est;* DS 311).

It seems rather clear that the wives' obligation to return to their former husbands is made contingent on one condition: husbands must want to resume life in common with them. But what if the husband does not want this? The pope's answer seems to indicate that the husband is entitled to renounce his rights if he so wishes. Does this mean that he is entitled to remarry? It certainly seems so. It follows that, in extreme cases, the pope did not deem it appropriate to insist all the way on the indissolubility principle. However, as we have said above, we should not exclude *a priori* the notion that some husbands might have preferred to live alone.

Letter to Rusticus, Bishop of Narbonne (*Written in 458–59; PL 54, 1204–05*)

In Roman law, concubinage refers to a simple liaison between two persons who do not want to marry or to appear in public as husband and wife. It differs from marriage because conjugal love (*affectio maritalis*) and life in common (*communio vitae*) are not part of it. Concubinage could exist simultaneously with marriage, but was always distinct from it: a husband was entitled to have a slave concubine in addition to his lawful wife. As a juridical insitition, concubinage began with postclassical Roman law, that is, at the time of the Christian emperors. Before that time, it existed in fact but was not subject to penalties. In 542, Justinian decreed that a married man was not to live in concubinage and that a single man was not to have more than one concubine.

About the year 458, Leo authorized the marriage of a man who had previously lived with a concubine. The pope did not regard concubinage as an indissoluble marriage. Therefore, he did not see it as an obstacle to a subsequent marriage. The pope's decision accorded with Roman law and had an additional advantage: it encouraged people to regularize a situation of which the Church disapproved. The pope made a clear distinction between the wife and the concubine and announced at the same time the conditions to be fulfilled if the marriage is to be valid. A woman is a wife (*uxor*) only if the marriage has been contracted between persons who are free, if it has been publicly celebrated, and if the dowry has been surrendered.

In order to justify his decision, the pope called on the authority of the bible rather than Roman law: "The Lord himself has decreed this long before Roman law came into existence." (*Multo prius hoc ipsum Domino constituente quam initium romani juris existeret.*) A free man would be entitled to marry a slave only if the slave had been freed. This meant that everything depended on the good will of the master.

Gregory the Great (590–604)

The Case of Those Who Enter Monastic Life

The letters of Gregory the Great (over 850 of them) are the largest contribution any pope made to Church law during the sixth and seventh centuries. Two of these letters pertain to the matter at hand. They state that marriage is not dissolved even by entry into monastic life.

The first of these was written in the year 601 to a patrician lady by the name of Teotista. In it, the pope lamented the fact that, on the strength of civil law, entry into monastic life on the part of one spouse is regarded by the other as a legitimate ground for dissolving the marriage and remarrying. The pope did not hesitate to brand this second marriage illicit and unclean. When one spouse enters monastic life, the other is obligated to practice continence, since the marriage is indissoluble. Of course, a serious temptation is there in the making. Speaking to the spouse who has entered monastic life, the pope asks: "What kind of conversion is this, where one and the same flesh moves partly into continence, while the other part persists in impurity?" (PL 77, 1161).

The second letter was written the same year to a notary of Palermo. It concerns the complaint of a woman by the name of Agathosa. She had written to the pope to complain that her husband had become a monk against her will. In the year 542, Justinian had decreed that entry into religious life must count *bona gratia,* that is, by way of benevolent concession, as grounds for divorce. Despite this law, the pope states that God's law must prevail: "Except in case of lewd conduct, a husband is not entitled to dismiss his wife since, once they have consummated their union, the spouses become one flesh. One part of that flesh cannot turn to monastic life, while the other remains in the world." Note that the pope was attempting to protect the rights of both parties against a unilateral decision imposed by one party upon the other. If life in common is to be interrupted, the spouses must freely agree to the interruption. Entry into monastic life should not serve as an excuse for dissolving marriage. Once the marriage has been consummated, a spouse is not permitted to enter monastic life, thus creating for the spouse who remains in the world an occasion of sin (PL 77, 1169).

Gregory II (715–31)

A Case of Impotency

In his letter *Desiderabilem mihi,* written in 726, St. Gregory II answered several queries of St. Boniface, Bishop of Mainz. The Bishop had raised the problem of a wife who was ill (*infirmitate correpta*) and could not fulfill the conjugal obligation. What was her husband to do?

The pope's reply is in two parts. He first mentions the solution he prefers: "It would be good if the husband would remain as he is and cultivate continence." (*Bonum esset, si sic permaneret ut abstinentiae vacaret.*) However, this solution is beset with difficulties. Perhaps the husband is not strong enough to live in continence. Continence is for strong people. (*Hoc magnorum est.*) Eventually, remarriage may be the solution: if he cannot restrain himself, let him marry. (*Qui si non potuit continere, nubat magis.*) However, he should not forget his obligations toward the woman who is deprived of conjugal life only because of illness, and has not lost her rights because of a detestable fault (PL 89, 525).

Gregory, then, showed tolerance toward human weakness, but tolerance did not abridge his sense of justice. All the same, we cannot help noticing that, as pope, he advised a husband to divorce his wife and remarry, which contradicts the constant teaching of the Western Church. It is imperative that we try to assess the precise import of this particular letter.

The text of this letter is often called the crux of canon lawyers; it has caused much ink to flow. The severest difficulty in the interpretation of the text, the one difficulty that cannot be removed on the basis of the available documents, has to do with the malady in question. Since we do not have the letter in which Boniface gives the particulars of the case, we do not know about the nature of the malady that occasioned the query. But no matter what malady was involved and what its consequences were, the important question is whether it was equivalent to what is known technically as impotency. Did it begin before the marriage or was it contracted after the marriage? Did it prevent consummation? Was it curable or incurable? None of these questions can be answered on the basis of either the text or the context. The text merely says: "afflicted by illness" (*infirmitate correpta*). In the absence of this information, how can we trust ourselves to make a judgment as to the pope's response? Was the marriage valid? Has it been consummated? The wording is so vague and the particulars so scanty that we are in no position to decide on the sense of the passage and make an interpretation which is proof against challenge.

The passage has generally been interpreted as referring to a case of impotency arising after the celebration of the marriage. The pope, then, would have been tolerating a custom contrary to the law of the gospel but current in Germany at that time. According to some commentators, the letter represents a concession to the Thuringians. Pope Gregory's position is that a man who discovers that his wife cannot have intercourse must resign himself to a life of continence. However, this solution could hardly have been applied to the Thuringians, for they had only recently converted to Christianity and were still unaccustomed to living an integral Christian life. The solution was simply too harsh for them. And so a concession seems to be in order, else they might have lost heart and turned away from Christianity. There is, however, no way of determining on what grounds the concession rested. Was it antecedent impotency, or nonconsummation because of consequent impotency? This text will always be a problem.

We cannot state, then, that the pope dissolved a marriage contracted and consummated (*ratum et consummatum*), even though we cannot exclude the possibility that he did so.[8]

Stephen II (752–57)

Pope Stephen II was consulted by English monks concerning the possibility of remarriage after separation. He replied by referring to the decisions of Pope Innocent I and Leo the Great. With regard to another question, his answer was as follows: "If a person contracts marriage and one of the spouses should happen to be unable to render the conjugal duty, separation is not permitted. Nor is any other malady a valid ground for separation, with the exception of the devil's malady and leprosy . . ." (PL 89, 1024).

Here we are dealing at least with a form of impotency or an illness that sets in after the celebration of the marriage, but perhaps also with an impotency that antecedes the celebration. According to the pope, neither is a valid ground even for separation. This text bears a great resemblance to that of Pope Gregory II, and yet the answer it contains is diametrically opposed to the answer given in that text. Either the two popes assessed the same situation differently, or the situations look the same but are different.

Nicholas the Great (856–67)

The popes of the second half of the ninth century, beginning with Nicholas I, endeavored to combat abuses and to reassert firmly the indissolubility principle, thus reinforcing the foundation of the institution of marriage. The popes were prompted to do so by some sensational marital cases. Also to be taken into account is the fact that Church discipline had already deteriorated in the churches of the Franks, and certain ecclesiastical judges had exhibited precious little firmness.

The Divorce of Boson and Engeltrude

The Count of Boson had dismissed his adulterous wife. Pope Nicholas I wrote a letter to Hincmar, Archbishop of Reims, invoked his apostolic authority (*praecipimus vobis apostolica auctoritate fulti*), and ordered him to have Engeltrude return to her husband. Should she refuse, Hincmar should not hesitate to excommunicate her (MGH: *Epistolarum* 6, 267). On March 7, 867, Pope Nicholas stated that Boson could not take another wife, even if he was not responsible for the fact that the efforts at reconciliation failed (MGH: *Epistolarum* 6, 333). In the end, the pope excommunicated the fugitive wife, but the Council of Metz (869) went over his head and removed the excommunication.

The Divorce of Lothair II

Lothair had divorced his barren wife and married Walrad, who had been his mistress. The divorce had been approved by the Council of Metz, but Pope Nicholas had the Lateran Council rescind this decision in the year 863. Walrad was excommunicated and so was the offending bishop. In the end, Lothair severed relations with the mistress and was reconciled with the pope.

Divorce and Remarriage

At the end of the year 861, Adon, Bishop of Vienne, consulted the pope to ascertain whether a husband might, without the approval of a general council, divorce a wife who has been charged with a crime, and remarry or take a mistress.

The wording of the query strongly implies that, in the matter of second marriages, some ecclesiastical judges tended to be rather accomodating. The pope's answer was firm, to say the least: "In the name of our apostolic authority and in accord with the mandate of the gospel, we resist them. We do not permit those who do things of this sort to enjoy sexual intercourse with another wife, nor do we give them permission to have a mistress." (MGH: *Epistolarum* 6, 618–19.)

It is clear that Nicholas is asserting here the primacy of jurisdiction of the see of Rome, which is competent to ratify or rescind decisions taken by local councils.

Alexander III (1159–81)

In response to a query by the Archbishop of Canterbury, Pope Alexander III explicitly asserted the indissolubility of marriage in case of leprosy. This disease is not adequate grounds for the separation of the spouses, even if custom often forces them to separate: "Since husband and wife are one flesh, the one may not be without the other for long." If they should separate, "you are to order them to practice continence, as long as the other partner lives. Should they refuse to obey, excommunicate them." (CJC: *Decretales Gregorii IX:* ed. Ae. Friedberg, col. 690–91).

In another passage, the pope declared that, should a wife leave her husband because of unfaithfulness on his part, she may not remarry, "because, even though they have separated, they still remain husband and wife." The pope asserted that the spouses are equal. He explicitly added: "This sentence applies in the same form even to men." (CJC: *Decretales Gregorii IX;* ed. Ae. Friedberg, col. 720).

Modern canonists quote far less frequently than their predecessors the interesting letter of Alexander III written in the year 1170 to a bishop named Vicentinus. The pope had been told that a certain bishop had issued a decree of divorce within the ecclesiastical assembly, then granted permission to remarry to a woman whose husband had been in foreign lands for over a decade. Taken to task, this bishop had refused to change his decision. In his letter, Alexander III first asked Vicentinus to conduct an investigation. If the investigation proves that the facts are as reported, the pope says, Vicentinus should simply legitimize the children, since the woman had remarried "on the authority of the aforementioned bishop, without resistance on the part of the Church" (*auctoritate praedicti episcopi, sine quaestione et contradictione Ecclesiae*). Considering that the ecclesiastical superiors had been themselves at fault and that the woman had obviously been in good faith, could the pope have gone further and insisted on indissolubility and its consequences? The pope obviously could not, and so he kept silent and merely requested that the situation of the children born of this union be regularized. (CJC: *Decretales Gregorii IX;* ed. Ae. Friedberg, col. 712).

Celestine III (1191–98) and Innocent III (1198–1216)

Celestine III extended the Pauline Privilege to cover cases of apostasy. An archdeacon had authorized a Christian woman to remarry after she had been forsaken by her husband who had apostatized. The pope was asked whether this had been a wise decision. He replied: "It seems to us that should the first husband return to the Church, the wife would not be bound to desert her second husband and go back to the first, since it is he who, in the eyes of the Church, has deserted his wife." According to Gregory, the contempt of the creator dissolves marriage for the spouse who has been deserted out of hatred for the Christian faith (. . . *teste Gregorio contumelia creatoris solvat jus matrimonii circa eum qui relinquitur odio fidei Christianae;* CJC: *Decretales Gregorii IX;* ed. Ae. Friedberg, col. 587–88).

In May 1199, Innocent III, Celestine's successor, repudiated this solution in his answer to a query from the Bishop of Ferrara. The bishop had inquired whether, if one spouse lapsed into heresy, the other could be permitted to allow the heretical spouse to remarry. The Pope replied that the Pauline Privilege did not apply to heresy or apostasy, "although a certain predecessor of ours seems to have entertained a different opinion." (. . . *licet quidam praedecessor noster sensisse aliter videtur;* CJC: *Decretales Gregorii IX;* ed. Ae. Friedberg, col. 722).

Pope Innocent III likewise resisted the demands of Philip Augustus, King of France (1180–1223), who wanted to divorce Ingeburg of Denmark.

3. ROME AND GREEK OR EASTERN CUSTOMS, 13TH CENTURY TO THE COUNCIL OF TRENT

The only pope who made pronouncements on the customs of the Greeks before the Council of Florence is Honorius III (1216–27). He was asked by John, the papal legate, what should be done about Greeks who divorced their wives and remarried. The pope answered on August 10, 1218: "The question of divorce cannot be settled, or a dispensation granted, since the bond is indissoluble both for the faithful, be they Greek or Latin, and for infidels." (*Regesta Pontificum Romanorum,* n. 5834).

A letter of Innocent IV, dated March 6, 1254, and addressed to the Greeks of Cyprus, recommends the adoption of Latin rites. It does not mention indissolubility (DS 830). A constitution *Ad Graecos et alios,* issued by Alexander IV (1254–61), does not mention divorce. (See *Constitutio instruens Graecos et alios,* 14, in *Pontificia Commissio ad redigendum Codicem Iuris Canonici orientalis; Fontes,* Series III, Vol. IV, Tomus 2, 111.)

In the year 1279, Gregory IX held the Council of Lyon in which Michael Palaeologus established full communion with the Church of Rome. However, the divergent discipline of the Eastern Churches, and particularly of the Byzantine Church, was practically ignored. We do find an implicit repudiation of the practice of divorce and remarriage when we are told about second marriages that death alone frees the spouses from the conjugal bond (DS 860).

The fathers of the Council of Sis in the year 1342 were invited by Pope Benedict XII (1334–42) to disavow a list of errors and abuses. They declared that abuses concerning divorce were still practiced in Armenia (which was not united with Rome), whereas in Cilicia bishops who granted divorces were deposed. The acts of this Council were brought to Pope Clement V (1342–52); he asked for further clarifications, but not precisely with regard to divorce.

At the Council of Florence, the Eastern custom of remarrying after separation due to adultery was mentioned in passing. However, by a sort of gentlemen's agreement, the question was not discussed. The union was established without any change being made in the discipline of either party; see the bull *Laetentur caeli,* July 6, 1439 (DS 1300–1308). The question was raised at the very last minute by Eugene IV (1431–47), but by that time the decree of reunion had already been signed. The Greeks replied that if they did at times permit divorce there was valid reason for doing so (*non sine iustis causis;* recognize here Origen's formula). The Latins did not press the point. (See Perrone, *De Matrimonio,* III, 364.)

On the contrary, when the Armenians signed the act of union a few months later, they were not allowed to retain the Eastern custom. The decree *Ad Armenos* explicitly declared that betrayed spouses may not remarry. In case of adultery, physical separation is in order, but divine right does not authorize a second marriage, "since the bond of marriage legitimately contracted is forever" (*cum matrimonii vinculum legitime contracti perpetuum sit;* see the bull *Exultate Deo,* November 22, 1439, DS 1327). This decree was imposed on the Syrian Jacobites united with Rome in 1442 (DS 1351).

If we except the interventions of Honorius III and Clement VI and the discussions at the Council of Florence, there are no other decisions of the Holy See prior to the Council of Trent concerning the practice of divorce among the Greeks and Easterners, both those united with Rome and those separated. We must conclude that, in spite of the rigidity of its doctrinal position, the Apostolic See thought it opportune to procrastinate. Undoubtedly it reserved the right to take action later, but the opportunity to do so did not arise.

4. Indissolubility at the Council of Trent

At the Council of Trent the situation with regard to the indissolubility of the conjugal bond was as follows. Catholic theologians were agreed that marriage is indissoluble even in cases of adultery. The only controversy concerned the theological note to be assigned to this assertion and what censure ought to be inflicted on those maintaining the opposite position. Parallel to this doctrine the three "great doubts" of Cajetan, Erasmus, and Catharinus had surfaced. The least we can say about their novel views is that they had not been well received by theologians. On the other side, Luther was accusing the Catholic Church of having lapsed into error. The Church, he contended, was a tyrant. She had usurped power. The pope has no authority to dissolve marriages or to interdict the dissolution of marriages any more than to erect impediments to marriage. All this belonged to the state. Finally, there was the tradition of the Eastern Churches, which permitted divorce at least in cases of adultery.

After many discussions, in the 24th session the council voted canon 7, which is the charter to which theologians and canonists refer when dealing with indissolubility: "Should anyone say that the Church commits error when she taught and teaches, in accordance with the doctrine of the gospel and of the apostles, that the bond of marriage cannot be dissolved because of the adultery of one of the spouses, and that neither spouse, including the innocent one who has not provoked the adultery, may contract another marriage while the other spouse is living, and that a man commits adultery who, after dismissing his adulterous wife, marries another woman, and that a woman commits adultery who, after dismissing her adulterous husband, marries another man, let him be anathema."[9]

This canon should not be considered in isolation, but in connection with canon 5, which disavows other grounds of divorce allowed by the Protestants: heresy, incompatibility of temperament, estrangement. Canon 7 should also be read in connection with canon 8, which defends the right of the Church to grant separation *quoad torum*. Finally, it should be interpreted in the light of the council's basic assertions on marriage (DS 1787–99).

Canon 7 came to the defense of Catholic teaching, even if it did not declare that this teaching in unchangeable in all its nuances. It simply said that the Church "has taught and teaches" (*docuit et docet*); it did not add "always" (*semper*). Therefore, the council did not deny the existence of practices and doctrines in the present and especially in the past that diverged from its own doctrine. All the same, the past was referred to in the verb *docuit*.

The teaching of canon 7 was not purely disciplinary in nature, that is, meant only to uphold canonical legislation. Neither was it purely doctrinal and theoretical, for it alluded to the Church's practice as presented and articulated in the documents of the teaching office.

As far as its content is concerned, canon 7 denied the possibility of dissolving the conjugal bond in case of adultery and the liceity and validity of remarriage. It made no distinction between intrinsic and extrinsic indissolubility. The context favors the view that intrinsic indissolubility was meant, but this was not explicitly stated. Nor did canon 7 make a distinction between consummated and nonconsummated marriages. It did not decide the question of whether the Church has any power over sacramental and consummated marriage.[10]

All the same, it is difficult to see how, both from a logical and a doctrinal point of view, anyone could object to the interpretation of Pius XI, who went beyond the limited opportunities of the sixteenth century and interpreted the teaching of the council by saying: "If the Church has not been, and is not mistaken, when she offered and offers this teaching, it is absolutely certain that marriage may not be dissolved, even on grounds of adultery. It is just as evident that the other and much weaker grounds of divorce that could be adduced are worth even less, and cannot be accorded any consideration at all" (see CC, December 31, 1930, AAS 22 (1930) 574; Latin text also in DS 1807, note 1).

Theological Note

We should not infer from this text more than hermeneutics allows. It is wiser to seek out from the didactic intention of the council, that is, what it intended to say and teach. It affirmed that the Church has not lapsed into error. This means that the council impressed upon its own statement the quality of a doctrine. However, when indissolubility is at stake, the council's assertion must be filtered through the indefectibility of the Catholic Church. We shall briefly say why this is so.

A council is under no obligation to say all that can be said about a given question. Obviously, it may not say more than it is entitled to say, but it also may say less for doctrinal and pastoral reasons. When an anathema is involved, is not a council obligated to restrict itself to the minimum? The consent of canon 7 does not exhaust what can be considered as theologically established in the doctrine and practice of the Church in the matter of indissolubility. It is only proper to situate the canon within the framework of the doctrine of the teaching office as such, considered in its totality.

What note should we assign to the general assertion that marriage is indissoluble? It is a Catholic doctrine (*doctrina catholica*), a firm assertion of the teaching office, even if it is not presented as a doctrine of defined faith.[11]

The Council of Trent and the Greek and Eastern Practices

The council chose to reaffirm Catholic doctrine and to formally condemn the error of the Protestants. However, it did not want to create yet another obstacle to the reunion of the Christian churches by explicitly and formally condemning the doctrine and practice of the Eastern Churches. Nor did it want to risk severing from Rome the Greek ecclesial communities which remained united with it by a bond which, all things considered, was not very sturdy. At the council the Venetians defended the practice of the Easterners, for at that time Venice occupied the islands of Crete, Cyprus, Corfu, Zante, and Cephalonia. For the sake of public peace, it was quite important that the Byzantine subjects of Venice not fall into formal heresy and be exposed to repression when they made use of the 'economy' of remarriage allowed by their Church. If they wanted to escape repression, they needed only to refrain from contending that Rome was mistaken and to practice pluralism and tolerance.

For reasons which anticipate somewhat the spirit of ecumenism, the Council of Trent preferred not to push the doctrine of indissolubility to its ultimate consequences and to stay on this side of what it could and perhaps wished to say.

To be sure, the council did not advocate a double evangelical and apostolic tradition, one element favoring indissolubility, the other favoring divorce in case of adultery. The doctrine of indissolubility which the council proclaimed is declared to be "in accordance with the doctrine of the gospel and the apostles" (*juxta evangelicam et apostolicam doctrinam*). And yet the council chose not to formally condemn the practice of the Eastern Churches and their faithful. Practically, then, the council faced what we call today a conflict of values. The value represented by an explicit definition of indissolubility, as distinct from an indirect proclamation, was less important in the mind of the council than values related to religious and public tranquillity. The council decided that it could take this course of action—that is, making an indirect proclamation—without betraying the gospel.

By deciding not to condemn the Easterners, Trent did tolerate a practice which, taken as it is, cannot be justified. Although it was prevented by its own interpretation of the gospel from adopting that practice, the council did countenance it.[12]

The Eastern practice remained contrary to the Scriptures. Even if it was not formally condemned, it was not justified as such. The only thing in its favor is that it was not entirely groundless—it could appeal for support to some patristic and medieval authorities. Trent looked upon it as something that can be conceded for the sake of avoiding greater mischief (*ad vitanda peiora*). To strike at the Greeks in the name of orthodoxy would have had an unpleasant result. They would have been deeply offended, and union with them would have become all the more difficult to achieve. For the sake of union, Trent chose to limit the obstacles as much as possible.[13]

We have here an official conciliar definition which resolved a value conflict. Is this the only conclusion we can draw? We cannot be sure *a priori*. Some will no doubt think that we have in the council's decision an indication of how to proceed, a pastoral attitude which could give us guidance even today. Can we further apply this indication? Could the Church, in order to safeguard more important values, refrain from always drawing the ultimate consequences from those doctrines which, according to Vatican II, do not occupy the first rank in the hierarchy of truths? It is not our responsibility to make this determination. But here one must also bear in mind that there is a difference between quiet tolerance and affirmation of principles, between closing an eye to existing situations on the one hand and letting abuses have their way on the other. Rome's long struggle against tolerating the remarriage of divorced persons in the uniate Churches is a theological argument which also deserves consideration.

Notes

1. We need not weigh down this presentation with a critical apparatus which readers can easily find in many fine recent works. How often have the same texts been quoted, commented upon, and discussed in the last fifteen years? Here we are interested less in documentation than in interpretation. The documentation can be found in the articles "Adultère" and "Mariage" in the DTC 1 (1930) 464–511 and 9 (1927) 2044–317, which retain all their value, as well as in recent publications, which likewise give rich bibliographies. Cf. particularly, P. Adnès, "Mariage et Vie Chrétienne," DS Fasc. 64–65 (Paris: Beauchesne, 1977) 355–88, and A.M. Henry, "Mariage," *Catholicisme: Hier, Aujourd'hui, Demain*, Fasc. 34 (Paris: Letouzey et Ané, 1977) 461–500.

2. 1 Cor. 7:10–11: " to those now married. . . . I give this command (though it is not mine; it is the Lord's) [cf. Mk 10:9–12 and parallels]: A wife must not separate from her husband. If she does separate, she must either remain single or become reconciled to him again. Similarly, a husband must not divorce his wife."

3. J. Masson, *Histoire des causes de divorce dans la tradition copte* ("Studia Orientalia Christiana-Collectanea") 14 (1970–71), 240–42.

4. A. Houssiau, "Le lien conjugal dans l'Eglise ancienne," AC 17 (1973) 570.

5. G. Pelland, *De Vinculo Matrimoniali apud Patres;* unpublished manuscript, 27–28.

6. Athenagoras, *Legation on Behalf of Christians*, 33 (PG 6, 965).

7. J. Masson, *Histoire des causes de divorce*, pp. 242–44.

8. W. Kelly, *Pope Gregory on Divorce and Remarriage* (Rome, 1976), 72–74; 285–86.

9. *Si quis dixerit, Ecclesiam errare, cum, docuit et docet, iuxta evangelicam et apostolicam doctrinam, propter adulterium alterius coniugum matrimonii vinculum non posse dissolvi, et utrumque, vel etiam innocentem, qui causam adulterio non dedit, non posse, altero coniuge vivente, aliud matrimonium contrahere, moecharique eum, qui dimissa adultera aliam duxerit, et eam, quae dimisso adultero alii nupserit: anathema sit* (DS 1807).

10. P. Adnès, *Histoire des conciles œcuméniques*, Vol. XI (to be published).

11. The theological note "of revealed truth" could also be suggested in view of the texts of Mk, Lk, and Paul. Obviously, we would stilll need to explain the Matthean clause *nisi fornicationis causa*. Another difficulty even more serious is created by the interpretaion given to this clause in some ancient Churches.

12. Lehman, "Unauflöslichkeit der Ehe und Pastoral für wiederverheiratete Geschiedene," IKZ 1 (1972) 364–65.

13. Ratzinger, "Zur Frage nach der Unauflöslichkeit der Ehe" in F. Heinrich and V. Eid (eds.), EE (Munich, 1972) 50–51.

18

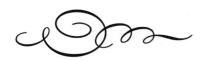

Divorce, Remarriage, and the Sacraments

Richard A. McCormick, S.J.

On November 27, 1985, at the Extraordinary Synod of Bishops, Archbishop Karl Berg (Salzburg, Austria) called for "more understanding" for divorced and remarried Catholics. He then suggested that "perhaps after a period of penance they might be re-admitted to the sacraments."[1] Archbishop Peter Seiichi Shirayanagi (Tokyo) stated that exclusion from the sacraments of the divorced and irregularly remarried "seemed an especially cruel measure." These people have not lost their faith and a way should be found "so that these people can fully participate in the life of the Church."[2]

A day later, November 28, Archbishop James Martin Hayes (Halifax, Nova Scotia) added his voice to those of the Austrian and Japanese prelates. Hayes said that "I feel a tremendous sympathy for persons in that situation, and I would certainly like to be able to reach out to them and come to their aid."[3] He then added at a press conference: "What I am asking for is that either the Synod or another group look at the theological principles involved there and see if the discipline we now have really interprets in the best way for the good of the persons concerned and especially the rights of the persons concerned."

These synodal interventions were not new. Similar suggestions had been made in the Synod of 1980. Archbishop Derek Worlock (Liverpool) asked: "Is this spirit of repentance and desire for sacramental strength to be forever frustrated?"[4] He noted that his own presynodal consultation would not accept the assertion that concession of the Eucharist to the irregularly remarried would scandalize Catholics and undermine the bond of marriage. At least fifteen of the 162 synodal fathers spoke to the question of finding a way to readmit Catholics in irregular second marriages to the sacraments. Archbishop Henri Legare (Grouard-McLennan, Alberta) went even further. The problem of the divorced-remarried, he said, cannot be faced merely at the pastoral level. The doctrine of marriage must be reexamined. It must be rethought "in a more existentialist and personalist framework" rather than out of an "essentialist philosophy."[5]

The response to such petitions is well known. It is contained in *Familiaris Consortio,* the apostolic exhortation of John Paul II that followed the 1980 synod. The pope, after insisting that the Church should make "untiring efforts to put at their disposal her means of salvation" and should "make sure that they do not consider themselves as separated from the Church," stated:

> However, the Church affirms her practice, which is based upon sacred scripture, of not admitting to eucharistic communion divorced persons who have remarried. They are unable

to be admitted thereto from the fact that their state and condition of life objectively contradict that union of love between Christ and the Church which is signified and effected by the Eucharist. Besides this there is another special pastoral reason: If these people were admitted to the Eucharist the faithful would be led into error and confusion regarding the Church's teaching about the indissolubility of marriage.[6]

John Paul II then adverted to the situation of remarrieds who cannot separate. They must "take on themselves the duty to live in complete abstinence, that is, by abstinence from the acts proper to married couples."

In summary, then, the pope reaffirmed the practice of excluding the divorced-remarried from the Eucharist unless they live as brother and sister. He did this on two grounds, one theological, one pastoral. Theologically, the pope argued that there is a contradiction between the state of the divorced-remarried and the union of love between Christ and the Church that is signified in the Eucharist. In other words, their state does not fully symbolize or correspond to what the Eucharist represents and what they profess by receiving it. The effect of this state is that those who are in it can receive the sacrament of penance, "which would open the way to the eucharist" only if they are "sincerely ready to undertake a way of life that is no longer in contradiction to the indissolubility of marriage." The obvious implication of this is that they are in a state of sin. Otherwise, why could they not receive penance? The heart of this "state of sin" is the intention to have sexual intercourse. For once the couple determines to live in complete abstinence, the obstacle to penance (and the Eucharist) disappears.

Pastorally, the pope argued that any other policy would cause scandal by confusing people about the Church's teaching on the permanence of marriage.

An analysis virtually identical to that of the pope was made in 1978 by the International Theological Commission. It stated:

> From the incompatibility of the state of the divorced-remarried with the command and mystery of the risen Lord, there follows the impossibility for these Christians of receiving in the Eucharist the sign of unity with Christ.[7]

This analysis is far from unanimously shared. Indeed, over the past twenty years or so, there has developed a theological consensus that the divorced-remarried may, in individual instances and under certain conditions, receive the sacraments. One of those conditions is *not* that they abstain from sexual relations. An example would be the statement of a committee of the Catholic Theological Society of America published in 1972. After mentioning the traditional demand of a brother-sister relationship, the committee stated:

> It is the judgment of this committee that, whatever may have been its theological justification or benefits in the past, there is serious reason to modify this practice. From the many reasons we have already cited for questioning the validity of marriages that have broken down, and the powerlessness of any human community to judge so many of these cases with certainty, one can reasonably conclude that there are Catholics whose marital status in the eyes of God does not correspond to their legal status. Also, there are unions, e.g., where children are involved, where it may be morally wrong to terminate the relationship. Many will not understand how it will be possible for them to sustain this relationship without marital union. We do not think these people should be excluded from the sacraments or participation in the life of the church. If a couple decides after appropriate consultation, reflection and prayer that they are worthy to receive the sacraments, their judgment should be respected. If the

consultation and the judgment that takes shape around it are to be responsible, they must center on the quality of the present union, its fidelity and stability, the state of conscience of the couple, the quality of their Catholic lives in other respects, their acceptance by the community, etc.

Some might object that this solution would be a source of scandal. It would arise from the fact that these people are accepted into full participation in the life of the Church without any change in their present status. But we believe that if the reasons we have given are properly explained to the Catholic people, fear of scandal is unjustified. Moreover, when these couples are leading otherwise responsible and religious lives, their standing in the community is usually very good.[8]

In this chapter I want to respond to Archbishop Hayes' suggestion that we "look at the theological principles involved there and see if the discipline we have really interprets in the best way" the implications of the Church's teaching on indissolubility.

In order to clarify the exact question I want to discuss, I must say a word about both indissolubility and reception of the sacraments. By indissolubility I mean the doctrine *in itself* and its pastoral implications. The term "in itself" is used to distinguish the notion from any prevailing understanding of it at a particular time. In all matters doctrinal and moral we must always distinguish the substance of a teaching from its formulation at a particular point in history. That is a burden I wish the term "indissolubility in itself" to carry. Concretely, one particular understanding of indissolubility might join it inseparably with reception of the Eucharist by the divorced and force the conclusion that the two are but one issue. Another understanding might yield a different conclusion. To make the distinction between substance and formulation where indissolubility is concerned will, of course, clearly require an attempt on my part to state what I believe to be the substance of that teaching. That I hope to do, delicate and even arrogant as the attempt may appear.

As for reception of the Eucharist, I wish to understand a reception warranted by public teaching in the Church, a teaching stated in and controlled by public norms whereby at least some divorced-remarried persons can be allowed to receive the Eucharist. I put the matter this way, not because it is desirable or even tolerable that there be a policy of exceptions of equal valence with the demand of indissolubility, but because I do not wish the main emphasis to fall on internal forum solutions. Why? For two reasons. First, such pastoral solutions include the condition *secluso scandalo* and therefore when properly implemented should not, or at least need not, raise the indissolubility issue. Second, and more importantly, one instance of an internal forum solution is one where a conclusion of nullity of the first marriage is drawn on prudent and probable, but legally nondemonstrable or unacceptable grounds. If this is the case, the issue is not truly indissolubility itself as commonly understood, but the sufficiency of the legal structures whereby it is supported and adjudicated.

Within the confines of the above clarifications, the issue is the following: are those in a second canonically irregular marriage (and one that cannot be regularized and is not patient of an internal forum solution) necessarily to be excluded by policy from the reception of the Eucharist, the necessity being the demand of indissolubility? Or put differently, would the doctrine of indissolubility be intolerably undermined if the Church adopted a policy that allows some divorced-remarried to receive the Eucharist? Or again, can the Church maintain the doctrine of indissolubility and still administer the Eucharist to those whose life-status represents a violation of this teaching? Is not the indissolubility of marriage so fundamental to the gospel and the Church's proclamation of it that violation of indissolubility implies rejection of a substantial element of the gospel (and the faith) and therefore excludes one from celebration of the sacrament that is preeminently the celebration of unity in faith? The question can be worded in many ways, some more tendentious than others. My pleonasms here are simply an attempt to formulate the problem as it might be formulated by a variety of publics.

The answer given to this question *at the level of practice* varies. While this is to be regretted, it must not be the prime focus of concern here. For what is theologically enlightening is not only one's ultimate posture or conclusion, important as it may be, but how one got there. It is just as theologically (and canonically) irresponsible to be warm-hearted but wrong-headed as it is humanly irresponsible to be cold-hearted and right-headed. A healthy pastoral policy can exist only if a warm heart is guided by a right head, in this case one that does not betray the Lord's teaching.

My reflections on this matter will be grouped under three subheadings: (1) the negative response (that is, the position that holds that reception of the Eucharist and indissolubility are a single issue in the sense that the Church cannot allow the Eucharist to the divorced-remarried without fatally undermining her commitment to indissolubility); (2) the affirmative response; (3) personal reflections.

The Negative Response

To the best of my knowledge this position is not widely defined in recent theological writing but is found chiefly in the manualist tradition and episcopal statements. It is therefore what is properly known as "the official doctrine and policy."

First I shall state what I believe is the position itself, then the strongest arguments possible for it. A marriage that is sacramental and consummated is indissoluble by any human authority, be it the partners themselves (internal indissolubility) or any other authority (external indissolubility). In such a marriage, a bond comes into being that is dissolved only with the death of one of the partners. If the marriage factually breaks up and a partner to it remarries, his or her marriage is in violation of this existing bond. Such a partner, should he desire to remain in eucharistic communion with the Church, has but two options. Either he or she must abandon the second marriage, or if he or she cannot (because of obligations that have arisen within it), he or she must live as brother-sister. That is a brief, but, I believe, accurate summary of the official understanding of indissolubility and its pastoral concomitants. It was restated by John Paul II.

There are three major arguments used to support this official position on the Eucharist for the divorced-remarried: the state of sin, imperfect symbolization, scandal. A word about each.

The state of sin. It has been, and indeed still is, common teaching that one may not remain in the free proximate occasion of serious sin. If he does so, he may not be absolved "for the will to remain in the proximate occasion of sin constitutes a new grave sin."[9] Obviously, if the person's very determination indisposes him for the sacrament of penance, it also indisposes him for the Eucharist. This indisposition is acknowledged both in the treatise on the recipient of the sacraments and that covering the duty to deny the sacraments to the unworthy (*indigni*). They are described as those who are indisposed, "that is one who will receive a valid sacrament but not the grace of the sacrament."[10]

Applied to the divorced-remarried, this means that unless they are determined to forego sexual relations, they are in a permanent state of grave sin (a free proximate occasion of the grave sin of adultery). Their sexual relations are adulterous as long as the first spouse is still alive. Therefore, their remaining together without the determination to live as brother-sister is persistence in the free proximate occasion of adultery.

Imperfect symbolization. This argument was used recently by the bishops of the Ivory Coast. They first reject the full impact of the state-of-sin argument as follows: "actually God alone fathoms depths and hearts and knows the real spiritual condition of men. It would be, for priests and members of the community, an error and a sin against fraternal charity to consider those to whom church law forbids access to the sacraments as in a state of grave sin."[11]

Why, then, may the divorced-remarried not receive the sacraments? The bishops note that the sacraments have as one of their purposes "to build up the Body of Christ." Now in the Body of Christ, the divorced-remarried "cannot witness fully to the sanctity of the Church. It is because the sacraments are signs of the People of God for the world that those may not receive them who do not fulfill all the conditions required for being signs of the Church." Others might word the matter differently, but the substance of the argument is the witness or symbolization involved in sacramental participation. This seems to be the heart of the argument found in *Familiaris Consortio* as well as in the analysis of the International Theological Commission.

Obviously, this argument did not originate on the Ivory Coast. It is a concise statement of the rather traditional teaching on the obligation to administer the sacraments. Let me recall the highlights of that teaching. Moralists maintain that the "one who has the care of souls *ex officio* is obligated in justice to administer the sacraments to those under his care who reasonably request them."[12] This means that the faithful have a right to the Eucharist, a right reflected in the duty or office undertaken by the minister. This right is conditioned by the phrase "who reasonably request them" (*rationabiliter petentibus*). When, then, do persons "reasonably request" the sacraments? Genicot answers somewhat broadly: "This is to be judged by the laws of the Church and local customs." I think it can be said that apart from the laws of the Church and local customs, the reasonableness of this request is determined by a combination of the need of the recipient and the inconvenience to the minister.

However, at this point we must, by extrapolation, include among those who do not "reasonably request" the sacraments the so-called "unworthy" (those who would receive validly but not fruitfully). For if the minister ought to deny the sacraments to *indigni*, then clearly they do not request them reasonably. At this point, Josef Fuchs adds an extremely interesting sentence: "Equivalent to the unworthy are those who, though they are personally disposed for a fruitful sacramental reception, are however not to be admitted (to the sacraments) because of the common good of the Church and because of its concern for discipline and unity."[13]

In applying this to heretics and schismatics who are in good faith and personally well disposed, Fuchs notes: "The reason for the prohibition in this instance is different; it is that the sacraments are the greatest signs of ecclesial unity. Therefore, administration of the sacraments would easily promote indifferentism. And as a general rule (per se) unity in the sacraments supposes full unity in faith and discipline."[14]

If Fuch's reasoning were applied to the divorced-remarried, it would go as follows: since the sacraments are the greatest signs of ecclesial unity, their administration to the divorced-remarried would easily undermine that unity by undermining the permanence of marriage. For the permanence of marriage is indisputably a substantial element of the gospel. He who rejects such a substantial element rejects the Christ who demanded it. But since the Church must maintain unity in faith and discipline, she must not tolerate practices that undermine it. This is, in slightly different words, the argument used by the bishops of the Ivory Coast. And it is found widely in the manualist tradition. It is forcefully stated by Karl Lehmann as follows: "As regards admission to the eucharist anyone who publicly and permanently intends to persist in this state publicly contradicts the Lord's commandment by his adulterous life, while by taking part in the Lord's supper he would simultaneously make a profession of faith in Jesus Christ. This intolerable discrepancy publicly displayed contradicts the meaning of faith of the ecclesiastical community, and of the function of the sacraments as symbols effecting what they signify."[15] At this point Lehmann is stating the argument, not necessarily endorsing its every aspect or implication.

Scandal. This is but an explication of an argument already present in the second argument. But it is so important at the practical level that it deserves separate consideration. It would run as follows. If the divorced-remarried are allowed to receive the Eucharist, others will conclude that it is not wrong to remarry after divorce, that the Church is changing her teaching on indissolubility, that the Church is approving second marriages, etc. If this is the way the faithful would respond to a change in pastoral policy, then clearly we are dealing with a policy that would undermine the permanence of marriage by eroding the determination to permanence from the very beginning. Briefly, a policy that would constitute scandal in the theological sense.

The cumulative force of these three arguments is that indissolubility and reception of the Eucharist by the divorced and remarried are not separate or separable issues. A change in traditional pastoral policy will necessarily affect corrosively the teaching on indissolubility. For instance, if the second marriage (while the first spouse still lives) is *not* a "state of sin," then precisely what is wrong with entering this state? And if there is nothing wrong with entering this state, then what is left of the traditional notion of indissolubility? The same deductions could be drawn from the second and third arguments.

The Affirmative Response

Contemporary moral writing that adopts the position that the right to the Eucharist and indissolubility are separate issues usually proceeds in two steps. First, it shows the weakness of the arguments for the opposite position. Second, it attempts to show in a variety of ways that it would be for the overall good of the Church's mission of reconciliation and mercy were she to adopt a policy that allowed some divorced-remarried access to the sacraments. A word should be said about each to fill out the theological state of the question.

The state of sin. Clearly, there are some couples in a second marriage whose situation and personal awareness could be described as "the state of sin." But to say this of all second marriages that are canonically irregular labors under many telling, even fatal weaknesses. The following points are frequently made.

1. Some, even many couples are factually convinced that they are not living in sin, whatever may have been the sinfulness in the rupture of the first marriage and the entry into the second. The second union is stable, characterized by mutual respect and profound affection, and is often supported by deep Christian attitudes in all other spheres of life. To stigmatize this as a "state of sin" is to speak a language with little or no resonance in the couples' experience.

2. The state-of-sin argument identifies in the term "unworthy" the external state of irregularity with a subjective and personal sinful will. Of this facile identification Karl Lehmann says: "This seems to be one of the really problematic presuppositions of the traditional argument."[16]

3. In some instances the Church admits that it is humanly and Christianly better for the couple in the second marriage to remain together, deepen their Christian life, attend Mass, etc. This all supposes that they are living the life of grace and are not precisely in a state of sin. As a group of French moral theologians state it: "From the moment that the Church recognizes that the Christian divorced-remarrieds have the human and even Christian duty to live their second union, and not to ruin it or to attempt to revive the first marriage, she cannot impute sin to them or consider as a *state* of sin that which in other respects she considers their *state* of life and even as their obligatory *state*."[17]

4. The state-of-sin argument supposes the adequacy of the present tribunal system in determining the status of the first marriage and the freedom (or its absence) to enter the second marriage. It is canon lawyers themselves who have raised the most serious objections to this supposition. It further supposes a sufficiently well-developed theology of marriage to undergird any adjudicative system, a supposition denied widely within the theological community.

5. The official policy which sees the second marriage as a state of sin also sees this state of sin dissolved by a brother-sister relationship. But the notion of such a relationship has its own serious problems. First of all, there are the grave disorders that can arise for a couple and their children from an intimate life together without any sexual expression. *Gaudium et Spes* recognized this when it stated: "But where the intimacy of married life is broken off, it is not rare for its faithfulness to be imperiled and its quality of fruitfulness ruined. For there the upbringing of the children and the courage to accept new ones are both endangered" (no. 51). Second, there is an attitudinal contradiction in the brother-sister relationship. On the one hand, the Church views sexual intimacy as so essential to marriage that the marriage is not consummated without it (and is indeed dissoluble). On the other hand, this intimacy is denied to the divorced-remarried at the very time the Church urges them (at times) to remain together and deepen conjugal affection.[18]

6. The state-of-sin argument seems to suppose that the morality of sex relations depends solely on the recognition of the legal validity of the union. This is not compatible with canon 1161's express admission that even in invalid or irregular unions there can be a true marital intention. If such a marital intention were not present, the notion of a radical sanation (convalidation of marriage without renewal of consent retroactive to the moment the marriage was celebrated) would be empty and erroneous.

7. To view all irregular second marriages as involving a state of sin is to make the rupture of the first marriage an unforgivable sin. The Church does this with no other failures, even though the objective effects of the sins are irreparable (e.g., murder). An analogy may help enlighten what is the true state of sin in this matter. It is not the thief who repents who is in a state of sin. It is the thief who intends to continue to thieve who is. His very mentality and outlook constitutes a state of sin. Similarly, it is not the divorced-remarried person as such who is in a state of sin; it is the divorced-remarried person who is unrepentant and intends to continue to allow his second union to go stale and to remarry. If we say anything else, we have made divorce and remarriage an unforgivable sin.

8. Finally, and quite tellingly, it is argued that if indissolubility is denied by reintegration of the divorced-remarried, it is because one concludes that no matter what the state of the second union, *the first still exists.* And thus the state of sin. There are two weaknesses to this conclusion. First, this means that indissolubility assures the existence of a reality with no other content, no other properties. This is an unacceptably essentialist notion of marriage and indissolubility. Second, this notion of indissolubility contradicts official pastoral practice. For this practice often and rightly attempts to promote the Christian life of the couple in the second union. The Church demands of the divorced-remarried a life of faith, attendance at Mass, the fulfillment of all familial obligations. This she does not do with bigamists as the term is popularly used. In other words, the Church acts as if the first marriage no longer existed.

In summary, then, the present official pastoral policy which sees the second union in which sexual intimacy occurs as a state of sin is, it is argued, impaled on contradictory attitudes. It both recognizes the marriage, but does not recognize it. It both recognizes the necessity and desirability of a Christian life for these Christians, but does not recognize it completely. The French moral theologians have summarized very trenchantly the difficulties in the state of sin approach.

The single thing apropos of which one can speak of a personal actual sin, according to presently admitted pastoral practice, would be the practice by the partners of sexual union. This is why it is demanded of them that they abstain from the sacraments. But we have repeatedly underlined the paradoxical character of this demand. On the one hand, what notion of marriage and sexuality underlies the position of the Church that demands of Christians that they honor all the dimensions of their union with the exception of the sexual? On the other hand, what conception of the sacraments and of sexuality leads us to the notion that the sacraments would be compatible with the exercise of all the other dimensions of the conjugal union but that they would not be compatible with that of sexuality?[19]

This type of inconsistency is present in *Familiaris Consortio*. The document (no. 84) states that "the Church will therefore make untiring efforts to put at their [divorced-remarrieds] disposal her means of salvation." Clearly, among the most important "means of salvation" are penance and the Eucharist, the very means denied the divorced-remarried by the same document.

Imperfect symbolization and the Church's concern for unity in faith and discipline. The answer to this second argument is not the denial of the Church's concern for unity in faith and discipline. It is rather that the form this concern takes can and must vary, depending especially on one's assessment of two factors: the nature and purpose of the Church (and of the sacraments as actions of the Church), the cultural and theological perspectives on lack of full integration with the Church. In other words, the argument supposes that administration of the Eucharist to those who do not fulfill all the conditions for complete ecclesial integration will de facto undermine unity in faith and discipline, and thus undermine the common good of the Church. If that were true, the Church would have little choice in her pastoral response to the problem of the divorced-remarried. But whether it is true is highly questionable, so it is argued, and the determination of this revolves especially around the two factors just mentioned.

First, the nature and purpose of the Church. In the mind and words of the Second Vatican Council, the Church has a double finality which it expresses in its sacramental life: the unity of the Church (the only Body of Christ), the indispensable means of grace and salvation.[20] Just as the Church is both the sacrament of unity and the means of salvation, so her ministry has the twofold finality. As Ch. Robert has pointed out, neither of these finalities can be suppressed or forgotten. In concrete circumstances it is necessary to balance and compromise to do justice to both finalities. Concretely, the Church judges it appropriate at times to renounce the fullness of the conditions of integration which she imposes in principle in order to extend more widely the means of grace.

This she does, for example, when dealing with common worship. In the Decree on Ecumenism, the Council stated: "Such worship (common) depends chiefly on two principles: it should signify the unity of the Church; it should provide a sharing in the means of grace. The fact that it should signify unity generally rules out common worship. Yet the gaining of a needed grace sometimes commends it" (no. 8).

This dialectical balance was applied explicitly to common worship with the Eastern churches. In the *Decree on Eastern Catholic Churches* (no. 26), we read:

> Divine Law forbids any common worship (*communicatio in sacris*) which would damage the unity of the Church, or involve formal acceptance of falsehood or the danger of deviation in the faith, of scandal, or of indifferentism. At the same time pastoral experience clearly shows that with respect to our Eastern brethren there should and can be taken into consideration various circumstances affecting individuals, wherein the unity of the Church is not

jeopardized nor are intolerable risks involved, but in which salvation itself and the spiritual profit of souls are urgently at issue.

Hence, in view of the special circumstances of time, place, and personage, the Catholic Church has often adopted and now adopts a milder policy, offering to all the means of salvation and an example of charity among Christians through participation in the sacraments and in other sacred functions and objects.

Therefore, once the Church's double finality is acknowledged, there is nothing *in principle* that prevents sacramental reception by those who are incompletely integrated into the Church. If that is true of our seperated brethren, is it not at least as true of those who are not separated but have encountered marital tragedy or failure?

Whether there is *in fact* (in our present circumstances) something that would prevent reception of the sacraments by the divorced-remarried is closely associated with our cultural and theological attitudes toward those who do not fulfill all the conditions for full integration in the Church. For example, whether granting the sacraments to heretics (in good faith) and schismatics will foster indifferentism and undermine unity in the faith, depends heavily on the prevailing attitudes toward heretics and schismatics. If the age is unecumenical and the atmosphere is one of religious distance and warfare between Protestants and Catholics—the Protestant being viewed dominantly in terms of what he/she does *not* share with Catholics—and if the atmosphere is one of suspicion, fear and rather low-grade apologetics, common sharing in the sacraments will more readily lead to practical indifferentism. If, however, our Protestant brethren are viewed as believing, good-faith separated *brothers and sisters* who share in most of our beliefs and with the Spirit's help and guidance are seen as struggling with us toward unity, then the atmosphere is such that common worship could not involve the same degree of danger of indifferentism. This the Council itself clearly concluded.

Something similar can be said of the divorced-remarried. What are the dominant notions or perspectives that lead to the conclusion that unity in faith and discipline would be threatened if some divorced-remarried could receive the sacraments? They are above all two: (1) the "state of sin" view of the second union; (2) the implication that the ability to receive the sacraments is tantamount to full legal good standing—scil., legal approbation of the second marriage with connotation of its validity before God—with the further connotation that marriage is dissoluble, a connotation at odds with the basic Catholic understanding of marriage.

However, if we have changed our perspectives on these two dominant notions, then the danger of undermining unity in faith and discipline by undermining marital permanence is profoundly lessened. Enough has been said about the "state of sin" to indicate that at least theologically the designation is, as a generalization, unsupportable.

The second notion needs attention here. The implication that the ability to receive the Eucharist is tantamount to full legal good standing or integration is an implication with roots in a widespread popular and highly legal mentality. That is, this is how many people think about the sacraments. They believe that going to communion is a sign to themselves and others that their marriage is accepted and approved by the Church. And obviously, they want this to be the case since their own peace of mind is closely connected with such acceptance and approval. In this sense, it is a popular mentality that makes this indissolubility and reception of the Eucharist a single, nonseparable issue.

However, with a fresh awareness in the postconciliar Church that we are a pilgrim Church, in need of sacramental sustenance not because of our sanctity and wholeness but precisely because we are weak, are sinners, are only more or less possessed by the faith we profess, are only more or less led by the charity that defines our being, we are well positioned to distinguish between sacramental nourishment at the Eucharistic table and full legal integration into the Church. Thus, though it can be admitted that the integration of the divorced-remarried into the Church is incomplete (as whose is not in one way or other?), still this incompleteness is, in a pilgrim Church, hardly reason for denial of the sacraments, sacraments of whose need and importance to the Christian life the Church herself has spoken so eloquently.

Briefly, a policy allowing some divorced-remarried to receive the sacraments would undermine unity in faith and discipline only if we (quite unrealistically and inconsistently) demanded full integration into the Church as a condition of sacramental life, and if we (quite legalistically) allowed participation in the sacraments to be viewed as the equivalent of complete integration or legal good standing. Since we need do neither—though some popular mind changing might be called for—the argument from imperfect symbolization is no insuperable obstacle to a change in pastoral policy.

Scandal. The third argument uniting inseparably indissolubility with sacramental reception was scandal. That is, people would conclude that, if the second union is a "state of sin" and the partners may receive the Eucharist, it is not wrong to remarry after divorce, that the Church is abandoning indissolubility, etc.

The answer given to this type of objection in the literature is simple, perhaps too simple. It is insisted that forgiving and reconciling need not and does not imply approval of what has gone before and even now come to be. Thus, the objection centers on the wrong thing. The precept of permanence is what the Church proclaims and what the couple must live. *That* is not affected by forgiving those who have failed, even sinfully, to live that command and find themselves in a position of irregularity as a result. Therefore, if the people are properly prepared for this change of approach by a careful explanation of its meaning, no scandal need occur. Recall again Archbishop Derek Worlock's statement cited earlier that his people would not be scandalized by a modified policy.

Once the weakness of the arguments uniting inseparably indissolubility and reception of the sacraments has been shown, the theologians who espouse the position of separability of issues develop other arguments to show why the Church ought to adopt a cautious policy of readmission to the sacraments. Some of the arguments are the following: (1) The need of the partners for sacramental sustenance. The faith of the individuals is imperiled without such sustenance. (2) Readmission to the sacraments better manifests the reconciling role of the Church in a sinful world and her message that it is always possible to begin anew. (3) An open juridically practicable policy avoids the confusion, abuses and disarray associated with the clandestinity of internal forum approaches. (4) The right to marry is a very fundamental right. Given the many doubts about the extent and meaning of Christ's injunction against divorce and remarriage, and of its practical consequences in the contemporary world, the Church ought to honor the fundamental character of this right by leaving the validity and dissolubility of the first marriage to God and put more emphasis on "the present dispositions and good consequences of those second-marriage Catholics who meet the four conditions I have described."[21]

This is the way the discussion has proceeded. It is fair to say that recent writing (at least of my acquaintance) favors a policy of *cautious* readmission of *some* divorced-remarried to the sacraments. In this sense, it constitutes a rather massive dissent from *Familiaris Consortio*. I say "cautious" because the literature lists in detail the conditions that ought to be observed. I say "some" because I know of no serious literature that proposes a kind of conditionless and indiscriminate "amnesty" for all divorced-remarried persons. In this sense, then, it is true to say that contemporary theological writing moves in the direction of answering the question posed at the beginning of this chapter as follows: indissolubility and the reception of the Eucharist are separate issues, at least in some cases. The reasons for this conclusion are, I believe, substantially the ones I have reported here.

There is one word in the above paragraph I would like to highlight. It is "policy" (as in "favors a policy of cautious readmission," etc.). In *Familiaris Consortio,* John Paul II referred (no. 84) to the exclusion of divorced-remarrieds from the Eucharist as "her [Church's] practice." It seems clear that he is speaking of a *public teaching* about the implications of indissolubility; for he refers to a "state and condition," a "way of life," that is an *objective* contradiction to the indissolubility of marriage. Such a teaching would not, it should be noted, exclude all internal forum solutions, even though it would restrict them to judgments about the validity of the first marriage.

At a key point, *Familiaris Consortio* states:

> Reconciliation in the sacrament of penance, which would open the way to the Eucharist, can only be granted to those who, repenting of having broken the sign of the covenant and of fidelity to Christ, are sincerely ready to undertake a way of life that is no longer in contradiction to the indissolubility of marriage.[22]

Much recent literature has pointed out that the ecclesial juridical status of a marriage cannot simply be identified with the real status of marriage before God. In other words, there will be some couples whose first marriage was invalid but who cannot establish this with the type of evidence required in the tribunal system of the Church. When parties to such a "marriage" remarry, it cannot be said of them that they have "broken the sign of the covenant and of fidelity to Christ" nor that their second marriage is "in contradiction to the indissolubility of marriage." In this sense, they are not indisposed for penance and the Eucharist. The "practice" reaffirmed by *Familiaris Consortio* does not, indeed cannot, exclude this possibility, unless it assumes the perfect adequacy of the tribunal system to determine the real status of the first marriage. Such an assumption is clearly unwarranted.

When, therefore, recent literature speaks of a *"policy* of *cautious* readmission of *some* divorced-remarried to the sacraments," it should not be read as referring to internal forum solutions of the kind mentioned. Rather it is discussing the consistency and persuasiveness of the type of analysis found in *Familiaris Consortio.* This analysis is directed toward those in a second marriage whose first marriage was clearly valid. The nature of the papal argument indicates this (i.e., indisposed for penance). It is this analysis which is appealed to to found a practice, i.e., a public policy. It is such a teaching and subsequent policy that is questioned in the theological literature.

Some might want to keep the papal teaching in place and "adapt" it in pastoral practice. But I believe this is not possible. For the very nature of John Paul II's analysis makes adaptation impossible. He has equivalently turned a prima facie duty (to refrain from the Eucharist) into an *actual and absolute one.*

Personal Reflections

This chapter began with the threat that it would conclude with some personal reflections. Let me now make good that threat. I believe that indissolubility and reception of the sacraments by the divorced-remarried are separable issues. That is, a practicable public policy of admission of some divorced-remarried persons to the sacraments need not constitute a challenge to the teaching on indissolubility of marriage, and thereby weaken the Church's unity in faith and discipline.

I use the words "separable" designedly. For at present, at the popular level and in the public mind, so to speak, they are possibly not separate issues. What does this mean? It means that for many decades, even centuries, the Church had interpreted the indissolubility of marriage in a particular way and drawn certain consequences from it with regard to pastoral policy. This has had the effect of inculcating a mentality in the faithful, a mentality that views indissolubility as open to but one pastoral policy where the divorced-remarried are concerned. Change the pastoral policy and you have changed or revoked the teaching. I may be wrong in this assessment of public attitudes, but if this is actually the popular understanding of things, then obviously a change in policy will indeed harm the common good of the Church by seeming to deny or weaken one of its substantial teachings. Therefore, some readjustment of perspectives is called for, first theologically, then at more popular levels, before indissolubility and reception of the sacraments by the divorced-remarried can become actually *separate* issues at the practical level.

What is this adjustment? In other words, what is the basic theological justification for saying that indissolubility and reception of the sacraments by divorced-remarried are separable issues? I believe it lies in the understanding of indissolubility. For many centuries marriage and its indissolubility were understood in highly "essentialist" terms, to use the wording of Archbishop Henri Legare. When a marriage was sacramental and consummated, a bond (*vinculum*) was said to come into existence which no human power, neither the pope (extrinsic indissolubility) nor the marriage partners themselves (intrinsic indissolubility), could untie. Thus, one form of pastoral accommodation for marital distress was "invalidation of the bond." Once indissolubility is conceived in this way, it seems to dictate inexorably certain practical conclusions—the "state of sin" being one of them.

But should indissolubility be conceived in this way? Or better, is this the only way indissolubility can be conceived if we are to be true to the Lord's command? (Here I refer back to my suggestion that we talk of indissolubility in itself.) I think not. I would like to suggest that indissolubility ought to be thought of above all and primarily as an absolute moral precept, a *moral ought* inherent in the marriage union. Because marriage represents the most intimate union of man and woman and is inseparably tied to the procreation and education of children, it ought to be one and permanent. That is, from the very beginning there is a most serious obligation upon the couple to support and strengthen this marriage. They are absolutely obliged not to let the marriage fall apart and die. This is particularly binding on those who have made their marriage a sacrament to the world because they have undertaken a true ministry to the world: to mirror Christ's love for and fidelity to his Church. The moral ought of which I speak, in its imposing urgency, is rooted in faith in the redemption. With Christ's redeeming grace we know we can do what might appear to be impossible to sinful persons.

Indissolubility as a moral ought implies two things: (1) the couple must strengthen and support their union and not allow it to die; (2) when the relationship has fallen apart and separation occurs, they must resuscitate it. A too quick conclusion that the marriage is dead is itself a violation of this ought, just as a premature pronouncement of death in a heart donor is a violation of his life.

If indissolubility is thought of in this way, then when a marriage irretrievably breaks down it can be said that at least one of the partners (whether through weakness or sinfulness can be left, indeed must be left, to God's merciful understanding) has failed to live up to the precept of indissolubility. What ought not be has come to be. A serious disvalue, both personal and social, has occurred.

But when a marriage is truly dead, then it seems meaningless to speak of the moral ought of not letting the marriage die. If indissolubility is conceived in highly essentialist and juridical fashion, the unbreakable bond (*vinculum*) continues, and subsequent remarriage is in violation of this *vinculum,* is an objective state of sin, etc.

What I am suggesting, therefore, is that it may be quite possible to conceive of the permanence of marriage in a way compatible with Christ's command without viewing it in terms of a continuing moral and legal bond (*vinculum*). And if this *vinculum* is not present, then the basic reason preventing reception of the sacraments disappears. Another way of wording this would be the following: the indissolubility of sacramental and consummated marriage prevents the institutional possibility of another *sacramental* marriage, but not of another nonsacramental marriage. This seems to be the direction of the Church's pastoral practice when she advises some couples to stay together rather than break up the second union. But her recognition of this second union is incomplete and inconsistent, as noted. To circumvent this inconsistency the Church would have to abandon her teaching that every true marriage between the baptized is thereby a sacrament.

If this notion of indissolubility is viable, then it seems quite clear that indissolubility and reception of the sacraments by the divorced-remarried are separable issues. Is it a viable notion? John Donahue, S.J., believes that it is. Explicitly adverting to my suggestion, he writes:

> The teaching of the historical Jesus is cast in the form of such a "moral ought", but it is not in the legal form of a declarative pronouncement about a bond which cannot be broken.[23]

Clearly, the Eastern Orthodox Church does not believe it has abandoned or compromised Jesus' teaching on marital permanence by its practice of *oikonomia*.[24] Behind such a pastoral practice there must be an understanding of indissolubility similar to the one I propose.

The understanding of indissolubility proposed here corresponds, I believe, to Archbishop Legare's plea for a more personalist and existentialist (in contrast to an essentialist) approach to the matter. If the indissolubility of marriage is understood as I have suggested—as a serious precept, and the bond as an obligation—then a readjustment of our theological and juridical concepts would occur. In impoverishing outline, it might build as follows.

1. Marriage is a "community of love," an "intimate partnership" (Vatican II). Inability to establish such a community is lack of capacity for marriage. Inability to achieve it is the death of marriage.

2. The capacity to establish this "community of love" plus the public determination to do so, generates the *bond* between two people, scil., the serious and absolute *obligation* to continue growing in the total "community of love." Thus: (a) this "intimate partnership is rooted in the conjugal covenant of irrevocable personal consent."[25] (b) "As a mutual gift of two persons, this intimate union, as well as the good of the children, imposes total fidelity on the spouses, and argues for an unbreakable oneness between them."[26] The capacity and the public determination (consent) *constitute* the bond. The spouses are *bonded* to each other. They *ought not* allow the bond to be broken and must do everything possible to protect it when it is imperiled.

3. Christ's absolute precept is merely an affirmation about the nature of marriage, of this particular perpetual covenant between men and women. It does not add "from outside" a characteristic not already there. It is marriage which is indissoluble, not a particular kind of marriage. If the Church can "dissolve" a marriage, this means and must mean that the *bond* was no longer there, the obligation rooted in the capacity. A *bond* is absent only when capacity is gone. Otherwise, *any* dissolution is an abuse. It is also an admission that the *bond* is not a metaphysical-juridical entity independent of the human reality.

4. Therefore, when the capacity to live in a "community of love" with a particular person is gone, is irretrievably lost, the *bond* is no longer there. For we should not speak of an obligation without a capacity. The bond remains only in so far as the capacity remains. The mere existence of a spouse is not a bond unless that existence carries with it the possibility of a "community of love."

5. Where there is no bond, a subsequent marriage cannot be a violation of that bond. A subsequent marriage can have a genuine human reality (not merely the "psychological relationship" admitted by the International Theological Commission)—though there may be good reasons why a divorced individual should remain unmarried. For instance, the individual would want to avoid undermining the permanence others are trying to lead. However, there may be reasons that lead an individual to a second marriage, e.g., the spiritual good of the individual. ("Let him accept this teaching who can" [Mt 19:12]. "Dissolution of the marriage *in favor of the faith*.") The Church may choose not to celebrate second marriages for pedagogical and other reasons.

The above five paragraphs contain an entire theology of marriage and a corresponding jurisprudence. In happy abandon I shall leave it to others to spell out the implications of such a theology and jurisprudence—indeed more basically, to pass on its merits. But the general lines of development do seem to me to be entailments of the idea of indissolubility as a precept.

Whatever the case, the Church must continually review its pastoral practices in the light of a new historical consciousness. . . . In doing so, it can derive guidance from biblical scholars. At this point recall the statement of Joseph Fitzmyer, S.J. [cited below].[27]

If Matthew under inspiration could have been moved to add an exceptive phrase to the saying of Jesus about divorce that he found in an absolute form in either his Marcan source or in "Q," or if Paul likewise under inspiration could introduce into his writing an exception on his own authority, then why cannot the Spirit-guided institutional church of a later generation make a similar exception in view of problems confronting Christian married life of its day, or so-called broken marriages (not really envisaged in the New Testament), as it has done in some situations?

Let me add to it a paragraph of Bruce Vawter.

The Christian communities which have accepted divorce as a deplorable but an inevitable fact of life have taken some guidance admittedly from the New Testament exegesis, but far more they have taken their guidance from other indices to the realities of the human condition in their times, and this is perhaps partly as it should be. I speak here not particularly of the Protestant churches, for of no Christian community is this fact truer than of the Roman Catholic Church, which despite its reputation for an adamantine opposition to divorce in any form yet has asserted to itself more than any other Christian body the prerogative of dissolving—that is, divorcing—practically every conceivable bond of marriage save one; and that one, as it happens, which should be the chief focus of its pastoral concern, the sacramental marriage *ratum et consummatum*.[28]

One final remark to this admittedly tentative probe. If indissolubility and reception of the sacraments are not only *separable* issues, but are to be practically *separate*, then it is clear that the validity of the slightly dejuridicized notion of indissolubility I have proposed must not only be established in the academic community. It must be prepared for, understood, and accepted at the popular level. Otherwise, at the level where scandal and division ought not to be, it will continue to be and grow. As Charles Whelan noted: a modified pastoral practice "would require careful explanation to the membership of the Church of the reasons for the change in discipline.

It must be abundantly clear that the purpose of the change is to show compassion and to do justice, not to introduce another form of divorce into the Church."[29]

"Abundantly clear." For if this is not the case, the Church will be seen, in adopting a more lenient policy on reception of the sacraments for divorced-remarrieds, to be adjusting not her partial and historically conditioned grasp of the consequences of indissolubility, but she will be seen as revoking the very notion of indissoluble marriage. That I think she cannot do, nor can she tolerate the conclusion by the faithful that this is what she is doing.

Notes

1. *New York Times*, 29 November, 1985.
2. Ibid.
3. Ibid.
4. Derek Worlock, "Marital Indissolubility and Pastoral Compassion," *Origins* 10 (1980), 273–75.
5. Henri Legare, "Current Situations: Value, Risk, Suffering," ibid., 280–82.
6. John Paul II, *Familiaris Consortio* (Washington: United States Catholic Conference, 1982), 83.
7. "Christological Theses on the Sacrament of Marriage," *Origins* 8 (1978): 200–04. These theses were composed by Gustave Martelet, S.J.
8. Cf. *America* 127 (1972): 258–60.
9. E. Genicot, S.J., *Institutiones Theologiae Moralis* II (Bruxelles: L'Edition Universelle, 1951), 17th ed., no. 357.
10. Genicot, loc. cit., no. 20.
11. *Documentation catholique* 69 (1972): 739.
12. Genicot, loc. cit., no. 18.
13. Josef Fuchs, S.J., *De Sacramentis in Genere. De Baptismo. De Confirmatione* (Rome: Gregorian University, 1963), 50.
14. Fuchs, loc. cit., 51.
15. Karl Lehmann, "Indissolubility of Marriage and Pastoral Care of the Divorced Who Remarry," *Communio* 1 (1974): 219–42, at 222–23.
16. Lehmann, loc. cit., 223.
17. "Le problème pastoral des Chrétiens divorcés et remariés," *Vie Spirituelle: Supplement* 109 (1974): 124–54, at 146.
18. "Le problème . . ." loc. cit., 136.
19. Loc. cit., 145.
20. Ch. Robert, "Est-il encore opportun de priver des sacrements de la reconciliation et de l'eucharistie indistinctement tous les divorcés remariés?" *Revue de droit canonique* 24 (1974): 152–76, at 169.
21. Charles Whelan, "Divorced Catholics: A Proposal," *America* 131 (1974): 363–65, at 365. It should be noted that similar proposals have been made by Joseph Ratzinger, Bernard Häring, Franz Böckle, Karl Hörmann, Johannes Gründel, Hans Rotter, Walter Kasper and many others in other countries. Cf. R. A. McCormick, S.J., *Notes on Moral Theology 1981–84* (Lanham: University Press of America, 1984), 101.
22. Loc. cit., no. 84.
23. John Donahue, S.J., "Divorce: New Testament Perspectives," *Month* 14 (1981): 113–20.
24. Cf. Bernard Häring, "Pastorale Erwägungen zur Bischofssynode über Familie und Ehe," *Theologie der Gegenwart* 24 (1981): 71–80.
25. *Documents of Vatican II*, ed. Walter M. Abbott, S.J. (New York: America Press, 1966), 250.
26. *Documents*, 251.
27. Joseph Fitzmyer, S.J., "The Matthean Divorce Texts and Some New Palestinian Evidence," *Theological Studies* 37 (1976):197–226, at 224–25.
28. Bruce Vawter, "Divorce and the New Testament," *Catholic Biblical Quarterly* 39 (1977): 542.
29. Loc. cit., 365.

19

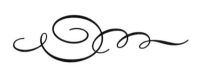

Pastoral Care of the Divorced and Remarried

Kenneth R. Himes, O.F.M., and James A. Coriden

On July 10, 1993, the three bishops of the ecclesiastical province of the Upper Rhine in Germany issued a pastoral letter calling for increased dialogue with divorced and remarried Catholics. It was read in all the churches of the three dioceses in September that year. The letter stated that a pastoral dialogue was needed to determine whether the "generally valid" prohibition against the remarried receiving the Eucharist "applies also in a given situation."[1] The German letter was noteworthy for several reasons, not least being the reputation of the three ordinaries who signed it. Walter Kasper of Rottenburg-Stuttgart is a theological scholar of international repute, Karl Lehmann of Mainz, also a distinguished theologian, is president of the German episcopal conference, and Archbishop Oskar Saier of Freiburg, a canon lawyer, is vice-president of the conference.

On October 14, 1994, the Congregation for the Doctrine of the Faith (CDF) sent a letter to the worldwide episcopacy entitled "Concerning the Reception of Holy Communion by Divorced-and-Remarried Members of the Faithful."[2] Written after a series of meetings between the German bishops and Cardinal Ratzinger, head of the CDF, the curial letter reaffirmed the traditional ban on reception of the Eucharist for those living in irregular unions. The three German prelates responded to the CDF letter with a public message to the people of their dioceses in which they noted that in regard to their position and that of the CDF "we do not find ourselves in any doctrinal disagreement," but "the difference has to do with the question of pastoral practice in individual cases." The bishops maintained that there does "exist room, beneath the threshold of the binding teaching, for pastoral flexibility in complex individual cases that is to be used responsibly."[3]

This extraordinary series of public statements by the CDF and members of the German episcopacy raises a number of issues. Also, the exchange takes place in a context which should be examined if the breadth of the issues is to be understood. We shall first comment on the remote and proximate contexts for the discussion. Then we will examine the substance of the German bishops' position as well as the CDF letter. Following that we will survey representative responses from other episcopal and theological quarters. Finally, we shall offer comments upon the many issues raised by this exchange of viewpoints between members of the German hierarchy and the Roman Curia.

CONTEXTS FOR THE DISCUSSION

At the beginning of this century the options available to the divorced and remarried was a settled matter. There was widespread agreement among Catholic canonists and moralists that the options in dealing pastorally with those whose marriage was invalid due to the existence of a prior bond were four: (1) declare the nullity or secure the dissolution of the first marriage, and then validate the present union; (2) advise the remarried couple to separate to remove them from cohabitation as a proximate occasion of sin; (3) leave the couple in good faith, i.e. dissimulate, decide not to inform them of their canonical status or moral situation; (4) permit the couple to live as brother and sister, i.e. to continue cohabitation but without any sexual relationship, in those rare instances where this arrangement seemed possible.[4]

The presumption behind these pastoral options was that those whose marriages were invalid due to the existence of a prior bond of marriage were living in a sinful situation, an adulterous union. Their lives together placed them in the proximate occasion of serious sin, thus endangering their salvation. Moreover, it was intolerable because it could be a source of scandal to the faithful.

The Church's marriage tribunals functioned ponderously, and declarations of nullity were slow and very few. The tribunals could respond to only a tiny fraction of the pastoral need. Often couples could not separate, since their obligations to their children, their dependence on one another, or their economic condition simply did not permit it. Living together as brother and sister was an arrangement "full of dangers" and to be suggested only in the rarest of cases.[5]

Then, in the 1940s in the U.S., partly because of northward migration of African Americans, the "good faith" option began to expand and be more frequently utilized.[6] When the validity of the prior marriage, after investigation, remained in doubt, the marriage tribunal issued a written "decree of good faith," which permitted prospective converts to be received into the Church while continuing in their existing marriage.[7] The decree was issued only if the existing marriage seemed stable, if the parties gave assurance that they were in good faith when they entered the marriage, and if there seemed to be no danger of scandal from the continuance of the union.[8]

The "decree of good faith" was not a judicial decision; it declared neither the nullity of the former marriage nor the validity of the existing marriage.[9] It provided a process of consultation for the parish priest, and the assurance of an official-looking document for the couple. The procedure was administrative, and the decision was seen as "canonico-moral."[10] In the late 1960s, tribunals began to question the issuance of the decrees, and asked whether the parish priest could not more simply assist the couple in making what is essentially a moral decision about receiving the sacraments, consulting the tribunal by phone when help or advice were needed.[11]

The "good faith solution" which at first was used for the marriages of two non-Catholics, was then extended to marriages which involved one Catholic party. The Catholic could have entered the second marriage in good faith if he or she thought the first marriage in question was invalid but was unable to establish that fact canonically. The suggestion arose whether this solution could be extended even to situations in which the first marriage was clearly valid, in view of the harm that would be done to the couple, their children, and to society, if they were obliged to separate before returning to the sacraments.[12]

Here we should note a basic distinction, made by Ladislas Orsy in 1970, which is still widely used in analyzing individual circumstances: (a) "conflict situations" refer to contexts where the internal and external forums are in conflict, that is, an earlier marriage was invalid but cannot be proved to be so canonically, for any of a variety of reasons including physical or moral impossibility; in this situation the fundamental human right to marry can override the merely ecclesiastical law which requires that the nullity be established before another marriage can be contracted (cc. 1060, 1085.2); (b) "hardship situations" are those situations where a first marriage, presumably valid, has in fact broken down, and one of the parties has remarried and desires to return to sacramental and ecclesial communion without abandoning the second union.[13]

In 1971, a committee of the Catholic Theological Society of America submitted its study of the "problem of second marriages." In the section dealing with "second marriages and participation in the life of the Church," the committee endorsed a reconsideration of the Church's pastoral practice by stating that respect for a couple's conscience should permit reception of the Eucharist by those who present themselves "after appropriate consultation, reflection and prayer."[14]

In June 1972, Bishop Robert Tracy of Baton Rouge, motivated by a desire to have a uniform pastoral practice in his local church, wrote a pastoral letter on "Good Consciences Cases" to be read in all of the churches of the diocese. His plan envisioned that an administrative procedure, i.e. a "decree of good conscience," would be issued by the tribunal. But he also called it "an internal forum solution."[15] The Baton Rouge process extended this internal forum solution to those whose previous marriage was of doubtful validity, on the presumption that its invalidity was not canonically provable. The solution was proposed as well to Catholics who believe in their consciences that their first marriage was not a true marriage, but that their present one is, and that they have a serious moral obligation to maintain the second union.[16]

On August 17, 1972, Cardinal Krol of Philadelphia, the president of the NCCB, issued a statement saying that the issue of the reception of the sacraments by divorced and remarried Catholics was under study by the Holy See and by the NCCB's Committee on Pastoral Research and Practices. He referred to a letter from the Holy See which made clear that "dioceses are not to introduce procedures that are contrary to current discipline" while the studies are under way.[17] The September 1972 meeting of the NCCB Administrative Board decided to send to the Vatican its study of the issue of permitting the sacraments to divorced and remarried Catholics.[18]

On April 11, 1973, Cardinal Seper, the prefect of the CDF, wrote back to the president of the NCCB. His letter spoke of "new opinions which either deny or attempt to call into doubt the teaching of the Magisterium of the Church on the indissolubility of matrimony" and which are used as arguments "for justifying abuses against current discipline on the admission to the Sacraments of those who are living in irregular unions." The final paragraph of the letter stated:

> In regard to admission to the Sacraments the Ordinaries are asked on the one hand to stress observance of current discipline and, on the other hand, to take care that the pastors of souls exercise special care to seek out those who are living in an irregular union by applying to the solution of such cases, in addition to other right means, the Church's approved practice in the internal forum.[19]

The leadership of the NCCB was uncertain about the meaning of "approved practice in the internal forum." Did it include "internal forum solutions" as they were being used in the U.S.? Was it limited to the brother-sister arrangement? Did it include some form of "good faith" or dissimulation? The NCCB president wrote back to the CDF for an official interpretation.

On March 21, 1975, Archbishop Hamer, the secretary of the CDF, wrote to Archbishop Bernadin, who had become the NCCB president:

> I would like to state now that this phrase [*probata praxis Ecclesiae*] must be understood in the context of traditional moral theology. These couples [Catholics living in irregular marital unions] may be allowed to receive the sacraments on two conditions, that they try to live

according to the demands of Christian moral principles and that they receive the sacraments in churches in which they are not known so that they will not create any scandal.[20]

This response did not clarify the American pastoral scene, and the bishops continued to work toward guidelines which could command common agreement. A 29–page draft of January 1976, "Pastoral Care of Catholics in Irregular Marriages"[21] allowed for the "internal forum solution" in situations where the first marriage was invalid or doubtful but not provable in the external forum. In cases where the first marriage was presumably valid, the draft offered the possibility of leaving persons in "good faith" or "good conscience" about their continued cohabitation, and admitting them to the sacraments, even when their consciences were inculpably erroneous or perplexed. This was understood as an application of the principle of the lesser of two evils. The brother-sister arrangement could be permitted rarely for those who accept the invalidity of their present marriage. The work of the NCCB Committee came to naught; no guidelines were ever issued.[22] Pastoral practice regarding access to the sacraments by the divorced and remarried continued to be and still remains diverse in the U.S.

During the 1980 International Synod on the Family there was concern expressed to improve pastoral care toward the divorced and remarried. At the time there was criticism of the synod's final text for failing to catch the nuances of the discussion, i.e. not consistently distinguishing between conflict and hardship cases, and within the hardship category ignoring the difference between those who were abandoned and people in other situations. Overall, however, the tone of the synod discussions and the declared desire to provide a positive program of pastoral care was a big step forward in the Church's ministry to those in irregular unions.[23]

In 1981, John Paul II issued his apostolic exhortation *Familiaris consortio* which provided his thoughts on the synod topic. In paragraph 84 he addressed the situation of the divorced and remarried. There he made distinctions not found in the synod statement. The distinctions, however, did not make any practical difference in pastoral care—all divorced and remarried are to be extended pastoral care and all are to be excluded from the Eucharist. While gracious in tone and strong in his affirmation of the place of the divorced and remarried within the Catholic community, the pope repeated the synod's reasons for eucharistic exclusion—namely, a contradiction between the objective state of those in irregular unions and the unity which the Eucharist signifies. Furthermore, he asserted that admitting remarried persons to the Eucharist without resolving the issue of the first marriage would cause error and confusion among believers.

One of the principal authors of the draft of *Familiaris consortio* proposed a different approach to the divorced and remarried than the one found in the papal text. Immediately after the synod, Cardinal Ratzinger sent a pastoral letter to the priests of the Archdiocese of Munich-Freising in which he stated that those in conflict cases could receive the Eucharist provided no scandal was caused. He also called for further study of those in hardship cases who wished to receive the Eucharist. That call was echoed by other members of the hierarchy in the next two synods. The Japanese bishops' conference as well as several individual bishops attending the 1983 synod on reconciliation and penance called for a less strict norm than that articulated by John Paul II. At the time of the 1985 extraordinary synod, the Japanese bishops' conference again called for reconsideration of the treatment of the divorced and remarried. During the meeting other bishops made similar requests.

Evident in all this is that the positive tone and obvious concern for the divorced and remarried expressed by the pope in *Familiaris consortio* has been welcomed, but a number of bishops wish to press the issue beyond the papal position. As James Provost has stated, a "consensus supporting a more wholesome pastoral attitude to divorced remarrieds" exists, but the agreement "does not extend to the issue of access to the sacraments."[24] On this question the papal position is a firm stance of exclusion, whereas other bishops have been willing to give greater nuance to their position or have called for more discussion about the present discipline.

The German Bishops' Pastoral

It is within this ecclesial context that the letter of the three German bishops must be read: the official teaching has been restated without further refinement or additional argument and the pastoral practice exhibits a divergence of approaches, some going beyond the papal position. As they begin their letter the bishops comment on the characteristics of the situation of the divorced and remarried and then turn their attention to the teaching of the gospel on the topic. They note that with regard to pastoral care "the church is not simply free," for the standard of the Church must be "the word, will and example of Jesus."[25] Their conclusion makes two points. "The church cannot assume the right to disregard the word of Jesus regarding the permanence of marriage; but equally it cannot shut its eyes to the failure of many marriages. For wherever people fall short of the reality of redemption, Jesus meets them in mercy with understanding for their situation."[26]

The bishops do not question the Church's teaching on indissolubility but make clear the place of the divorced and the divorced remarried in the Church. For a person in the former category there is "no restriction with regard to his or her rights or position in the church." Concerning those persons who have civilly remarried after divorce they too "belong to the church and thus to the parish community in which they live." While "their membership rights are somewhat reduced, they are neither excommunicated nor excluded from the church"; in fact, the Church must "give them special care because of the difficult situation in which they find themselves." In this, the German prelates are in full accord with the papal viewpoint. Inevitably, the question arises whether giving "special care" to the divorced remarried includes permission to receive the Eucharist. The bishops warn that "one must not take an all-or-nothing stance here." They acknowledge, citing *Familiaris consortio*, that present official teaching declares "divorced and remarried people generally cannot be admitted to the eucharistic feast as they find themselves in life situations that are in objective contradiction to the essence of Christian marriage."[27] Quoting their own catechism, the German bishops go on to point out that canon law can "set up only a valid general order; it cannot regulate all of the often very complex individual cases."[28]

Quoting *Familiaris consortio*, the bishops distinguish between those abandoned and those culpable for destroying a valid marriage. Further, those who have entered into a second marriage for the sake of raising children and who believe their first marriage to be invalid are different than those who admit the validity of their first union. In differing with the papal exhortation the German bishops ask whether these different situations can lead to different treatment.

Unless there is a process of "spiritual and pastoral dialogue, which should include elements of repentance and conversion, there can be no participation in the eucharist." While the participation of a priest is necessary in this process "the priest does not pronounce any official admission in a formal sense." Rather the priest is present to insure that a serious and informed discernment occurs, and then he is to "respect the judgment of the individual's conscience." Respect here has "different degrees," and it "may be in a certain borderline situation that is extremely complex" the priest "cannot in the end forbid" a person's participation in the Eucharist.[29]

In an interview for the Italian magazine *Il Regno*, Cardinal Ratzinger noted the bishops' "pastoral intentions" but said their text "presents some problems."[30] Over a year later in its formal reaction, the CDF reaffirmed the position of *Familiaris consortio* that those who have left valid first marriages and have remarried may not receive communion. Such a stance is "not at all a punishment or a discrimination" against the remarried but merely expresses the reality of the situation, namely that "their state and condition of life objectively contradicts that union of love between Christ and his church which is signified and effected by the eucharist." The CDF document also adds the risk of "error and confusion regarding the church's teaching about the indissolubility of marriage" as a reason for denying communion to the divorced remarried. Only after sacramental absolution may such persons receive the Eucharist, and absolution is contingent upon a readiness "to undertake a way of life that is no longer in contradiction to the indissolubility of marriage." This means either separation or, in cases where that causes serious difficulties, the agreement to live according to the brother/sister solution.[31]

In the CDF's account of the discernment process, a priest has a different role than that suggested by the German bishops. Confronted by a couple in an irregular union who have decided they can in good conscience receive the Eucharist, "pastors and confessors, given the gravity of the matter and the spiritual good of the church, have the serious duty to admonish them that such a judgment of conscience openly contradicts the church's teaching."[32] In doing this the priest accompanies the couple, but only to the extent "compatible with the dispositions of divine law, from which the church has no power to dispense."[33] The argument concludes: "Sacramental communion with Christ includes and presupposes the observance, even at times difficult, of the order of ecclesial communion, and it cannot be right and fruitful if a member of the faithful, wishing to approach Christ directly, does not respect this order."[34]

On the same day the CDF statement was issued, the three German bishops made public their joint response. They began by stating "it was not and could not be our intent to introduce doctrinal innovations or a new canon law. Rather, we have attempted, even while upholding the doctrine and discipline of the church, to arrive at acceptable solutions in terms of their pastoral application."[35] After recounting the process of meetings they had with the CDF since their initial letter, the bishops emphasized the points of agreement which existed between their position and the congregation. They saw "no fundamental disagreement whatever" on fundamental matters of church teaching. What they reiterated, however, was that the issue for them was the "pastorally difficult" work of concrete application of the Church's teaching in "delicate and highly complex human situations." Admitting that the issue around which controversy swirls is reception of the Eucharist by the divorced and remarried, the bishops repeated that they made no call for "official admission, but rather of an approach to the table of the Lord under precisely stated conditions." For them, the "distinction between admission and approach is fundamental." A few lines later they state the matter as the difference between "approval" and "toleration." The bishops make clear that the Church "still has much to learn at all levels" in its pastoral care of the divorced and remarried but they also acknowledge that in light of the CDF response certain of the statements and principles in their letter "cannot be the binding norm of pastoral practice."[36]

Reactions

In a letter issued in July of 1994, before the CDF's reaction, the bishops of Pennsylvania addressed the pastoral care of the divorced and remarried. They reaffirmed the positive measures of pastoral concern which have become widely accepted since the 1980 synod. Those who are divorced and remarried are encouraged to be active members of the Church, and priests are instructed to "do everything possible to include to the extent allowed divorced Catholics in the life of their parishes." The bishops make distinctions between different situations but make it clear that "those who have remarried and live in a sexual relationship cannot be readmitted to holy communion."[37]

The Pennsylvania bishops continue with an extended commentary on the "internal forum" solution which they deem "unacceptable, unnecessary and pastorally unsound." They consider it pastorally unsound because such an approach "cannot bring about the full reconciliation of the couple to the church." They find it unnecessary because the 1983 Code of Canon Law has made tribunal procedures "responsive enough to declare invalid all marriages which truly are." Finally, it is unacceptable for a variety of reasons. First, such an approach, especially when applied beyond the conflict situation to include hardship cases, "has the effect of ratifying an erroneous judgment of conscience against the reality of objective moral truth"; second, it "undermines the teaching of the Lord and the church on indissolubility of marriage"; third, it risks scandal, so that "others will be confused, weakened and misled into immoral behavior themselves."[38]

During the same summer, Rene Gracida, Bishop of Corpus Christi, issued a pastoral letter in which he repeated the official teaching and urged people in irregular unions to seek the help of the marriage tribunal. Like the Pennsylvania bishops, Gracida is confident that the revised Code of Canon Law provides that "proof of nullity can be met whenever there really was something that prevented the relationship from being a valid marriage." For those whose first marriage was valid but now find themselves in a second civil marriage, the brother/sister alternative is recommended with the bishop's assurance that "with God's grace, a Christian can do everything God asks."[39]

On the day the CDF letter was released, Archbishop Francis Stafford of Denver made a brief statement which asserted that the congregation was clarifying a teaching, not judging people. Emphasizing that the Church "cannot serve human needs without first serving the truth about the human person," Stafford stated that the Church's position on divorce and remarriage is not of its own making but "comes directly from the words of Christ." To violate that teaching is to rupture a sacramental covenant. Since the "eucharist is the defining act, the central celebration of Christian unity and community," those who participate must not be living a life which violates the sacramental unity. One cannot simply exalt the individual's conscience over the Church's teaching, especially on a matter so central to the Church's life as marriage.[40]

The German prelates also evoked several replies from scholars. An open letter to the three Germans was published by Germain Grisez, John Finnis, and William E. May. Stating that while they "believe there are very serious problems" in the way that the bishops treat conflict cases, the authors of the open letter chose to focus on the Eucharist and hardship situations.[41] In their opinion, the options open to someone in such a situation who decides to receive Communion are three. First, the person admits that he or she is committing adultery and that adultery is a mortal sin but maintains that "persisting in mortal sin is not inconsistent with receiving Communion."[42] Second, that the person acknowledges the commission of adultery but does not consider it grave matter and thus not a mortal sin. Or the final option is that, although "the present relationship does not meet the Church's official, canonical requirements, it has come to have the moral reality of marriage, and so is valid."[43] Therefore there is no adultery, since the first marriage no longer binds; and if one follows the directives proposed by the three German bishops in reviewing one's conscience, the individual may receive Communion. It is this third option which Grisez-Finnis-May see the Germans espousing. They view such a position as "indefensible" since it puts the bishops in the contradictory position of saying both that they believe in the Church's teaching about indissolubility and that in some cases valid marriages dissolve.

Ladislas Orsy, in a brief article, observes that the bishops are "on solid ground" in upholding the general prohibition against eucharistic participation by the divorced and remarried while stressing the need to examine individual cases. In his mind such a posture is not advocacy of the arbitrary nor a weakening of the teaching on indissolubility. For Orsy, faithful observance of the law "ought to be coupled with the spirit of mercy" and this balance he believes the bishops have achieved.[44]

John Grabowski of the Catholic University of America comments on how the German bishops use the internal-forum approach to conflict cases. He is sympathetic to the bishops while raising questions about their proposal. "Specifically, they must clarify the relationship of their proposal to the already established annulment procedure, the authority of individual conscience vis-à-vis the power of jurisdiction with the ecclesial community and the theological status of second marriages." Despite these unresolved matters, Grabowski considers the German proposal as "at least a step toward a more nuanced pastoral approach."[45]

Moral theologian Kevin Kelly, writing after the CDF response, hears the Congregation's response as "saying nothing new," either in its arguments for the Church's position or in the practical pastoral advice offered. The argument about a civilly remarried couple being in a state which is an objective contradiction to the unity the Eucharist signifies "proves too much," according to Kelly, for it overlooks the objective sinfulness present in the lives of us all. That is why, Kelly maintains, we begin the Eucharist with a rite of penance and just before reception of the sacrament say, "Lord, I am not worthy." Regarding the other rationale for the Church's ban, the "argument about scandal is an argument from consequences" and "no empirical evidence is offered to prove the truth of this assertion." As for the approved pastoral solutions, separation or the brother/sister relationship, Kelly sees major difficulties. The first would frequently lead to great injustices as a result of new obligations, and the second "seems to imply that the heart of marriage lies in sexual intercourse rather than the whole loving relationship of shared life together." Since the Vatican letter does little to advance the pastoral question, Kelly does not believe those divorced and remarried persons who are already receiving the sacraments should change their minds.[46]

Issues at Stake

While certain items in this dispute merit comment regardless of how one reads the document by Kasper, Lehmann, and Saier, other items depend very much on what one thinks the German bishops intended. Grabowski interprets the document as concerned solely with conflict cases.[47] Given the common use of the internal forum in dealing with such cases, the fact that none of the pastoral principles offered by the bishops are new, the improving tribunal practice in many nations, and the enormity of the number of hardship cases, this interpretation seems too narrow. On such a reading the bishops' statement is largely a rehash of things said by them and others (including Cardinal Ratzinger) years earlier.

The broader reading of the German letter is the one taken under review by Grisez, Finnis, and May, namely, that the bishops were willing to consider hardship cases within the range of those pastoral solutions by which people might be able to receive the Eucharist. The broader reading is presumed in the CDF response, since it specifically cites three examples of cases in addition to those who believe their previous marriage to be null but not provably so.[48] Finally, the text of "Principles of Pastoral Care," the document accompanying the pastoral letter, clearly addresses the hardship case.[49] Including hardship cases in their pastoral approach raises the stakes considerably when assessing the letter of the German bishops and the subsequent reactions.

Brother/Sister Solutions

Matthäus Kaiser has argued that the present discipline of the Church is incompatible with the theology of marriage. He claims the present discipline reflects an understanding of marriage as contract (see c. 1012 of the 1917 Code). This contract gave to each partner the "life-long mutual right to sexual union oriented toward procreation" (see cc. 1110–1111). This legal relationship "existed independently of whether there was or was not a personal relationship between the partners." This way of viewing the matter led to three consequences. (1) No violation of a right exists "if it is mutually agreed that the right will not be exercised." Hence divorced persons are not excluded from the Eucharist. (2) If a divorced person remarries the legal right of the other person is violated since "the right to sexual union excludes any third party" and "this right cannot be transferred to another partner." Therefore, the divorced remarried person is excluded from the Eucharist since adultery is a sin. (3) Adultery "exists exclusively in sexual communion. Thus, nothing stands in the way of admission to the sacraments if the partners of the new marriage reject sexual union, even if they live together in personal community." In other words, the brother/sister relationship permits eucharistic participation.[50]

Kaiser argues that it is the contractual model of marriage which continues to shape our pastoral practice.[51] Moreover it is precisely the brother/sister solution which demonstrates this. For a couple may share all other aspects of married life—spiritual, emotional, psychological, financial, parental, intellectual—at an intimate level, and none of this violates the rights of the former spouse; but should there be the physical intimacy of sexual union, then the rights of the former partner have been transgressed. Such a viewpoint makes no sense, Kaiser argues, in a model of marriage as covenant, a partnership in the whole of life. In the theology articulated at Vatican II, "marriage is the personal living and loving community of husband and wife who mutually give and accept each other as persons and are bound together in a new reality so that they are no longer two but one." In this framework sexual union is not a right existing in isolation but is meant to give "expression and realization" to the "personal community of life and love" that is the marital union of husband and wife.[52] Precisely for this reason the bishops at Vatican II had to relinquish the claim that the primary end of marriage was procreation. Sexual union serves marital intimacy as well as procreation. Absent such intimacy no right to sexual union exists.

In this newer model of marriage three consequences result. (1) Marriage is not only attained through the consent of the partners, but the couple is bound by God into a unity. Such a community of love can be destroyed, "and this is confirmed by divorce." Once "there is no more personal community between divorced spouses, they no longer have the right to sexual union which is the expression of personal unity." (2) "The other component for the realization of marriage, union by God, cannot be annulled because what God does is irrevocable." Thus, the divorced spouses are not free to remarry, nor is the Church able to witness or solemnize a new marriage. (3) However, if the divorced person enters into a civil marriage, "there is a mutual personal self-sharing between husband and wife" and their sexual union is an expression of their loving community. There is no violation of the rights of previous spouses to sexual union, "because that right ceased to exist with the destruction of the personal living and loving community." In sum, once one accepts the Council's understanding of marriage as covenant, "the sexual union of divorced and remarried persons is judged differently than extra-marital, adulterous, sexual relationships."[53] This is because no spousal rights to sexual union perdure once the community of marriage has ended. Following Kaiser, one can conclude that the brother/sister relationship is a practice which should be explicitly abandoned by the Church in its ministry to the divorced and remarried.[54]

The Question of Sin

The issue of sin arises not only in regard to adultery. Kaiser makes the point that "not only the remarriage, but the divorce is an offense against God's command." Whether this offense is a sin must be judged not only by the objective situation but by personal culpability, for the present pope has "expressly acknowledged that not every divorced spouse lives in mortal sin." Each case must be examined. Some may not be sinfully culpable for their divorce, e.g. the abandoned. Yet other spouses may well have "destroyed the personal living and loving community of a marriage in a mortally sinful way." Such persons must earnestly undergo an examination of their actions and in "true repentance turn from sin" through the sacrament of penance. Such individuals are not excluded from the Eucharist, even if the divorce remains in effect, since reestablishment of the loving communion of the first marriage may no longer be possible. Divorced persons in this situation are free to receive the sacraments, although they were culpable in a serious way for the break-up of the marriage and their divorced state is not altered.

Remarriage must be assessed in the same way as divorce, according to Kaiser, for "in every instance remarriage of a divorced person is as objective an offense against God's command as divorce." Objective invalidity, however, "says nothing about whether the remarriage of the divorced person is also considered mortal sin." Some remarried may not be guilty of mortal sin, "for example, when a divorced person remarries for the sake of the children's education." Kaiser believes that due to "circumstances the moral guilt is diminished or entirely removed" in specific cases. Even those who have "mortally sinned through the remarriage can later earnestly repent of the sin and, after examining their conscience, come to the conviction that under the prevailing circumstances the marriage should be pursued."[55]

Once we move beyond the preconciliar understanding of marriage as contract, we find that the divorced and remarried are in no different a situation pastorally than the divorced. Divorce, like remarriage, objectively violates God's will for married life. In many cases sinful culpability is present when a marriage dies. Just as the divorced person may repent yet persist in the "objectively wrong" status of being divorced, so the remarried may honestly pursue a path of repentance and sacramental forgiveness yet remain in a canonically invalid second union. The Church acknowledges this to be so since it encourages a couple to live up to the obligations, both human and Christian, that derive from the new marriage. The Church cannot tell a couple that their present state in life is their duty while at the same time tell them that their present state of life entails persisting in sin. True, the official teaching presently maintains that the couple meet their obligations while living as brother and sister. But since, as has already been argued, no rights of former spouses are violated by the sexual sharing present in the new marriage, because no such right exists, the full intimacy of marriage at all levels can and should occur in the second marriage. Thus, provided the divorced and remarried honestly seek to build a life of personal self-giving and loving communion, their participation in the Eucharist should be permitted when they approach the table, irrespective of the canonical status of their marriage.

This conclusion is valid, we believe, even if the pastoral minister continues to question the nature of the second union. Canon 915 of the 1983 Code of Canon Law (for the Western Church) gives canonical criteria for "non-admission" to Holy Communion. Canon 915 says that those "who obstinately persist in manifest grave sin" are to be excluded. It places the burden of not admitting such persons on the one administering Communion. The norm is a general one, but it is tightly drawn. The Relator for the Commission for Revision of the Code and some commentators say that it refers to those living in irregular unions, specifically the divorced and remarried.[56]

However, as John Huels notes, the canon is restrictive of rights and therefore must be interpreted strictly (c. 18). Canons 213, 843.1, and 912 state strongly the right of the faithful to the sacraments, and to Communion in particular. Each word of the prohibition must be carefully weighed, and "a minister may doubt whether a baptized person in an irregular marriage who comes to Communion is *obstinately* persisting in *manifest, serious* sin."[57]

> The minister cannot assume, for example, that the sin of public concubinage arising from divorce and remarriage is always grave in the internal forum. Any prudent doubt about either the gravity or the public nature of the sin should be resolved by the minister in favor of the person who approaches the sacrament.[58]

Canon 712 of the 1990 Code of Canons of the Eastern Churches states the norm more broadly: "Those who are publicly unworthy are to be prohibited from the reception of the divine Eucharist."[59] The interpretation of *publici indigni* must take account of the same issues as those mentioned above. Following Kaiser, since adultery is not at issue and the failure to witness to the nature of marriage occurs with divorce, not remarriage, it does not seem that the unresolved canonical nature of the second marriage merits an absolute and universal ban on reception of Communion.

Eucharistic Unity

Ever since the International Theological Commission issued a document of 16 theses on the sacrament of marriage, magisterial pronouncements have repeated the argument found in Thesis 12: "In receiving the divorced and remarried to the eucharist, the church would let such parties believe that they can, on the level of signs, communicate with him whose conjugal mystery they disavow on the level of reality." The thesis continues with the statement that such a couple embodies an "objective contradiction" with the life and teaching of the Lord, thus making it impossible for the couple to share the sacrament of unity.[60] Appeal to an "objective contradiction" to eucharistic unity has replaced the more traditional "living in sin" argument in magisterial statements.[61] This emphasis on an objective contradiction between the state of life of the divorced and remarried and the unity celebrated in the Eucharist reflects a reluctance to impute subjective evil to couples in a second civil marriage. This is not surprising given the testimony of pastors and people about the graced dimension of so many second marriages. The argument from eucharistic unity is at the heart of the CDF rejection of the German bishops' proposal and it was the substance of John Paul II's reasoning in *Familiaris consortio*.

Does the present emphasis on this argument from unity do justice to the sacramental theology of the Church? A number of years ago the British Jesuit John Mahoney named two principles which must be held in tension regarding the Eucharist. On the one hand, the sacrament is for humankind and for our salvation. On the other hand, the Church must prevent the sacraments from being administered in a lax manner which undermines the integrity of the Eucharist. The early Church in developing its eucharistic discipline appealed to both the Matthean text, "do not give to dogs what is holy" (Matthew 7:6) and the Pauline warning to the Corinthians not to receive the body and blood of the Lord unworthily (1 Corinthians 11:27–29).[62] These texts have helped to shape a restrictive approach on the part of the Church concerning admission to the Eucharist. Nonetheless, we should remember that Paul himself warned against Christians judging one another. Paul called upon believers to examine themselves "and so eat of the bread and drink of the cup." This attitude has fostered the presumption that if persons present themselves to the minister, the Eucharist should not be refused.

Then there are examples of the other principle of eucharistic practice, namely, that the sacrament is for a weak and sinful humankind. In the "Decree on Ecumenism" the bishops acknowledged that the lack of unity within the Church generally ruled out eucharistic sharing, but the desire for grace "sometimes commends" the practice.[63] Evidently the concern for unity is not so great that it creates an absolute prohibition against all eucharistic sharing. Inevitably the question arises: If those not in full unity of faith with the Catholic Church can, by way of exception, share in the Eucharist, is it not possible that those lacking full conformity in public status with the Church may also share in the Eucharist, at least on an exceptional basis? The exclusion of the divorced and remarried from any reception of Communion is stated as an absolute, but this seems to go beyond what is necessary to maintain the necessary integrity of eucharistic symbolism, given the ecumenical experience.

Furthermore, there is the matter of the one-sided nature of the theory informing the present discipline. Sacraments not only celebrate what is already fulfilled, but they effect what they celebrate. The Church does not believe there must be no original sin before baptism, nor no mortal sin before penance. Rather, these sacraments bring about what they celebrate, the forgiveness of sin. Must the sacrament of the Eucharist presume unity in order to celebrate it? Or may it be the means whereby unity is effectively created? Because the present church discipline does not give sufficient weight to the concern expressed in the second question we do not appear to have a balanced view of sacramental effectiveness.

Behind the present policy there also lurks an understanding of the sacraments which suggests we have not fully appropriated the teaching of Vatican II about being a pilgrim people. The people who are the Church need the sacraments not only because they are holy but because they are sinful. Sacraments are not rewards for a life well lived but a means to deepen one's love of God and desire for conversion. Restricting the sacraments to those faithful who are completely integrated into the life of the Church overlooks the example of Jesus who seems to have been generous in sharing his table with all who approached him, even public sinners. "It may be that in our human and very understandable concern that God's gracious gift in Christ, and especially in his body and blood, be not abused, we risk forgetting Jesus' own retort that he came to share his earthly and heavenly table with those who needed him. . . . [W]e tend to think that because God gives his grace freely he gives it grudgingly."[64]

A remaining difficulty with the argument from unity is the tendency found in Martelet's original paper to objectify metaphors.[65] The unity argument tends to treat metaphorical language as if there is a one-to-one equivalency. But saying "the Church is the body of Christ" is a different sort of statement than saying, "you are sitting on a chair." The richness of the metaphor is precisely that it offers insight and meaning at many levels. To take one meaning from the metaphor and conclude this is all it means is to misunderstand the nature of metaphor.

A good example of the abuse of marital metaphor was provided years ago by Theodore Mackin. One cannot simply move from saying that the sacramental marriage of a man and woman is a symbol of Christ's love for the Church to the claim that such a marriage is thereby indissoluble. One can argue that because such a sacramental marriage should witness to Christ's love it needs to embody a faithful and permanent bond of love which does not end. That is to draw a reasonable implication, namely, that if marriage is to be a sign of Christ's love, then a couple should imitate the qualities of Christ's love. But to conclude that because Christ's love for the Church cannot end, then this couple's love for each other cannot end, is doing something more. In the first case we are drawing out moral implications, in the second we are making an ontological claim.⁶⁶ To state that indissolubility is a moral ideal, an ethical obligation, is a justifiable conclusion from the prior claim that sacramental marriage is meant to be a sign of Christ's love. Such a conclusion does not determine, however, what we are to do when people fail to live up to their moral obligation. At that point the Church may decide that the punishment should be severe, e.g. the exclusion of the divorced and remarried from the Eucharist. What the Church cannot say is that this is the only possible alternative because the metaphor requires it. Theology must be cautious when translating metaphorical language, as in speaking of marriage and the Eucharist, into simple assertions.

Scandal

Mentioned along with eucharistic unity in both the CDF response and previous magisterial statements is the danger of scandal if those who are divorced and remarried are admitted to eucharistic sharing. Scandal, like the oft-noted right of the faithful not to be disturbed, has a paternalistic tone and may be invoked where the risk is minimal. While scandal should not be dismissed as unimportant, over-frequent reference to the risk of scandal can make the Church and its ministers overly fearful and lacking in the initiative and fortitude which reflects a Spirit-filled community. The large number of annulments being granted in recent years makes it implausible for third parties to presume that those living in a second marriage and receiving the Eucharist are engaged in scandalous activity.

The possible scandal involved in the topic under review is that people will come to think that the Church no longer maintains that marriage is to be governed by permanence and fidelity. Surely if people come to think such is the case there will be a great loss for the Church. What is not at all certain, however, is that people will believe the Church has changed its teaching on marriage if one extends eucharistic hospitality to the divorced and remarried. For one thing, quite apart from the Church's teaching, people earnestly desire their marriages to be permanent and faithful. In reports from those regularly engaged in premarital-preparation programs there is little reason to conclude that couples enter into marriage indifferent to the ideals of permanence and fidelity. Every couple wants its marriage to be a success. Even as they admit that marriages often do not succeed, they want theirs to succeed. That is why divorce is a tragedy and many people who know nothing of Catholicism see it exactly that way. The actual legal decree of divorce may not be experienced by all as a tragedy since for some it is a relief, an end to wrangling, fear, and anger. But the existential process of the breakdown of a marriage leading to the legal judgment is deeply painful for all.

Even if the Church were to be silent about permanence and fidelity in marriage, the human yearning for a committed and exclusive love would remain strong. "Indissolubility is misunderstood if it is seen as an externally imposed law, it is rather a law written in the human heart: human relationships reach for permanence, long for communion."⁶⁷ To presume that a change in eucharistic discipline regarding the divorced and remarried will lead to people giving up their own commitment to the ideals of marriage or that they will no longer know that the Catholic Church teaches those ideals seems unlikely. Even many Catholics who have undergone the torment of divorce do not want the Church to change its teaching on permanence and fidelity in marriage. What they seek is understanding and support for themselves and others when their lived reality falls short of the beauty and truth of the teaching.

In the CDF response as well as earlier magisterial statements, no evidence is cited to gauge the risk of scandal that will result from permitting the remarried to receive the Eucharist. Therefore it is at least equally plausible that "an across-the-board denial of the sacraments to divorced people who have remarried gives scandal by weakening the witness of the Church to the compassion and forgiveness of Christ."[68] Indeed, testimony from a number of priests who work in programs with alienated Catholics indicates that the single biggest reason people cease active participation in the Church is that they have found themselves in irregular marital situations and feel unwanted and rejected by the Church. Exclusion from the Eucharist is the most commonly cited expression of how the Church manifests its nonacceptance of the divorced and remarried.[69]

In those situations where the risk of scandal is real, there is no insuperable obstacle to eucharistic sharing for the divorced remarried. After all, the Church permits the reception of the Eucharist by those living in a brother/sister relationship, yet this officially sanctioned solution does little in itself to resolve the danger of scandal. As Kelly remarks, "unless a couple had a 'brother and sister' logo on their doorpost, neighbours and fellow parishioners would be none the wiser and so the alleged scandal would presumably still be given."[70] If measures are available to avoid scandal caused by those living in a brother/sister relationship, similar means are at hand for other divorced and remarried persons.

Pastoral Care / Pastoral Solutions

One of the positive developments within the Church in recent decades has been the growing sensitivity to divorced and remarried Catholics. No longer is the language of bigamy or excommunication found in formal teaching. The Church has now reached out in a wide variety of ways to those who have suffered the break-up of a marriage, e.g. better tribunal practice, parish-based support groups, weekend retreat programs, welcoming attitudes among parish staff and congregations. The official teaching of the Church has encouraged such developments and both the CDF and the German bishops agree that many things can be done to support those who are divorced, whether single or remarried. People whose marriages have failed are still members of the Church and are entitled to pastoral care appropriate to their situation. In providing such care ministers ought not make the mistake of equating it only with the celebration of the sacraments. Even without admission to the Eucharist, much can and should be done for the divorced and remarried by pastoral leaders.

Undoubtedly, however, it is the question of reception of the Eucharist by those divorced in civil second marriages which occasioned the exchanges we have reported here. What can be done? In their second letter, the three German bishops emphasize that, when discussing reception of communion by those in noncanonical second marriages, the "distinction between admission and approach is fundamental for us." They go on to say that the model of pastoral care being proposed does not entail the "approval" of the divorced remarried participating in the Eucharist, but "a toleration of this."[71] Toleration within the tradition is an attitude which "first considers another's activity as threatening certain values, then disagrees with the activity, and refuses to approve or recommend the activity, but to prevent greater harm it permits the activity with which it disagrees."[72] The episcopal trio obviously believes that the greater harm to be prevented is that which is done to the person denied the Eucharist. The values being threatened are the indissolubility of marriage and the integrity of the Eucharist.

However, the proposal of the German bishops treats both conflict and hardship cases together, using the language of toleration to deal with situations in which what is being tolerated is quite different. In conflict cases, indissolubility is not truly at issue; only the adequacy of existing measures in the external forum is being questioned.[73] Nor is the integrity of the Eucharist at stake since there is good reason to think that the present, not the former union is the genuine marriage. Thus the person is not living in a state of life which objectively contradicts the symbol of unity which is the Eucharist.[74]

When the principle of toleration is employed in cases of hardship, however, the analysis changes, for now indissolubility and eucharistic integrity are arguably at greater risk. Here the conclusion is not that the validity of the first marriage is uncertain, but that the validity of the Church's policy is. The bishops avoid facing this by insisting on their agreement with the Church's teaching and treating the hardship case as if it asks no more of the Church than the conflict case, a pastoral attitude of tolerance. Joining hardship cases with conflict cases, as the bishops appear to do, does not advance the question. We maintain that making pastoral exceptions to existing policy is not fully adequate as a response to the situation. A new policy toward the divorced and remarried receiving the Eucharist is also needed.[75]

The language of pastoral care can obscure the true nature of what is involved. For example, describing the outcome of a discernment process as a "good faith" solution is, in our opinion, unsatisfactory. There is a tendency to link "good faith" with invincible ignorance and the pastoral practice of dissimulation. However, many couples are fully aware of what the Church teaches regarding indissolubility and marriage. In any number of instances people simply do not see why the ban on eucharistic participation must be absolute when it comes to those in canonically irregular marriages. None of the rationales presented, including the two most commonly cited—scandal and eucharistic unity—justify an absolute ban on eucharistic sharing.

Still, even as the debate about present policy continues, pastoral care must be accorded individual cases. Perhaps the first thing needed is an acknowledgement that admission to the sacraments of penance and Eucharist is essentially a moral, not canonical decision. This seemed to be the direction in which things were heading during the 1970s. Today, we continue to muddle the moral-discernment process necessary for eucharistic participation with canonical categories employed in marriage. "Laws are necessary but clumsy and limited ways of organizing human affairs; they never absolve us from the exercise of discernment or from the exercise of making responsible and conscientious decisions."[76] Terms like "valid" and "invalid," "internal forum" and "external forum," are not especially helpful in making the necessary moral choices.

More appropriate and accurate categories would be something similar to what the German bishops, following many others, propose.[77] Certainly an assessment of motivation is needed, i.e., that the person is seeking reconciliation for religious reasons, not for extrinsic reasons. Evidence of a sincere conversion of heart should also be manifest, i.e., that if the person was the cause (main or partial) of the breakdown of the first marriage, he or she has repented. Obviously the person should not be in a state of serious sin, but the pastoral minister cannot presume that a noncanonical marriage is demonstration of such a state. After all, if lack of canonical form can cause invalidity, then many baptized Catholics throughout the world are living in canonically invalid marriages, yet no one thinks all such persons are living in serious sin. Whatever obligations stem from the first union should be acknowledged and properly met. Finally, the present commitment should demonstrate the qualities of a genuine marriage, i.e., that the person and the new partner are living in a public and responsible family relationship as husband and wife, and that their union is stable and established, holding itself out to the community as a marriage, not a temporary or trial relationship. These are the sorts of concerns which should be assessed in a serious moral discernment process.

When this moral framework is employed and the couple maintains that the new marriage exists, then three pastoral options are possible: (1) convalidate their present marriage after seeking annulment or dissolution of the first marriage; (2) leave the couple in good faith, dissimulate; (3) admit them to penance and Eucharist, without any formal judgment about the first union. Separation is most often impossible, economically and morally, and may be inadvisable. As we have already suggested, the brother/sister arrangement should not be proposed. In following this approach a priest's intervention does not seem to be essential. It is an exercise of moral discernment, and a morally sensitive third party is advisable to assist in the honest formation of conscience. But there is no need to assume that a priest is the only person or even always the best one for such a task. A spiritual director, retreat master, pastoral associate, permanent deacon, or other similar pastoral minister may fulfill the role.

Important to remember, however, is that simply addressing this issue at the level of pastoral care is inadequate as a complete response to the topic of divorce, remarriage, and the Eucharist. Making exceptions to a general rule is too important an activity to leave the matter as is. As John Mahoney once put it: "[Exceptions] are the growth points of understanding. And to surrender before them as impenetrable moral mysteries is to abdicate all serious moral enquiry."[78] The community of the faithful must press on to ask why this is a legitimate exception, i.e. what makes it so. Unless we are willing to ask such questions we shall not achieve deeper insight into the realities of life as disciples. For several decades now the suggested pastoral practice which goes under the rubric of the "internal forum" relies on finding reasons to excuse people from culpability or to adapt a norm to a person's situation. This is clearly what the German bishops have in mind. What we are suggesting is that the questions arising in pastoral practice ought to compel us to open up the question at another level.[79] What is the moral obligation stemming from a failed first marriage? What is the moral reality of the second union? Unless our Church is willing to allow a free and honest dialogue on such matters, we will force pastors and couples to continue to search for adaptations to norms which should themselves be examined and open to revision.[80]

Need for a Church Dialogue

Just this sort of dialogue is what can be hoped for as a result of the German bishops' letter, although the public nature of the CDF response to the bishops may have dimmed this hope. As Kevin Kelly observed, "[I]n the present climate this makes it difficult for individual bishops, or groups of conferences of bishops, to beg to differ from the CDF line without seeming to challenge the authority of the Pope himself." What is dismaying is that although the relationship of the local ordinary's pastoral role to that of the pope or the episcopal college remains unresolved, any effort to assert the role of the local bishop is interpreted as a challenge to Rome. We may be grateful that the German bishops in their response to the CDF indicate that they do not think the matter is closed. This is important for matters beyond the pastoral care of the divorced and remarried. For several years now the atmosphere within the Church has been unreceptive to free inquiry and free expression, so that pastors and scholars are reluctant to risk exploring what is behind pastoral intuitions. The letter of the German hierarchs may provide an opportunity to overcome such reluctance.

Ladislas Orsy believes that the initial German text was "a model of what today a pastoral letter ought to be" and was an initiative by the bishops which took seriously the "power conferred on them directly through their sacramental ordination." The bishops "balanced their unfailing communion with the universal church with the quiet assertion of their own authority."[81] Addressing the present imbalance between the universal and local Church is an important ecclesiological concern. In Peter Hünermann's view, the bishops of the Upper Rhine were demonstrating "how bishops should function." They had taken up a pressing pastoral concern for the Church in Germany and had answered the frustration of many German Catholics who wondered if, in the present situation, "the bishops [are] any more than Vatican officials."[82] By exercising their rightful role as pastoral leaders in their local churches, the three Germans have signalled that they see themselves as more than Roman legates to the local church. Although the first stage of the conversation has ended with the Vatican reasserting a rigorist position on eucharistic participation, there remains reason for hope. As an editorial in the London *Tablet* suggested, both for the sake of the specific issue of the treatment of the divorced and remarried but also for the sake of the larger ecclesial issue of the authentic role of the local bishops, "what counts is that the matter has been raised at the episcopal level, responsibly and pastorally."[83]

Notes

1. "Pastoral Ministry: The Divorced and Remarried," *Origins* 23 (March 10, 1994) 670–73, at 673 (hereafter cited as "Pastoral Ministry"). The German letter was accompanied by a more detailed statement of "Principles of Pastoral Care" an excerpt of which appeared in translation in the same issue of *Origins* 673–76 (hereafter cited as "Principles").

2. *Origins* 24 (October 27, 1994) 337, 339–41 (hereafter cited as "Reception").

3. "Response to the Vatican Letter" (hereafter cited as "Response") *Origins* 23 (March 10, 1994) 341–44, at 341.

4. J. Krol, "Permission for Parties Invalidly Married to Live as Brother and Sister," *Jurist* 11 (1951) 7–32, at 11; B. Sullivan, *Legislation and Requirement for Permissible Cohabitation as Invalid Marriages: A Historical Synopsis and a Commentary,* Canon Law Studies 356 (Washington: Catholic University of America, 1954) 48, 81.

5. Sullivan, *Permissible Cohabitation* viii.

6. R. Carey, "The Good Faith Solution," *Jurist* 29 (1969) 428–38, at 428.

7. Carey describes the procedures and their development (ibid.).

8. Ibid. 432–33.

9. The decree was based on the solution very often given by the Holy Office: *relinquendi in bona fide* (ibid. 430). Some tribunals issued a *decretum non-inquietandi*, meaning that the parties are "not to be disturbed," their present marriage is to remain in peaceful possession.

10. Ibid. 434.

11. Ibid. 434–35.

12 Ibid. 436–37.

13. Ladislas Orsy, "Intolerable Marriage Situations: Conflict Between External and Internal Forum," *Jurist* 30 (1970) 1–14, at 10. The five articles in that issue of the *Jurist* are of lasting value.

14. "Divorce and Remarriage," *Origins* 2 (October 12, 1972) 251–54, at 254. The members of the CTSA committee were John Connery, S.J., Joseph Kerns, Richard McCormick, S.J., Brendan McGrath, O.S.B., James McHugh, John Thomas, S.J., and George Wilson, S.J.

15. "It is a recognition by the Church in an official way of the right of a party involved in a second marriage by reason of his [sic] good conscience in the matter to receive the sacraments with no official decision being rendered one way or the other as to the validity or invalidity of a previous marriage or marriages" (Robert Tracy, "Divorce, Re-Marriage and the Catholic," *Origins* 2 [July 27, 1972] 130, 135–36, at 135).

16. Ibid. 135–36.

17. John Krol, "Good Conscience Procedures," *Origins* 2 (September 7, 1972) 176–77.

18. See "On File," *Origins* 2 (September 28, 1972) 220.

19. The final words in the Latin original are *probatam Ecclesiae praxim in foro interno* (Protocol nos. 1284/66 and 139/69).

20. Prot. no. 1284/66.

21. A working draft from the subcommittee of the NCCB Pastoral Research and Practices Committee.

22. The fate of these efforts is described by James Provost, "Intolerable Marriage Situations Revisited," *Jurist* 40 (1980) 141–96, at 176–77.

23. This account of the synod relies upon James Provost, "Intolerable Marriage Situations: A Second Decade," *Jurist* 50 (1990) 573–612. This essay along with Provost's earlier article (see n. 22 above) are indispensable reading for those who wish to pursue the recent historical background of the present discus-

sion. An essay by Peter Hünermann, "A Church in Dialogue," *Tablet* 249 (1995) 896–98, offers useful background on the immediate context for understanding the German bishops' initiative.

24. For the post-1980 synod reactions, see Provost, "Intolerable Marriages: Second Decade" 586–90.

25. "Pastoral Ministry" 670. It does seem, however, that the present leaders of the Church are more conservative on this matter of the Church's freedom than need be. In an excellent essay, New Testament scholar Pheme Perkins concluded that on the matter of divorce, as well as in other areas, the early Church "did not assume that Jesus had formulated a universally binding rule that could be inserted into any context without modification" ("Jesus and Ethics," *Theology Today* 52 [1995] 49–65, at 63–64). See also the conclusion of Raymond Collins, "the fact that the tradition of Jesus' saying on divorce exists in so many different versions and that it is almost impossible to recover the most primitive versions of the saying with any surety . . . stands as evidence that the first generations of Christians experienced a need not only to pass along Jesus' teaching on divorce but also to adapt it to ever new circumstances" (*Divorce in the New Testament* [Collegeville: Liturgical, 1992] 231).

26. "Pastoral Ministry" 670.

27. Ibid. 672.

28. Ibid. 673, quoting *The Creed of the Church* (the Catechism for Adults of the German Bishops' Conference) 395.

29. "Pastoral Ministry" 675. The bishops suggest eight criteria for discernment: (1) responsibility for the collapse of the first marriage "must be acknowledged and repented"; (2) it must be clear "that a return to the first partner is really impossible"; (3) "restitution must be made for wrongs done"; (4) any "obligations to the wife and children of the first marriage" must be met; (5) "scandal should be taken into consideration"; (6) the second relationship "must have proved itself over a long period of time to represent a decisive and also publicly recognizable will to live permanently together"; (7) whether or not there exist moral obligations of "fidelity to the second relationship" should determined; (8) it should be clear that "the partners seek truly to live according to the Christian faith and with true motives" (ibid. 674).

30. As reported in *Origins* 23 (March 10, 1994) 670.

31. "Reception" 339.

32. Ibid.

33. Ibid. 340.

34. Ibid.

35. "Response" 341.

36. Ibid. 342–43.

37. "Pastoral Care of Divorced Catholics Who Remarry," *Origins* 24 (August 18, 1994) 205–08, at 206.

38. Ibid. 207–08.

39. Rene Gracida, "Pastoral Ministry to the Divorced and Remarried: A Pastoral Letter," *Fellowship of Catholic Scholars Newsletter* (June 1994) 16–19, at 18.

40. Francis Stafford, "The Ecclesial Dimension of Conscience," *Origins* 24 (October 27, 1994) 345.

41. Germain Grisez et al., "Letter to: Archbishop Saier, Bishop Lehmann, and Bishop Kasper,"*Fellowship of Catholic Scholars Newsletter* (June 1994) 20–27, at 22 (the same letter was also published in *New Blackfriars* 75 [1994] 321–30 under the title "Indissolubility, Divorce and Holy Communion").

42. Ibid. 22.

43. Ibid. 23.

44. Ladislas Orsy, "Divorce and Remarriage: A German Initiative,"*Tablet* 248 (1994) 787.

45. John Grabowski, "Divorce, Remarriage and Reception of the Sacraments," *America* 172 (October 8, 1994) 20–24, at 24.

46. Kevin Kelly, "Divorce and Remarriage: Conflict in the Church," *Tablet* 248 (1994) 1374–75, at 1374. Two scholarly replies from Italian authors should also be noted: G. Marchesi, "Un problema per la Chiesa: La cura pastorale dei divorziati," *Civiltà cattolica* 145 (1994) 486–95; and S. Consoli, "Il problema della partecipazione ai sacramenti dei fideli separati o divorziati," *Monitor Ecclesiasticus* 119 (1994) 84–94.

47. Grabowski, "Divorce, Remarriage and Reception" 21–22.

48. The three cases involve those unjustly abandoned, those who have gone through a period of penance, and those in a second union who for moral reasons cannot separate ("Reception" 339).

49. After discussing the conscience which is "convinced that the earlier, irreparably destroyed marriage was never valid" the bishops state, "the situation would be similar when those concerned already have come a long way in reflection and penance. Moreover, there could also be the presence of an insoluble conflict of duty, where leaving the new family would be the cause of grievous injustice" ("Principles" 674); note the similarity to the examples which the CDF document cites.

50. Matthäus Kaiser, "Why Should the Divorced and Remarried (not) be Admitted to the Sacraments?" *Theology Digest* 41 (1994) 8–14, at 9; original German text in *Stimmen der Zeit* 118 (1993) 741–51.

51. Anne Thurston makes a similar point: "One of the problems in the practice of the Roman Catholic Church is that the move towards a description of marriage as covenant rather than contract has not sufficiently penetrated pastoral practice when it comes to the breakdown of marriages" ("Living with Ambiguity," *Doctrine and Life* 44 [1994] 537–42, at 538).

52. Kaiser, "Why Should the Divorced and Remarried" 10.

53. Ibid. 11. This is a needed corrective to the assertion of the Catechism that the remarried spouse is "in a situation of public and permanent adultery" (*Catechism of the Catholic Church* [New York: Paulist, 1994] no. 2384).

54. Leading authors have long looked askance at the brother/sister arrangement. Bernard Sullivan began his doctoral dissertation on the subject by gathering their opinions: "... [C]anonists and theologians uniformly warn that the sanctioned cohabitation in the brother-sister arrangement is a '*res plena periculis*' and is seldom to be recommended; some say '*raro*' (Vermeersch-Creusen, Merkelbach, Sporer-Bierbaum); others say '*rarissime*' (DeSmet, Genicot, Coronata, Chretien, Payen); others say '*fere numquam*' (Gasparri, Vlaming-Bender, Capello). It is evident that all apparently mean to say as Chelodi and Wernz-Vidal put it: 'Cohabitation on the brother-sister basis is permissible only in extraordinary circumstances and when no other remedy is possible'" (Sullivan, *Permissible Cohabitation* viii). In the face of this extreme reluctance, American canonists like Sullivan and Krol continued to promote it as a pastoral option, suggesting detailed requirements and procedures, and constructing printed forms for requesting permission from the local ordinary to live as brother and sister (Sullivan, ibid. 81–171; John Krol, "Parties Invalidly Married" 22–32, and "Permissible Cohabitation in Invalid Marriages," *Jurist* 18 [1958] 279–306, at 299–306). By the late 1960s, canonical attitudes seemed to have changed: "As for the possibility of a brother-sister relationship, this is clearly unrealistic among the great majority of people" (Carey, "Good Faith" 432). It was astonishing to see this arrangement put forward as a pastoral option in *Familiaris consortio* no. 84, and again in the *Catechism* no. 1650.

55. Kaiser, "Why Should the Divorced and Remarried" 12.

56. "Certo certius textus respicit etiam divortiatos et renuptiatos," *Communicationes* 15/2 (December, 1983) 194. See also J. Manzanares, *Codigo de Derecho Canonico* (Madrid: BAC, 1985); A. Marzoa, *Codigo de Derecho Canonico* (Navarra: Eunsa, 1983); G. Damizia, *Commento al Codice de Diritto Canonico* (Rome: Urbaniana University, 1985)—all a propos of canon 915.

57. *CLSA Advisory Opinions 1984–1993*, ed. P. Cogan (Washington: CLSA, 1995) 285. It should also be noted that "questions of 'sin' and 'grave' are not canonical notions and need to be dealt with by confessors, not by those dispensing the Eucharist" (Provost, "Intolerable Marriages: Second Decade" 595).

58. *The Code of Canon Law: A Text and Commentary*, ed. J. Coriden, T. Green, and D. Heintschel (New York: Paulist, 1985) 653.

59. "Arcendi sunt a susceptione Divinae Eucharistiae publici indigni."

60. "Christological Theses on the Sacrament of Marriage," *Origins* 8 (1978) 200–04, at 203. Although released by the ITC, the document was written by an individual, Fr. Gustave Martelet, S.J., a member of the Commission.

61. One of the interesting consequences of such a shift is to raise in a different way the question of which marriage is truly the "objective contradiction" to Christ's teaching. As Thurston writes, "There are relationships which become destructive for all involved and where without stretching language far beyond what words can bear it is not possible to talk of such marriages as 'symbolizing the union between Christ and the Church.' Paradoxically the second union may in fact be the means of restoring faith, of renewing hope and of embodying love" ("Living with Ambiguity" 538).

62. John Mahoney, S.J., *Seeking the Spirit: Essays in Moral and Pastoral Theology* (London: Sheed and Ward, 1981) 158.

63. "Decree on Ecumenism" no. 8.

64. Mahoney, *Seeking the Spirit* 162.

65. Whether it be Origen's struggle with how to interpret Scripture or Aquinas's insistence on the analogical nature of theological discourse, there are numerous examples of the Church's wrestling with the problem of religious language. Within the contemporary English-speaking world of theology, a world profoundly shaped by Wittgenstein, there has been significant interest in what some have called the "linguistic turn"; see a number of the essays and reports in *Catholic Theological Society of America Proceedings* 42 (1987). Martelet's paper and subsequent magisterial usage of his argument do not reflect familiarity with the literature in this area.

66. Theodore Mackin, *Divorce and Remarriage* (New York: Paulist, 1983) 517. A related point can be made about how defenders of the present policy make reference to the words of Jesus in the Synoptic Gospels as if his teaching on the permanence of marriage is to be equated with the Church's claim that *ratum et consummatum* marriages cannot be dissolved even by the Church itself. Familiarity with the evolution of the Church's teaching on indissolubility should provide the lesson that the present position has been achieved only after considerable and long development. Acting as if further development now is impossible due to the teaching of Jesus seems to ignore the historically conditioned nature of the present teaching.

67. Thurston, "Living with Ambiguity" 538.

68. Kelly, "Divorce and Remarriage: Conflict" 1374.

69. This statement is based on interviews conducted by K. Himes of priests working with alienated Catholics in Bergen County, N.J., Boston, Mass., New York, N.Y., Providence, R.I., and Wilmington, Del.

70. Kelly, "Divorce and Remarriage: Conflict" 1374.

71. "Response" 343.

72. James Keenan, S.J., "Toleration, Principle of," in Judith Dwyer, ed., *The New Dictionary of Catholic Social Thought* (Collegeville, Minn.: Liturgical, 1994) 951–52, at 951.

73. Despite the confidence of the Pennsylvania bishops in the tribunal system, Provost documents the many concerns which still remain. After examining the evidence he concludes, "The conflict situation continues to exist in many parts of the Church, even those with well functioning tribunals" ("Intolerable Marriages: Second Decade" 599–603, at 603). See also the comments of Tim Buckley, C.Ss.R. "Many have found the tribunal process one of growth and healing but, for all the pastoral relief which the annulment process has brought to these people, it remains a sad fact that for many others it is not the solution" ("Caring for the Remarried," *Priests and People* 9 [1994] 325–30, at 328). The reasons the author mentions as to why the tribunals are inadequate for many are not first of all canonical but emotional and psychological. Buckley recently spent five years investigating pastoral care of the separated, divorced, and divorced and remarried at the request of the bishops of England and Wales.

74. We believe that the language of toleration is inadequate. If the pastoral minister and the individual, having engaged in dialogue, conclude there is probable cause to believe that a first marriage was invalid, then reception of Communion by the person should not just be tolerated but encouraged. In such a conflict case, the harm is a matter of allowing some marriage situations to remain unresolved canonically while denying the Eucharist to those seeking it in good conscience. Since the legal irregularity is a considerably lesser evil than the denial of the Eucharist, we believe ministers should recommend eucharistic participation. Toleration toward eucharistic participation may be the apt term when a minister remains dubious of the initial marriage's invalidity but the individual in good faith concludes that it was null. The pastor's practice is described by the traditional term of dissimulation.

75. Even an ideal tribunal system is not the best answer. We agree with Thurston when she writes that too often "attempts to extend the concept of nullity seem to me inappropriate here." Our present pastoral procedures require "that the failed marriage is negated rather than taken up in the human experience of the gap between what we desire and what we realize." We need a process in which "the fragile nature of all human relationships" is sufficiently recognized ("Living with Ambiguity" 539).

76. Ibid. 541.

77. See n. 28 above.

78. *Seeking the Spirit* 42. See also the comment by Tim Buckley, "It is said that hard cases make bad law but, in this arena, there are so many hard cases that of necessity we must ask whether the law as it stands truly represents the will of God for his people" ("Caring for the Remarried" 326).

79. In this we are in agreement with Buckley. "The three German bishops chose to address the problem in the practical pastoral arena, which is where so much of the debate has centered in recent times. This is understandable in view of the continuing urgency of the problem for so many people, but I believe the time is long overdue when the more fundamental systematic theological questions must be addressed" (ibid. 329). Buckley maintains that "the evidence from [his] research suggests that the *sensus fidelium* would be totally in harmony with the teaching that marriage *per se* is a sacred and permanent union as expressed in the *Catechism* (1614), but not with the discipline the Church employs to defend its concept of the indissolubility of the bond as expressed in the same *Catechism* (1640)" (ibid.).

80. Because the German letter did not directly address the question of indissolubility, indeed explicitly affirmed the present understanding and teaching on it, we did not survey the literature on this topic. Since the last time this topic was addressed in these "Notes" several worthwhile essays on indissolubility have appeared, including Bernard Cooke, "Indissolubility: Guiding Ideal or Existential Reality?" in *Commitment to Partnership*, ed. William Roberts (New York: Paulist, 1987) 64–75; and four papers by Cooke, John Erickson, Theodore Mackin, and Margaret Farley in *Divorce and Remarriage*, ed. William Roberts (New York: Paulist, 1990).

81. Orsy, "A German Initiative" 787.

82. Hünermann, "A Church in Dialogue" 898.

83. "Dialogue on Divorce," *Tablet* 248 (1994) 1335–36, at 1335.

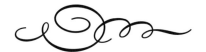

Contraception

20

Contraception: The Doctrine and the Context

John T. Noonan, Jr.

The period from 1880 to the present—in which contraception spread throughout the world, the planning of births became a generally accepted ideal in Western and Western-influenced cultures, and the Catholic Church waged war on contraception—was also marked by changes whose impact on the Catholic position was inescapable. The changes created a new context for the teaching on contraception. At the same time developments within the Church and an internal evolution of doctrine on marriage affected the inner constituents of the teaching. The question of permissible means of regulating birth could not be decided by the simple inspection of alternatives. It was set within the context of a changed environment and an evolved theology of marriage.

The Changed Environment

Population. Until about 1650, the population of the world had increased at an annual rate of no more than .1 percent. At this date the world population was about 500 million. The annual rate of growth then began to increase and rose to about .5 percent. By 1850 the world population had doubled to one billion. The rate of growth now began to accelerate. By 1900 it was nearly 1 percent per year. By 1930 the world population had, in eighty years, doubled to two billion. In 1964 the rate of growth was nearly 1.75 percent, or double the rate in 1880. It was predicted that, unless there were major checks, the world population would reach four billion by 1980, and that the rate of growth would probably continue as high as 2 percent.[1]

The principal factor bringing about these increases in the total world population and in its rate of increase was the control of disease. The creation of healthful environments, the development of public health measures, a vast improvement in the care of infants and young children, and the discovery and use of means to cure infectious diseases first increased life expectancy in western Europe and North America, and then, in the twentieth century, had the same beneficent effect in eastern Europe and much of Asia, Latin America, and Africa. The preservation of millions of human beings through childhood into child-producing ages meant that the population grew not only because people were living longer, but because there were more child-producing people. In areas where modern health measures were suddenly introduced, such as Ceylon and Brazil, there were dramatically sharp climbs in life expectancy and in population.

The changes in western Europe occurred more gradually; but a comparison of nineteenth- and twentieth-century mortality and life expectancy rates is equally dramatic. From a crude death rate of 30 per year per thousand in western Europe in 1800, the death rate fell to 11 by 1960. Even between 1913 and 1955 there was an impressive gain in life expectancy for Western countries. In 1913 life expectancy at birth in the Netherlands was 52; in 1956 it was 75; in the same period in Italy it rose from 45 to 70, and in Canada from 45 to 70. By 1964 life expectancy in northwestern Europe, North America, Oceania, and the U.S.S.R. was nearing 75.[2]

The rate of growth, projected, created a hypothetical situation in which avoidance of procreation could seem mandatory: "a two percent growth rate will result in one square yard of land area per person 600 years hence, an obvious absurdity."[3] But most moralists probably did not feel bound to deal with this hypothetical, believing that against it could be played off other hypothetical possibilities, such as the colonization of outer space. In short, immediate moral judgments were difficult to obtain on a situation in a remote and contingent future.[4]

The real bite of the population increase was in its effect on the countries characterized as underdeveloped because of their low per capita incomes, low rate of saving and investment, and low industrial output. In these African, Latin American, and Asian countries the drastic reduction of mortality by modern health measures resulted in expansions of population which consumed their resources and made economic accumulation and improvement difficult or impossible. In some of these countries, dependent on forestry, mining, or primitive agriculture, the diminution of space per person had an immediate impact which it would not have in a modern industrial society. In countries with millions of very poor workers, such as India, the increase of people was accompanied by a danger of malnutrition which would not have threatened a population whose density was greater but whose wealth was more equitably divided.[5] In the underdeveloped countries, the increase of population also sometimes overloaded inefficient educational systems to the point of endangering them. In none of these countries could the influx of numbers alone be said to be causing the disappointment of educational and economic aspirations. Existing systems of economic allocation, political patterns, social organizations, cultural ideals, were also responsible. But given the existence of these factors, the influx had serious consequences. In specific underdeveloped countries, "overpopulation" acquired a meaning and became a menacing reality.[6]

The status of women. The same period, from the last part of the nineteenth century to the present, in which population so enormously expanded, was independently characterized by the emancipation of women. This emancipation was embodied in four remarkable changes. Economically, women in the West became income-earning members of society on a large scale. Husbands lost most of their earlier legal controls over their wives' property. In capitalistic countries like the United States women came to own a major share of the national wealth. Equality with men in the economic world, if not totally attained, was in the way of being realized. Politically, in most of the democracies by the mid-twenties, women had acquired the right to vote. Intellectually, women gained access to higher education, and by the 1960's countries like the United States and the U.S.S.R. were educating many girls at a college level and beyond. Women begn to write on a variety of subjects, including contraception, hitherto man's exclusive domain. Finally, with a substantial effect on a wife's position in marriage, divorce became easier for women to obtain and less socially disastrous if obtained.[7]

These familiar phenomena of freedom, characteristic in varying degrees of Western or Westernized cultures, gave women a status of near or complete equality with men, and necessarily affected the relationship possible in marriage. No longer was the average wife bound by economic chains and condemned to educational inferiority. More often than was objectively possible before, marriages could be the meeting of equal persons. What was true of marriage itself was also true of courtship. The meeting of reltively free and relatively equal persons became possible on a large scale. Modern Western society became the first society in history where individual decision consciously played a major role in the choice of a spouse. In the great slave systems of Greece and Rome, a large segment of the population could not marry; in feudalism, much of the population had little choice as to marriage; in aristocratic and bourgeois Europe, and even in the class- and property-conscious Victorian era, personal choice was largely fettered; only in the twentieth century did personal decision become predominant. The confining influences of religion, race, wealth, social status, family, were not eliminated, but while they frequently guided decision they were infrequently strong enough to override personal choice, and were seldom set forth as ideals more important than personal response. Marriage by personal choice was the system. The "great mystery" of St. John Chrysostom's day and La Tour Landry's day and St. Alphonsus Liguori's day—how two persons who had never met before could love each other for life—was replaced by more complex mysteries of personal interaction.[8]

With women relatively free and equal, rules for marriage developed in an age of slave concubinage and continued in a feudal era when women generally lacked education, were put in a new setting. Much of the traditional teaching had tried to prevent exploitation of the wife as an object. Much of the teaching had tried to safeguard personal values in unions formed with a minimum of personal consent. The assumptions, the social framework, of the rules had altered.

Methods of education. Partially as a corollary of feminine independence, partially as the result of urban industrial life, Western families became "single-cell" units, rather than including ancestors and collaterals. The early care and raising of children became the task for man and wife alone with little help from other kin. Western man was usually the sole material and moral support of his children.

The raising and eduction of children not only became a more personal responsibility, it became a more expensive one. A technical society required more education, and democratic society made it possible, at some cost to the family, for every child to attend grammar school and for many children to attend high school and college. The stage reached by the United States, where in 1964 over 4,500,000 students were engaged in higher education after twelve years of school, could be seen as the one likely to become common. Formal education could be expected to last sixteen or more years.[9]

The medieval theologians had seen education as an essential constituent of parental duty to offspring, and they had meant by education a spiritual training. They had not envisaged a formal process of sixteen years as the norm. Yet nothing in the old teaching had limited the parental obligation to a stationary minimum; on the contrary, implicit in the notion of education was that it be such as would meet the spiritual and intellectual needs of a man of age. As the age set higher standards of education, so a new content was given the requirement of education. In the medieval and Counter-Reformation theologians, the tension between the demands of procreation and the demands of education had already been evident. Yet the formula had been unchanged: the primary purpose of marriage was the procreation and education of offspring. The new substance to "education" in the old formula gave a different weighting to the issues where the two duties clashed.

Scientific knowledge and philosophy. The sheer physical number of people increased, one of the two sexes emerged from inequality to equality as persons, the education of millions became better—not only did these well-known changes in the social environment occur, but the most relevant physical data changed. The ovum had been discovered in 1827, but an understanding of the joint role of spermatozoa and ovum in generation was obtained only in 1875. The existence of several hundred thousand potential ova in the ovaries of every woman was established only in the twentieth century. That fecundation was possible in only a fraction of the menstrual cycle was known only in 1923. Only very recently have studies been made of the number of children women were likely to have who made no effort to restrain their fecundity.[10]

These facts, discovered since 1875, were relevant to what the purposes of sexual intercourse could be said to be. The theologians had shaped their arguments and conclusions in the light of the biology of their day. Relying on erroneous biological data, they had made intercourse in menstruation or in pregnancy mortal sin. Their arguments against contraception had also been constructed in the light of the biology they knew. Until well into the twentieth century, some theologians continued to believe that their predecessors, who had known nothing of the basic constituents of generation, spermatozoa and ova, had been enlightened as to the only way in which the natural law of reproduction could be observed. There were signs, however, as will be observed, that this confidence in ancient misconceptions was becoming obsolete.

Psychology also presented relevant fresh data—less unassailable than the biological information, but better verified than the casual observations of human behavior made before empirical psychology existed. The penetration of personality by sexuality was suggested. The focus of the old theological approach on distinct genital acts as the chief criterion of marital virtue was implicitly challenged. A greater understanding of the interaction of persons in marriage and the place of sexual intercourse in their relationship was obtained.[11]

Sociology, another science to develop only at the end of the nineteenth century, brought information on the growth and decline of populations where rough guessing had formerly sufficed. Anthropology provided new information on human sexual behavior. The kinds of data these new sciences offered were not to be mistaken for moral judgments. In trying to prescind from their own prejudices, the sociologists and anthropologists often claimed to offer only statistics or observations. Moral theologians could not determine the good way of behavior merely from the average way that was described. But neither could they make judgments about the ideal requirements of man without attention to these data. "Before the age of sociology," wrote Canon Jacques Leclerq, professor of moral and social philosophy at Louvain, "the questions have never been studied"; and by "these questions" he said he meant "the natural conditions of the family order."[12]

It is platitudinous to remark that the modern consciousness is historical. But it may not be superfluous to observe that the development of this consciousness was of immense importance for a subject so immersed in history as moral theology. Sensitive as a writer like Liguori had been to differences of opinion among his predecessors, he treated the differences as though they were talking of the same case. In his introduction to his *Moral Theology* he reviewed earlier works of moral theology from patristic times to his own day. He noted that the scholastic treatment of moral topics was "by far better and fuller" than that of the penitentials; he rebuked the rigorists of his age who "boast much of the Fathers, value the Popes little, and esteem more recent theologians not at all" (*Moral Theology,* Prolegomena, 1.66). But although he was aware that methods had changed, and although he defended the right of modern theologians to contribute modern solutions, Liguori ignored the environmental context. For him all writers of the past stood on the same flat line; all were supposed to have sought the same abstractly rational result. In the nineteenth century, moral theology had immunized itself from excesses of German historicism by conceding nothing to history, first opying eighteenth-century casuistry, then attempting a literal restatement of St. Thomas. Occasional apologetical necessities led to historical discriminations, as in the case of Francis X. Funk's *Zins und Wucher,* which tried to explain the evolution of the doctrine on usury. But moral theology in general, and the sexual ethic in particular, were proof against the historical spirit. Only when Western society was saturated by it, only when no respectable intellectual process could be undertaken without it, did the moral theologians succumb. The consequence began to be clear in the books which, beginning with *Der Usus matrimonii* of Lindner in 1929, sought to explore historically the development of doctrine on sexual ethics.[13]

Developments in philosophy also had a substantial effect on the framework of the old prohibition. About 1850 Thomism began to be thought of by some Italian ecclesiastics as a solution to the evils of the day. After the encyclical *Aeterni Patris* of Leo XIII, issued August 4, 1879, Thomism was the cry in Catholic circles. At Louvain in 1882 Désiré Mercier instituted a course in Thomistic philosophy, capping it with the establishment in 1895 of the Higher Institute of Philosophy.[14] The 1917 Code of Canon Law represented the apogee of the movement Leo XIII had launched. Canon 1366, sec. 2, prescribed that the teaching of philosophy and theology must be "according to the arguments, doctrine, and principles of St. Thomas, which they [the professors] are to hold inviolately." The Catholic University of America was committed to a literal Thomism and remained so, as did the Angelicum and the Lateran University in Rome. In other parts of Europe, however, in the 1920's the phenomenology of Edmund Husserl and Max Scheler and the existentialist personalism of Gabriel Marcel became fecund influences on Catholic thought. A personalist conception of natural law came to compete with a literally Thomistic view. Thus, by 1962, a contemporary Dutch Dominican, M. Plattel, could note that natural law at one time was conceived of by analogy with a static world order in terms which emphasized the givenness of biological imperatives. Today, in a personalist perspective, natural law "appeals to the authentic choice of man, who, from his very being as a person, must fashion a concrete universal image of man, more in the manner of a creator than of a conformist ... [It possesses] a dynamic, functional character because of its active orientation toward the ideal personal community." As biological regularity became less emphasized than the freedom of the spiritual person, so, Plattel said, it became more difficult to insist that biological norms should completely govern human acts.[15] As this concept of natural law was advanced, so the most basic concepts in the analysis of the law prohibiting contraception were affected.

All of this intellectual development—biological, medical, psychological, sociological, historical, and philosophical—created a world of data and of mental attitudes very different from the world in which contraception had been analyzed since the second century after Christ. Both the facts and the methods of analyzing them were fresh.

The internal structures of the Church. The teaching on contraception might have remained static, immunized against the social and intellectual changes, if the institutional life of the Church had not also been modified. This modification, itself partially the product of the new environmental forces, made it more probable that the Church would consciously respond to the environmental developments.

Catholic higher education began to recover from the nadir of 1800. In the 1820's Catholic faculties of theology were established at Tübingen and Munich. In the 1830's Louvain was refounded with some claim to moral continuity with the medieval university. It was only in 1876, however, that Catholic universities became legal in France and only in 1876 that the Institut Catholique was founded. In the United States a beginning was made in 1889 with the founding of the Catholic University of America as a center for graduate study. In the nineteenth century, Louvain and the theological faculties at the German universities proved the most fruitful institutions. The French centers were first buffeted by the fierce anticlerical battles of the 1880's and 1890's, then shaken by the crisis of the Modernist errors from 1900 to 1908. The Catholic University of America became, for the most part, an enlarged seminary. None of these institutions had much immediate impact on the work of moral theology; its status in 1900 was almost as low as in 1800.[16] The problems engaging attention seemed more fundamental: the existence of God, the truth of the Catholic claim, the relation of the Church to society. Lecomte's work on ovulation stands out as an exception. It was not until the 1920's that much influence of the German and French faculties, Louvain, and the Catholic University of America on moral theology could be discerned. The consequences were more indirect than direct. The universities did provide bases where the advances in knowledge could be related to Catholicism. The universities did form a community of men interested in developing the self-consciousness of the Church in its incarnation in the world. Only in the 1960's, however, did the existing Catholic universities, joined now by Nijmegen in the Netherlands, St. Michael's College at Toronto, and Notre Dame, St. Louis, and Georgetown in the United States, contribute substantially to what had been the province of the seminaries. The importance for the development of moral doctrine of Catholic institutions not encumbered by the job of providing practical training for priests became evident. The universities showed promise of bringing an academic detachment, a speculative boldness, and an historical perspective to matters where pastoral and apologetical needs had played a dominant role.

The slow and uncompleted growth of the Catholic universities was intimately connected with another growth within the Church, the expression of loyal, critical, and free opinion. The counter forces within the Church were strong. Even before the Reformation, ecclesiastical authority had been suspicious of a free press. Since the Fifth Lateran Council in 1515, a form of prior restraint on books had existed in the requirement that any book bearing on Catholic doctrine carry the imprimatur of the bishop of the diocese of the publisher; the old rule was continued in substance, but without the earlier severe penalties, in canon 1385 of the 1917 Code of Canon Law.[17] In addition to this theoretical commitment to the right of authority to restrain free expression by any Catholic, there were special restrictions on members of religious orders. Members of a religious order were subject not only to the bishop's imprimatur but, according to the law established by Trent and reaffirmed by canon 1385, to censorship from their own order. Not only were they bound to respect Catholic dogma; often they were prevented from writing anything which would disturb the posture or image which their superiors believed appropriate to their order. Beyond the canonical requirements of censorship, administrative sanctions existed. Removal from a teaching position could be used by a bishop or a religious superior against any priest teaching in a seminary if he expressed unsound or unwelcome opinion. The mere existence of this power of removal, subject to little practical restraint, was generally sufficient to impose silence on priests with dangerously new ideas. The effect of this censorship was especially severe on moral theology because so much of it was written by members of the orders. With a few exceptions at Paris and Louvain—Le Maistre, Major, Sinnich—almost all the moral theology on sexual matters from the second quarter of the thirteenth century to the first quarter of the twentieth was written by priests under the special discipline of a religious order.

Administrative control of theological speculation produced a situation in which no one could pretend that what was written represented what was thought by all theologians. The result was not insincerity on the part of those who wrote openly with a strong conviction of the rightness of their views, but silence, involuntary or voluntary, from those who disagreed. An unhealthy climate for discussion was created when it was not certain that all the thinking of theologians was being communicated. This climate, characteristic of many seminaries in which university influences were absent, prevailed particularly from 1800 to the very recent past. It was notable that in the controversy over the progesterone pill Van der Marck could remark that "many opinions" on the issue did not appear in print, and that Bishop Reuss found it necessary to begin his article with a strong plea for candor: "Despite all the fidelity which is due the common doctrine, the theologian should teach nothing as absolutely valid when he is not himself convinced that it is legitimate."[18] It was common knowledge that in private some theologians were freer and bolder in their expressions on the subject of contraception than they dared to be in any publication.[19]

Despite the continuation of restraints on discussion, a new trend in the theological defense of freedom was apparent. A pioneer essay was "On Consulting the Faithful in Matters of Doctrine," by John Henry Newman. Writing in 1859, Newman drew on the process by which Pius IX had reached the decision to promulgate the dogma of the Immaculate Conception: "Pope Pius has given us a pattern, in his manner of defining, of the duty of considering the sentiments of the laity upon a point of tradition, in spite of whatever fullness of evidence the bishops had already thrown upon it."[20] Newman added that in the fourth century it was the faithful who had preserved the true doctrine on the Trinity when the majority of the bishops had gone over to the Arian heresy. This occasional piece, designed to vindicate an expression of Newman's, necessarily vindicated the freedom of all members of the Church. In the pontificate of Pius IX it was received with cold hostility in Rome.[21]

Newman was the outstanding Catholic theologian of the nineteenth century. His thesis was neglected in his time. But, as often in the history of theology, a principle was reasserted by the Church when the world had most absolutely denied it. In reaction to the totalitarian Nazi and Communist regimes, the idea of freedom was vindicated. Speaking on February 17, 1950, to an International Congress of Writers of Catholic Newspapers, Pius XII brought out the evil of a totalitarian society in which only the opinion of the leaders is heard. To reduce citizens to silence is, he said, "an attack on the natural right of man, a violation of the order of the world as God has established it." He concluded with a word on "public opinion in the very breast of the Church (naturally, in matters left to free discussion)." The Church, he said, "is a living body, and something would be lacking in its life if public opinion defaulted in it, a default for which the pastors and the faithful would be responsible" (*AAS* 42:251, 256). Pius XII's reservation, "naturally, in matters left to free discussion," was an exception that could have swallowed the rule. But a new note had been sounded by a Pope: a free public opinion was a natural part of every society. The Pope also recognized that "the Church" could not be identified with the authorities—Pope, bishops, theologians. The laity, he told the college of cardinals on February 20, 1946, "are the Church" (*AAS* 38:141).

Using the remarks of Pius XII to the press as a springboard, a leading Catholic theologian of the twentieth century, the Austrian Jesuit Karl Rahner, in 1953 wrote *Free Speech in the Church*. Fifty years before, he noted, one would hardly have expected the words of Pius XII on the lips of a Pope. Rahner went on to distinguish two kinds of opinion within the Church. First, he noted that the Holy Spirit "can breathe upon whomsoever he will in the Church—even the poor, the children, those who are 'least in the kingdom of God.'" The Church which teaches and the Church which is taught are the same Church. "The 'Church taught' has its own understanding of the Faith, its own kind of 'infallibility'—in the sense that not only the teaching Church but the 'Church taught,' as a whole, will always remain within the orbit of divine truth, safe under the power of the Holy Spirit."[22] This kind of supernaturally protected opinion, of which Newman wrote, was to be distinguished from another kind of public opinion to which Rahner addressed himself, which was not necessarily the effect of the guidance of the Holy Spirit: "Its justification is simply that this is the sole means of discovering what is really going on. If there is any real desire to know the current situation—spiritual, psychological, social, etc.—then Catholics must be allowed (within the limits already laid down) to talk their heads off."[23] The limits of discussion were what "comes into conflict with the Church's dogma and her divinely willed constitution." But, Rahner added, "there is always a strong tendency to narrow down far too closely the range of what parts of the Faith can be legitimately discussed." He observed, "If there is, as there should be, a real public opinion within the Church, not merely an unthinking reflection of the Church's official views, a certain tension is likely to exist around all those matters that are subject to change and hence to free discussion."[24]

With some theological and ecclesiastical encouragement, then, free speech became more prized in the Church. The universities embodied the principle and at the same time provided persons capable of exercising the right. Finally, "the spirit of Pope John," and the climate of freedom from bureaucratic surveillance created by the open discussion at the Second Vatican Council, produced an atmosphere in which frank discussion of the basic prohibition of contraception could occur. Whether the speakers were only Catholics talking their heads off, or whether their witness constituted the *consensus fidelium,* the divinely protected expression of Christian faith, was not immediately determinable.

The emergence of the universities and the later development of articulate discussion were closely associated with an increasing role for the laity in the Church. Before the founding of magazines edited by Catholic laymen but not under ecclesiastical control, there was no institutional form designed to express the opinion of the laity on matters in the Church. In the United States, the way was led by *Commonweal,* founded in 1924, followed by *Cross Currents, Jubilee, The Critic,* and *Ramparts.* These magazines were both symbols of and outlets for an educated Catholic laity which was seriously concerned with the teaching of the Church. The articulation of lay sentiment had special significance for the analysis of contraception.[25]

In declaring evil an act of contraception performed by lawfully wedded persons, the theologians had condemned an act which was literally beyond their experience. The number of married men who had written as Catholic theologians on contraception could be numbered on a hand—Joannes Andreae is the only prominent name. Obviously, experience is not a precondition for judging the morality of an act intelligently. All condemn murder, though few are murderers. Observation, empathy with the experience of others, reasoning, can be the process of moral judgment. At the same time the characteristic problems and joys of one occupation or state of life are usually more acutely perceived and feelingly expressed by those who experience them. To judge rightly of the morality of particular acts may require close listening to those who have had experience of the way of living in which the questions arise.

The theologians of the past had heard the sins of many married folk recounted in confession, but the context in which communication occurred did not invite impartial evaluation of the experience. The theologians may also have had limited and probably inhibited conversations on the subject with spiritual advisers, friends, and kin. But there is a uniqueness to random individual testimony that could easily cause it to be discounted in the face of any strong official position. The lay voice on marriage was never entirely lost after the late fifteenth century, when it played a part in framing the new doctrine on the purposes of marital intercourse. It was not much listened to. When Bishop Bouvier cited the belief of the younger couples of Le Mans that contraception was not a sin, the testimony of the laity never rose to the dignity of an argument that contraception was lawful, but was used to support the plea that their good faith not be unsettled. The laity spoke, but their testimony was individual, oral, unsystematic, and not expressed in theological categories. To most theologians it failed to be persuasive or even relevant.

It was, then, a capital event in the development of testimony when in the fall of 1964 there appeared *The Experience of Marriage,* edited by Michael Novak, in which thirteen Catholic couples stated their own experiences in attempting to observe the theological doctrines on contraception and on rhythm. There had been harbingers within the preceding twelve months in the form of magazine articles by laymen. The book, open to criticism from all sides, was a limited pledge that the experiences reported were not idiosyncratic. It preserved in a form available to all future theologians the voices of educated married American Catholics in 1964.

Not only did the direct written testimony of laymen add new data. The testimony of women was added. In twenty centuries no Catholic woman had written on contraception. The emancipation of women in the late nineteenth century was particularly resisted by some Catholic churchmen who identified a given social structure with the Gospel; as late as 1930 a portion of *Casti connubii* gave a caricature of feminine emancipation and deplored the consequences. But by the 1960's there were many Catholic women who had been sufficiently emancipated by education to be able to articulate their views on marriage and contraception. There was testimony now not only of the experience of the married, but of those who bore the children.

Finally, a factor, partly external, partly internal, began to be of importance in the light of ecumenical developments. This was the testimony of the other Christian churches. As long as hostility to "the heretics" marked Catholic relations with these bodies, there was a negative reaction to doctrinal development by Protestants. But with the inauguration of a new approach by John XXIII and the institution in 1961 of the Secretariat for Christian Unity as a Roman office, a new appreciation became apparent of the many Christian beliefs, signs, and values shared by Catholic and non-Catholic Christians. In this era of dialogue, the testimony of the other churches became important.

Beginning with the Anglican decision in 1929, a large number of churches publicly abandoned the absolute prohibition of contraception by married couples. What was especially striking was the change in position of the bodies whose general theology was closest to Catholic thought: the Anglican, Lutheran, and Calvinist communions. The bodies changing their stand were as follows: the Congregational Christian General Council (1931); the General Council of the United Church of Canada (1936); the Methodist Conference of Great Britain (1939); the British Council of Churches (1943); a special commission of the Church of Scotland (1944); the bishops of the (Lutheran) Church of Sweden (1951); the General Synod of the Netherlands Reformed Church (1952); the Augustana Evangelical Lutheran Church (1954); the General Conference of the Methodist Church in the United States (1956); the United Lutheran Church in the United States (1956); the National Council of the Reformed Church of France (1956); the (Lutheran) Church of Finland (1956); the International Convention of the Disciples of Christ (1958); the World Council of Churches (1959). A similar position against any absolute prohibition of contraception was taken by such leading theologians as Derrick Sherwin Bailey, Karl Barth, Emil Brunner, Jacques Ellul and Reinhold Niebuhr.[26] A substantial consensus of Christian thought in the West outside the Catholic Church now approved of some form of contraception.[27]

The consciousness of the Church itself could not but be affected by the new institutional forms, the new voices, the new freedom within it, and the Christian testimony outside it. These developments produced new data on the question of contraception; they brought into being new attitudes; they created a demand for greater clarity and rationality in the rules against contraception.

The Development of Doctrine

Between 1850 and 1964 the teaching of the Church on the purposes of marital intercourse experienced substantial evolution. The process partly reflected the environmental changes, partly reflected the new voices speaking in the Church, partly represented a work of self-criticism by the theologians. This evolution reached the point where the question was asked: Is contraception sometimes permissible? And the broad question met the technical question raised by surgery and the pill: When is sterilization permissible?

Pleasure and Love as Values in Coitus

In the age of St. Alphonsus Liguori, pure Augustinianism, represented by writers like Billuart, still held a strong position. By 1850 the triumph of St. Alphonsus had banished Augustinian doctrine on the sole lawful intent with which intercourse might be initiated. But the Augustinian distrust of pleasure and indifference to love as purposes of intercourse remained. A new step was taken by the humble compendium of Gury.

Gury declared that marital intercourse was lawful for any one of four purposes: "the generation of offspring"; "the satisfaction of the obligation"; "the avoidance of incontinence in oneself or one's partner"; "the desire of fostering or bringing about decent friendship, of manifesting or promoting conjugal affection, and so forth." No reasons were given for this conclusion, but authority was cited as follows: "So commonly with Liguori, n. 881, Sanchez, and others, against others who eliminate the last two ends."[28] The names cited suggest how Gury had proceeded. He had taken the approach hesitantly adopted by Liguori himself of looking to the purposes of marriage to determine the purposes of intercourse. In his *Moral Theology* 6.881, Liguori had listed among the lawful extrinsic reasons for marrying the purpose "to effect peace among kingdoms and illustrious families." This social motive for marriage was the slender basis for Gury's "fostering or bringing about decent friendship." The awkwardness of the phrase came from its transfer from being the description of a motive for marriage to being the description of purpose of intercourse. By the 1874 edition the inappropriate term "friendship" had been replaced by "love." Gury's other inspiration had been the proposition set out by Sanchez, and accepted by Liguori, that some acts short of coitus were lawful among spouses "to foster or show mutual love" (above, pp. 325, 329). This thesis was boldly, but logically, applied to coitus itself.

If the fostering of love or the manifesting of conjugal affection could be a lawful purpose of coitus, the old dispute over pleasure as a purpose lost some of its significance. As long as only procreation and avoidance of concupiscence were recognized as lawful purposes, the spontaneous desire for intercourse was suspect. The new theory meant that there were no longer only three possible categories, of which two were dutiful and virtuous and one was pleasure-seeking and mortally or venially sinful. Gury himself said of the pleasure purpose merely that the condemnation of Innocent XI applied to intercourse sought for pleasure alone. His reviser, Anthony Ballerini, developed this point by saying that to act for pleasure meant "positively excluding" the other ends of action so that one placed one's "last end" in the pleasure. Without such positive exclusion of other ends, it was lawful to seek pleasure in marital intercourse (Gury-Ballerini, *Compendium of Moral Theology* 1.28; 2.908). This almost complete acceptance of pleasure was attacked by the anonymous Redemptorist authors of the *Vindiciae Alphonsianae;* they urged that the old authorities stood to the contrary.[29] Ballerini answered them with a thorough defense of pleasure, joy, and enjoyment as proper human ends (Gury-Ballerini, *Compendium,* 1887 ed., 2.908). Ballerini was then followed in substance by the leading moralist of the day, Augustine Lehmkuhl (*Moral Theology* 2.850).

At the turn of the century a long review of the controversy by John Becker concluded with a vigorous defense of pleasure as a proper purpose in sexual intercourse—as proper a purpose as seeking pleasure in intellectual activity. But there was one caveat: to seek pleasure, excluding other objectives, was mortally sinful, because this rare state of mind excluded any relation of the act to God.[30] That pleasure was a proper end in marital intercourse, if other ends were not willfully excluded, was then supported by Jesuits such as Jerome Noldin and Arthur Vermeersch, Dominicans such as Dominic Prümmer and Benedict Merkelbach, and secular priests such as Alois de Smet. It would be fair to describe the position as common after 1900.[31]

The position was still subject to qualification. In his address to the Italian Catholic Society of Midwives on October 29, 1951, Pius XII said, "The Creator who in His goodness and wisdom has willed to conserve and propagate the human race through the instrumentality of man and woman by uniting them in marriage has ordained also that, in performing this function, husband and wife should experience pleasure and happiness in body and spirit. In seeking and enjoying this pleasure, therefore, couples do nothing wrong. They accept that which the Creator has given them" (*AAS* 43:851). This passage was followed by a strong warning against attributing a value to sexuality as such independently of the end of the procreation of a new life. The Pope's words taken alone could be read as saying that pleasure might be sought only when man and wife were performing "this function" of propagating the species. However, this reading would not be justified by the larger context of the allocution; the Pope had already admitted the lawfulness of intercourse on the basis of rhythm. His words were simply a rebuke to "anti-Christian hedonism" which would "obey blindly and without check the caprices and impulses of nature."

In the *Law of Christ*, the German Redemptorist Bernard Häring drew a different distinction. If one generally sought only pleasure in marital intercourse, one would be behaving with sinful hedonism; such was the teaching of Innocent XI's condemnation of the proposition on intercourse for pleasure alone. But the "sudden need" of pleasure might be the "occasion" for intercourse, and intercourse to meet this need was lawful.[32]

In 1963, the American Jesuit theologians John C. Ford and Gerald Kelly made this wry comment:

> If sexual pleasure is to serve as an inducement to propagate, then God must want men to choose the act because of pleasure, not the other way round. If they were to choose the pleasure because of the act (a process psychologically difficult to envision), the pleasure would not be an inducement at all. The older authors seemed oblivious of this psychological aspect of the matter.

Ford and Kelly concluded that

> those who consciously act for the pleasure of sexual intercourse, apprehended as something permissible, need no further explicit legitimating motive to escape the imputation of acting *ob solam voluptatem*. In other words, if their conduct in marital intimacies is such that it preserves the inherent purposes or values which belong to conjugal intimacy, the pleasure they seek is well-ordered.[33]

Pleasure was not unqualifiedly recognized as an independent value. But the opinion dominant from 1880 to the present was closer to Le Maistre and Major than to Augustine.

Pleasure as a purpose, then, received guarded acceptance. Love was to be given complete recognition. Gury's adaptation of Sanchez had been made without theoretical underpinning. In the later nineteenth century a more reasoned development was attempted. In Germany in 1850 Ferdinand Probst, in his vernacular *Moral Theology*, spoke of the sharing of life by husband and wife and said, "In the conjugal act alone this sharing finds its highest expression. By it the principal end of marriage becomes other [than procreation], to wit, precisely the sharing of undivided life of the spouses."[34] In 1878, also writing in the vernacular, Francis X. Linsenmann, professor of theology at Tübingen, distinguished between the subjective and objective purposes of coitus. Objectively, the primary purpose was procreation. Subjectively, the primary purpose was that "through the ordered appeasement of the natural drives the spiritual union of the spouses be consolidated." Making these distinctions, Linsenmann sought to integrate the end usually expressed as "satisfaction of concupiscence" into an account which found a positive spiritual value in intercourse.[35] At the turn of the century De Smet spoke as Trent had spoken of love in marriage, but added the un-Tridentine thought, "The marriage act itself, by which the partners are made one flesh, cultivates and nourishes this love" (*Les Fiançailles et le mariage* 2.1.3.1.4).

It was only after World War I, however, that there was a substantial development of the relation of intercourse to love. This advance in speculation occurred principally in Germany, and principally under the influence of the phenomenology of Edmund Hussrl and Max Scheler. The most prominent of the early writers on the relationship was Dietrich von Hildebrand, professor of philosophy at the University of Munich, the first married layman to make a substantial contribution to Catholic doctrine on marriage. In lectures delivered to the Federation of Catholic Students at Innsbruck in 1925, Von Hildebrand spoke in lyrical terms of coitus. He rejected "the purely biological approach." The intention to propagate would not, by itself, "organically unite physical sex with the heart and spirit." The marital act, he declared, "has not only a function, the generation of children; it also possesses a significance for man as a human being (*in quantum homo*)—namely to be the expression and fulfillment of wedded love and community of life—and, moreover, it participates after a certain fashion in the sacramental meaning of matrimony." For the first time, a Catholic writer taught that love was a requirement of lawful, marital coition. He tied this novel demand to an ancient term—*fides*, fidelity. Fidelity required that person meet person in a giving of self. The old and long-used Augustinian comparison of intercourse to eating was rejected. The significance of eating was exhausted by its objective end. In eating it made no difference if one paid attention to the process of eating. But, in the marital act, "a fully deliberate, conscious attention is demanded." "The act of wedded communion has indeed the end [*Zweck*] of propagation, but in addition, the significance of a unique union of love."[36]

This evaluation of marital intercourse, where ideal aspirations were set out as guides, made an extreme contrast with Augustine and the whole patristic and medieval tradition. Yet Von Hildebrand was not an advocate of sexual activity deprived of religious criteria. His position was linked to the Catholic tradition by the special, sacral value assigned to the act of coition. The tradition had made coitus a sacral act free from human interference; Von Hildebrand first fully emphasized its content of love. With St. Albert, he saw a sacramental value in it; but, unlike St. Albert, he cut away completely from the Augustinian and scholastic approach that made procreation and a remedy for concupiscence the only values present. Not confusedly like Abert, not grudgingly like Gury, but enthusiastically, with conviction coming from the heart, Von Hildebrand made love central to the moral meaning of conjugal coitus.

The new approach, if not warmly accepted, was not attacked by *Casti conubii*. The encyclical quoted the Roman Catechism that "matrimonial fidelity" demanded a union in love. Love held in Christian marriage "a kind of primacy of excellence." The encyclical added that the "especial task" of this union was that "the spouses aid each other in more fully perfecting and conforming the interior man" (*AAS* 22:548). The emphasis on interior spiritual perfection scarcely responded to Von Hildebrand's emphasis on coitus as expressive of love. But love, even if not considered in its physical expression, was given a place in marriage which the sixteenth-century teaching had ignored. Where the Roman Catechism had said that the primary reason for marriage was mutual aid in bearing the burdens of life, the encyclical made a reinterpretation and enlarged the teaching: "This mutual interior formation of the partners, this earnest desire of perfecting one another, can be said in a very true sense, as the Roman Catechism teaches, to be the primary reason and cause for marriage, if marriage is not considered strictly as instituted for the proper procreation and education of children, but is more broadly taken as a sharing, way, and partnership of all of life."

To this point, the encyclical had exalted the importance of love, but only in relation to spiritual development. It went on: "This same charity ought to harmonize with all the rest of the rights and duties of the spouses; and so it is not only the law of justice, it is the rule of charity that must be recognized in the word of the Apostle, 'Let the husband render to his wife the debt, and equally the wife to her husband'" (*AAS* 22:548–549). In this restrained reference to charity and "the debt," the thesis of Von Hildebrand, that love must animate intercourse, was faintly reflected. No attempt was made to develop the relation between coitus and the perfection of the other spouse and the communion of lives. But, for the first time in a papal document, coitus and love were linked. The propostion owed to Gury and ultimately to Sanchez was restated, if not emphasized: among the "secondary ends" of marital intercourse was "the fostering of mutual love." Provided "the intrinsic nature" of coitus was safeguarded, spouses were "not forbidden" to have this secondary end in view (*AAS* 22:561). This lukewarm teaching marked a stage in the absorption of the new approach. The encyclical was not a vigorous affirmation of the personal values attainable in intercourse, and in stressing that procreation was the primary end of intercourse it ran counter to some personalist thought. But it was only the beginnng of discussion.

Five years later Von Hildebrand's ideas were restated and enlarged by Herbert Doms in *The Meaning and End of Marriage*.[37] Doms was to have, in a different way, as great an influence on the next quarter century of Catholic thought on marriage as Vermeersch had had on the first quarter. Doms, born in 1890 in Regensburg, had been a student of zoology before becoming a priest; he earned doctorates in both philosophy and theology; and in 1935 he was a *Privatdozent* teaching Catholic theology at the University of Breslau. In his book he said eloquently what serious Catholic laymen were waiting to hear: not only marriage, but marital intercourse, was a means of achieving holiness. The theory sketched by Von Hildebrand was given solidity and buttressed by scholarship. Doms provided biological data; a critique of St. Thomas' analysis of marriage; an explicit evocation of the passages from St. Albert on the sacramental significance of intercourse; and a discussion of the related ideas of Max Scheler. *The Meaning and End of Marriage* was the most comprehensive attempt yet made to develop a theory of Catholic marriage different from that of Augustine. It did not succeed in wholly winning the professional moral theologians, but its influence on later Catholic writing on marriage was inescapable.

The biological end, Doms argued, could not be the primary end. The sperm might or might not meet the egg, whose production did not depend on the sexual act. The Thomistic theory rested on the belief that the active form, the male seed, immediately acted on the female matter; of course, this was a biological misconception (*The Meaning and End of Marriage* [French edition, 1937], pp. 73–74). Doms's own thesis was as follows: "In the perfect act, worthy of human beings, the two partners grasp each other reciprocally in intimate love; that is, spiritually they reciprocally give themselves in an act which contains the abandonment and enjoyment of the whole person and is not simply an isolated activity of organs" (ibid., p. 27). The act of marital coitus was an ontological act, that is, an act affecting the being of the persons who interacted; a true, not symbolic, abandonment of oneself; a completion of oneself in the other. The elementary human desire to have relationship with a person was realized in the actuation and completion of the two partners (ibid., pp. 48, 54–55).

Doms's theory was comprehensive enough to account for at least seven practices in the life of the Church which the Augustinian-Thomistic theory made imcomprehensible. Four of these practices related to sterile intercourse. If ontological completion of the person, not procreation, was the end of marriage, the marriage and the intercourse of the sterile could be understood. Similarly coitus in pregnancy had an understandable end. Sterile marriages were indissoluble, because the ontological union held although procreation was impossible. The fornication of the sterile was illicit, for ontological union could be realized only in the way ordained by God, although no offspring would result (ibid., pp. 104, 97, 101, 191). The rule on sterility was explicably different from that on impotency; for the impotent, union was impossible (ibid., p. 172). The Pope's long-recognized power to dissolve sacramental unconsummated marriages when one spouse wanted to enter religious life was also given a rationale: the absence of completed ontological union made dissolution possible (ibid., p. 107). Finally, the ancient and still existing disfavor for remarriage on the death of a spouse was also accounted for: the second ontological completion was unnecessary and in a sense diminished the first (ibid., p. 172). All of these common practices in the Church were anomalies in a theory which said that procreation was the primary purpose of marriage. All were at least harmoniously explained by Doms. Again and again Doms offered a better explanation of the treatment of sterility; again and again he hit the weakness of the Augustinian position. To touch the keys of an organ when the pipes are not working, he observed, is not to play the organ; nor can one pressing the soundless keys be said to have the primary purpose of playing. To say coital acts were directed to offspring by persons who because of their physical condition could not have offspring was, Doms declared, nonsense (ibid., p. 180).

The theory of Doms had four additional merits. The old approach treated pleasure like bait, and the spouse seeking intercourse like an animal lured by the bait to procreate. Doms said that the pleasure and sentiment experienced were great, not as bait to action, but as reflections of the profound ontological change involved. The old theory took little account of the ordinary absence of a conscious desire to procreate in any given act of intercourse. Doms's position reflected the primacy of the consciousness of personal fulfillment. Even when spouses consciously desired children, he observed, the emphasis on personal accomplishment was often reflected by the statement "I am becoming a parent." The old theory treated the generative organs as though they had a finality of their own apart from the human person. Doms's theory rested on the fact that sexuality marked the whole human person. What was involved in the sexual exchange was not the finality of the genital organs alone, but the finality of the person. Finally, the old theory had nothing to say on the sacramental structure of marital intercourse. Doms boldly developed the parallel with the Eucharist. The physical union in marriage completed the moral participation in the life of the other just as physical union with Christ in the Eucharist completed the believer's moral union with Christ (ibid., pp. 23–27, 127).

Doms proposed an integrated new approach to Catholic marriage. No one would have supposed that anything so new and so complete would win instantaneous acceptance. In fact, Doms was met by one of those official reactions which so often have checked enthusiasm without fundamentally stopping progress. Doms had discarded the classic terminology of "primary" and "secondary" ends in marriage. Marital intercourse had an "immanent" end or meaning, the realization of interpersonal union. It had a procreative end, which Doms called the *finis operis* and treated as the end for which coitus might be accomplished. In the work of another personalist writer, Bernhardin Krempel, a Swiss Passionist, marriage was said to have only one essential end, the perpetual union of the lives of two persons of opposite sex. On April 1, 1944, the Holy Office noted that in some recent writings "a meaning is attached to words which occur in the teaching of the Church (for example, *end, primary, secondary*) which is not appropriate to these words according to their common use among theologians." With this word of explanation, the Holy Office answered the question: "Can the opinion of certain modern writers be admitted, who either deny that the primary end of marriage is the generation and education of children or teach that the secondary ends are not essentially subordinate to the primary end, but are equally principal and independent?" (*AAS* 36:103). The answer was, No. There was no note of doctrinal censure attached. Doms was not mentioned by name, and, arguably, Krempel's book rather than his contained the propositions criticized. Nonetheless, Doms was asserted to be the object of the decree by the *Nouvelle revue théologique* (67:839), which seemed to have access to unidentified but highly placed sources. The official rebuke addressed to a particular aspect of his book weakened its prestige as a whole. In the long run, however, the moral theology of the Church is determined not by decrees but by a more complicated process of reasoning by the theologians and response by the faithful. In the evaluation of marriage and marital intercourse after 1944, the book of Doms continued to play a preeminent part.

Reinforcement of the personalist position came in an unexpected way and from an unexpected quarter only seven years after the action of the Holy Office. To understand the development, it is necessary to return to 1897. In this year the Inquisition had acted on a very simple question, "May artificial insemination be applied to a woman?" The answer of the Congregation, approved by Leo XIII on March 26, 1897, had been negative (*AAS* 29:704). The question put was extraordinarily abstract; it did not introduce the supposition that the semen came from the woman's husband. At this time theologians such as Lehmkuhl (*Moral Theology* 2.835) and Ballerini and Palmieri in the revision of Gury (*Compendium* 6.1304) were teaching that semen resulting from marital coitus might lawfully be placed by instrument in the vagina, while it was unlawful to obtain semen by the ejaculation of the husband apart from intercourse. An anonymous commentator in the *Nouvelle revue théologique* (29:324) observed that the decision did not change this teaching.

In his book Doms argued that the 1897 decrees supported his position. The sexual act was there regarded not merely as a means to a biological end. It was regarded as an act meaningful in itself; and this meaning imposed restraints even upon an action which achieved the biological end of generation (*The Meaning and End of Marriage*, p. 187). Doms had an argument. But could the decree be accounted for only by a personalist theory of intercourse? Francis Hürth, who had succeeded Vermeersch as the leading Jesuit authority on sexual matters, thought not. Artificial insemination was immoral because nature had determined the manner of reproduction "in the smallest details," and "it would be absurd to abandon to the good pleasure of man the right of choosing this manner or of replacing it by another he has invented." His line of reasoning barred even the insertion by instrument of semen emitted in lawful coitus.[38] The insistence on the rigidity of the natural order paralleled the Thomistic argument against contraception based on the natural structure of the act, and avoided any concession to the personalist perspective.

In the light of this rejection of Doms by an influential Roman theologian, the evolution of teaching by Pius XII was instructive. In 1949 Pius XII condemned artificial insemination, not mentioning insemination by semen obtained in normal coitus (Address to the Fourth International Congress of Catholic Doctors, September 29, 1949, *AAS* 41:559). Two years later, in his comprehensive Address to the Midwives, he explained that his objection had been based on personalist considerations. Referring to the 1949 statement, he said that in it he had "formally excluded" artificial insemination, because the family is not "a biological laboratory." He continued, "The conjugal act, in its natural structure, is a personal action, a simultaneous and immediate cooperation of the two spouses, which, by the nature of the participants and the quality of the act, is the expression of the reciprocal gift, which, according to the word of the Scriptures, effects the union 'in one flesh alone'" (*AAS* 43:850). This language sounded more like Doms than Hürth. Five years later, on May 19, 1956, Pius XII repeated his personalist objections to artificial insemination. The biological result cannot be lawfully separated, he declared, from "the personal relation of the married couple," who "surrender themselves to each other and whose voluntary self-donation blossoms forth and finds its true fulfillment in the being which they bring into the world" (Address to the Second World Congress on Fertility and Sterility, *AAS* 48:470). In both talks the Pope insisted that the personal purposes of the spouses were subordinate to "what surpasses them, paternity and maternity." But the papal statements aimed at the manipulation of nature by insemination had the effect of emphasizing the personal values of intercourse and giving official approval at least to the personalist rejection of a narrow interpretation of procreative purpose. The significance of intercourse for the person had been expounded by the Pope. The self-donation of the spouses had been championed by him as a value of coitus.

The leading theologians on marriage in the 1950's also embraced a qualified personalist understanding of intercourse. Bernard Häring said in 1954 that he did not agree with Doms that "conjugal love was the first end of marriage." But he formally abandoned Doms only to combine a modified version of Doms's theory with the old teaching on procreation. Love was seen as the fundamental, although not the final value, in every act of the spouses (Häring, *The Law of Christ* 2–2.4.3.2.3.a). It was a love sacramentally established and vivified: conjugal love he described as "the accomplishment of a sacramental mission in virtue of a sacramental grace" (ibid. 2–2.4.3.2.6.c). In this perspective marital intercourse itself became "a fundamental mediation of charity." Apart from procreation, one of its permissible purposes was "the augmentation of love" (2–2.4.3.2.6). The loving union of spouses was not directed, however, to their own completion but to the child, whose "virtual presence" was somewhat vaguely said to be "inscribed in the ontological act of total union." But while this orientation to the child was acknowledged, Häring spoke in Doms's terms of a "completion of persons" in coitus. Only, he added, the completion was not ultimate; it "surpasses the dyad and in the image of the Trinity produces a third" (2–2.3.2.1.1.a). The old insistence on "the debt" was transcended in a statement which carried the seeds of development: as a sacramental community of persons, marriage was "infinitely richer than all categories of personal justice" (2–2.3.2.1.3.a).[39]

A new stage was reached when the new doctrine was expounded in 1960 by Joseph Fuchs, who had succeeded to the mantle of Vermeersch and Hürth as the leading Jesuit authority in Rome on marital morality. Fuchs found the expression of love to be an objective purpose of intercourse as much as procreation was an objective purpose: "Sexual actuation is in itself ordered to the generation of offspring"; it is also "in itself ordered to the intimate expression of love between joined persons of different sexes." At last the neglected thought of St. Thomas that fidelity (*fides*) was an objective end of intercourse was revived, with "love" substituted for fidelity. To have intercourse without love was declared to violate the objective order or purpose of the marital act. Like Häring, Fuchs did not formally abandon the teaching that the good of the offspring was primary. But he added a considerable gloss to the statement of this purpose in documents such as *Casti connubii:* "This love, together with all the consequences of common life, entirely (although not solely or as a mere means) serves and is subordinated to the education of offspring, to whose generation such an act expressive of love is evidently ordered" (*Chastity and the Sexual Order* 2.4.1). The good of the offspring was maintained as primary by pointing to the relation of conjugal love to the education of the children. This love itself was no longer seen "solely or as a mere means" at the service of the child.

The doctrine now seemed solidly established. It was vigorously affirmed in 1963 by Ford and Kelly in their book in the vernacular: "Marital intercourse is immoral when love has ceased," because conjugal acts are properly "expressions of love." They added, "It is hardly stressing sex too much to say that in the ordinary providence of God, the marriage act is one of the chief means by which Christian spouses are to attain God together, just as it is the central act of that state of life to which God has called them."[40]

At Vatican II in 1964 four major addresses by fathers of the Council related the new theory of love to the question of contraception. They spoke on Schema 13, "The Church and the Modern World," drafted by a commission of which Bernard Häring had been the secretary. Cardinal Leger, archbishop of Montreal, said that the schema was too hesitant in affirming the place of conjugal love: "It should clearly present human conjugal love—I stress human love which involves both the soul and the body—as a true end of marriage, as something good in itself, with its own characteristics and laws." The schema should "proclaim the two ends of marriage as equally good and holy. Once that is done, the moral theologians, doctors, psychologists, and other experts can much more easily determine for particular cases the duties both of procreation and of love." Cardinal Alfrink, archbishop of Utrecht, stated that conjugal love was essential both to the motive for procreation and to the education of one's children. This love was "sustained and increased by sexual intercourse." It was endangered if abstinence was the only way of regulating offspring. The Church must examine if "the only efficacious, moral and Christian solution to such conflicts" is continence. Maximos IV, patriarch of Antioch, declared, "The development of personality and its integration into the creative plan of God are all one. Thus, the end of marriage should not be divided into 'primary' and 'secondary.' This consideration opens new perspectives concerning the morality of conjugal behavior considered as a whole." The patriarch added that there was now a "break between the official doctrine of the Church and the contrary practice of the immense majority of Christian couples."[41]

Cardinal Suenens, archbishop of Malines-Brussels, spoke with particular authority. As an auxiliary bishop in 1956 he had already suggested a new approach to the old doctrine on the primary end. The end of generation, he had written, was "objective and inherent in all genital activity." This end could be characterized as "primary" in the sense of "the most important." "On the psychological plane, the immediate end, experienced as first, will be the mutual perfection and complementation of the couple." In this view of intercourse, he had stated, "God's first demand of the act of love is that it be based on love."[42] Now, in the Council, Suenens asked if the Church had maintained "a perfect balance" between "Increase and multiply" and "they will be two in one flesh." These scriptural doctrines must illuminate each other. "This 'two in one' is a mystery of interpersonal communion given grace and sanctified by the sacrament of marriage." Suenens urged that the commission set up by the Pope "tell us whether we have excessively stressed the first end, procreation, at the expense of another equally important end, that is, growth in conjugal unity."

Schema 13 itself, as circulated to the Council Fathers in April 1964, adopted Häring's position that love was linked to procreation. "Such is the nature of conjugal love that matrimony is essentially ordered to the procreation and education of offspring." At the same time it was recognized that "the good of the offspring requires that the spouses truly love each other." In procreation the spouses were not to be "bound by blind instinct" but to act "with full and conscious responsibility." It was further recognized that there might be a serious conflict between responsible procreation and the demands of love. "In particular," the schema recognized "the frequent difficulty of harmonizing the responsibility of not being able, at least for a time, to increase one's offspring, and of the tender cultivation of love; and if love ceases, the spouses often become as strangers to each other, and the good of fidelity is called into question and the good itself of offspring is subverted, either in relation to the education of the existing offspring or in relation to the live and open spirit to be kept toward offspring to be later procreated in less adverse circumstances." The treatment of the schema concluded with a plea to anthropologists, psychologists, sociologists, and experienced and virtuous couples to collaborate with the theologians in seeking "practical solutions for many conflicts" by exploring more profoundly "the complex order given to nature by Providence." In its frank admission of conflicts, in its insistence on inquiry, in its deliberate avoidance of any specific statement on contraception, Schema 13 marked a new era in the history of the church's thought on the subject.[43]

Changes in Discipline

Three modifications or mitigations of the law enforcing the teaching on contraception reflected resistance by some of the faithful. Each change was a reason for re-examination of the theory being enforced. They occurred as to the duty of inquiry, the treatment of cooperation, and the annulment of marriages.

Pius XI had inculcated a duty of inquiry about contraception in the confessional so that confessors would not leave the faithful in good faith practicing contraception. The instruction of the Holy Office in 1943 entitled "Certain Rules for Action by Confessors About the Sixth Commandment" did not withdraw from this position; neither did it reaffirm it. Its studied avoidance of a stand, however, might be read as a retreat. It told confessors not to interrogate about "material sins" (that is, acts committed in good faith) "unless the good of the penitent himself or the averting of the danger of a common evil requires or prompts admonition."[44] Confessors were not told that contraception was such a "common evil."

In 1960 the German Jesuit Joseph Fuchs, teaching at the Gregorian University in Rome, observed that "conjugal onanism" was found almost everywhere, even in "truly Christian homes" (*Chastity* 5.16.1).[45] Yet he suspected that the practice of contraception in good faith was rare. True, "not a few faithful" took the position that "onanism, exercised because of difficulties which are, in some fashion, real," cannot be a serious sin. It was hard to say whether these Catholics were in good faith. However, for the common good, "lest this opinion be spread," their good faith, if it exists, must be destroyed by telling them the true Catholic doctrine (ibid. 5.16.3). Fuchs added that many theologians held that in some regions contraceptive practices might be so prevalent that "all married persons" were to be treated as suspect of committing contraception, unless the confessor had reason to believe to the contrary. In these areas, there was an obligation on the confessor to interrogate those who were silent about the sin (ibid. 5.16.3).

On the other hand, there was still dissent on the meaning of "founded suspicion." John J. Lynch, an American Jesuit teaching at the Jesuit college in Weston, Massachusetts, held that "founded suspicion" did not rest on statistics. Rather, he wrote, "It seems to me that the references of the Sacred Penitentiary to a founded suspicion or prudent doubt in this matter of birth control are not only legitimately, but far more prudently, understood as applying to the individual penitent and not to married people in general."[46] If Lynch's theory was followed, as it probably was by many priests, there was little inquiry about contraceptive practice in the confessional. There was created a situation where contraception might be practiced without challenge to the good faith of the penitent. This possibility was particularly likely to be realized in countries when there had been public debate about the progesterone pill, and many persons might in good faith take the pill to prevent pregnancy.

A second disciplinary change had been realized earlier. The canon law had committed itself to the proposition that any intention to exclude "any essential property of marriage" was a ground of nullity of marriage (canon 1086, above, p. 435). Theoretically, an antecedent intention to avoid procreation even for a period of time was an exclusion of an essential property of marriage. The Rota in 1931 said, "What is said as to the invalidity on account of the exclusion of the right to procreation and education of offspring or to conjugal acts applies equally whether the exclusion happens perpetually or for a time."[47] If this logic were followed, many marriages where the couples intended to avoid offspring for a year or two might be considered void. The Rota was unwilling to come to this conclusion, and, in the same case in which the dictum quoted occurs, it went on, "In practice, however, exclusion of offspring or of the conjugal act for a limited time is regarded as a proposal [*propositum*] of abstaining from the use of the conjugal right or of abusing or violating conjugal obligations, and so is no obstacle to the validity of marriage."[48] In fact, not only has the intention to avoid procreation for a period usually been labeled a mere proposal to violate the conjugal right, but the intention to avoid offspring permanently has also been customarily analyzed as something less than an intention to exclude an "essential property of marriage."[49] One may conclude that, in order to prevent fraud on the court and to favor the stability of marriages, the Rota has refused to annul some marriages which are theologically invalid.[50] Alternatively, one might draw a theological conclusion from the living law of the Rota: the intention to exclude offspring is not necessarily destructive of the essence of marriage.

A third development occurred as to cooperation. The early thirties had been the high point not only of active teaching against contraception, but of an absolute stand against cooperation with instruments. The next thirty years saw questioning and modification of the position. Vermeersch's teaching on the diaphragm was the first to be challenged. In 1936 the Dominican moralist Merkelbach argued that intercourse by the husband when his wife used a diaphragm could not be intrinsically evil: coitus took place, and in pregnancy coitus was lawful although the passage to the uterus was closed. Hence, cooperation by the husband in his wife's sin was lawful for him on the usual grounds permitting material cooperation (*Questions of Chastity and Lechery* 8.2.2). Merkelbach's views received limited Roman support twenty years later in a letter dated April 21, 1955, from the Holy Office to certain unnamed bishops. The letter dealt with the case of a husband "cooperating materially" with a wife using a diaphragm. Material cooperation, the Holy Office warned, could not itself be regarded as lawful as a matter of course. "Ordinaries shall not permit the faithful to be told or taught that no serious objection may be made [to it] according to the principles of Christian law."[51] Yet the very description of the act as "material cooperation" accepted Merkelbach's contention that formal participation in an evil act was not at issue.

The shift from Vermeersch on cooperation with a diaphragm can be explained in terms of lines drawn centuries ago between inability to ejaculate semen and inability to impregnate. The doubts and difficulties experienced over implementing the rules on cooperation by a wife with a husband using a condom pointed to more fundamental weaknesses of theory. Almost all moral theologians who wrote on the subject felt bound to maintain the analogy with rape. Resistance by the wife was required unless it was impossible "without very grave physical consequences to her here and now."[52] Yet the communication of this apparently logical but strangely harsh rule was difficult. It was noted by an English priest that the analogy with rape "was not intended to be used as a direct pastoral admonition to the wife."[53] In this view the analogy was merely a technical device for bringing out the principles involved. But if theologians needed a dramatic illustration to understand that something terribly serious was involved in cooperation, how could housewives get the principle without the illustration? It seems entirely probable that in practice most confessors felt that it went beyond the bounds of prudential decency even to inquire about the resistance to cooperation offered.

The emotional difficulty in enforcing the principle caused doubt about the principle itself among those who were not professional moral theologians. A London priest, Wilfred Stibbs, probably spoke for many when he wrote, in the course of a running discussion in *The Clergy Review*, "One cannot but feel that anyone, even when dealing formally with the *finis operis* of the act of intercourse, who seriously equates a loving wife with a virgin in danger of rape, is out of touch with real people and real human problems."[54]

In 1956 a questioning of the casuistic on cooperation was suggested by Suenens. He noted that a survey of a "large number" of wives who were practicing Catholics had found that they considered "repugnant" the "moral distinction" permitting their cooperation in coitus interruptus. He added, "They are the more offended by this oral 'dualism' because the passivity in question implies a minimum of active cooperation. They know they are not sinning mortally, but they are unanimous in saying that the solution seems to be spiritual mediocrity." Suenens suggested that the theologians reexamine the whole question of cooperation. As a guide to such reconsideration, he quoted with approval the statement of one spouse: "I accuse us of my partner's sin, and we must do all we can together to leave it behind us."[55]

At first glance, the thrust of Suenens' remarks would seem to favor a more stringent rule on cooperation. But was he not, in effect, pointing to the lack of realism in the existing rule? The distinctions drawn to permit cooperation by one spouse in the contraceptive act of the other were of an abstract kind which seemed to ignore the psychological realities of the situation, and to define as "passivity" what most people would call "activity." The teaching, moreover, was of a character so repugnant to the emotions of ordinary married couples that it was evident that many priests felt unable to communicate it. The practical difficulty of making reasonable distinctions, the practical difficulty of communicating the doctrine, raised the possibility that there was some defect in the analysis which made everything turn on whether or not in a given sexual act ejaculation was completed within the vagina. The narrow focus on this aspect of conjugal relations seemed to distort the more fundamental question of love between the spouses.

Controversy

The April 1964 draft of Schema 13 of Vatican II not only avoided any direct condemnation of contraception; it also said that the number of children to have was the decision of each couple, to be made not by blind instinct, but "with full and conscious responsibility." In an Appendix, circulated with the draft of the schema, some issues were amplified or explained without seeking to put conciliar authority behind the proposals. Under the heading "Fecundity of Matrimony" it was observed, "And if according to the ordination of nature not each and every conjugal act is directly destined to lead to procreation, yet the character and expression of this act and the mind of the spouses ought to be such that the generous disposition to procreate and educate children is favored." This language was only another way of saying that love between the spouses had a link to procreation. The Appendix went on to say that the Council warned all men of good will: "Every deliberate intervention of men which vitiates the work proper to the conjugal act of the person is contrary to divine law and the order of matrimony; nor can such a way of acting be consonant with the integrity of conjugal love." Here was an explicit but very carefully qualified condemnation of some forms of contraception. What were condemned were means affecting "the act of the person," that is, coitus interruptus and the condom. It was not clear whether pessaries, douches, diaphragms, or pills were included in these words. A proposed footnote referred to methods "falsifying the conjugal act itself, which *Casti connubii* had in contemplation, to wit, deliberate interruption of copulation, the condom, and so forth"; the footnote added that no judgment was given as to the use of progesterones. The entire footnote was struck from later versions of the text.[56]

The draft of Schema 13, with its emphasis on love in marriage, and its clear but qualified condemnation of contraceptives put in a subordinate document, suggested that development of doctrine was about to receive conciliar approval. The suggestion created tension. New stages have rarely been reached in the life of a doctrine without partisans of the old position insisting that the ancient letter be preserved, while partisans of the new point to a spirit whose law is organic growth. The commitment of the papacy, hierarchy, and theologians to a condemnation of contraception made the crisis particularly acute. The momentum of the great campaign which had been climaxed with *Casti connubii* had carried over into the allocutions of Pius XII. John XXIII, in *Mater et magistra,* issued May 15, 1961, had included a rejection of the solution of the population problems of underdeveloped countries by measures "by which, in addition to violation of the discipline of morals determined by God, there is violation of the procreation of human life itself." He described these measures as "means and plans [*rationes*] which are alien to the dignity of man; which those are not ashamed to advocate who think man himself and his life can entirely be reduced to matter" (*AAS* 53:446–447). The Pope's words, to be sure, did not have the same juridical cast as *Casti connubii,* and the methods he condemned were unspecified; but, taking account of the pastoral, paternal style in which John XXIII couched his strongest rebukes and bearing in mind the background of the theological description of contraceptive methods, it would be a feat of reinterpretation to say that at least some forms of contraception were not in his mind. The present Pope, Paul VI, when Prosecretary for Ordinary Affairs in the Secretariat of State under Pius XII, had also written strongly against "the diffusion of Neo-Malthusian practices which violate the divine laws presiding at the transmission of life."[57]

Not only the papacy but several national hierarchies had also taken strong stands in the late 1950's and early 1960's when the population problem was already altering the context of the question. In November 1957, the bishops of India, gathered at Bangalore, solemnly warned the faithful of India against Communism, immoral movies, and contraception: "Family limitation by unnatural means is an offense against natural and divine law. It is against the primary ends of the holy state of matrimony. The deliberate destruction of life in potency is a crime close to murder, as St. Thomas stated in the thirteenth century." After disuse for over a century, a reminiscence of the homicide analysis appeared again. The Indian bishops added to St. Thomas a statement of Mahatma Gandhi in *Harijan,* March 28, 1936, where Gandhi spoke of procreation as the sole end of intercourse. The bishops closed with an evocation of "the traditions of our country and the sacred character of family life."[58]

On March 3, 1961, the Assembly of Cardinals and Archbishops of France issued a statement on contraception. The Church was not "nataliste à tout prix." The primary end of marriage, it reminded the faithful, is "not only the procreation but the education of children." Responsible regulation of birth was lawful and desirable. But man is forbidden "to violate the natural order established by God, who is the sole Master of human lives." "That is why it is necessary to reject every manipulation which, by contraceptive procedures or sterilizing products, has the purpose of artifically preventing the coming of children into the world."[59]

In the United States, the hierarchy acted after the President's Committee to Study the U.S. Military Assistance Program (the Draper Committee) had issued a report on July 13, 1959, recommending cooperation with underdeveloped countries in "plans designed to deal with the problem of rapid population growth." This vague statement caused much speculation that the United States government would aid birth control programs abroad.[60] At the annual meeting of the bishops of the United States, November 26, 1959, a strong statement was issued in the name of all the bishops by the five cardinals and cardinals-designate and ten bishops constituting the Administrative Board of the National Catholic Welfare Conference. The bishops stated that the population increase in the underdeveloped countries should be met by international economic measures, not programs of artificial birth control, abortion, or sterilization. They deplored the propagandist use of the term "population explosion." They rebuked persons who had stated that "artificial birth prevention within the married state is gradually becoming acceptable even in the Catholic Church." "This," they said, "is not true." "The Catholic Church has always distinguished artificial birth control, which is a frustration of the conjugal act, from other forms of birth regulation which are morally lawful." The only true solutions were "those which are morally acceptable under the natural law of God."[61]

The statement of the hierarchy of England and Wales on May 7, 1964, quoted the condemnations of contraception of St. Augustine in *Adulterous Marriages,* of Pius XI in *Casti connubii,* of Pius XII in the Address to the Midwives. Contraception, they concluded, "is not an open question, for it is against the law of God."[62]

In the debate in the Council, the statements of Leger, Alfrink, Suenens, and Maximos IV in favor of re-examination of the doctrine drew a strong reaction. Three cardinals, identified with the conservative wing of the curia, and opposed to the liberal majority on issues ranging from methods of biblical exegesis to the collegial constitution of the church to freedom of conscience from coercion by the state, challenged these speakers who, on the other issues too, had been their opponents. Cardinal Browne, an Irishman who had been general of the Dominicans, appealed to classic scholastic theology, to *Arcanum Divinae Sapientiae,* to *Casti connubii,* and to the Address to the Midwives. He brought into play an old Thomistic distinction between two kinds of love, the love of friendship (*amor amicitae*) and the love of concupiscence (*amor concupiscentiae*), "concupiscence" being used here in a morally neutral sense. By the love of concupiscence one used another person for one's own good; by the love of friendship one sought the good of another. In the analysis of St. Thomas both forms of love are good, although the love of friendship is higher (*Summa theologica* 1–2.26.41). In Cardinal Browne's application, he suggested that intercourse involved the love of concupiscence, and that this use of one's spouse was destructive of the love of friendship that should develop between man and wife. Cardinal Browne's exercise in the application of a Thomistic text was supported by Cardinal Alfred Ottaviani, the head (under the Pope) of the Holy Office. Speaking now, as he said, as the eleventh of twelve children, he declared, forthrightly, "The freedom granted by the schema to married couples to determine for themselves the number of their children cannot possibly be approved." He expressed his amazement at hearing doubt expressed about whether until now a correct stand had been taken on the principles governing marriage. He asked if the inerrancy of the Church was being called into question. Cardinal Ottaviani was followed by Cardinal Ernest Ruffini, archbishop of Palermo. He noted critically the passages in the schema leaving the number of offspring to the judgment of the parents. He then quoted, not by name, *Aliquando,* the famous text on contraception in Augustine's *Marriage and Concupiscence,* which had been the canon of Gratian, the locus classicus of Peter Lombard, the law of the Church from 1150 to 1917, the inspiration of *Effraenatam.* Once more the words "Sometimes lustful cruelty or cruel lust" were employed to describe the motives for contraception, and the ancient formula rang in the basilica of St. Peter and in the councils of the Church.[63]

Battle had been joined. Popes, cardinals, and bishops had, from 1951 to 1964, reaffirmed that contraception was against God's law; they had pointed to no exceptions. Some of the leading fathers of the Council had asked for re-examination. No Catholic writer before 1963 had asserted that the general prohibition of contraception was wrong. In late 1963 and in 1964, however, in addition to the writers favoring the direct use of the progesterone pills, in addition to Bishop Reuss's defense of sterilization, there appeared Catholic writers challenging the doctrine itself. Of these the most prominent was Thomas D. Roberts, a leading English Jesuit, who, as former archbishop of Bombay, was free of the censorship of his order and now acted as a gadfly in the Church. In his article in *Search,* which alarmed the English hierarchy, Roberts said that he was constrained by the authority of the Church, but that he could not see any rational argument against contraception. In the fall of 1964, Archbishop Roberts introduced a collection of essays, *Contraception and Holiness,* and declared, "on the grounds of reason alone, one can conceive of many cases in which a husband and wife might, after having examined their consciences, decide that contraception was the only means for preserving the health of one or the other spouse, or for preserving the marriage itself. If that is so, then, with the most spiritual of motives such a husband and wife might be convinced that contraception was necessary for the growth in holiness which is the aim of the sacrament of matrimony."[64] Finding no reason for the Church's absolute prohibition, Roberts asked the Church to clarify and reconsider its position.

The possibility and rationality of a less than absolute prohibition were urged by the other contributors to *Contraception and Holiness*: E.R. Baltazar, assistant professor of philosophy at the University of Dayton; Gregory Baum, an Augustinian of St. Michael's College at the University of Toronto; Kieran Conley, a Benedictine professor of dogmatic theology at St. Meinrad's Seminary, Indiana; Wlliam V. D'Antonio, associate professor of sociology at the University of Notre Dame; Elizabeth A. Daugherty a zoologist; Leslie Dewart, associate professor of philosophy at St. Michael's College at the University of Toronto; Justus George Lawler, professor of humanities, St. Xavier College, Chicago; Julian Pleasants, research associate in the Lobund Laboratory, University of Notre Dame; Rosemary Reuther, a teacher of classics at Scripps College, California. In another book appearing in the fall of 1964, *Contraception and Catholics*, Louis Dupré, a layman who was associate professor of theology at Georgetown University, also criticized the existing arguments for an absolute prohibition.[65] In a third work of the same date, *What Modern Catholics Think About Birth Control*, entirely written by married laymen, the existing rule was upheld by Vernon Bourke, professor of philosophy at St. Louis University, but criticized by William Birmingham, an editor of *Cross Currents*, Mary Louise Birmingham, an editor of a publishing house, Sydney Cornelia Callahan, a writer, Eugene Fontinell, an editor of *Cross Currents* and teacher at Queens College, New York, James Finn, editor of *Worldview*, Michael Novak, author of *The Open Church*, and Sally Sullivan, a writer. Daniel Sullivan, a student at the Institut Catholique, outlined the development of Catholic thinking on the subject; Frederick E. Flynn, professor of philosophy at the College of St. Thomas, Minnesota, showed how the natural law was capable of development.[66] A fourth book, *The Experience of Marriage*, edited by Michael Novak, was composed of statements by thirteen anonymous Catholic couples, American and mostly engaged in intellectual work; the book was a compelling presentation of injury and strain in the marital relation by the attempt to regulate birth by the use of rhythm.[67] The devotion of these writers to the Church was evident. They wrote not as enemies or as rebels, but as witnesses. Only one couple in *The Experience of Marriage*, only two contributors to *What Modern Catholics Think About Birth Control*, used contraceptive methods which had been condemned; these asserted respectfully their free right to obey their consciences when it seemed wrong to have more children, wrong to abstain from intercourse altogether, and impracticable to use rhythm. While some attention was given to population pressures, the main thrust of the critics of the absolute rule was to justify in theory what these two couples had done in practice. As the good of parents and of existing children demanded both family planning and sexual intercourse, and as rhythm was unreliable and destructive of the free expression of love, the critics urged the Church not to condemn all forms of contraception.

The success of the critics' pleas for revision depended, at least in part, on the strength of the rational arguments supporting an absolute prohibition. Rational arguments in moral matters are, perhaps, never absolutely decisive. Too many intuitions, too many sentiments, escape articulation. It is possible to be wise without arguments to justify one's wisdom. Yet arguments are the usual means for examining doctrinal position, and, if only as indices, they point to the health of a teaching. Of the arguments against all contraception, Dupré quoted La Fontaine's words on the animals in the plague, "They did not all die, but they were all struck." The arguments had been affected by the changes in environment. They had undergone some criticism by the theologians. They were now subjected to direct attack by the advocates of modification.

The arguments purported to show that contraception was injurious to society, family, and self, and against the will of God. Did they still hold?

Injury to Particular Populations and to the Human Race

The argument that contraception injured society had a double aspect. Sometimes it was viewed as endangering particular groups, sometimes the race as a whole. In the declarations of the German hierarchy in 1913 and the French hierarchy in 1914 the notion appeared that it was good to procreate citizens for the state; the standard was a nationalistic one. Similarly, depopulation of a particular nation appeared to be the evil evoked by Belgian theologians like De Smet and Merkelbach, and by an American like Ryan, who pointed to the French example.[68] What weakens the national state was, in these presentations, assumed to be evil. This assumption was least likely to be challenged between 1870 and 1940. Thereafter, in a world increasingly conscious of its unity, a yardstick based on the nation, although not wholly abandoned, did not have much status as a moral guide.

An interesting variant of this argument, substituting the Church for the state, was doubtless often enough in the back of some ultraclerical minds. The position was that contraception would deprive society of a fair share of Catholics, or, put more imperially, that the Church might grow if Catholics controlled their procreative activities less than other people. The traditional doctrine that the purpose of marital intercourse is the generation and *religious* education of offspring could be given this emphasis; and such emphasis does occur in *Casti connubii*, with its language on procreation as a way of making "the people of God increase day by day." Similarly, the argument seemed to Ryan a reason to restrict the use of rhythm: "A large proportion of Catholic couples would be under specific and particular obligation to discard the practice of periodical abstinence so far as would be necessary to maintain at least the previously existing proportion between Catholics and non-Catholics."[69]

As nationalism declined, so also did competition of this kind among the churches; and within religiously divided areas like Canada and the Netherlands, ecumenicism softened competitive anxieties. It was doubtful if a respectable moral theologian could have been found in 1964 to maintain that contraception was forbidden to Catholics because they had a duty to increase their numbers by births in order to best other religions or irreligious groups.

A mutation of these arguments was based on the observation that in a typical underdeveloped country contraception was more often practiced by the urban elite than by the least educated. The practice thereby effected a disproportionate reduction in offspring of the leading elements in a society.[70] This argument, however, might be read as merely suggesting the need to intensify propaganda for contraception among the uneducated. At most, it showed that contraception practiced without a sense of social responsibility might harm a particular nation.

The argument directed to the social evil of depopulation was given a more metaphysical attire by some writers. Arthur Vermeersch argued in 1919 that the person practicing contraception violated the subordination of his act to the species: "The human race, as it is a moral person, provides for its perpetuity by conjugal copulation. The onanists positively exclude this perpetuity by the manner in which they couple" (*Chastity and the Contrary Vices*, no. 258). Here each act of contraception was treated as an act against the species. In 1946 the same argument appeared in Iorio's revision of Gury: the contraceptive act "tends *per se* to the extinction of society" (*Moral Theology*, no. 1206). A Kantian variant of the argument was chosen by Creusen: if contraception became "a general principle" of action—that is, if everyone practiced it—the human race would be destroyed.[71]

This metaphysical form of the argument was criticized by Herbert McCabe, an English Dominican, in 1964. What the race required was "a whole complex of acts which go to make possible the birth and survival of a child." Not every sexual act in this complex had to be generative. Using an analogy which only an English writer would invoke, he compared the complex of required acts to the complex of acts necessary to score in a game. Not every single act had to tend toward the goal: the player may be "occasionally making a move which is the opposite of the crucial one—making a move which if invariably employed would make success impossible."[72] *On recule pour mieux sauter,* both in games and in the preservation of the race, was McCabe's suggestion.

A difficulty in the older theology which had indirectly lent plausibility to the "race suicide" argument was removed by a theological development. The old theory, in its anxiety to preserve the lawfulness of virginal marriages, had recognized no obligation in marriage to procreate. A marriage was lawful and valid in which intercourse, and consequently procreation, were abstained from. "The Anglicans assuredly err," taught Vermeersch in 1934, when they say there is a duty for married persons to have children: "The multiplication of the human race is sufficiently provided for so that no precept is given that it be undertaken."[73] In this traditional analysis, the obligation to procreate attached to the exercise of the marital act, not to the entrance into matrimony. It might have seemed, if this analysis were pursued, that to eliminate the absolute obligation not to render particular acts of intercourse infertile would mean that married couples would be morally free to have intercourse without ever having children, and in the long run the preservation of the race would be threatened.

The same child-avoiding result was also possible, in the old analysis, merely by the use of rhythm. To reach a more acceptable conclusion, some theologians in the 1940's, led by Gerald Kelly, found an affirmative obligation for married persons engaging in intercourse to have some children.[74] This tentative theory was accepted by Pius XII in his discussion of the sterile period in the Address to Midwives:

> On partners who make use of matrimony by the specific act of their state, nature and the Creator impose the function of providing for the continuance of the human race. This is the characteristic debt [*prestazione*] from which their state of life derives its peculiar value, the *bonum prolis*. The individual and society, the people and the state, the Church itself, depend for their existence, in the order established by God, on fertile marriage. Consequently, to embrace the state of matrimony, to use continually the faculty proper to it, and allowed in it alone, and on the other hand to withdraw always and deliberately, without a grave motive, from its primary duty, would be to sin against the very meaning of conjugal life. (*AAS* 43:845–846)

Some questions concerning the extent of the duty to procreate were left open; Kelly and Ford, for example, found a limit to the duty in the population needs of a time and country: "a family of three children would sufficiently provide for the needs of the United States." But while analysis remained to be done, the theologians followed the papal lead, and the new position seemed accepted.[75] It provided a moral basis for opposing contraceptive practice which made a couple completely childless. The indirect result was to put less weight on the argument that every act of intercourse must be immune from human interference if the race was to survive.

Arguably, society still might be endangered by the attitudes bred of contraception. The old fear that if there were approval of contraception there would be approval of other forms of nonprocreative sexual activity was voiced in 1960 by Stanislas de Lestapis. He asked, as a rhetorical question, "If in fact erotic activity between two persons has a complete meaning in itself, if its purpose is purely psychological in the service of the couple, if the reference to the work of the flesh is only incidental, why should we wish at all costs to limit mutual erotic activity to heterosexuality?"[76] This question had already been answered by theologians like Fuchs and Häring who had refused to treat "erotic activity" and "conjugal love" as identical. It was also answered by the new critics like Michael Novak, who defined lawful intercourse as "that act of two persons which physically symbolizes the permanent union of their mutual good will, and which, when the biological imperative so commands, is apt for the generation of children."[77] The new answers were, in fact, more satisfactory than the old position, which could never explain why the fornication of the sterile was wrong or why the intercourse of the pregnant was right.

The heart of the "race suicide" argument was removed by the demographic changes since 1850. Vermeersch and Creusen had come from Belgium; the popes had come from Italy. Yet none of these inhabitants of densely populated areas had remarked that a high density of population in relation to economic resources might threaten society or race as much as avoidance of procreation. Indeed, the Belgian bishops in their 1909 Instructions told priests to combat contraception by blessing large families.[78] Pius XII, on January 20, 1958, told the Association of Large Families, an Italian society, that large families were "those most blessed by God and specially loved and prized by the Church as its most precious treasures" (*AAS* 50:90). In the 1960's, however, the impact of population growth was evident in the theological discussion. Joseph Fuchs rejected Creusen's contention that "if everyone practiced it, the human race would be destroyed." The argument failed to show why, under particular circumstances, particular acts of contraception were not permissible. Moreover, he said drily, that the existence of the race would be threatened if every sexual act was not per se generative "could be doubted" (Fuchs, *Chastity and the Sexual Order* 5.2). In the United States, at the annual meeting of the Catholic Theological Society in 1963, Gerald Kelly dismissed the race suicide argument as obsolete.[79]

A different kind of argument from social consequences was provided by the statistics on abortion. It was alleged that dissemination of contraceptive methods with official sanction brought about a "contraceptive state of mind": parents who did not want a child, who therefore practiced contraception, and who failed in their effort at avoidance, were often led to resort to abortion. In England, for example, the Royal Commission on Population noted that in 1949 the proportion of procured abortions was 8.7 times as high among couples who habitually practiced contraception as among the others. In Sweden, after contraception had been fully sanctioned by law, legal abortions increased from 703 in 1943 to 6,328 in 1951.[80] In Switzerland, where contraception was almost unrestricted, abortions by 1955 were alleged to equal or outnumber live births.[81] In Hungary, a Communist country with a Catholic tradition of eight hundred years, legal abortions rose from 1,600 in 1949 to 163,700 in 1962; in 1962 legal abortions, at the rate of 16.3 per thousand, exceeded the birth rate of 12.9 per thousand. In Poland, a country with a large Catholic population, legal abortions rose from 1,400 in 1955 to 140,400 in 1962. Japan was the chief example. Under the influence of the United States army of occupation, the Japanese Diet passed the Eugenic Protection Law in 1948. Overtly eugenic in purpose, its actual intent was to control the population. It permitted legal abortions for reasons of health, and it set up Eugenic Protection Consultation Offices, to be run in conjunction with governmental health centers or private associations, to furnish contraceptive advice and train midwives and nurses in the methods of contraception. From 1948 to 1955, contraception, already known and practiced to some extent by the more educated Japanese, spread rapidly through urban Japan and with some difficulty in rural Japan. But much more dramatic was the rise in abortions. The law was amended in 1949 to permit legal abortion if the mother's health was endangered "for economic reasons," and by a 1952 amendment a requirement that the operating physician first consult an official medical committee was eliminated. Legal abortions rose as follows: 1949—246,104; 1950—489,119; 1951—638,350; 1952—798,193; 1953—1,068,066; 1954—1,143,059; 1955—1,170,143. The numbers were a minimum, because legal abortion required the disclosure of income, which could be used for tax purposes; it was consequently estimated that the actual number of abortions might be twice that reported. The number of abortions was higher in the higher income groups, and the total number increased as Japan experienced economic prosperity.[82]

It was, of course, impossible to conclude from the case of Japan that "a contraceptive mentality" led to abortion on a mass scale. What would have happened if abortion had received no official encouragement could not be determined. The figures did show that availability of contraceptive means was not necessarily a substitute for abortion.[83] Beyond that, they suggested on a grand scale what the Hungarian, Swiss, and Polish statistics suggested on a smaller scale: it was dangerous to create the idea that offspring were to be avoided. Japan could be written off as a "pagan civilization"; Switzerland was more difficult to explain. The statistics suggested that the evil dreaded in the Roman Empire had still to be feared in the modern world: the greatest threat to the life of a human being was his own parents. In the presence of this evil, any revision of the universal and absolute prohibition of contraception had to take into account the degree to which it might be a necessary outer protection to fetal human life.

Injury to the Family

Children in a small family grow up spoiled, selfish, effete. This result is true especially of the child who is an only child, but to a lesser degree of children in families with two or three children. Considerations of this kind were advanced in the nineteenth century by Michael Rosset. They were given a homely American presentation in the twentieth century by John A. Ryan. Their authors did not attempt to establish their observations by any statistical survey of small families. Ryan anticipated the obvious rejoinder, What of families who were small because the couple practiced sexual continence? His answer was that in these families the discipline and self-control of the parents was exemplary and counter-balanced the lack of many children.[84]

This kind of guessing, unsupported by systematic empirical inquiry, was never indulged in by the major theologians. The flimsiness of a case for an absolute prohibition of contraception built on this ground was evident. By 1964 the argument was no longer used.

Some writers urged that contraception was a factor leading to divorce. They cited statistics showing dissolution of a higher number of marriages with one child or none than with two or more children.[85] This argument suffered from several defects. It was not established how often the sterility of the divorced was due to natural causes and the divorce sought because of the sterility. It was not clear whether, in a country like France where the women were more often practicing Catholics than the men, the refusal of the women to practice contraception did not result in contention, making divorce more probable. It was not shown to be more likely that the absence of children was the reason for the divorce than that other causes producing tension in the family had led to the avoidance of children. Moreover, divorce allowed less time for a family to have children.

A third argument, advanced by Anthony Zimmerman, an American priest of the Society of the Divine Word, asserted that contraception injured the family by increasing the number of sins of extramarital intercourse.[86] Like the other two arguments, this one suffered from a lack of supporting evidence. It was also unconvincing unless comparative statistics were obtainable on the extramarital sins committed in a society where contraception was not practiced but the birth rate was kept low by late marriages. Such statistics—short of an Irish Kinsey report—were not likely to be obtained.

More specific injury to the family was claimed by many writers who found contraception to inflict an injury on a spouse. One argument invoked medical testimony to show that contraception inflicted injuries on the health of the wife. Coitus interruptus was said to cause nervous difficulties and pelvic disorders; other contraceptives were vaguely connected with uterine cancer. This kind of argument was never used by the leading theologians, but it does appear in writers such as Rosset and Roelandts.[87] As late as 1930, Richard de Guchteneere, a Belgian doctor, devoted an entire chapter of his *Judgment on Birth Control* to reports of medical injury.[88] In the light of the acceptance of contraception by the medical profession in most countries, the theological concern on grounds of health seemed misplaced, and this line of attack was largely abandoned.

More subtle psychological damage to a spouse was argued by many theologians. Characteristically they assumed that the injured spouse was the wife, and that the contraceptive act was performed against her will. Thus John A. Ryan restated the ancient Augustinian contention in mild American terms: contraception involved a "loss of reverence" for one's spouse.[89] In 1954 Bernard Häring quoted Augustine himself: in the contraceptive act a wife was treated as a harlot. In such an act, Häring added, a wife "was not loved as a companion for salvation, but rather sought as an instrument for the release of passion" (*Das Gesetz Christi* 2–2.4.3.6.7. [5th ed., p. 1093]).

The old Augustinian approach, as indeed was evinced by Häring's acceptance of it, was strikingly close to the position taken by the Catholic personalists. Von Hildebrand had indirectly touched on this point when he declared that the act of married intercourse was "perfect self-surrender and self-revelation"; any other use was a "desecration of the other person."[90]

The most influential of all the writers of the new school, Herbert Doms, wrote in 1935:

> Every artificial alteration of the normal biological act, which ends in making impossible the biological end of generation inscribed in the form of the sexual organs and processes, constitutes a falsification of an act which is profoundly mysterious and extremely complex, an act which carries with it the mutual abandonment of the persons and the consequences of this abandonment . . . If a person mutilates the biological process anatomically or physiologically, before, during, or after the act, he gives himself only with an arbitrary reservation, which is contrary to the immutable meaning of the sexual act and the most profound intention of conjugal love.[91]

In this exposition by Doms, the focus was not on "the desecration of the other person," but on the destruction of love. A closely related contention was made by Suenens: "Contraception is an essential denial of conjugal communion, which it secretly disintegrates and turns into self-seeking."[92]

Another variant of this approach was developed in an essay written in 1961 by an American Jesuit, Paul Quay. Coitus, he argued, is a natural, not conventional, symbol of love. As a "natural symbol," the structure of the coital act cannot be altered without violence to the truth. When contraception is practiced, the communication which coitus should be is distorted; coitus becomes "lying," in the sense of telling an untruth. The partners "take that which says perfect union and corrupt it till it can express only mutual pleasure."[93]

Contraception was thus variously characterized as selfish, as an exploitation of the spouse, as a denial of love, as a destruction of the natural meaning of coitus. The characterizations may be distinguished in the consequences they focused on and the perspectives from which they were made. They shared a common ground: from Augustine to Suenens the essential contention was that contraceptive intercourse violated love. To reject this line of argument as did André Snoeck, with the statement that "the moralists have considered this value as important only in the last twenty-five years,"[94] was to fail to perceive the identity of principle in the development of doctrine.

The various forms of the contention that contraception violated love did, however, share one weakness. It was not evident who was injured. In an approach like Häring's, a psychological aspect seemed to predominate: the wife, it was implied, was humiliated. In Suenens the emphasis was an injury to the husband himself: he became "self-seeking." Yet no demonstration was attempted of why the wife was injured if she consented, or why the husband was self-seeking if he had good reason to avoid more offspring. Neither writer showed why intercourse which was intentionally rendered sterile was more degrading or selfish than intercourse which was naturally sterile. In an approach like Doms's or Quay's an ontological injury was alleged; the entitative completion of the act, or its structure, was said to be denied. This contention was puzzling. In terms of the usual Christian approach, an act was a sin only if it hurt oneself, one's neighbor, or God. If the arguments centered on love were to hold, either injury to oneself or one's neighbor, or violation of some order directly identified with the will of God, had to be shown. The alleged ontological injury seemed to be no injury to self or neighbor. If injury there was, it was offense to the will of God, and the argument resolved itself into the contention, soon to be examined, that coitus was sacral.

The experimental basis of the arguments appealing to love was also open to question. They appeared to assume that the only lawful intercourse was that in which the person gave himself totally. Michael Novak commented on this assumption: terms such as "'total surrender' or 'total self-donation' are not the language of ordinary human life. We learn to love only gradually. Perfect love is not attained so easily as the invocation of the simple criterion of the nonuse of contraceptives seems to imply. The language of 'total surrender' concludes to a sense of moral superiority that perhaps has not been earned. Some who use contraceptives may love one another more than some who do not."[95] Somewhat similarly, Louis Dupré observed that no single act could express the gift of self in marriage; the gift was necessarily made in a repetition of acts over a period; there could be no "total" expression in a single act of intercourse, and hence there was no contradiction of a total expresion of love if contraception were occasionally practiced.[96]

Another argument analyzable in terms of injury to the family was the Augustinian statement that contraception violated the purposes of marriage. The statement was retained in the later editions of Gury, and was invoked by such a writer as Rosset (*Marriage,* V, no. 3333). It was used in the 1909 Instructions of the Belgian bishops. *Casti connubii* affirmed, "First place among the goods of marriage is held by offspring"; and the Pope quoted from St. Augustine on Genesis (*AAS* 22:543).

Again, the question was presented, Who was injured by violation of the primary purpose: self, neighbor, or God? If neither injury to self nor to neighbor appeared, the argument, to be successful, had to assert that in the institution of marriage God had set up an order inviolable even when violation would injure no man. Moreover, it was not evident how the primary purpose of marriage became the necessary purpose of every marital act. Once it was admitted that no procreative purpose was required for lawful coitus, it became extremely difficult to find in the primary purpose doctrine any absolute barrier to contraception. At most the doctrine created a state of mind in which contraception was regarded as undesirable; no complete prohibition was established, and, as an argument against contraception, the primary purpose rule was invoked with increasing rarity.

Injury to Self

The Christian tradition of asceticism is strong: "If anyone wishes to come after me, let him deny himself and take up his cross, and follow me" (Mark 8:34; cf. Matthew 10:38, 16:24; Luke 14:27).

In describing the contribution of different factors in shaping the doctrine on contraception, I have alluded to this tradition only as it was embodied in the exaltation of virginity. Now Christian asceticism was brought into more direct relationship with the prohibition of contraception. Contraception was opposed because of the materialistic, unascetic reasons often adduced for practicing it. Remind the faithful, said the Belgian bishops in 1909, that Christian life is "a way to the fatherland," that is, to the Christian fatherland which is heaven. Contraception, said the German bishops in 1913, is "the consequence of luxury."[97] The run-of-the-mill theologians sounded the same note. Materialism was at the root of the desire to practice contraception, wrote Bishop Rosset in 1898. "The impelling principle" of contraception is "dislike of sacrifice," said John A. Ryan in 1915.[98]

To the person not holding Christian convictions this appeal to sacrifice, asceticism, and the cross was foolishness. Even for the Christian it was difficult to see that failure to practice self-sacrifice, either through continence or through raising a large family, necessarily constituted a mortal sin. If the Christian was *homo viator,* a wayfarer in "a vale of tears," carrying his cross, it was not established that refraining from contraception was the particular cross inflicted on every married Christian under pain of serious sin. The refusal to sacrifice might be injurious to one's spiritual welfare; but specific sacrifices were not shown to be mandatory. The argument based on Christian asceticism was a counterargument to bourgeois reasons for practicing contraception. It did not attempt, by itself, to show that every act of contraception was a mortal sin.

Injury to Nature

A new and substantial form of the Stoic and Thomistic contentions that contraception was contrary to nature was made in 1964 by Germain G. Grisez, a married layman and associate professor of philosophy at Georgetown University. Grisez postulated in man's rational constitution the prescription, "Procreation is a good which should be pursued." This principle, like the principle, "Life is a good which is to be sought," or "Truth is a good which is to be sought," was a first principle of human action and therefore indemonstrable; it was postulated because demanded by the fact that rational beings did, in fact, procreate. Basic principles of this kind were not rules externally imposed by a superior, nor were they always being implemented. Man was not always engaged in truth-seeking activity; man was not always procreating. But because these principles were part of the radical, rational constitution of man, the goods they set for human action could not be directly attacked by man without his doing violation to his rational nature. To act against truth, to act against life, to act against procreation, was to deny part of man's rational nature.[99]

In distinguishing from the lawful use of rhythm a contraceptive act which attacked the procreative first principle, Grisez was compelled to distinguish between "individual acts" and "policy acts." Individual acts of contraception were always evil; acts setting a policy to practice rhythm might be good.[100] It was not clear, however, why a decision to avoid conception, executed by a series of acts, was less directly opposed to the procreative principle than a decision to perform a discrete contraceptive act. Moreover, in concentrating purely on a philosophical presentation of what his system postulated in the human constitution, Grisez did not focus on the requirement of Christian morality that for an act to be sinful it must be shown to be contrary to charity. In criticizing "situationist" ethics for selecting a "controlling value," which was treated as "an absolute end in itself," Grisez seemed to ignore the implication his criticism had for Christian ethics based on love as the absolute value.[101] At one point, however, he seemed to posit an unconceived entity as the neighbor to whom love was not shown: "The objection that the unconceived child has no actual rights is narrow-minded legalism."[102] But generations of Catholic theologians had taken that position: there are no souls waiting to be born; if a being has not been conceived there is no "unconceived child" to talk about. The current of thought which held contraception to be homicide had been itself a legal, rhetorical way of speaking. To emphasize the protection of life, the prevention of conception had been "interpretively" homicide. But when the canon law was codified in 1917 most rules of substantive morality had been dropped from the code; *Si aliquis* was among the provisions eliminated. Nothing now in the canon law supported, even rhetorically, the notion that the child-to-be-conceived had rights that justice or charity should lead a potential parent to take into account.

It appeared, in fact, in Grisez's analysis, that the person injured by the contraceptive act was the person performing it. But to maintain this analysis Grisez was required to suppose that a conflict could not exist for a parent between procreation and education. His statement of principle, "Procreation is a good which should be pursued," omitted one element which Christian moralists had traditionally insisted on: procreation and education had always been linked as the good of Christian intercourse. By omitting the educational element Grisez's analysis suppressed the tension built into the traditional statement. If man were not free to ignore the basic postulate which Grisez's analysis attributed to him, it had to be because God himself would be offended by the departure from His order. Offense against nature, then, became analyzable as offense to God.

Offense to God

Some theologians, assuming that contraception was evil, argued against its practice because of the punishments that would overtake its perpetrators. They seem to have believed that they had found a punishment peculiarly suited to the crime and that God would back them up: the perpetrators would be punished by the premature death of their children. The contentio was made by Bishop Rosset and by Adam Tanquerey, the Sulpician author of a manual for seminaries. It was recommended by the Belgian Roelandts as a threat to be used by confessors, and Tanquerey was cited with approval by Merkelbach as late as 1944.[103] Most strikingly of all, the threat was endorsed by the Belgian bishops in their 1909 instructions to confessors. The somewhat similar approach of Ferreres, predicting other evils for the children of those who practice contraception, was cited with approval by Thomas Iorio as recently as 1946 (*Moral Theology*, no. 1221).

Most reputable theologians have never engaged in these efforts to anticipate divine justice. I should suppose that almost eveyone today who read them would feel keenly the cruelty of these arguments *ad terrorem* and be struck by the absurdity of men assuming that they were privy to the judgments of God. But I can imagine one pressing further: Is it essentially different for the theologians to proclaim that they know God's will as to the purpose of coitus? Is not there here an equally farfetched claim to be the spokesman for God, and is not the result as arbitrary and cruel as the more primitive case of the preaching *ad terrorem*? For one who did not share the convictions of Catholics as to the authority of the Church, there would be no answer to the claim that here man presumed to know what God wanted. A Catholic, however, might discriminate between the first case of men playing God, and the second case, where he believed the Church indeed spoke with divine authority. Nor would the assertion of such authority be either arbitrary or cruel if it was necessary in a given environment to safeguard human life and protect the holiness of marriage. The question would remain, How does the Church know it is God's will? It makes no claim to a "pipeline to God," no claim to a crude infusion of knowledge. What it has, it has from a revelation which closed with the Apostles.

That contraception was a direct offense to God might, theoretically, be proved by a text of Scripture saying so. This was the way, in fact, that many Catholic exegetes in all ages had read

Genesis 38:8–10. It continued to be the reading of late-nineteenth-century writers such as Rosset and the revisers of Gury. Two of the leading theologians of the mid-twentieth century followed this ancient path. Häring, in 1954, cited Genesis 38 to condemn contraception and described Onan's act as constituting sacrilege, a sin against the Creator, and a display of lack of love for his wife. Hürth, in 1955, asserted that Onan was punished for his contraceptive act.[104] The most authoritative interpretation of Genesis 38 was given by Pius XI in *Casti connubii:* "It is, therefore, not remarkable that Holy Writ itself testifies that the Divine Majesty pursued this wicked crime with detestation and punished it with death, as St. Augustine recalls" (*AAS* 22:559).

The argument from Genesis was not used by a good many theologians, including St. Jerome, St. Thomas, St. Albert, St. Alphonsus. It was not used by all twentieth-century theologians. The term "onanism" was itself not an exegesis; it was merely the conventional term for the sin of contraception. The difference of exegetical opinion was clear in the early twentieth century. De Smet wrote, "From the text and context it seems that the criticism of the sacred author is less directly and formally attached to the spilling of the seed than to the frustration of the levirate law which Onan intended to achieve" (*Les Fiançailles et le mariage* 2.1.3.1.1, annex 2, n.5). It seems unlikely that *Casti connubii* intended to resolve definitively a point of exegesis where there was respectable exegetical authority on both sides. The interpretation given by Pius XI was by quotation of Augustine, not by independent papal determination.

In 1953 André Snoeck, professor of theology at the Jesuit scholasticate at Louvain, rejected the controlling force of Genesis. The sin of Onan "obviously consisted in the fact that he did not observe the levirate law."[105] The argument was dismissed with similar brusqueness on the same grounds by Louis Janssens in 1963.[106] More cautiously, Joseph Fuchs said in 1960 that many modern exegetes "understand Onan to have been condemned only for his failure to observe the Mosaic law" (*Chastity and the Sexual Order* 2.6.2.2). Fuchs did not endorse these opinions; neither did he reject them. In the present state of exegetical opinion, it would not seem that the argument based on Genesis is heavily relied on to sustain the condemnation of all contraception.

That an act offends God, though not man, might be proved by reason alone. An unspoken blasphemous thought is at least one case of an act offensive to God, although arguably doing harm to no man. Analogously, desecration of the Eucharist would be principally an offense against God and demonstrably so by reason, once the premise of Catholic faith was accepted that the Eucharist contained the Body and Blood of Christ. Was contraception an act which reason alone or reason in conjunction with the premises of faith showed to be offensive to God?

A medieval line of thought had stressed the value of procreation as a way of replenishing heaven, which had lost the fallen angels. A more modern form of this thought contended that God was given glory by the multiplication of men. Thus in 1933 John A. Ryan commented on the command of Genesis to increase and multiply: "And the purpose of this injunction was not merely that the earth should be populated but that God should be increasingly glorified both on earth and in heaven."[107] If this view were taken literally, it would be an offense to God to limit the number of beings glorifying Him. The trouble with this contention was that it proved too much: if glory was given by the multiplication of men, then the value of virginity and the condemnation of extramarital procreation were both drawn in question. Granted that God was glorified by man, it was evident that the main line of Catholic thought held that mere multiplication of men was no absolute value, that other values were higher, and that among the higher values was the perfection of existing men.

There was, however, one argument which offered an absolute bar to contraception because of its departure from the order established by God. As has already been shown, the Thomistic argument that intentional prevention of generation is unnatural essentially embodied this contention: to interfere with the procreative act is to offend God, although no injury is done to man.

The essence of this argument was frequently obscured by its rhetoric, which focused on the injury to "nature." But, as was observed by thousands of skeptical critics, "nature" as such possessed no special immunity from interference; dams and irrigation projects were never considered immoral. Nor was human nature itself ordinarily regarded as immune from improvement or from mutilation for the good of the person; the principles permitting surgery were deeply embedded in Catholic moral thought. If, in the one case of the sexual act, nature could not be interfered with, it was because in this one case the natural order was treated as special, as sacral, as in some extraordinary way God's.

The new critics subjected this argument to three basic attacks. Julian Pleasants took it at face value as a defense of what was natural in man. The argument, he said, "implies that inhibiting one purpose of an act while achieving another is unnatural." But biology shows that "a biological action is ordinarily multifunctional, and that inhibition of a function which is not needed is the typical means of achieving the integrated control required by living things." He gave as examples the action of the kidneys and the action of the nervous system: in their functioning action was initiated and then frustrated in some of its effects. On the contrary, the body commonly overdoes things, and then inhibits or frustrates any excessive results. If this seems untidy, it certainly cannot be called unnatural."[108] If such frustration of some effects was the ordinary biology of man, what was unnatural in frustrating the procreative function of intercourse while permitting the achievement of its purpose of expressing love?

Secondly, the critics observed that no showing had been made that procreation was the natural purpose of each act of intercourse. The evidence was just the other way. "Nature" sought to achieve its end by a plurality of acts, of which only a few could be meant to be procreative. Once more in the history of this doctrine animal behavior was invoked to explain a point, but this time the invocation was made after close observation. "Conception as a result of mating," Elizabeth Daugherty noted, "holds primacy of purpose only among the subprimate forms." The freedom of human beings from physiologically dominated sexual desires related to procreation was a human characteristic.[109]

A third line of criticism was tellingly developed by Louis Dupré and Michael Novak. To treat the act of intercourse as absolute, Dupré argued, was to isolate it from its normal context in a marriage. There was no reason to value the attainment of the biological end of the act as absolute, and to sacrifice to it the welfare of spouse or existing children. "To absolutize one particular value, even the most basic, at the expense of all the others is precisely what we call moral evil."[110] Similarly, Michael Novak objected to the narrow focus of the moralists on the integrity of the biological act: "The act of intercourse is not only defined by its biological externals; it reaches out into the total texture of our lives. This total texture is a 'good of the whole' more important than the good of any part—i.e. the biological placement of the act. The part must sometime yield to the good of the whole."[111]

These criticisms left the defenders of the Thomistic argument in this position: they could accept the characterization of their position made by Dupré: "To build an argument against contraception on the sacredness of nature (understood in such a way that the 'natural' course of the marriage act excludes any deliberate interference) is to withdraw the act from the sphere of the properly human, even for the attainment of its natural, biological end."[112] They could say, that is exactly what we mean. The act of coitus is sacred, is invested with a nonhuman immunity. It is sacramental for Christians and non-Christians alike. Why is it thus? Because by means of it God permits two human beings to join in the creative task of producing human life. The unique power of this act is such that every instance of its exercise must be treated reverently, as one would treat a sacrament. The criticisms based on the function of the biological system, the analogies drawn from animal behavior, even the arguments showing that to absolutize this value destroys other marital values—all these miss the point. This act is absolute, interference with its natural function is immoral, because it is the act from which life begins.

It would be possible to read the teaching of the theologians and canonists, popes and bishops, for over seventeen hundrd years, as embodying this position. To do so would require isolating a single strand of the teaching from other reasons and treating it, abstracted from all contexts, as dispositive of the morality of any act which, in the exercise of coitus, "intentionally deprives it of its natural power and strength." This interpretation of the requirements of the tradition would reaffirm the teaching of *Casti connubii*. It would, however, be consistent with a position which permitted the use of anovulants as agents not affecting the sacral act of coitus itself. To predict that this position would not be the option adopted by the Church would be to presume beyond the purview of history.

A sense of option was a least present. Paul VI had summed up the state of thought in the Church when on June 23, 1964, he addressed the cardinals on "the problem which everyone is talking about, that is, birth control." "The problem," he said,

> is extremely complex and delicate. The Church recognizes in it multiple aspects, multiple competencies, among which certainly the first is that of the spouses, their liberty, their conscience, their duty. But the Church has also to affirm her own competency, which is that of the laws of God. The Church has to proclaim such laws of God in the light of scientific, social, and psychological truths which, in recent times, have received new and most ample studies and documentation. It will be necessary to pay attention to this development of the question both in its theoretical and practical aspects. And this is precisely what the Church is doing.[113] (*AAS* 56:588)

The recorded statements of Christian doctrine on contraception did not have to be read in a way requiring an absolute prohibition. The doctrine had been molded by the teaching of the Gospels on the sanctity of marriage; the Pauline condemnation of unnatural sexual behavior; the Old Testament emphasis on fertility; the desire to justify marriage while extolling virginity; the need to assign rational purpose and limit to sexual behavior. The doctrine was formed in a society where slavery, slave concubinage, and the inferiority of women were important elements of the environment affecting sexual relations. The education of children was neither universal nor expensive. Underpopulation was a main governmental concern. The doctrine condemning contraception was formulated against the Gnostics, reasserted against the Manichees, and established in canon law at the climax of the campaign against the Cathars. Reaction to these movements hostile to all procreation was not the sole reason for the doctrine, but the emphases, sweep, and place of the doctrine issued from these mortal combats.

The environmental changes requiring a reconsideration of the rule accumulated only after 1850. These changes brought about a profound development of doctrine on marriage and marital intercourse: love became established as a meaning and end of the coital act. Before women were emancipated and marriages in the West came to be based on personal decision, writing like that of Von Hildebrand, Doms, Häring, Suenens, Fuchs, Ford, and Kelly would have seemed chimerical. Their work responded to the change in conditions. Their teaching on marriage was in many ways different from that of older theologians. Huguccio would have marveled at the teaching of Ford and Kelly, Jerome would have been astounded at Häring. Suppose the test of orthodoxy were, Would Augustine or Thomas be surprised if he were to return and see what Catholic theologians are teaching today? By this criterion, the entire development on the purposes of marital intercourse would have been unorthodox. But it is a perennial mistake to confuse repetition of old formulas with the living law of the Church. The Church, on its pilgrim's path, has grown in grace and wisdom.

That intercourse must be only for a procreative purpose, that intercourse in menstruation is mortal sin, that intercourse in pregnancy is forbidden, that intercourse has a natural position—all these were once common opinions of the theologians and are so no more. Was the commitment to an absolute prohibition of contraception more conscious, more universal, more complete, than to these now obsolete rules? These opinions, now superseded, could be regarded as attempts to preserve basic values in the light of the biological data then available and in the context of the challenges then made to the Christian view of man.

At the core of the existing commitment might be found values other than the absolute sacral value of coitus. Through a variety of formulas, five propositions had been asserted by the Church. Procreation is good. Procreation of offspring reaches its completion only in their education. Innocent life is sacred. The personal dignity of a spouse is to be respected. Marital love is holy. In these propositions the values of procreation, education, life, personality, and love were set forth. About these values a wall had been built; the wall could be removed when it became a prison rather than a bulwark.

Notes

1. M. Cépede, F. Houtart, and L. Groud, *Population and Food* (New York, 1964), pp. 10–12; Julian Huxley, *The Human Crisis* (Seattle, 1963), p. 50.

2. Cépède, Houtart, and Groud, *Population and Food*, pp. 152–156.

3. Hudson Hoagland, "Mechanisms of Population Control," *Daedalus* 93 (1964), 814.

4. The point was also made that "overpopulation" in the sense of too many persons per unit surface was not, in the present context, "very useful, except in situations where the primary resources are extractive, such as mining, the most primitive types of agriculture (independent of industry for fertilizers, machines, etc., and hence essentially dependent on area), and forestry" (Jean Mayer, "Food and Population: The Wrong Problem?" *Daedalus*, Summer 1964, pp. 835–836). Mayer also points out that as to food shortage, the problem now is not lack of production, but lack of rational distribution and even destruction of food "surpluses." There seems to be little correlation between population density and present shortages. The 14,000–square-mile area from Boston to Washington has more than 2000 persons per square mile, more often suffering from overweight than starvation. A small poulation is not necessarily a better fed one. In the foreseeable future, moreover, no absolute shortage of food appears probable. Only 3.4 billion acres, or less than 11 percent of the total land area, is now cultivated; 13 to 17 billion acres could be made arable. Increase in the use of fertilizers could easily double the low yield now realized in underdeveloped countries. The possibilities of making synthetic food from oil have been recently enhanced. Food through the photosynthesis of algae appears to be a likely possibility. "A breakthrough in this field [of photosynthesis] could for centuries altogether remove food as a limiting factor to population growth" (ibid., pp. 836–842).

5. See Ansley J. Coale and Edgar M. Hoover, *Population Growth and Economic Development in Low-Income Countries* (Princeton, 1958).

6. A vigorous presentation of the dangers of overpopulation was given by Huxley in *The Human Crisis*, pp. 50–80.

7. See *The Potential of Women*, a symposium held at the University of California San Francisco Medical Center January 25, 26, and 27, 1963, ed. Seymour M. Farber and Roger H. L. Wilson (New York, 1963); Eric J. Dingwall, *The American Woman: An Historical Study* (New York, 1956).

8. For sociological study of this change, see Alain Girard, *Le Choix du conjoint: Une enquête psychosociologique en France* (Paris, 1964); for an interpretive study, see Denis de Rougement, *Love in the Western World*, rev. ed., trans. Montgomery Belgion (New York, 1956), pp. 291–302.

9. For a development of the points in the two paragraphs above, see Cépède, Houtart, and Grond, *Population and Food,* pp. 216–227.

10. See Paul Vincent, "Etude d'un groupe de familles nombreuses," *Population* 16 (1961), 105–112 (report of a study of 14,000 families who had been candidates for the Prix Cognacq-Jay, a French prize for fertility).

11. E.g., Ignace Lepp, *The Psychology of Loving,* trans. Bernard B. Gilligan (Baltimore, 1963), pp. 21–24, 133–166.

12. Jacques Leclerq, "Natural Law the Unknown," *Natural Law Forum* 7 (1962), 10–13.

13. The pioneer work was Dominikus Lindner's *Der Usus matrimonii: Eine Untersuchung über seine sittliche Bewertung in der katholischen Moraltheologie alter und neuer Zeit* (Munich, 1929).

14. On the slow rebirth of Thomism and the work of Mercier at Louvain, see Louis de Raeymaeker, *Le Cardinal Mercier et l'Institut Supérieur de Philosophie de Louvain* (Louvain, 1952), pp. 40, 47–62.

15. M.G. Plattel, "Personal Response and the Natural Law," *Natural Law Forum* 7 (1962), 36–37.

16. By the end of the nineteenth century the state of Catholic moral theology was not perceptibly improved in comparison with its state in 1800. Cardinal d'Annibale could observe, "What the old theologians considered broadly and at length we scarcely touch with our fingertips" (*Summula theologiae moralis,* 3rd ed., Rome, 1892, I, 12). An anonymous reviewer in the Jesuits' *Civiltà Cattolica* could agree, adding that "with few exceptions, we have a mass of compendiums made and fashioned with a somnolency almost senile" (*Civiltà Cattolica,* series 14, 6 [1890], 443). Thomas Bouquillon (1840–1902), a professor at the Catholic University of America, found that moral theology had "failed to put itself in touch with new currents of thought, failed to anticipate problems of life." "Moral Theology," he concluded, "is all but an outcast." Bouquillon, "Moral Theology at the End of the Nineteenth Century," *Bulletin of The Catholic University of America,* April 1899, pp. 246–248.

17. The bull of Leo X, *Inter sollicitudines,* May 4, 1515, after rejoicing in the benefits of printing, observed that a number of books were being printed which led people into errors of faith or morals. The Pope, with the approval of the ecumenical council, decreed, under penalty of the burning of the book and the fining and excommunication of the author, that no book should be published without the approval of the bishop of the diocese and the approval of the inquisitor of the diocese (*Inter sollicitudines,* in *Codicis iuris canonici fontes,* ed. Peter Gasparri. Rome, 1923. I. 115–116). This legislation was renewed as to the requirement of approval of the bishop by the Council of Trent, April 8, 1546, Session IV, *De editione et usu sacrorum librorum,* as to books "on sacred matters," in a context which arguably restricted the law to books on sacred scripture, but was more broadly interpreted by the canonists. This legislation also made it mandatory for members of religious orders to have the approval of their superiors (Mansi 33:22–23). The penalty of excommunication was renewed in the same terms, as to "books treating of sacred matters," by Pius IX in the constitution *Apostolicae Sedis moderationi, Fontes* III, 28. The Constitution of Leo XIII, *Officiorum ac munerum* (*Fontes* III, 502–512), of January 25, 1897, expanded the term to include explicitly "books regarding the sacred Scriptures, sacred theology, ecclesiastical history, canon law, natural theology, ethics, and other religious and moral disciplines of this kind, and generally all writing of special interest to religion and decent morals." The penalty of excommunication was dropped. The 1917 Code followed this approach, eliminating the phrase "all writing of special interest to religion and decent morals." The license could be given by the bishop of the diocese of the author or of the printer or of the place of publication. Laymen were explicitly included by the canon. The additional obligation of permission from their major superior was imposed on members of religious orders (canon 1385). As recently as 1941, the Holy Office exhorted bishops to be more careful in granting permission for publication (*AAS* 33:121), and in 1943 the Holy Office called attention to the obligation imposed by canon 1397 on all the faithful, but especially clerics, to report pernicious books to the local bishops or the Apostolic See (*AAS* 35:144). There is no express penalty now provided for disobedience to canon 1385, and in practice in the last twenty years it has often been ignored by Catholic laymen.

18. Willem van der Marck, "Vruchtbaarheidsregeling," *Tijdschrift voor Theologie* 3 (1963), 378; Josef Maria Reuss, "Don mutuel des époux," *La Vie spirituelle* 17, Supplement (1964), 104.

19. Cf. Louis Dupré, *Contraception and Catholics: A New Appraisal* (Baltimore, 1964), p. 86: "In their personal convictions, many moralists are far more advanced than in their publications. It is regrettable

that at least the technical publications do not reflect more of the doubts concerning the traditional position which are so widespread in theological circles."

20. John Henry Newman, "On Consulting the Faithful in Matters of Doctrine," *Rambler,* July 1859; reprinted and amended in Newman, *The Arians of the Fourth Century* (London, 1879); separately published, ed. John Coulson (London, 1961). The quoted passage is on p. 104 of the Coulson edition.

21. John Coulson, Introduction to *On Consulting the Faithful in Matters of Doctrine,* pp. 36–42.

22. Karl Rahner, *Das freie Wort in der Kirche* (Einsiedeln, 1953); English translation, *Free Speech in the Church* (New York, 1959). The quotation is on pp. 18–19 of the English translation.

23. Ibid., p. 25.

24. Ibid., pp. 27–42.

25. On the new phenomenon of an educated, articulate, and concerned laity in the United States, see Daniel Callahan, *The Mind of the Catholic Layman* (New York, 1963); Donald Thorman, *The Emerging Catholic Layman* (New York, 1963); Michael Novak, *A New Generation: American and Catholic* (New York, 1964). The Christian Family Movement, an essentially lay organization designed to study Christian principles and apply them to family life, numbered 11,000 couples in 1956 (John L. Thomas, S.J., *The American Catholic Family,* Englewood Cliffs, N.J., 1956, pp. 428–430). By 1965 it numbered over 40,000.

26. The positions of the churches and the theologians is set out in Richard M. Fagley, *The Population Explosion and Christian Responsibility* (New York, 1960), pp. 195–208. An international study group, convened at the instance of officers of the World Council of Churches and the International Missionary Council, met at Mansfield College, Oxford, April 12–15, 1959, and adopted a statement on "Responsible Parenthood and the Population Problem," otherwise known as the Mansfield Report. The Report said that married persons in deciding how many children to have should act after deliberation together in love, valuing children as persons in their own right, recognizing the witness a Christian family offered of the fruit of the Spirit even in the most adverse physical conditions, and taking into account the social needs, including the population pressures, of the region in which they lived. If the decision was reached not to have a child, there was no moral difference between use of the infertile period, artificial barriers to the meeting of the sperm and ovum, and drugs regulating ovulation ("Responsible Parenthood and the Population Problem," paragraphs 19 and 22, printed in Fagley, pp. 231–233).

The Lambeth Conference in 1958 also emphasized the duty of responsible parenthood in the light of "a thoughtful consideration of the varying population needs and problems of society and the claims of future generations" (The Lambeth Conference, 1958, resolution 115). Nothing was said as to means of contraception. The Committee which had prepared the report which led to the resolution had said, "The *means* of family planning are in large measure matters of clinical and aesthetic choice, subject to the requirement that they be admissible to the Christian conscience." The Anglican bishops did not go so far as the Committee.

27. On the other hand, the Greek Orthodox Church, as far as can be judged, still opposes all contraception. A letter of the hierarchy of the Church of Greece in October 1937 condemned the "unnatural evil" of "escape from begetting children and nurturing them." In 1956 Archbishop Michael of the American archdiocese also condemned contraception (Fagley, *The Population Explosion,* pp. 164–166).

28. Gury, *Compendium of Moral Theology* (Turin, 1852), "Marriage," no. 688.

When Bouvier is reciting the arguments of the married laity in favor of coitus interruptus, he notes that it is said to "favor mutual love" (*Supplement to the Treatise on Marriage* 2.1.3.4).

29 "Certain Redemptorist Theologians," *Vindiciae alphonsianae* (Rome, 1873), 7.8.

30. Becker, "Die moralische Beurteilung des Handelns aus Lust," *Zeitschrift für katholische Theologie* 26 (1902), 679, 689.

31. De Smet, *Les Fiançailles et le mariage* 2.1.1.3.1.1.; Noldin, *De sexto praecepto et de usu matrimonii,* 19th ed. (Innsbruck, 1923), no. 78.2; Vermeersch, *Theologiae moralis principia, responsa, consilia* (Bruges, 1922–1923), vol. IV, no. 53; Merkelbach, *Questions on Chastity and Lechery* 8.1.2.; Dominic Prümmer, *Manuale theologiae moralis* 3.701.5 (Freiburg im Breisgau, 1923).

32. Bernard Häring, *Das Gesetz Christi,* 5th ed. (Freiburg im Breisgau, 1961).

33. Ford and Kelly, *Contemporary Moral Theology,* vol. II: *Marriage Questions* (Westminster, Md., 1963), pp. 192–193.

34. Ferdinand Probst, *Katholische Moraltheologie* (Tübingen, 1848–1850), II, 180.

35. Francis X. Linsenmann, *Lehrbuch der Moraltheologie* (Freiburg im Breisgau, 1878), p. 630.

36. Dietrich von Hildebrand, *Reinheit und Jungfräulichkeit* (Munich, 1928); English translation, *In Defense of Purity* (New York, 1931), pp. 20, 22. Quotations are from the English translation.

37. Herbert Doms, *Vom Sinn und zweck der Ehe* (Breslau, 1935); French translation by Paul and Marie Thisse, *Du sens et de la fin du mariage,* revised and augmented by the author (Paris, 1937); English translation, *The Meaning of Marriage* (New York, 1941). Citations are to the French edition. A brief biography of Doms is given at the end of a second book by him, *Dieses Geheimnis ist gross* (Cologne, 1960).

38. Francis Hürth, "La Fécondation artificielle: Sa value morale et juridique," *Nouvelle revue théologique* 68 (1946), 415, 406.

39. The first three citations are to the fifth edition of *Das Gesetz Christi;* the last two are to the French translation of the fourth edition. The translators, Francis Bourdeau, Armand Danet, and Louis Vereecke, have, with Häring's approval, made additions to the original text (*La Loi du Christ,* Paris, 1959).

Doms himself in his new work in 1960 synthesized the doctrine on love and procreation: "Conjugal coitus intends not simply offspring, but a new human person as the direct, substantial reproduction of the permanent community of life of the spouses, who have become a bodily unity—a new human person who is by this engendering through unity a faint image of the Incarnation, that is, of the relation of Christ to Church" (*Dieses Geheimnis ist gross,* p. 112).

40. Ford and Kelly, *Contemporary Moral Theology,* II, 117–119, 157. For an analysis of marriage in philosophical terms, finding in it a "vertical" finality of love, see Bernard Lonergan, S.J., "Finality, Love, Marriage," *Theological Studies* 4 (1943), 477–510.

41. English translations of the speeches of Leger, Alfrink, Maximos IV, and Suenens appeared in *The National Catholic Reporter,* November 11, 1964, p. 6.

42. Leo Joseph Suenens, *Un problème crucial: Amour et maîtresse de soi* (Bruges, 1956), trans. George J. Robinson, *Love and Control* (Westminster, Md., 1961). Quotations are from the English translation, pp. 68, 94–95.

43. Documents of the Second Vatican Council, Schema 13, "The Church and the Modern World," chapter 4 (draft, April 1964). The idea that the number of children in a family should depend on the family's circumstances, and that the decision should be made by the family, had been strongly urged by Bernard Häring in his book *Ehe in dieser Zeit* (Salzburg, 1960), p. 365.

44. *Periodica de re morali, canonica, liturgica* 33 (1944), 131.

45. Two Italian priests observed that "conjugal onanism" was almost universal in Italy; *Perfice munus* 36 (1961), 555. In Spain, too, it was believed that a majority of couples practiced contraception (Bernard Häring, *Ehe in dieser Zeit,* p. 374). A study of a southern Dutch group of Catholic churchgoers found that a majority practiced contraception, almost always by coitus interruptus (L. A. G. J. Timmermans, *Huwelijksbeleving van Katholicke Jonggehuwden,* Utrecht, 1964).

46. Lynch, "Notes on Moral Theology," *Theological Studies* 17 (1956), 192.

47. *Sacrae Romanae Rotae decisiones seu sententiae* (Rome, 1912–), 23.30, before Francis Morano, June 23, 1931.

48. The theory was applied in a case begun in 1903 where the Rota first held the marriage valid (14.14, before Parillo, April 29, 1922); and then determined that nullity existed on the grounds of a premarital intention of the wife not to have intercourse with her future husband, for whom she felt antipathy, until she came to love him (16.14, before Chimenti, March 14, 1924). However this was a short-lived victory for the principle that intention to exclude offspring temporarily nullifies a marriage. On March 23, 1925, the Rota held finally for the validity of the marriage (17.18, before André Julien).

49. The policy has been given practical effect by the application of a distinction as old as Sanchez. Sanchez had taught that there was a distinction between an intention contrary to the obligation of having children and an intention contrary to the execution of this obligation. According to this distinction one can intend to assume the obligation and at the same time intend to violate it. Comparison is made with someone taking an oath intending to violate it. He sins in his intention, but he is bound by the oath. Similarly, he who intends to assume the obligations of marriage, but to violate them, sins; yet he is held to the obligations assumed, and his marriage is valid (Sanchez, *The Holy Sacrament of Matrimony* 2.29.11).

This distinction has been criticized as unintelligible when the question is one of internal assent. Gerard Oesterle, O.S.B., "Animadversiones in sententiam S.R.R. diei 23 Februarii 1951 coram Staffa," *Il Diritto ecclesiastico* 62 (1951), 730, defending the judgment of nullity given by him as a member of the tribunal for the vicariate of Rome and published in *Il Diritto ecclesiastico* 60 (1949), 159–169. This decision had been overruled by the Rota. For a response by the Rota auditor responsible, see Dino Staffa, "De iure et eius exercitio relate ad bonum prolis," *Il Diritto ecclesiastico* 62 (1951), 1059. Staffa cited as decisive the words of Pius XII quoted below. Oesterle reasoned that marriage demands internal consent, and one cannot at the same time intend to assume an obligation and intend to violate it. The intention not to have offspring contradicts the intention to assume the obligation of having offspring. The comparison with oath-taking does not hold, because there a man is held by what he externally manifests: if he swears, then his subsequent falsehood will be punished as perjury, whatever his state of mind in taking the oath. On the other hand, Pius XII adopted the distinction in his celebrated talk to the midwives. He said that a premarital agreement to practice periodic continence did not vitiate matrimonial consent, for it did not exclude the perpetual marriage right, but only "the use of the marriage right" during certain periods (Address to the Italian Catholic Society of Midwives, *AAS* 43:845 [1951]).

50. This is the conclusion of Raoul Naz, "Les Empêchements de mariage improprements dits (can. 1081–1103 d'après la jurisprudence de la Rote)," *L'Année canonique* 1 (1952), 126. According to the statistics published annually in *L'Année canonique* since 1952 there has been a small rise since the 1920's in the number of annulments for a condition against offspring, but the increase does not seem large enough to establish a trend.

51. See Ford and Kelly, *Contemporary Moral Theology*, II, 214.

52. See the survey of authorities by Lawrence L. McReavy, "Cooperatio in Copula Condomistica," *The Clergy Review* 48 (1963), 119.

53. Maurice O'Leary, Letter to the Editor, *The Clergy Review* 48 (1963), 651. Father O'Leary is a leading member of the Catholic Marriage Advisory Council of London.

54. Letter, *The Clergy Review* 48 (1963), 322.

55. Suenens, *Love and Control*, p. 72, p. 67.

56. Schema 13, "The Church and the Modern World," appendix 2 (draft, April 1964).

57. Letter of G. B. Montini to Cardinal Siri, September 19, 1954, trans. in *Les Enseignements pontificaux: Le mariage,* ed. the Monks of Solesmes (Le Mans, 1956). In 1939, in one of the first acts of his reign, in congratulations addressed to the American hierarchy on its sesquicentennial, Pius XII noted that among the evils flowing from neglect of the law of God was "avoidance of the procreation of offspring" (*Sertum laetitiae, AAS* 31:639).

58. "Birth Control," Declaration of the Bishops of India, *Documentation catholique* 55 (1958), 210.

59. "La Limitation des naissances: Déclaration de l'Assemblé des cardinaux et archévêques de France," *Documentation catholique* 58 (1961), 371.

60. See, e.g., *America* 101 (1959), 583.

61. Statement of the administrative board of the National Catholic Welfare Conference, in *The New York Times,* November 26, 1959, p. 43.

62. Statement of the hierarchy of England and Wales in *The Universe,* May 7, 1964, reprinted in *The Pill and Birth Regulation,* ed. Leo Pyle (Baltimore 1964), pp. 95–98.

63. English translations of the speeches in the *National Catholic Reporter,* December 16, 1964.

64. *Contraception and Holiness,* by Archbishop Thomas D. Roberts et al. (New York, 1964), p. 10.

65. Louis Dupré, *Contraception and Catholics: A New Appraisal* (Baltimore, 1964).

66. *What Modern Catholics Think About Birth Control,* ed. William Birmingham (New York, 1964).

67. *The Experience of Marriage,* ed. Michael Novak (New York, 1964).

68. De Smet, *Les Fiançailles et le mariage* 2.1.3.1.1, annex 2; Merkelbach, *Questions on Chastity and Lechery* 8.4; John A. Ryan, "Family Limitation," *Ecclesiastical Review* 54 (1915), 693.

69. John A. Ryan, "The Moral Aspects of Periodical Continence," *Ecclesiastical Review* 89 (1933), 34.

70. Stanislas de Lestapis, *La Limitation des naissances,* 2nd ed. (Paris, 1960), p. 69. De Lestapis urged this phenomenon not as a general argument against birth control, but as an objection to the claim that birth control could help the population of underdeveloped countries.

71. Joseph Creusen, "L'Onanisme conjugal," *Nouvelle revue théologique* 59 (1932), 308–309.

72. Herbert McCabe, "Contraceptives and Natural Law," *The New Blackfriars* 46 (1964), 89, 93.

73. Arthur Vermeersch, "De prudenti ratione indicandi sterilitatem physiologicam," *Periodica de re morali, canonica, liturgica* 23 (1934), 242.

74. Gerald Kelly, "Notes on Moral Theology, 1949," *Theological Studies* 11 (1949), 74.

75. See the discussion by Ford and Kelly, *Contemporary Moral Theology,* II, 400–430. Ford and Kelly pointed out that Pius XII left open four questions: Is the obligation to procreate derived from the state of marriage or from habitual intercourse? Is the obligation traceable to the virtue of legal justice or to some other virtue? Is there a limit to the duty? Is violation of the duty a mortal sin? Francis Hürth, clearly desirous of preserving a place for virginal marriage, taught that the duty to procreate arose only from exercise of the marital act (Hürth, *De re matrimoniali* [Rome, 1955], pp. 112–115). Ford and Kelly rejected this analysis, believing it to be a reminiscence of the Augustinian view that intercourse needed an excuse. They held that the obligation arose from the state of marriage, and that the higher good of a virginal marriage could excuse from this kind of affirmative precept (pp. 404–409). On the second question Ford and Kelly found it unlikely that society had, in legal justice, a right to require procreation, and suggested that the governing virtues were piety toward family and fatherland, and chastity (pp. 411–417). On the fourth question, the gravity of the obligation, Fuchs held that "the more probable opinion" was that the practice of rhythm without justification, for the duration of the marriage constituted mortal sin (*Chastity and the Sexual Order* 10.4.2). Hürth held that use of the sterile period "sometimes" became serious sin. Ford and Kelly, however, argued that omission of the duty "in any individual instance would rarely have any damaging effect." They continued, "It may be objected that if everyone refused to have children the common good would suffer grave damage. Therefore it is necessary to impose a grave obligation on individuals even if individual omissions would not of themselves be seriously damaging. This line of reasoning is not conclusive. If everyone lied habitually, the common good would suffer grave damage; if everyone refused to go to the polls, the common good would suffer grave damage. Yet individuals do not ordinarily sin gravely by lying (even habitually) or by failing to vote (*Contemporary Moral Theology,* II, 427–428).

76. De Lestapis, *La Limitation des naissances,* p. 97.

77. Novak, "Toward a Positive Sexual Morality," in *What Modern Catholics Think About Birth Control,* p. 113.

78. "Instructions," *Nouvelle revue théologique* 41 (1909), 623.

79. Gerald Kelly, "Contraception and Natural Law," *Catholic Theological Society of America, Proceedings of the Eighteenth Annual Convention* (St. Louis, 1963), p. 38.

80. De Lestapis, *La Limitation des naissances,* pp. 63–65.

81. "Le Droit à la vie," Pastoral Letter of the Bishops of Switzerland, *Documentation catholique* 55 (1958), 205.

82. The figures and description of the developments in Japan are taken from Irene B. Taeuber, *The Population of Japan* (Princeton, 1958), pp. 269–276. The figures on Hungary and Poland are taken from Christopher Tietze, "The Demographic Significance of Legal Abortion in Eastern Europe," *Demography* 1 (1964).

83. This was the main purpose for which such statistics were cited by De Lestapis, *La Limitation des naissances,* pp. 63–66. A sharp conflict had been going on since 1955 in France to revise the French laws against the promotion of birth control. The claim had been advanced that more contraception would reduce the number of abortions. This claim, in particular, many Catholic spokesmen doubted. For an account of the French controversy in 1955 and 1956 see *Documentation catholique* 53 (1956), 873–887.

84. Michael Rosset, *De sacramento matrimonii* (Saint-Jean-de-Maurienne, 1895), V, no. 3336; Ryan, "Family Limitation," pp. 691–692.

85. Suenens, *Love and Control,* pp. 16–17; De Lestapis, *La Limitation des naissances,* pp. 98–99. De Lestapis argued that the Netherlands, France, and Belgium, whose laws did not permit the promotion of contraception, had lower divorce rates than the United States, Sweden, Switzerland, and Denmark. But his argument did not hold, as he failed to show that contraception was practiced less in fact in one set of countries than in the other.

86. Anthony Zimmerman, *Catholic Viewpoint on Population* (Garden City, N.Y., 1961), p. 148.

87. Rosset, *De sacramento matrimonii*, V, no. 3336; L. Roelandts, "Théologie pastorale," *Nouvelle revue théologique* 38 (1906), 316.

88. Raoul de Guchteneere, *Judgment on Birth Control* (New York, 1931), pp. 152–165. There is still some medical opinion supporting the contention that the practice of coitus interruptus can result in serious emotional disturbances; William S. Kroger and S. Charles Freed, *Psychosomatic Gynecology* (Glencoe, Ill., 1956), p. 276.

89. Ryan, "Family Limitation," p. 690.

90. Von Hildebrand, *In Defence of Purity*, p. 36.

91. Doms, *Du sens et de la fin du mariage*, pp. 177–178.

92. Suenens, *Love and Control*, p. 103.

93. Paul Quay, "Contraception and Conjugal Love," *Theological Studies* 22 (1961), 35.

94. André Snoeck, "Morale catholique et devoir de fécondité," *Nouvelle revue théologique* 75 (1953), 898.

95. Novak, "Toward a Positive Sexual Morality," in *What Modern Catholics Think About Birth Control*, p. 117.

96. Dupré, *Contraception and Catholics*, pp. 77–78.

97. "Instruction de Evêques de Belgique sur l'onanisme," *Nouvelle revue théologique* 41 (1909), 618. Letter of the bishops of Germany, quoted in Joseph Laurentius, "Das Bischofswort zum Schutze der Familie," *Theologish-praktische Quartalschrift* 67 (1914), 519.

98. Rosset, *De sacramento matrimonii*, V, no. 3336; Ryan, "Family Limitation," p. 691.

99. Germain G. Grisez, *Contraception and the Natural Law* (Milwaukee, 1964), pp. 78–86.

100. Ibid., pp. 162–163.

101. Ibid., p. 56.

102. Ibid., p. 95.

103. Roelandts, "Théologie pastorale," p. 315; Benedict Merkelbach, *De castitate et luxuria* 8.4.3 (Bruges, 1944).

104. Häring, *Das Gesetz Christi* 2.2.4.3.6.6 (5th ed., p. 1093); Hürth, *De re matrimoniali*, pp. 101–103.

105. Snoeck, "Morale catholique et devoir de fécondité," p. 909.

106. Louis Janssens, "Morale conjugale et progestogènes," *Ephemerides theologicae lovanienses*, 39 (1963), 816.

107. Ryan, "The Moral Aspects of Periodical Continence," pp. 33–34.

108. Julian Pleasants, "The Lessons of Biology," in Roberts et al., *Contraception and Holiness*, pp. 97–98.

109. Elizabeth A. Daugherty, "The Lessons of Zoology," in Roberts et al., *Contraception and Holiness*, pp. 112–126.

110. Dupré, *Contraception and Catholics*, p. 44.

111. Novak, "Toward a Positive Sexual Morality," in *What Modern Catholics Think About Birth Control*, p. 114.

112. Dupré, *Contraception and Catholics*, p. 87.

113. The Pope was referring to the commission on problems of population, the family, and natality set up to advise the Holy See. Established under John XXIII with a membership of six, it had been expanded to fifteen by May 1964, and to fifty-two by March 1965. The commission was international. There were nine members from the United States, seven from France, six from Germany, five from Belgium, five from Italy, two apiece from Canada, England, India, Japan, the Netherlands, and Spain, one apiece from Brazil, Chile, Jamaica, Madagascar, the Philippines, Senegal, Switzerland, and Tunis. Theologians—nineteen in all—were a plurality, but not a majority; there were fifteen demographers or economists, a dozen doctors, six representatives of the married laity, including the leaders of the Christian Family Movement. There were five women. The first plenary session of the commission was held March 25–28, 1965, in Rome. Addressing this group, Pope Paul VI pointed to the Church's guardianship of life and of love, and said, "In the present case, the problem posed may be summarized as follows: in what form and according to what norms ought spouses to accomplish in the exercise of their mutual love that service of life to which their vocation calls them?" (*L'Osservatore romano*, March 29, 1965, p. 2).

21

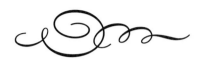

Humanae Vitae
(On the Regulation of Birth)

Pope Paul VI

To His Venerable Brothers the Patriarchs, Archbishops, Bishops and other Local Ordinaries in Peace and Communion with the Apostolic See, to the Clergy and Faithful of the Whole Catholic World, and to All Men of Good Will.

Honored Brothers and Dear Sons, Health and Apostolic Benediction.

The transmission of human life is a most serious role in which married people collaborate freely and responsibly with God the Creator. It has always been a source of great joy to them, even though it sometimes entails many difficulties and hardships.

The fulfillment of this duty has always posed problems to the conscience of married people, but the recent course of human society and the concomitant changes have provoked new questions. The Church cannot ignore these questions, for they concern matters intimately connected with the life and happiness of human beings.

I. Problem and Competency of the Magisterium

2. The changes that have taken place are of considerable importance and varied in nature. In the first place there is the rapid increase in population which has made many fear that world population is going to grow faster than available resources, with the consequence that many families and developing countries would be faced with greater hardships. This can easily induce public authorities to be tempted to take even harsher measures to avert this danger. There is also the fact that not only working and housing conditions but the greater demands made both in the economic and educational field pose a living situation in which it is frequently difficult these days to provide properly for a large family.

Also noteworthy is a new understanding of the dignity of woman and her place in society, of the value of conjugal love in marriage and the relationship of conjugal acts to this love.

But the most remarkable development of all is to be seen in man's stupendous progress in the domination and rational organization of the forces of nature to the point that he is endeavoring to extend this control over every aspect of his own health—over his body, over his mind and emotions, over his social life, and even over the laws that regulate the transmission of life.

New Questions

3. This new state of things gives rise to new questions. Granted the conditions of life today and taking into account the relevance of married love to the harmony and mutual fidelity of husband and wife, would it not be right to review the moral norms in force till now, especially when it is felt that these can be observed only with the gravest difficulty, sometimes only by heroic effort?

Moreover, if one were to apply here the so-called principle of totality, could it not be accepted that the intention to have a less prolific but more rationally planned family might transform an action which renders natural processes infertile into a licit and provident control of birth? Could it not be admitted, in other words, that procreative finality applies to the totality of married life rather than to each single act? A further question is whether, because people are more conscious today of their responsibilities, the time has not come when the transmission of life should be regulated by their intelligence and will rather than through the specific rhythms of their own bodies.

Interpreting the Moral Law

4. This kind of question requires from the teaching authority of the Church a new and deeper reflection on the principles of the moral teaching on marriage—a teaching which is based on the natural law as illuminated and enriched by divine Revelation.

No member of the faithful could possibly deny that the Church is competent in her magisterium to interpret the natural moral law. It is in fact indisputable, as Our predecessors have many times declared,[1] that Jesus Christ, when He communicated His divine power to Peter and the other Apostles and sent them to teach all nations His commandments,[2] constituted them as the authentic guardians and interpreters of the whole moral law, not only, that is, of the law of the Gospel but also of the natural law. For the natural law, too, declares the will of God, and its faithful observance is necessary for men's eternal salvation.[3]

In carrying out this mandate, the Church has always issued appropriate documents on the nature of marriage, the correct use of conjugal rights, and the duties of spouses. These documents have been more copious in recent times.[4]

Special Studies

5. The consciousness of the same responsibility induced Us to confirm and expand the commission set up by Our predecessor Pope John XXIII, of happy memory, in March, 1963. This commission included married couples as well as many experts in the various fields pertinent to these questions. Its task was to examine views and opinions concerning married life, and especially on the correct regulation of births; and it was also to provide the teaching authority of the Church with such evidence as would enable it to give an apt reply in this matter, which not only the faithful but also the rest of the world were waiting for.[5]

When the evidence of the experts had been received, as well as the opinions and advice of a considerable number of Our brethren in the episcopate—some of whom sent their views spontaneously, while others were requested by Us to do so—We were in a position to weigh with more precision all the aspects of this complex subject. Hence We are deeply grateful to all those concerned.

The Magisterium's Reply

6. However, the conclusions arrived at by the commission could not be considered by Us as definitive and absolutely certain, dispensing Us from the duty of examining personally this serious question. This was all the more necessary because, within the commission itself, there was not complete agreement concerning the moral norms to be proposed, and especially because certain approaches and criteria for a solution to this question had emerged which were at variance with the moral doctrine on marriage constantly taught by the magisterium of the Church.

Consequently, now that We have sifted carefully the evidence sent to Us and intently studied the whole matter, as well as prayed constantly to God, We, by virtue of the mandate entrusted to Us by Christ, intend to give Our reply to this series of grave questions.

II. Doctrinal Principles

7. The question of human procreation, like every other question which touches human life, involves more than the limited aspects specific to such disciplines as biology, psychology, demography or sociology. It is the whole man and the whole mission to which he is called that must be considered: both its natural, earthly aspects and its supernatural, eternal aspects. And since in the attempt to justify artifical methods of birth control many appeal to the demands of married love or of responsible parenthood, these two important realities of married life must be accurately defined and analyzed. This is what We mean to do, with special reference to what the Second Vatican Council taught with the highest authority in its Pastoral Constitution on the Church in the World of Today.

God's Loving Design

8. Married love particularly reveals its true nature and nobility when we realize that it takes origin from God, who "is love,"[6] the Father "from whom every family in Heaven and on earth is named."[7]

Marriage, then, is far from being the effect of chance or the result of the blind evolution of natural forces. It is in reality the wise and provident institution of God the Creator, whose purpose was to effect in man His loving design. As a consequence, husband and wife, through that mutual gift of themselves, which is specific and exclusive to them alone, develop that union of two persons in which they perfect one another, cooperating with God in the generation and rearing of new lives.

The marriage of those who have been baptized is, in addition, invested with the dignity of a sacramental sign of grace, for it represents the union of Christ and His Church.

Married Love

9. In the light of these facts the characteristic features and exigencies of married love are clearly indicated, and it is of the highest importance to evaluate them exactly.

This love is above all fully *human*, a compound of sense and spirit. It is not, then, merely a question of natural instinct or emotional drive. It is also, and above all, an act of the free will, whose trust is such that it is meant not only to survive the joys and sorrows of daily life, but also to grow, so that husband and wife become in a way one heart and one soul, and together attain their human fulfillment.

It is a love which is *total*—that very special form of personal friendship in which husband and wife generously share everything, allowing no unreasonable exceptions and not thinking solely of their own convenience. Whoever really loves his partner loves not only for what he receives, but loves that partner for the partner's own sake, content to be able to enrich the other with the gift of himself.

Married love is also *faithful* and *exclusive* of all other, and this until death. This is how husband and wife understood it on the day on which, fully aware of what they were doing, they freely vowed themselves to one another in marriage. Though this fidelity of husband and wife sometimes presents difficulties, no one has the right to assert that it is impossible; it is, on the contrary, always honorable and meritorious. The example of countless married couples proves not only that fidelity is in accord with the nature of marriage, but also that it is the source of profound and enduring happiness.

Finally, this love is *fecund*. It is not confined wholly to the loving interchange of husband and wife; it also contrives to go beyond this to bring new life into being. "Marriage and conjugal love are by their nature ordained toward the procreation and education of children. Children are really the supreme gift of marriage and contribute in the highest degree to their parents' welfare."[8]

Responsible Parenthood

10. Married love, therefore, requires of husband and wife the full awareness of their obligations in the matter of responsible parenthood, which today, rightly enough, is much insisted upon, but which at the same time should be rightly understood. Thus, we do well to consider responsible parenthood in the light of its varied legitimate and interrelated aspects.

With regard to the biological processes, responsible parenthood means an awareness of, and respect for, their proper functions. In the procreative faculty the human mind discerns biological laws that apply to the human person.[9]

With regard to man's innate drives and emotions, responsible parenthood means that man's reason and will must exert control over them.

With regard to physical, economic, psychological and social conditions, responsible parenthood is exercised by those who prudently and generously decide to have more children, and by those who, for serious reasons and with due respect to moral precepts, decide not to have additional children for either a certain or an indefinite period of time.

Responsible parenthood, as we use the term here, has one further essential aspect of paramount importance. It concerns the objective moral order which was established by God, and of which a right conscience is the true interpreter. In a word, the exercise of responsible parenthood requires that husband and wife, keeping a right order of priorities, recognize their own duties toward God, themselves, their families and human society.

From this it follows that they are not free to act as they choose in the service of transmitting life, as if it were wholly up to them to decide what is the right course to follow. On the contrary, they are bound to ensure that what they do corresponds to the will of God the Creator. The very nature of marriage and its use makes His will clear, while the constant teaching of the Church spells it out.[10]

Observing the Natural Law

11. The sexual activity, in which husband and wife are intimately and chastely united with one another, through which human life is transmitted, is, as the recent Council recalled, "noble and worthy."[11] It does not, moreover, cease to be legitimate even when, for reasons independent of

their will, it is foreseen to be infertile. For its natural adaptation to the expression and strengthening of the union of husband and wife is not thereby suppressed. The fact is, as experience shows, that new life is not the result of each and every act of sexual intercourse. God has wisely ordered laws of nature and the incidence of fertility in such a way that successive births are already naturally spaced through the inherent operation of these laws. The Church, nevertheless, in urging men to the observance of the precepts of the natural law, which it interprets by its constant doctrine, teaches that each and every marital act must of necessity retain its intrinsic relationship to the procreation of human life.[12]

Union and Procreation

12. This particular doctrine, often expounded by the magisterium of the Church, is based on the inseparable connection, established by God, which man on his own initiative may not break, between the unitive significance and the procreative significance which are both inherent to the marriage act.

The reason is that the fundamental nature of the marriage act, while uniting husband and wife in the closest intimacy, also renders them capable of generating new life—and this as a result of laws written into the actual nature of man and of woman. And if each of these essential qualities, the unitive and the procreative, is preserved, the use of marriage fully retains its sense of true mutual love and its ordination to the supreme responsibility of parenthood to which man is called. We believe that our contemporaries are particularly capable of seeing that this teaching is in harmony with human reason.

Faithfulness to God's Design

13. Men rightly observe that a conjugal act imposed on one's partner without regard to his or her condition or personal and reasonable wishes in the matter, is no true act of love, and therefore offends the moral order in its particular application to the intimate relationship of husband and wife. If they further reflect, they must also recognize that an act of mutual love which impairs the capacity to transmit life which God the Creator, through specific laws, has built into it, frustrates His design which constitutes the norm of marriage, and contradicts the will of the Author of life. Hence to use this divine gift while depriving it, even if only partially, of its meaning and purpose, is equally repugnant to the nature of man and of woman, and is consequently in opposition to the plan of God and His holy will. But to experience the gift of married love while respecting the laws of conception is to acknowledge that one is not the master of the sources of life but rather the minister of the design established by the Creator. Just as man does not have unlimited dominion over his body in general, so also, and with more particular reason, he has no such dominion over his specifically sexual faculties, for these are concerned by their very nature with the generation of life, of which God is the source. "Human life is sacred—all men must recognize that fact," Our predecessor Pope John XXIII recalled. "From its very inception it reveals the creating hand of God."[13]

Unlawful Birth Control Methods

14. Therefore We base Our words on the first principles of a human and Christian doctrine of marriage when We are obliged once more to declare that the direct interruption of the generative process already begun and, above all, all direct abortion, even for therapeutic reasons, are to be absolutely excluded as lawful means of regulating the number of children.[14]

Equally to be condemned, as the magisterium of the Church has affirmed on many occasions, is direct sterilization, whether of the man or of the woman, whether permanent or temporary.[15]

Similarly excluded is any action which either before, at the moment of, or after sexual intercourse, is specifically intended to prevent procreation—whether as an end or as a means.[16]

Neither is it valid to argue, as a justification for sexual intercourse which is deliberately contraceptive, that a lesser evil is to be preferred to a greater one, or that such intercourse would merge with procreative acts of past and future to form a single entity, and so be qualified by exactly the same moral goodness as these. Though it is true that sometimes it is lawful to tolerate a lesser moral evil in order to avoid a greater evil or in order to promote a greater good,[17] it is never lawful, even for the gravest reasons, to do evil that good may come of it[18]—in other words, to intend directly something which of its very nature contradicts the moral order, and which must therefore be judged unworthy of man, even though the intention is to protect or promote the wefare of an individual, of a family or of society in general. Consequently, it is a serious error to think that a whole married life of otherwise normal relations can justify sexual intercourse which is deliberately contraceptive and so intrinsically wrong.

Lawful Therapeutic Means

15. On the other hand, the Church does not consider at all illicit the use of those therapeutic means necessary to cure bodily diseases, even if a foreseeable impediment to procreation should result therefrom—provided such impediment is not directly intended for any motive whatsoever.[19]

Recourse to Infertile Periods

16. Now as We noted earlier (no. 3), some people today raise the objection against this particular doctrine of the Church concerning the moral laws governing marriage, that human intelligence has both the right and responsibility to control those forces of irrational nature which come within its ambit and to direct them toward ends beneficial to man. Others ask on the same point whether it is not reasonable in so many cases to use artificial birth control if by so doing the harmony and peace of a family are better served and more suitable conditions are provided for the education of children already born. To this question We must give a clear reply. The Church is the first to praise and commend the application of human intelligence to an activity in which a rational creature such as man is so closely associated with his Creator. But she affirms that this must be done within the limits of the order of reality established by God.

If therefore there are well-grounded reasons for spacing births, arising from the physical or psychological condition of husband or wife, or from external circumstances, the Church teaches that married people may then take advantage of the natural cycles immanent in the reproductive system and engage in marital intercourse only during those times that are infertile, thus controlling birth in a way which does not in the least offend the moral principles which We have just explained.[20]

Neither the Church nor her doctrine is inconsistent when she considers it lawful for married people to take advantage of the infertile period but condemns as always unlawful the use of means which directly prevent conception, even when the reasons given for the latter practice may appear to be upright and serious. In reality, these two cases are completely different. In the former the married couple rightly use a faculty provided them by nature. In the latter they obstruct the natural development of the generative process. It cannot be denied that in each case the married couple, for acceptable reasons, are both perfectly clear in their intention to avoid chidren and wish to make sure that none will result. But it is equally true that it is exclusively in the former case that husband and wife are ready to abstain from intercourse during the fertile period as often as for reasonable motives the birth of another child is not desirable. And when the infertile period recurs, they use their married intimacy to express their mutual love and safeguard their fidelity toward one another. In doing this they certainly give proof of a true and authentic love.

Consequences of Artificial Methods

17. Responsible men can become more deeply convinced of the truth of the doctrine laid down by the Church on this issue if they reflect on the consequences of methods and plans for artificial birth control. Let them first consider how easily this course of action could open wide the way for marital infidelity and a general lowering of moral standards. Not much experience is needed to be fully aware of human weakness and to understand that human beings—and especially the young, who are so exposed to temptation—need incentives to keep the moral law, and it is an evil thing to make it easy for them to break that law. Another effect that gives cause for alarm is that a man who grows accustomed to the use of contraceptive methods may forget the reverence due to a woman, and, disregarding her physical and emotional equilibrium, reduce her to being a mere instrument for the satisfaction of his own desires, no longer considering her as his partner whom he should surround with care and affection.

Finally, careful consideration should be given to the danger of this power passing into the hands of those public authorities who care little for the precepts of the moral law. Who will blame a government which in its attempt to resolve the problems affecting an entire country resorts to the same measures as are regarded as lawful by married people in the solution of particular family difficulty? Who will prevent public authorities from favoring those contraceptive methods which they consider more effective? Should they regard this as necessary, they may even impose their use on everyone. It could well happen, therefore, that when people, either individually or in family or social life, experience the inherent difficulties of the divine law and are determined to avoid them, they may give into the hands of public authorities the power to intervene in the most personal and intimate responsibility of husband and wife.

Limits to Man's Power

Consequently, unless we are willing that the responsibility of procreating life should be left to the arbitrary decision of men, we must accept that there are certain limits, beyond which it is wrong to go, to the power of man over his own body and its natural functions—limits, let it be said, which no one, whether as a private individual or as a public authority, can lawfully exceed. These limits are expressly imposed because of the reverence due to the whole human organism and its natural functions, in the light of the principles We stated earlier, and in accordance with a correct understanding of the "principle of totality" enunciated by Our predecessor Pope Pius XII.[21]

Concern of the Church

18. It is to be anticipated that perhaps not everyone will easily accept this particular teaching. There is too much clamorous outcry against the voice of the Church, and this is intensified by modern means of communication. But it comes as no surprise to the Church that she, no less

than her divine Founder, is destined to be a "sign of contradiction."[22] She does not, because of this, evade the duty imposed on her of proclaiming humbly but firmly the entire moral law, both natural and evangelical.

Since the Church did not make either of these laws, she cannot be their arbiter—only their guardian and interpreter. It could never be right for her to declare lawful what is in fact unlawful, since that, by its very nature, is always opposed to the true good of man.

In preserving intact the whole moral law of marriage, the Church is convinced that she is contributing to the creation of a truly human civilization. She urges man not to betray his personal responsibilities by putting all his faith in technical expedients. In this way she defends the dignity of husband and wife. This course of action shows that the Church, loyal to the example and teaching of the divine Savior, is sincere and unselfish in her regard for men whom she strives to help even now during this earthly pilgrimage "to share God's life as sons of the living God, the Father of all men."[23]

III. Pastoral Directives

19. Our words would not be an adequate expression of the thought and solicitude of the Church, Mother and Teacher of all peoples, if, after having recalled men to the observance and respect of the divine law regarding matrimony, they did not also support mankind in the honest regulation of birth amid the difficult conditions which today afflict families and peoples. The Church, in fact, cannot act differently toward men than did the Redeemer. She knows their weaknesses, she has compassion on the multitude, she welcomes sinners. But at the same time she cannot do otherwise than teach the law. For it is in fact the law of human life restored to its native truth and guided by the Spirit of God.[24]

Observing the Divine Law

20. The teaching of the Church regarding the proper regulation of birth is a promulgation of the law of God Himself. And yet there is no doubt that to many it will appear not merely difficult but even impossible to observe. Now it is true that like all good things which are outstanding for their nobility and for the benefits which they confer on men, so this law demands from individual men and women, from families and from human society, a resolute purpose and great endurance. Indeed it cannot be observed unless God comes to their help with the grace by which the goodwill of men is sustained and strengthened. But to those who consider this matter diligently it will indeed be evident that this endurance enhances man's dignity and confers benefits on human society.

Value of Self-Discipline

21. The right and lawful ordering of birth demands, first of all, that spouses fully recognize and value the true blessings of family life and that they acquire complete mastery over themselves and their emotions. For if with the aid of reason and of free will they are to control their natural drives, there can be no doubt at all of the need for self-denial. Only then will the expression of love, essential to married life, conform to right order. This is especially clear in the practice of periodic continence. Self-discipline of this kind is a shining witness to the chastity of husband and wife and, far from being a hindrance to their love of one another, transforms it by giving it a more truly human character. And if this self-discipline does demand that they

persevere in their purpose and efforts, it has at the same time the salutary effect of enabling husband and wife to develop to their personalities and to be enriched with spiritual blessings. For it brings to family life abundant fruits of tranquility and peace. It helps in solving difficulties of other kinds. It fosters in husband and wife thoughtfulness and loving consideration for one another. It helps them to repel inordinate self-love, which is the opposite of charity. It arouses in them a consciousness of their responsibilities. And finally, it confers upon parents a deeper and more effective influence in the education of their children. As their children grow up, they develop a right sense of values and achieve a serene and harmonious use of their mental and physical powers.

Promotion of Chastity

22. We take this opportunity to address those who are engaged in education and all those whose right and duty it is to provide for the common good of human society. We would call their attention to the need to create an atmosphere favorable to the growth of chastity so that true liberty may prevail over license and the norms of the moral law may be fully safeguarded.

Everything therefore in the modern means of social communication which arouses men's baser passions and encourages low moral standards, as well as every obscenity in the written word and every form of indecency on the stage and screen, should be condemned publicly and unanimously by all those who have at heart the advance of civilization and the safeguarding of the outstanding values of the human spirit. It is quite absurd to defend this kind of depravity in the name of art or culture[25] or by pleading the liberty which may be allowed in this field by the public authorities.

Appeal to Public Authorities

23. And now We wish to speak to rulers of nations. To you most of all is committed the responsibility of safeguarding the common good. You can contribute so much to the preservation of morals. We beg of you, never allow the morals of your peoples to be undermined. The family is the primary unit in the state; do not tolerate any legislation which would introduce into the family those practices which are opposed to the natural law of God. For there are other ways by which a government can and should solve the population problem—that is to say by enacting laws which will assist families and by educating the people wisely so that the moral law and the freedom of the citizens are both safeguarded.

Seeking True Solutions

We are fully aware of the difficulties confronting the public authorities in this matter, especially in the developing countries. In fact, We had in mind the justifiable anxieties which weigh upon them when We published Our encyclical letter *Populorum Progressio*. But now We join Our voice to that of Our predecessor John XXIII of venerable memory, and We make Our own his words: "No statement of the problem and no solution to it is acceptable which does violence to man's essential dignity; those who propose such solutions base them on an utterly materialistic conception of man himself and his life. The only possible solution to this question is one which envisages the social and economic progress both of individuals and of the whole of human society, and which respects and promotes true human values."[26] No one can, without being grossly unfair, make divine Providence responsible for what clearly seems to be the result of misguided governmental policies, of an insufficient sense of social justice, of a selfish accumulation of material goods, and finally of a culpable failure to undertake those initiatives and responsibilities which would raise the standard of living of peoples and their children.[27] If only all governments which were able would do what some are already doing so nobly, and bestir themselves to renew their efforts and their undertakings! There must be no relaxation in the programs of mutual aid between all the branches of the great human family. Here We believe an almost limitless field lies open for the activities of the great international institutions.

To Scientists

24. Our next appeal is to men of science. These can "considerably advance the welfare of marriage and the family and also peace of conscience, if by pooling their efforts they strive to elucidate more thoroughly the conditions favorable to a proper regulation of births."[28] It is supremely desirable, and this was also the mind of Pius XII, that medical science should by the study of natural rhythms succeed in determining a sufficiently secure basis for the chaste limitation of offspring.[29] In this way scientists, especially those who are Catholics, will by their research establish the truth of the Church's claim that "there can be no contradiction between two divine laws—that which governs the transmitting of life and that which governs the fostering of married love."[30]

To Christian Couples

25. And now We turn in a special way to Our own sons and daughters, to those most of all whom God calls to serve Him in the state of marriage. While the Church does indeed hand on to her children the inviolable conditions laid down by God's law, she is also the herald of salvation and through the sacraments she flings wide open the channels of grace through which man is made a new creature responding in charity and true freedom to the design of his Creator and Savior, experiencing too the sweetness of the yoke of Christ.[31]

In humble obedience then to her voice, let Christian husbands and wives be mindful of their vocation to the Christian life, a vocation which, deriving from their Baptism, has been confirmed anew and made more explicit by the Sacrament of Matrimony. For by this sacrament they are *strengthened* and, one might almost say, *consecrated* to the faithful fulfillment of their duties. Thus will they realize to the full their calling and bear witness as becomes them, to Christ before the world.[32] For the Lord has entrusted to them the task of making visible to men and women the holiness and joy of the law which united inseparably their love for one another and the cooperation they give to God's love, God who is the Author of human life.

We have no wish at all to pass over in silence the difficulties, at times very great, which beset the lives of Christian married couples. For them, as indeed for every one of us, "the gate is narrow and the way is hard, that leads to life."[33] Nevertheless it is precisely the hope of that life which, like a brightly burning torch, lights up their journey, as, strong in spirit, they strive to live "sober, upright and godly lives in this world,"[34] knowing for sure that "the form of this world is passing away."[35]

Recourse to God

For this reason husbands and wives should take up the burden appointed to them, willingly, in the strength of faith and of that hope which "does not disappoint us, because God's love has been poured into our hearts through the Holy Spirit who has been given to us."[36] Then let them implore the help of God with unremitting prayer and, most of all, let them draw grace and charity from that unfailing fount which is the Eucharist. If, however, sin still exercises its hold over them, they are not to lose heart. Rather must they, humble and persevering, have recourse to the mercy of God, abundantly bestowed in the Sacrament of Penance. In this way, for sure, they will be able to reach that perfection of married life which the Apostle sets out in these words: "Husbands, love your wives, as Christ loved the Church... Even so husbands should love their wives as their own bodies. He who loves his wife loves himself. For no man ever hates his own flesh, but nourishes and cherishes it, as Christ does the Church... This is a great mystery, and I mean in reference to Christ and the Church; however, let each one of you love his wife as himself, and let the wife see that she respects her husband."[37]

Family Apostolate

26. Among the fruits that ripen if the law of God be resolutely obeyed, the most precious is certainly this, that married couples themselves will often desire to communicate their own experience to others. Thus it comes about that in the fullness of the lay vocation will be included a novel and outstanding form of the apostolate by which, like ministering to like, married couples themselves by the leadership they offer will become apostles to other married couples. And surely among all the forms of the Christian apostolate it is hard to think of one more opportune for the present time.[38]

To Doctors and Nurses

27. Likewise we hold in the highest esteem those doctors and members of the nursing profession who, in the exercise of their calling, endeavor to fulfill the demands of their Christian vocation before any merely human interest. Let them therefore continue constant in their resolution always to support those lines of action which accord with faith and with right reason. And let them strive to win agreement and support for these policies among their professional colleagues. Moreover, they should regard it as an essential part of their skill to make themselves fully proficient in this difficult field of medical knowledge. For then, when married couples ask for their advice, they may be in a position to give them right counsel and to point them in the proper direction. Married couples have a right to expect this much from them.

To Priests

28. And now, beloved sons, you who are priests, you who in virtue of your sacred office act as counselors and spiritual leaders both of individual men and women and of families—We turn to you filled with great confidence. For it is your principal duty—we are speaking especially to you who teach moral theology—to spell out clearly and completely the Church's teaching on marriage. In the performance of your ministry you must be the first to give an example of that sincere obedience, inward as well as outward, which is due to the magisterium of the Church. For, as you know, the pastors of the Church enjoy a special light of the Holy Spirit in teaching the truth.[39] And this, rather than the arguments they put forward, is why you are bound to such obedience. Nor will it escape you that if men's peace of soul and the unity of the Christian people are to be preserved, then it is of the utmost importance that in moral as well as in dogmatic theology all should obey the magisterium of the Church and should speak as with one voice. Therefore We make Our own the anxious words of the great Apostle Paul and with all Our heart We renew Our appeal to you: "I appeal to you, brethren, by the name of our Lord Jesus Christ, that

all of you agree and that there be no dissensions among you, but that you be united in the same mind and the same judgment."[40]

Christian Compassion

29. Now it is an outstanding manifestation of charity toward souls to omit nothing from the saving doctrine of Christ; but this must always be joined with tolerance and charity, as Christ Himself showed in His conversations and dealings with men. For when He came, not to judge, but to save the world,[41] was He not bitterly severe toward sin, but patient and abounding in mercy toward sinners?

Husbands and wives, therefore, when deeply distressed by reason of the difficulties of their life, must find stamped in the heart and voice of their priest the likeness of the voice and the love of our Redeemer.

So speak with full confidence, beloved sons, convinced that while the Holy Spirit of God is present to the magisterium proclaiming sound doctrine, He also illumines from within the hearts of the faithful and invites their assent. Teach married couples the necessary way of prayer and prepare them to approach more often with great faith the Sacraments of the Eucharist and of Penance. Let them never lose heart because of their weakness.

To Bishops

30. And now as We come to the end of this encyclical letter, We turn Our mind to you, reverently and lovingly, beloved and venerable brothers in the episcopate, with whom We share more closely the care of the spiritual good of the People of God. For We invite all of you, We implore you, to give a lead to your priests who assist you in the sacred ministry, and to the faithful of your dioceses, and to devote yourselves with all zeal and without delay to safeguarding the holiness of marriage, in order to guide married life to its full human and Christian perfection. Consider this mission as one of your most urgent responsibilities at the present time. As you well know, it calls for concerted pastoral action in every field of human diligence, economic, cultural and social. If simultaneous progress is made in these various fields, then the intimate life of parents and children in the family will be rendered not only more tolerable, but easier and more joyful. And life together in human society will be enriched with fraternal charity and made more stable with true peace when God's design which He conceived for the world is faithfully followed.

A Great Work

31. Venerable brothers, beloved sons, all men of good will, great indeed is the work of education, of progress and of charity to which We now summon all of you. And this We do relying on the unshakable teaching of the Church, which teaching Peter's successor together with his brothers in the Catholic episcopate faithfully guards and interprets. And We are convinced that this truly great work will bring blessings both on the world and on the Church. For man cannot attain that true happiness for which he yearns with all the strength of his spirit, unless he keeps the laws which the Most High God has engraved in his very nature. These laws must be wisely and lovingly observed. On this great work, on all of you and especially on married couples, We implore from the God of all holiness and pity an abundance of heavenly grace as a pledge of which We gladly bestow Our apostolic blessing.

Given at St. Peter's, Rome, on the 25th day of July, the feast of St. James the Apostle, in the year 1968, the sixth of Our pontificate.

†

LATIN TEXT: *Acta Apostolicae Sedis,* 60 (1968), 481–503.

ENGLISH TRANSLATION: *The Pope Speaks,* 13 (Fall, 1969), 329–346.

Notes

1. See Pius IX, encyc. letter *Qui pluribus: Pii IX P.M. Acta,* 1, pp. 9–10; St. Pius X, encyc. letter *Singulari quadam:* AAS 4 (1912), 658; Pius XI, encyc. letter *Casti connubii:* AAS 22 (1930), 579–581; Pius XII, address *Magnificate Dominum* to the episcopate of the Catholic world: AAS 46 (1954), 671–672; John XXIII, encyc. letter *Mater et Magistra:* AAS 53 (1961), 457.

2. See *Mt* 28. 18–19.

3. See *Mt* 7. 21.

4. See Council of Trent Roman Catechism, Part II, ch. 8; Leo XIII, encyc. letter *Arcanum: Acta Leonis XIII,* 2 (1880), 26–29; Pius XI, encyc. letter *Divini illius Magistri:* AAS 22 (1930), 58–61; encyc. letter *Casti connubii:* AAS 22 (1930), 545–546; Pius XII, Address to Italian Medico-Biological Union of St. Luke: *Discorsi e radiomessaggi di Pio XII,* VI, 191–192; to Italian Association of Catholic Midwives: AAS 43 (1951), 835–854; to the association known as the Family Campaign, and other family associations: AAS 43 (1951), 857–859; to 7th congress of International Society of Hematology: AAS 50 (1958), 734–735 [TPS VI, 394–395]; John XXIII, encyc. letter *Mater et Magistra:* AAS 53 (1961), 446–447 [TPS VII, 330–331]; Second Vatican Council, *Pastoral Constitution on the Church in the World of Today,* nos. 47–52: AAS 58 (1966), 1067–1074 [TPS XI, 289–295]; Code of Canon Law, canons 1067, 1068 §1, canon 1076, §§1–2.

5. See Paul VI, Address to Sacred College of Cardinals: AAS 56 (1964), 588 [TPS IX, 355–356]; to Commission for the Study of Problems of Population, Family and Birth: AAS 57 (1965), 388 [TPS X, 225]; to National Congress of the Italian Society of Obstetrics and Gynecology: AAS 58 (1966), 1168 [TPS XI, 401–403].

6. See *1 Jn* 4. 8.

7. *Eph* 3. 15.

8. Second Vatican Council, *Pastoral Constitution on the Church in the World of Today,* no. 50: AAS 58 (1966), 1070–1072 [TPS XI, 292–293].

9. See St. Thomas, *Summa Theologiae,* I–II, q. 94, art. 2.

10. See Second Vatican Council, *Pastoral Constitution on the Church in the World of Today,* nos. 50–51: AAS 58 (1966), 1070–1073 [TPS XI, 292–293].

11. See ibid., no. 49: AAS 58 (1966), 1070 [TPS XI, 291–292].

12. See Pius XI, encyc. letter *Casti connubii:* AAS 22 (1930), 560; Pius XII, Address to Midwives: AAS 43 (1951), 843.

13. See encyc. letter *Mater et Magistra:* AAS 53 (1961), 447 [TPS VII, 331].

14. See Council of Trent Roman Catechism, Part II, ch. 8; Pius XI, encyc. letter *Casti connubii:* AAS 22 (1930), 562–564; Pius XII, Address to Medico-Biological Union of St. Luke: *Discorsi e radiomessaggi,* VI, 191–192; Address to Midwives: AAS 43 (1951), 842–843; Address to Family Campaign and other family associations: AAS 43 (1951), 857–859; John XXIII, encyc. letter *Pacem in terris:* AAS 55 (1963), 259–260 [TPS IX, 15–16]; Second Vatican Council, *Pastoral Constitution on the Church in the World of Today,* no. 51: AAS 58 (1966), 1072 [TPS XI, 293].

15. See Pius XI, encyc. letter *Casti connubii:* AAS 22 (1930), 565; Decree of the Holy Office, Feb. 22, 1940: AAS 32 (1940), 73; Pius XII, Address to Midwives: AAS 43 (1951), 843–844; to the Society of Hematology: AAS 50 (1958), 734–735 [TPS VI, 394–395].

16. See Council of Trent Roman Catechism, Part II, ch. 8; Pius XI, encyc. letter *Casti connubii:* AAS 22 (1930), 559–561; Pius XII, Address to Midwives: AAS 43 (1951), 843; to the Society of Hematology: AAS 50 (1958), 734–735 [TPS VI, 394–395]; John XXIII, encyc. letter *Mater et Magistra:* AAS 53 (1961), 447 [TPS VII, 331].

17. See Pius XII, Address to National Congress of Italian Society of the Union of Catholic Jurists: AAS 45 (1953), 798–799 [TPS 1, 67–69].

18. See *Rom* 3. 8.

19. See Pius XII, Address to 26th Congress of Italian Association of Urology: AAS 45 (1953), 674–675; to Society of Hematology: AAS 50 (1958), 734–735 [TPS VI, 394–395].

20. See Pius XII, Address to Midwives: AAS 43 (1951), 846.

21. See Pius XII, Address to Association of Urology: AAS 45 (1953), 674–675; to leaders and members of Italian Association of Cornea Donors and Italian Association for the Blind: AAS 48 (1956), 461–462 [TPS III, 200–201].

22. *Lk* 2. 34.

23. See Paul VI, encyc. letter *Populorum progressio:* AAS 59 (1967), 268 [TPS XII, 151].

24. See *Rom* 8.

25. See Second Vatican Council, *Decree on the Media of Social Communication,* nos. 6–7: AAS 56 (1964), 147 [TPS IX, 340–341].

26. Encyc. letter *Mater et Magistra:* AAS 53 (1961), 447 [TPS VII, 331].

27. See encyc. letter *Populorum progressio,* nos. 48–55: AAS 59 (1967), 281–284 [TPS XII, 160–162].

28. Second Vatican Council, *Pastoral Constitution on the Church in the World of Today,* no. 52: AAS 58 (1966), 1074 [TPS XI, 294].

29. Address to Family Campaign and other family associations: AAS 43 (1951), 859.

30. Second Vatican Council, *Pastoral Constitution on the Church in the World of Today,* no. 51: AAS 58 (1966), 1072 [TPS XI, 293].

31. See *Mt* 11. 30.

32. See Second Vatican Council, *Pastoral Constitution on the Church in the World of Today,* no. 48: AAS 58 (1966), 1067–1069 [TPS XI, 290–291]; *Dogmatic Constitution on the Church,* no. 35: AAS 57 (1965), 40–41 [TPS X, 382–383].

33. *Mt* 7. 14; see *Heb* 12. 11.

34. See *Ti* 2. 12.

35. See *1 Cor* 7. 31.

36. *Rom* 5. 5.

37. *Eph* 5. 25, 28–29, 32–33.

38. See Second Vatican Council, *Dogmatic Constitution on the Church,* nos. 35, 41: AAS 57 (1965), 40–45 [TPS X, 382–383, 386–387]; *Pastoral Constitution on the Church in the World of Today,* nos. 48–49: AAS 58 (1966), 1067–1070 [TPS XI, 290–292]; *Decree on the Apostolate of the Laity,* no. 11: AAS 58 (1966), 847–849 [TPS XI, 128–129].

39. See Second Vatican Counci, *Dogmatic Constitution on the Church,* no. 25: AAS 57 (1965), 29–31 [TPS X, 375–376].

40. *1 Cor* 1. 10.

41. See *Jn* 3. 17.

22

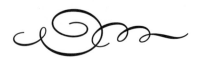

Humanae Vitae 25 Years Later

Richard A. McCormick, S.J.

Reactions to the silver anniversary of *Humanae Vitae* (July 25, 1968) will predictably vary as much as the recent reactions of two cardinals. At the 12th Human Life International World Conference held in Houston (spring 1993), Alfonso López Trujillo, the president of the Pontifical Council for the Family, referred to the teaching of the encyclical as a "gift of God." In a debate with Cardinal Joseph Ratzinger (published in the monthly periodical, *Jesus*, in May 1992), Franz König, the retired Cardinal Archbishop of Vienna, referred to the "irritating distinction between 'artificial' and 'natural' contraception." Cardinal König stated: "Here [on birth regulation] we have ended up in a bottleneck above all because of the distinction (cast into doubt even by medicine) between 'artificial' and 'natural,' as if even from the moral viewpoint what is important is the 'trick' of cheating nature."

It is quite possible to endorse both of these statements. The encyclical had many beautiful things to say about marriage and marital love. In this sense it was a gift. But its most controversial and "irritating" aspect was its rejection of every contraceptive act as intrinsically disordered.

When *Humanae Vitae* first appeared it caused a furor. My yellow and crumbling copy of the *National Catholic Reporter* for August 7, 1968, carries the headline: "Paul Issues Contraceptive Ban: Debate Flares on His Authority." Tom Burns, then the editor of the *London Tablet*, has said the encyclical was "the greatest challenge that came my way." Burns opposed the encyclical. He surmised that "never in the 150 years of the paper's existence has an editor of *The Tablet* been presented with a problem of conscience and policy so grave as that which confronted me with the publication of *Humanae Vitae*."

With that sentence Burns probably summarized the anguish of many bishops, priests, theologians and lay people around the world. Episcopal conferences began issuing pastoral letters on the encyclical. These ran the gamut from celebration to qualification. For instance, the Belgian bishops stated: "Someone, however, who is competent in the matter under consideration and capable of forming a personal and well-founded judgment—which necessarily presupposes a sufficient amount of knowledge—may, after a serious examination before God, come to other conclusions on certain points. In such a case he has the right to follow his conviction provided that he remains sincerely disposed to continue his inquiry." Of those who arrived at conclusions different from *Humanae Vitae*, the Scandinavian bishops stated: "No one should, therefore, on account of such diverging opinions alone, be regarded as an inferior Catholic." The Canadian bishops made a similar statement: "These Catholics should not be considered, or consider themselves, shut off from the body of the faithful."

Charles Curran composed a statement critical of the ecclesiology and methodology of *Humanae Vitae*. The statement concluded that "spouses may responsibly decide according to their conscience that artificial contraception in some circumstances is permissible and indeed necessary to preserve and foster the value and sacredness of marriage." This statement was eventually signed by over 600 theologians and other academics, including well-known theologians such as Bernard Häring, David Tracy, Richard McBrien, Walter Burghardt, Raymond Collins, Roland Murphy and Bernard McGinn. A group of European theologians met in Amsterdam on Sept. 18–19, 1968, and issued a dissenting statement. The signatories included some of the best known theologians in Europe: J. M. Aubert, A. Auer, T. Beemer, F. Böckle, W. Bulst, P. Fransen, J. Groot, P. Huizing, L. Janssens, R. van Kessel, W. Klijn, F. Klostermann, E. McDonagh, C. Robert, P. Schoonenberg, M. de Wachter.

These were heady days indeed. Overnight, dissent became a front-burner issue. Any number of episcopal conferences mentioned its possibility and legitimacy. The American bishops in their pastoral letter, "Human Life in Our Day" (Nov. 15, 1968), even laid out the norms for licit dissent. Expression of dissent is in order "only if the reasons are serious and well founded, if the manner of the dissent does not question or impugn the teaching authority of the Church and is such as not to give scandal." Paul VI himself, in a letter to the Congress of German Catholics (Aug. 30, 1968), stated: "May the lively debate aroused by our encyclical lead to a better knowledge of God's will."

Summarizing in these pages (*America*, 9/28/68) what had been said by several European hierarchies, Avery Dulles, S.J., issued this warning:

> In view of the American tradition of freedom and pluralism, it would be a serious mistake to use the encyclical as a kind of Catholic loyalty test. Nothing could so quickly snuff out the spirit of personal responsibility, which has done so much to invigorate American Catholicism in the past few years.
>
> Nothing could be more discouraging to young people and intellectuals, upon whom the future of our Church so greatly depends. Nothing could be more destructive of the necessary autonomy of Catholic universities and journals, which have begun to prosper so well. Nothing, finally, could be more harmful to the mutual relations of trust and cordiality that have recently been established between bishops and theologians.

So what has happened in the past 25 years? Father Dulles's worst fears have become reality. Five years after the publication of *Humanae Vitae* I wrote in these pages that the encyclical "produced shock and/or solace, suspension, silence—pretty much in that order" (7/2/73). I added that the matter of contraception provokes a yawn of public boredom, and I worried aloud that the church, by doing nothing, was playing the ostrich in face of massive dissent and thereby compromising the credibility of the teaching office. I argued that "if dissent is to be taken seriously within the community, it cannot be viewed as simply legally tolerable, a kind of paternal eye-shutting to the errors or immaturities of a child." It must be viewed as a source of new reflection in the church. Otherwise, personal reflection has been ruled out of order in the teaching-learning process of the church.

A source of new reflection? That has not happened. The uneasy silence continued, abetted by the fact that many bishops and priests just did not have their hearts in it.

On Sept. 26, 1980, the fifth Synod of Bishops began. Its subject: the family. There were several interesting interventions touching birth regulation. Cardinal Basil Hume of England insisted that those who experience the sacrament of marriage constitute "an authentic *fons theologiae* [theological source]." For some, the problem of *Humanae Vitae* remains a real problem not because of their frailty and weakness. "They just cannot accept that the use of artificial means of contraception in some circumstances is *intrinsece inhonestum* [intrinsically disordered]." Hume concluded that "if we [the Synod fathers] listen to all the different points of view," a right way will be found.

The most interesting intervention was that of Archbishop John R. Quinn of San Francisco. He noted that many men and women of good will do not accept the "intrinsic evil of each and every use of contraception." This conviction is shared by a majority of priests and theologians, a conviction found among "theologians and pastors whose learning, faith, discretion, and dedication to the church are beyond doubt." Archbishop Quinn argued that this cannot be dismissed. He noted that the church "has always recognized the principle and fact of doctrinal development." There, he proposed three things: 1) a new context for the teaching; 2) a widespread and worldwide dialogue between the Holy See and theologians on the meaning of this dissent; 3) careful attention to the process by which magisterial documents are written and communicated. He then elaborated these three points.

This was a careful, realistic and courageous statement. Careful—because the problem was stated accurately. For instance, Archbishop Quinn noted that the problem of many theologians is not that they view contraception as "simply something good, desirable or indifferent." The problem is the usage of "intrinsically evil" to apply to every contraceptive act. Realistic—because Archbishop Quinn was absolutely correct in saying that "this problem is not going to be solved or reduced merely by a simple reiteration of past formulations or by ignoring the fact of dissent." Courageous—because the suggestions were made in the presence of the Pope, whose views on this matter were well known and who therefore could not be thought to have called the Synod to have them questioned. I say "questioned" because Archbishop Quinn did refer to "doctrinal development" in areas such as biblical studies and religious liberty. In these contexts development meant change.

Archbishop Quinn's remarks were widely publicized and bluntly rejected by some American prelates of a more immobilist caste of mind. Interventions like those of Cardinal Hume and Archbishop Quinn got nowhere. The interesting intervention of Durban's Archbishop Denis Hurley ("the act of artificially limiting the exercise of one faculty of life is intrinsically evil while the act of exterminating life itself is not") never even made the published synopses of the Synod. It finally appeared in *The Tablet* (1980, pp. 1105–1107).

Thomas Reese, S.J., a reporter at the Synod, summarized events of the time as follows:

> The lay auditors were not representative of the church, but were in fact firm promoters of natural family planning. The majority of Catholic families, which practice birth control, were not represented. Nor were dissenting theologians welcome at the Synod. As a result no true dialogue was really possible. Any criticism of *Humanae Vitae* was considered scandalous. The final message ignored the population crisis. Some bishops were afraid to say what they really thought because they feared they would be misrepresented by the press or seen as challenging positions held by Pope Paul VI and John Paul II (*America*, 11/8/80).

The Tablet referred to "foregone conclusions virtually imposed on a so-called consultative body" (1980, p. 1059). In a word, the Synod was orchestrated, and perhaps that was a sign of things to come.

What things? The well-known fact that for some years now acceptance of *Humanae Vitae* has become one of the litmus tests for episcopal appointment. The fact that theologians who question it are excluded from speaking in some dioceses and seminaries, and are regularly denounced by the right wing press as "dissidents" and "disloyal." The fact that great numbers of Catholics no longer look to the church for enlightenment in the area of sexual morality. The fact that bishops do not feel free to state their opinions honestly.

At the present, therefore, we are far from Archbishop Quinn's proposed worldwide dialogue between theologians and the Holy See, and from Cardinal Hume's listening "to all the points of view." Rather, the atmosphere in the church on the matter of birth regulation is one of coercion. Bishop Kenneth Untener of Saginaw, Mich., adverted to this at the November 1990 U.S. bishops' meeting. Of the church's teaching on birth regulation, he said: "Many would compare us [bishops] to a dysfunctional family that is unable to talk openly about a problem that everyone knows is there."

John Paul II has become increasingly absolute and intransigent on the matter. On June 5, 1987, he stated to a conference on responsible procreation: "The Church's teaching on contraception does not belong to the category of matter open to free discussion among theologians. Teaching the contrary amounts to leading the moral consciences of spouses into error" (*L'Osservatore Romano*, English edition, July 6, 1987).

Indeed, the Sovereign Pontiff raises the stakes by tying the teaching to central truths of the faith (e.g., God's goodness), a move often described in Germany as "dogmatization" (*Dogmatisierung*). This was protested by 163 theologians from Germany, Austria, the Netherlands and Switzerland in the so-called "Cologne Declaration" (Jan. 27, 1989). The concerns of this declaration were subsequently endorsed by 130 French theologians, 60 Spanish theologians, 63 Italian theologians and 431 members of the Catholic Theological Society of America (*Origins*, Dec. 27, 1990).

Bernard Häring, C.SS.R., the eminent moral theologian, has pointed out that there are in the church today *two schools of thought* (*Commonweal*, Feb. 10, 1989).

The *first* is that the contraceptive act is always a grave moral wrong regardless of circumstances. This is God's law inscribed in human persons and confirmed by revelation. Those who doubt or deny this deny God's holiness and reject the teaching of the church as well as of their own conscience.

The *second* position insists that the basic issue is not primarily one of method, but of attitude. Spouses are called to generous but responsible openness to new life. Where methods are concerned, more intrusive forms of contraception will not be used where less intrusive ones (natural family planning) satisfy the needs of marital love and responsible parenthood. But artificial methods cannot be ruled out as intrinsically morally wrong.

These positions have hardened over the years, and reasoned discourse has often been replaced by the accusatory rhetoric of intolerance, especially by proponents of the first school of thought. The inability—or refusal—of the magisterium to deal with this problem except by repetition has resulted in a debilitating malaise that has undermined the credibility of the magisterium in other areas.

The anniversary of *Humanae Vitae* provides the occasion to raise two questions: 1. What is the issue? 2. What can the church do about the present impasse?

1. What is the issue?

There are, of course, any number of important issues inseparable from *Humanae Vitae*: the role of the pope and the other bishops in so-called "natural law" teaching; the sources of such teaching; the place of experience and human reflection; the binding force of the teaching; the reformability of such teaching, and so on. But the single issue that provoked the hailstorm of reactions was the teaching that every contraceptive act is intrinsically disordered (*intrinsece inhonestum*, No. 14). It is clear that Paul VI meant by this phrase intrinsically morally wrong. Absent that teaching, *Humanae Vitae* would be bannered as a beautiful contemporary statement on conjugal love and responsible parenthood.

At this point it would be helpful to emphasize what is *not* the issue. Certain apologists for *Humanae Vitae* assert that those who disagree with its central assertion "promote contraception" and by implication denigrate natural family planning. That is seriously to misplace the contemporary debate. Natural family planning is highly method-effective for highly motivated couples. For some, perhaps many, people it might be the method of choice, though how many can sustain the high motivation is a legitimate concern. But its desirability is not in question. The basic issue is the moral wrongfulness of some other methods. "Each and every marriage act must remain open to the transmission of life," the encyclical states. That teaching is elaborated as follows:

> That teaching, often set forth by the magisterium, is founded upon the inseparable connection, willed by God and unable to be broken by man on his own initiative, between the two meanings of the conjugal act, the unitive meaning and the procreative meaning. Indeed, by its intimate structure, the conjugal act, while most closely uniting husband and wife, capacitates them for the generation of new lives, according to laws inscribed in the very being of man and woman. By safeguarding both these essential aspects, the unitive and the procreative, the conjugal act preserves in its fullness the sense of true mutual love and its ordination toward man's most high calling to parenthood (No. 12).

Paul VI believed that people of our day "are particularly capable of seizing the deeply reasonable and human character of this fundamental principle." That has not happened. Indeed, the negative reaction was so widespread and intense that Bishop Christopher Butler stated that the encyclical was not received by the church, a phenomenon he viewed as "invalidating" the teaching (reported in *The Tablet*, March 13, 1993).

In *Familiaris Consortio* (1981), John Paul II repeated Paul VI's condemnation of contraceptive interventions, but in more personalistic terms. Sexual intercourse is presented as a language that "expresses the total reciprocal self-giving of husband and wife." But by contraceptive intervention this language is overlaid and contradicted by another language, "that of not giving oneself totally to the other."

The hidden supposition of this analysis is that *self*-giving is determined by the *physical* openness of the individual act. The burden of the discussion since *Humanae Vitae* has been precisely the question of whether the *giving of self* can be tied so closely with the physical structure of the act. As Lisa Sowle Cahill put it in her John Courtney Murray Forum lecture: "I am confident that most Catholic couples would be incredulous at the proposition that the use of artificial birth control necessarily makes their sexual intimacy selfish, dishonest and unfaithful. Nor is their valuing of parenthood based on their experience of isolated sex acts as having a certain 'procreative' structure" (*America*, 5/22/93). This consideration points us back to earlier history.

In commenting on the single controversial issue of *Humanae Vitae*, the late Bernard Lonergan, S.J., a renowned theologian, remarked: "The traditional views [on contraception] to my mind are based on Aristotelian biology and later stuff which is all wrong. They haven't got the facts straight" (*Catholic New Times*, Oct. 14, 1984).

What Lonergan was referring to was the analysis of the sexual act found in Aristotle's *De generatione animalium*. Male seed was viewed as an efficient cause that changed the nutritive material supplied by the female. According to this view every act of insemination (intercourse) is of itself procreative.

We now know, of course, that Aristotle was wrong. It must be recalled here that it was only in 1827 that Karl Ernst von Baer published his discovery of the ovum. The relation of insemination to procreation, we now know, is not that of a per se cause to a per se effect. The relation of intercourse to procreation is statistical, the vast majority of acts not leading to conception. Paul VI stated that "the conjugal act . . . capacitates them for the generation of new lives." That is true of only very few conjugal acts.

Humanae Vitae correctly acknowledges that sexual intercourse has a "unitive sense"; it expresses and nourishes mutual love. But it argues that each act also has a "procreative sense." This Lonergan, together with many others, contests. Even the encyclical seems shaky on this point. It notes that acts of sexual intercourse remain lawful during foreseen infertile periods "since they always remain ordained towards expressing and consolidating their union" (No. 11). The rather clear implication is that there is no ordination towards procreation, no procreative sense. A procreative sense in every act would be understandable if one accepted Aristotle's biology. In this light phrases such as "an act per se apt for procreation" and "open to procreation" are linear descendants and contemporary remnants of Aristotle's view. Lonergan would argue, however, if the relation of intercourse to procreation is only statistical, then one must ask if this statistical relationship is inviolable. If it is, then even natural family planning is excluded. If it is not, then artificial contraception can be permissible under certain conditions.

In summary, most theologians now argue that all forms of birth regulation—including natural family planning—contain negative elements. These could be psychological, medical aesthetic, ecological. What they have denied is that introducing such elements in our conduct is always morally wrong. Attempts to establish this moral wrongfulness have been and still are viewed as unpersuasive. As Cardinal König noted, a "bottleneck." We could say that many theologians accept the inseparability of the unitive and procreative if this inseparability is applied to the relationship, not each act. Couples bind themselves to a covenant that unites the conjugal and parental vocation. Their love is generously open to life, and procreation is the result of their deep personal love.

This raises the interesting question of the relation of a conclusion to the analyses available to support it. Paul VI was aware of this problem, for in No. 28 of the encyclical he exhorted priests to obedience "not only because of the reasons adduced, but rather because of the light of the Holy Spirit, which is given in a particular way to the pastors of the Church." It is certainly true that a teaching can be correct even when the reasons are faulty. But it is quite a different thing to propose a teaching of natural law as certain when, after many years, most theologians can find no persuasive reasoning to support its absoluteness.

Several bishops at the 1980 Synod asserted that *Humanae Vitae* was "certainly correct" but that "better reasons" had to be found to validate its conclusions. But what if after many years "better reasons" have not been found, at least as most theologians view the matter? To continue to maintain the conclusion as certainly correct is perilously close to saying that the formulation is correct regardless of the reasons. Catholic theological tradition will not, in my judgment, support this. And that brings us to the second point.

2. What should the church do about the present impasse?

Undoubtedly, there are those who would say that there would be no impasse and all would be well if theologians would fall in line and support the teaching of *Humanae Vitae,* or at least remain silent. Yet many would—and correctly, I believe—regard this as an abrogation of theological responsibility and an act of disloyalty to the church and the Holy Father. As the late and eminent Karl Rahner put it: "What are contemporary moral theologians to make of Roman declarations on sexual morality that they regard as too unnuanced? Are they to remain silent, or is it their task to dissent, to give a more nuanced interpretation?" Rahner's response is unhesitating: "I beieve that the theologian, after mature reflection, has the right, and many times the duty, to speak out against (*widersprechen*) a teaching of the magisterium and to support his dissent" (*Stimmen der Zeit,* Vol. 198, 1980).

Bernard Häring proposed that the Pope establish a special commission and charge it with the task of inquiring of bishops, theological faculties and important lay people which of the two schools of thought mentioned above should prevail in the church. Theologian André Naud of the University of Montreal believes that Häring's proposal is far more acceptable than the paralyzed status quo, but he finally rejects it for two reasons. First, he believes it represents an investment disproportionate to the importance of the matter, and one very likely to obscure the hierarchy of truths and to deepen the painful existing polarization. Second, it would rehash what is already known, since the issues have been on the table for many years (*L'Église Canadienne,* April 6, 1989).

Whether one sides with Häring's or Naud's solution will very likely depend on where one locates the question. If the basic question is judged to be the problem of the means of birth regulation, Naud is probably right. No commission is going to affect the practice of Catholics. They have quietly taken this matter into their own consciences. But if the question is above all an authority problem, then something close to Häring's proposal seems essential if the magisterium hopes to regain any credibility. Such a blue-ribbon commission would constitute a symbol of the church's openness and willingness to discuss the matter afresh. It would renew hope in many alienated Catholics.

I view the matter of the church's teaching on birth regulation as dominantly an authority problem. By that I mean that any analysis, conclusion or process that challenges or threatens previous authoritative statements is by that very fact rejected. Any modification of past authority is viewed as an attack on present authority. Behind such an attitude is an unacknowledged and historically unsupportable triumphalism, the idea that the official teaching authority of the church is always right, never errs, is always totally adequate in its formulations. Vatican II radically axed this idea in many ways, but nowhere more explicitly than in its November 1964 "Decree on Ecumenism": "Therefore, if the influence of events or of the times has led to deficiencies in conduct, in Church discipline, or *even in the formulation of doctrine* (which must be carefully distinguished from the deposit of faith itself), these should be appropriately rectified at the proper moment" (my emphasis, No. 6).

But on this question that remains unthinkable. Thus Paul VI rejected the recommendations of his commission to modify church teaching because he was led to fear that his teaching authority would be eroded. Subsequent attempts (e.g., the Synod of 1980) to reopen the issue have been summarily rejected and the church's teaching declared not "open to free discussion among theologians." A similar fear seems to lurk behind such assertions. What would happen if national episcopates would hold truly open consultations on birth regulation similar to those that led to the pastorals on peace and the economy? I think the answer is only too clear. We would have a replay of the deliberations of the Birth Control Commission, and, if we did, authority would see itself as threatened. Therefore it cannot happen. As Bishop Untener puts it: "a dysfunctional family." The lesson of the open procedure of the pastoral letters has not been learned: The best and only way to enhance authority in the modern world is to share it. To save our lives, so to speak, we must lose them. Catholics above all should know this.

On the 25th anniversary of *Humanae Vitae* it is important to point out, with Naud, that there are abiding substantial values that all disputants share and want to protect: the holiness of marriage, generous and responsible openness to life, the human character of the expression of married love, the fidelity and stability of marriage and respect for life. If these get lost in debates about the means of birth regulation, as I fear they may have, then to the malaise of polarization will have been added the tragedy of irrelevance. The means-question will have smothered the more basic message, a state of affairs from which only the Spirit can deliver us.

23

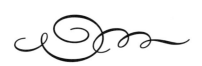

Some Theological Considerations on *Humanae Vitae*

Janet E. Smith

Humanae Vitae 4 states that the teaching of the Church concerning marriage is a teaching "rooted in natural law, illuminated and made richer by divine revelation." This chapter takes up a few of the theological considerations of the encyclical. First, it examines briefly the scriptural foundations for *Humanae Vitae* and shows how these "illuminate and enrich" (HV 4) its natural law foundations. Then follows a theological discussion of a very different sort. The word *munus* (which means variously, "gift," "reward," "duty," "task," and "mission," among other possibilities) and the concept it captures, as shaped in the documents of Vatican II, are explored. We shall see that this concept greatly enriches our understanding of the Church's valuation of childbearing and its consequent condemnation of contraception. The final portion of this chapter is on the questions of conscience and infallibility. Conscience is not strictly a theological concept, but insofar as violation of conscience in the Catholic tradition constitutes not simple wrongdoing, but sin, that is, an offense against God, it seems appropriate to discuss conscience along with other theological matters. And certainly, if the teaching of *Humanae Vitae* has been proclaimed infallibly, special constraints will be felt by the Catholic conscience to accept this teaching.

SCRIPTURAL FOUNDATIONS FOR THE TEACHING OF *HUMANAE VITAE*[1]

Scripture, of course, does not provide any statement that explicitly states, "Thou shalt not contracept."[2] Those in the Protestant tradition may be troubled by this, but in the Catholic tradition lack of explicit condemnation is no insuperable barrier to claiming that a teaching has scriptural foundation. Scripture also says nothing, for instance, about the morality of directly bombing civilian sites, but such an action clearly violates the Fifth Commandment, "Thou shalt not murder (that is, directly and deliberately kill the innocent)." The Church argues that both natural law and Scripture make clear the immorality of such an action.

The scriptural basis for the condemnation of contraception is not quite so straightforward as the example just given. Nonetheless, there are at least four themes in Scripture that provide strong evidence that contraception does not fit within God's plan for human sexuality. These are (1) the extreme value given to procreation, (2) the portrayal of sterility as a great curse, (3) the condemnation of all sexual acts that are not designed to protect the good of procreation, and (4) the likening of Christ's relationship to His Church to that of a bridegroom to his bride, a union that is meant to be a fecund relationship, one that will bring forth many sons and daughters of God. There is a wealth of scriptural material on all these issues; here it will be sufficient simply to sketch out how this evidence works to show the immorality of contraception. And let this caution be stated: Scripture is always open to various interpretations; particular readings of various texts here may be controversial and perhaps on occasion, highly questionable, though every effort has been made to offer interpretations that are not speculative but altogether straightforward. The hope is that the general thrust of the argument is not without warrant.

It is of no small significance that the first relevant texts are located at the very beginning of Scripture, in the very first chapters of Genesis. There we see God first as a creator, as one who brings about the existence of everything, as one who produces life. What we first learn about Man is that he is made in the image and likeness of God when "male and female He created them." It would not seem that the male alone images God, but that "male and female" do. In the context this suggests that Man images God in His creative powers as much as in any of His other powers. Indeed, once God has created male and female and thus brought about the actuality of human sexuality, His first directive to Man is "Be fertile and multiply; fill the earth and subdue it" (Gen. 1:27). We also quickly learn that man and woman are to become "one flesh." This seems to refer to the union that they achieve through having a child, which is one flesh of their two, as much as to the conjugal act itself, which makes two "one flesh."

Man is to share in God's abundance and fruitfulness through his procreative power. Thus, fertility and fruitfulness seem to be part of the covenant that Man has with God. When God renews His covenant with Man through Noah (and again when He makes a covenant with Abraham), He repeats His initial mandate: "Be fertile and multiply and fill the earth" (Gen. 9:1). Certainly, the other creatures are to multiply, too, but they are under the dominion of Man whereas Man is under the dominion of God. Animals reproduce, but Man procreates.

Throughout the Old Testament, fertility and family are portrayed as great goods, as evidence of faithfulness to God, as rewards for faithfulness to God. One of God's promises to Abram was "I will make your descendants like the dust of the earth; if anyone could count the dust of the earth, your descendants too might be counted" (Gen. 13:16). God was not quick to deliver on this promise; Abram's wife Sarai was barren until her old age. When Abram was ninety-nine years old, God made a covenant with him and made this His first promise: "I will render you exceedingly fertile; I will make nations of you . . ." (Gen. 17:6). Sarah at this point was ninety, but she bore Abram a son. God clearly wanted to show that He was lord of life, that fertility was His great gift. Children were not viewed as a burden but as a sign of favor and wealth. This is so throughout the Old Testament. Perhaps Psalm 127 says it best:

> Unless the Lord build the house, they labor in vain who build it.
> Unless the Lord guard the city, in vain does the guard keep vigil.
> It is vain for you to rise early, or put off your rest,
> You that eat hard-earned bread for he gives to his beloved in sleep.
> Behold, sons are a gift from the Lord; the fruit of the womb is a reward.
> Like arrows in the hand of a warrior are the sons of one's youth.
> Happy the man whose quiver is filled with them; they shall not be put to shame when they contend with enemies at the gate.[3]

In this context contraception could be seen as a rejection of a gift from God, as an action stunting the growth of God's chosen people, for which reason, to this day, Orthodox Judaism rejects contraception.

Passages indicating and singing the praises of fruitfulness could be multiplied abundantly, but let us here turn to the point that the opposite of fruitfulness, sterility or barrenness, is considered a great hardship and even a curse. Many of the key figures in Scripture suffered from infertility. Sarah's story has been told; Hannah, eventual mother of Samuel, prayed day and night to bear a child; Rachel was finally "remembered by God" and bore Joseph; Elizabeth in her old age bore John the Baptist. Since fruitfulness was so much a part of participation in the work of the chosen people, in God's plan, sterility was often considered a sign of disfavor or sinfulness; thus women begged God to relieve them, not of the burden of childbearing but of the burden of childlessness. Psalm 113 praises the Lord in this way:

> He raises up the lowly from the dust; from the dunghill he lifts up the poor
> To set them with princes, with the princes of his own people.
> He establishes in her home the barren wife as the joyful mother of children.

Again, contraception does not fit into this picture of the value of fertility; insofar as contraception renders one at least temporarily infertile, users of contraception would seem to be voluntarily putting themselves in a highly unenviable position.

Scripture does not explicitly condemn contraception, but it does condemn sexual relationships that are not designed to serve the good of procreation. Fornication, adultery, homosexual acts, and bestiality are typically included on the list of serious sins. In Romans 1:2 homosexuality is called an unnatural act, seemingly because the sexual acts of homosexuals are not ordained to procreation, the natural end of the sexual organs. Followers of Yahweh are not to participate in such acts; those who worship false gods regularly do. Misuse of sexuality seems to result whenever Man severs his relationship with God. Reestablishing right sexual relationships is part of the work of getting right with God again.

Finally, the great good of marriage is sung repeatedly throughout Scripture. The prophets regularly liken God's relationship to His people to a marital one: it is to be fruitful. It is jarring to think of contraception being a part of that relationship, to think of God's withholding His creative power from His chosen one. When He does, it is as a punishment for sin. Hosea at 4:7–10 warns:

> One and all they sin against me, exchanging their glory for shame.
> They feed on the sin of my people, and are greedy for their guilt.
> The priests shall fare no better than the people: I will punish them for their ways, and repay them for their deeds.
> They shall eat but not be satisfied, they shall play the harlot but not increase,
> Because they have abandoned the Lord to practice harlotry.

The new covenant instituted by Christ is, as were all the covenants, a marital one, to be marked by great fruitfulness. We might note that the first miracle that Christ performed, the changing of water into wine, was at a wedding feast. It was a miracle that celebrates abundance, as were many of the miracles of Christ (think, too, of the multiplication of the loaves and fishes). There is not a hint in Scripture that marriage or sexuality used properly is bad. Marriage, especially fruitful marriage, is a great good. Again, just as it is jarring—not to say scandalous—to think of contraceptives coming between God and the Israelites, so, too, is it jarring to think of any obstacle to the loving union of Christ and his Church. Insofar as married couples are to image that relationship (compare Ephesians 5), it would seem that the use of contraception violates the image they are to be.

Marriage, procreation, fertility, and fruitfulness, then, are all values sung in various ways throughout Scripture. Sterility and barrenness are not marks of those with God but of those separated from Him. Where is there room for contraception in this picture of God's plan for human sexuality, of God's plan for marriage, of God's plan for His people?

Scriptural Foundations for Specific Natural Law Arguments

Chapter 4 [of the author's *Humanae Vitae: A Generation Later*] set forth four different arguments based on natural law principles that purport to show the immorality of contraception. All these versions—the intrinsic worth of human life argument, the special act of creation argument, the contraception is contralife argument, and the violation of the unitive meaning of the conjugal act argument—all can be greatly strengthened by reference to Scripture. The value that Scripture puts on human life because of both its nature and its destiny, the view of God as author of life, the view of God as author of nature, and the understanding of God as an "unconditional" lover all illumine and enrich natural law arguments.[4]

Natural law can certainly establish the intrinsic value of human life, since there are rational grounds for valuing human beings above all else. But Scripture gives us even further warrant for treating human life as something of great intrinsic worth. For instance, it teaches us that Man is made in the image and likeness of God. God also has great plans for Man, namely eternal union with Him. The Christian view of God as one who created a universe precisely because He wanted to share His goodness with others puts a value on fertility far beyond what natural reason can readily discover. God clearly wants multitudes with whom to share His goodness, to be with Him in eternal union. In this light, contraception can be seen as being a kind of denial of God's plan that Heaven be populated through love, His love and the love of spouses. *Humanae Vitae* 8 states: "Conjugal love most clearly manifests to us its true nature and nobility when we recognize that it has its origin in the highest source as it were, in God, Who 'is Love' and Who is the Father, 'from whom all parenthood in heaven and earth receives its name.'" Footnote references to this passage cite 1 John 4, "The man without love has known nothing of God, for God is love," and the passage from Ephesians cited previously. The relationships of God, love, and family, then, are greatly underscored by Scripture. Thus by respecting Man we are respecting God.

The story of creation and all the revelations of God's special intervention in the creation of new life, in the miraculous conceptions of infertile women, all portray God as the Lord of Life. Through Scripture God is referred to as the Lord of Life. *Humanae Vitae* 8 cites Ephesians 3:15: "[God, Who is Love] is the Father from whom every family in heaven and earth is named." Psalm 139 gives beautiful testimony to God's interest in life long before birth:

> Truly you have formed my inmost being: you knit me in my mother's womb.
> I give you thanks that I am fearfully, wonderfully made; wonderful are your works.
> My soul also you knew full well; nor was my frame unknown to you
> When I was made in secret,
>   when I was fashioned in the depths of the earth.
> Your eyes have seen my actions; in your book were they all written; my days were limited
>   before one of them existed.
> How weighty are your designs, O God; how vast the sum of them!
> Were I to recount them, they would outnumber the sands; did I reach the end of them, I
>   should still be with you.

As Psalm 139 manifests, the God of Scripture is not the distant God of the philosophers, who is the God behind nature, an unmoved mover who set this ordered world in motion. The Judeo-Christian God is a "hands-on" creator, who pronounces His creation "good" and who takes an ongoing interest in it. The miracles of Scripture, such as the parting of the Red Sea, Christ's calming of the wind and sea, multiplication of loaves and fishes, and healings, all suggest a God who is master of nature. Thus, again, by respecting nature we are respecting God.

The natural law argument (version F), which argues that contraception is wrong because it violates the unitive meaning of the conjugal act, is also much strengthened by Scripture. The concept of marriage as requiring total self-giving is one that Man may be able to grasp through his reason. Scripture, however, manifestly portrays marriage in this light, especially in the portrait (given previously) of God's covenantal relationship with His people. Several sections of *Humanae Vitae* assure spouses that grace is available to them in their attempt to live their marital life in accord with God's will.[5] God gives totally and abundantly to His people and will assist them in giving totally to one another. Again, it seems difficult if not impossible to consider contraception a part of a relationship of total giving.

Scripture, then, illuminates and enriches the natural law understanding of marriage, sexuality, and contraception in many different ways. If the preceding interpretations of Scripture are correct, those who accept Scripture as a revelation of God's will should be greatly strengthened in their reasoned conviction that contraception is immoral. Catholic theology, though, works with more than Scripture. Through the tradition of the Church certain themes are developed in such a way that they greatly illumine the proper role of a Christian in this world. In fact the concept of *munus* is one of those very concepts that clarify how we are best to live a Christ-centered life.

The Concept of *Munus*[6]

Let us draw on the concept of *munus* to assist us in understanding the claim that spouses are turning their back on God when they use contraception. This concept may "enrich and illumine" our understanding of the natural law arguments against contraception. First we shall need to establish the meaning of this concept and to suggest how it weaves together some of the themes of earlier Church documents on marriage and *Humanae Vitae*. Then we shall make a particular application of this concept to the condemnation of contraception.

The word *munus* has a fairly technical meaning in the documents of the Church. One appearance, most relevant to our concerns, helps to close the section of *Gaudium et Spes* pertaining to marriage. "Let all be convinced that human life and [the *munus* of] its transmission are realities whose meaning is not limited by the horizons of this life only; their true evaluation and full meaning can only be understood in reference to man's eternal destiny" (GS 51).[7] The first line of *Humanae Vitae* speaks of "the most serious duty [*munus*] of transmitting human life," a phrase that clearly picks up this final portion of GS 51. Here let us first determine the meaning of this word and then consider how it might shed light on the relationship between the procreative values of marriage and the personalist values. This word seems to give us access to a dimension of the encyclical often neglected, a dimension that stresses the positive aspect of having children.

As we have seen, childbearing is a very important part of the responsibility of spouses. It flows not only out of the love that the spouses have for each other but from the love that God has for spouses and for the new life they bring forth. Childbearing is, in fact, a "special assignment," a *munus*, which God has entrusted to spouses. A proper understanding of this term should help illuminate the claim that childbearing is not only an act that spouses perform as a natural outcome of their love for each other but at the same time a service they perform for God. It will also assist us in understanding how the personalist values of marriage are intimately linked with the procreative good of marriage and how, by fulfilling the *munus* of having children, the spouses are advancing the perfecting of their persons.

As noted, the word "*munus*" appears in the very first line of *Humanae Vitae* (*Humanae Vitae tradendae munus gravissimum*...). This line is usually rendered "The most serious duty of transmitting human life...." The translation "duty" for *munus* is not incorrect, but it is inadequate, as is any one word, to capture all its important connotations. (Indeed, there is good reason to believe that the translation "duty" is not of *munus* but of the Italian *dovere*, for most English translations are primarily from the Italian text.)[8] The chief problem with the translation "duty" is that for many modern English-speaking people the word has a negative sense. A duty is often thought of as something that one ought to do and something that one often is reluctant to do; those who are responsible will perform their duties and may enjoy so doing, but they are thought to transcend what is negative about duties. The word *munus*, though, truly seems to be without negative connotations; in fact, a *munus* is something that one is honored and, in a sense, privileged to have. "Duty" is more properly the English translation of *officium*, one of the possible synonyms of *munus*.[9] It seems fair to say that a *munus* often confers or entails *officia*; that is, when one receives a *munus* one also is then committed to certain duties. What, then, is a *munus*? (Throughout most of the following analysis "*munus*" [plural, *munera*] is used, rather than any single English word or a multiplicity of words; for the references to the documents of Vatican II, both Flannery's[10] and Abbott's[11] translations are given in parentheses, in that order.)

One who knows classical Latin would as readily translate *munus* as "gift," "wealth and riches," "honor," or "responsibility" as "duty." Other English translations commonly used are "role," "task," "mission," "office," and "function"; indeed all of these are on occasion legitimate translations, and on a few occasions the word embraces all of these connotations. One common classical Latin use of the word that captures most of these connotations designates a public office or responsibility that has been bestowed on a citizen. Being selected for such an office would entail certain duties, but ones that the recipient willingly embraces. The word is also often used synonymously for "gift" or "reward";[12] It is something freely given by the giver and often, but not always, with the connotation that the recipient has merited the gift in some sense; it is given as a means of honoring the recipient. In Scripture and in the writings of Aquinas *munus* refers both to gifts that Men consecrate to God and to gifts and graces that Men receive from God. For instance, Ephesians refers to the different gifts (*diversi status et munera*), such as being an apostle, prophet, or teacher, with which Men are endowed to serve the Church and God. Rather than being a burdensome duty, a *munus* is much closer to being an assignment or mission that is conferred as an honor on one who can be trusted and who is chosen to share the responsibility of performing good and important work.

The words *vocation* (*vocatio*), *mission* (*missio*), *ministry* (*ministerium*), (which seems often to be a synonym for *apostolate* [*apostolatus*]), *munus*, and *duty* (*officium*) are often linked and occasionally interchangeable; the order of the list just given suggests a possible ranking of these words as far as comprehensiveness is concerned: that is, all Christians have the mission of bringing Christ to the world; they do so through different ministries or apostolates that involve various *munera* and carry certain duties. The second section of *Apostolicam Actuositatem* (*On the Apostolate of Lay People*) illustrates well one variation of the interconnection of these terms:

> The Church was established for this purpose, that by spreading the kingdom of God everywhere for the glory of God, she might make all men participants in Christ's saving redemption, and that through them the whole world might truly be ordered to God. All apostolic [*apostolatus*] activity of the Mystical Body of Christ is directed to this end, which the Church achieves through all of its members, in various ways; for the Christian vocation [*vocatio*], by its very nature is a vocation [*vocatio*] to an apostolate [*apostolatus*]. Just as in the make-up of a living body, no member is able to be altogether passive, but must share in the operation of the body along with the life of this body, so too, in the body of Christ, which is the Church, the whole body must work towards the increase of the body, "according to the function and measure of each member of the body" (Eph. 4, 16). Indeed in this body the connection and union of the members is so great (cf. Eph. 4, 16), that the member which does not contribute to the increase of the body according to its own measure, is said to benefit neither itself nor the Church.
>
> There is in the Church a diversity of ministries [*ministerii*] but a unity of mission [*missionis*]. The *munus* of teaching, sanctifying, and governing in the name and with the power of Christ has been conferred by Christ on the Apostles and their successors. But the laity, having been made participants in the priestly, prophetic, and kingly *munera*, are to discharge their own share in this mission of the whole people of God, in the Church and in the world. (AA 2)[13]

The documents of Vatican II make liberal use of the word *munus*; the index lists 248 appearances of it. One primary reference of the word is seen in the preceding passage; it is to the triple *munera* of Christ as being Priest, Prophet, and King (LG 31). Christians, in their various callings, participate in these *munera*; they do so by fulfilling other *munera*, specifically entrusted to them. For instance, Mary's *munus* (office, role) is being the Mother of God (LG 53), which also confers on her a maternal *munus* (function, duty) toward all Men (LG 60). Christ gave Peter several *munera*: for instance, Peter was given the *munus* (office, power) of binding and loosening and the *grande munus* (office, special duty) of spreading the Christian name, which was also granted to the apostles (LG 20). The apostles were assigned the *munera* (exalted functions, great duties) of "giving witness to the gospel, to the ministration of the Holy Spirit and of justice for God's glory" (LG 21). To help them fulfill these *munera*, they were granted a special outpouring of the Holy Spirit (LG 21). By virtue of his *munus* (office), the Roman pontiff has "full, supreme, and universal power" in the Church (LG 22), and also by virtue of his *munus* (office) he is endowed with infallibility (LG 43). Bishops, by virtue of their episcopal consecration, have the *munus* (office) of preaching and teaching (LG 21). The laity, too, sharing in the priestly, prophetic, and kingly *munera* of Christ, have their own *missio* (mission); they are particularly called (*vocantur*) by fulfilling their *munera* (own particular duties, proper functions) of to "contribute to the sanctification of the world, as from within like leaven. . . . Thus, especially by the witness of their life, resplendent in faith, hope and charity they must manifest Christ to others" (LG 31). *Munera* are conferred by one superior in power on another; it is important to note that Christ is routinely acknowledged as the source of the *munera* for each of the groups mentioned. *Munera* are not man-made but God-given.

Forms of *munus* appear ten times in the five sections of *Gaudium et Spes* that speak about the role of married people in the Church. There we learn that spouses and parents have a *praecellenti . . . munere* (lofty calling) (GS 47); that conjugal love leads spouses to God and aids and strengthens them in their *sublimi munere* (lofty role, sublime office) of being a mother and father (GS 48); that the sacrament of marriage helps them fulfill their conjugal and familial *munera* (role, obligations); that spouses are blessed with the dignity and *munus* (role, office) of fatherhood and motherhood, which help them achieve their *officium* (duty) of educating their children (GS 48); that young people should be properly and in good time instructed about the dignity, *munus* (role, duty), and *opere* (expression) of conjugal love (GS 49). The next occurrence appears in a paragraph that brings together several of the terms that are of concern here: "Married couples should regard it as their proper mission [*missio*] to transmit human life [*officio humanam vitam transmittendi*, etc.] and to educate their children; they should realize that they are thereby cooperating with the love of God the Creator and are, in a certain sense, its interpreters. This involves the fulfillment of their role [*munus*] with a sense of human and Christian responsibility..." (GS 50). Later in the same section, there is a mention of "the *munus* [duty] of procreating"; of fulfilling "this God-given *munus* [mission, task, *commissio a Deo*] by generously having a large family" (GS 50). And we meet again the passage at the close of GS 51: "Let all be convinced that human life and its transmission [*munus eam transmittendi*] are realities whose meaning is not limited by the horizons of this life only..." (GS 51).

The Interiority of *Munus*

To this point the discussion of munus has focused largely on its external dimensions, on its status as a task bestowed as an honor on Man by God. What is needed now is a consideration of the kind of internal benefits gained by one who eagerly embraces and seeks to fulfill his or her vocation, mission, or *munus*. What we need to do is focus on the interior changes, the growth in virtue and perfection, in the individual who lives his or her married commitment faithfully. And we wish to place particular emphasis on the role of children in fostering these interior changes. When *Humanae Vitae* 9 asserts that one of the defining characteristics of marriage is its fruitfulness, it states: "[Conjugal] love is fruitful since the whole of the love is not contained in the communion of the spouses, but it also looks beyond itself and seeks to raise up new lives." *Humanae Vitae* 9 cites further from *Gaudium et Spes* (50): "Marriage and conjugal love are ordained by their very nature to the procreating and educating of children. Offspring are clearly the supreme gift of marriage, a gift which contributes immensely to the good of the parents themselves."

Let us elaborate on this claim of *Gaudium et Spes* and *Humanae Vitae* that children contribute immensely to the good of the parents. The fundamental point is that having children and raising children are sources of great good for the parents, that having to meet the responsibilities entailed in the *munus* of transmitting human life works to transform individuals into more virtuous individuals and also works an attitudinal change that enables them to be better Christians. Here we will be drawing on the work of John Paul II, in particular from passages in his book *Sources of Renewal,* which he wrote (as Karol Wojtyla) as a commentary on Vatican II, and from *Familiaris Consortio,* itself, in some parts, a marvelous commentary on *Humanae Vitae.* In these works, John Paul puts a great deal of emphasis on Man's internal life, on his need for transformation in Christ.

The focus on interiority is characteristic of John Paul; it flows from his emphasis on personalist values, from his interest in the kind of self-transformation one works on one's self through one's moral choices. John Paul has labored hard to draw the attention of moralists to personalist values, the values of self-mastery and generosity, for instance, that are fostered by moral choices. He repeatedly depicts life as a continuous process of transformation. For instance, in *Familiaris Consortio* he states, "What is needed is a continuous, permanent conversion which, while requiring an interior detachment from every evil and an adherence to good in its fullness, is brought about concretely in steps which lead us ever forward. Thus a dynamic process develops, one which advances gradually with the progressive integration of the gifts of God and the demands of His definitive and absolute love in the entire personal and social life of man" (FC 9).[14] The task of life, then, is to become ever more like Christ through fidelity to the demands of one's calling in life.

In *Sources of Renewal*, Wojtyla places great stress on the "attitude of participation" required from Christians in Christ's mission, which he calls the "central theme of the Conciliar doctrine concerning the People of God."[15] There he refers to Christ's threefold power or *munus* as priest, prophet, and king in which Christians must participate. He maintains that sharing in this power of *munus* is not simply a matter of sharing in certain tasks; rather it is more fundamentally a participation in certain attitudes. He tells us that Man has the power or "'task' or 'office' (cf. Latin *munus in tria munera Christi*) together with the ability to perform it [the Latin is cited in Wojtyla's text]." He goes on to observe: "In speaking of participation in the threefold power of Christ, the Council teaches that the whole People of God and its individual members share in the priestly, prophetic and kingly offices that Christ took upon himself and fulfilled, and in the power which enabled him to do so.... The Conciliar teaching allows us to think of participation in Christ's threefold office not only in the ontological sense but also in that of specific attitudes. These express themselves in the attitude of testimony and give it a dimension of its own, as it were an interior form derived from Christ himself—the form of his mission and his power."[16] The claim that participating in a *munus* not only involves the power to act and the responsibility to complete an external act but also requires an internal attitudinal change by Christians adds another dimension to the complexity of this word. In *Sources of Renewal* Karol Wojtyla outlines the different attitudinal changes required to be faithful participants in Christ's threefold *munus*. He identifies a certain attitude associated with each of the three *munera* of priesthood, prophet, and king.

It is possible to crystallize these attitudes in the following way. In conjunction with the *munus* of *priesthood* shared by the laity, the attitude needed is a sacrificial one, whereby "man commits himself and the world to God." To explain this attitude, he cites part of a key passage in *Gaudium et Spes:* "It follows, then, that if man is the only creature on earth that God has wanted for its own sake, man can fully discover his true self only in a sincere giving of himself" (GS 24). Sharing in the *prophetic munus* of Christ requires that spouses work to bring the truth of Christ to the world, through evangelization. And the *kingly munus* is best exercised by Man not in rule over the world but in rule over himself. Thus, to be a priest, one must be self-sacrificing; to be a prophet, one must evangelize; and to be a king, one must govern—and govern one's self above all.

It is in *Familiaris Consortio* that we find more detailed instruction about how spouses are to participate in the threefold *munera* of Christ; how they are to be priests, prophets, and kings; or how they are to be self-sacrificing, evangelical, and self-mastering. *Familiaris Consortio* speaks specifically about the family's part in the threefold *munus* of Christ:

> The Christian family also builds up the Kingdom of God in history through the everyday realities that concern and distinguish its *state of life*. It is thus in *the love between husband and wife and between the members of the family*—a love lived out in all its extraordinary richness of values and demands: totality, oneness, fidelity, and fruitfulness—that the Christian family's participation in the prophetic, priestly, and kingly mission of Jesus Christ and of His Church finds expression and realization. Therefore love and life constitute the nucleus of the saving mission of the Christian family in the Church and for the Church. (FC 50)

In the remainder of *Familiaris Consortio,* he explains how the family fulfills their participation in Christ's threefold *munus*. He identifies the *prophetic* office with the obligation of the family to evangelize, especially to its own members. The pope rehearses the obligation of parents to be educators of their children, especially in matters of the faith. *Familiaris Consortio* refers to the evangelization of children as an original and irreplaceable ministry (FC 53): "The family must educate the children for life in such a way that each one may fully perform his or her role [*munus*] according to the vocation received from God." For the family, the *priestly* office is fulfilled by engaging "in a dialogue with God through the sacraments, through the offering of one's life, and through prayer" (FC 55). And the *kingly* office is fulfilled when the family offers service to the larger community, especially to the needy. Note this powerful passage:

> While building up the Church in love, the Christian family places itself at the service of the human person and the world, really bringing about the "human advancement" whose substance was given in summary form in the Synod's Message to families; "Another task for the family is to form persons in love and also to practice love in all its relationships, so that it does not live closed in on itself, but remains open to the community, moved by a sense of justice and concern for others, as well as by a consciousness of its responsibility towards the whole of society." (FC 64)

The family participates in the threefold *munus* of Christ by being true to its own *munus*. In the previous sections of *Familiaris Consortio,* which laid the foundation for the discussion of the family's participation in the threefold *munus* of Christ, John Paul sketched out the interior changes to be gained when the family is true to its *munus*. What John Paul hopes for from marriage is that it will result in the formation of a new heart within the spouses, the children, and ultimately all of society. This heart will be one that is loving, generous, and self-giving (FC 25). The family serves to build up the kingdom of God insofar as it is a school of love; as John Paul puts it, "The essence and role [*munus*] of the family are in the final analysis specified by love" (FC 17). He goes on, "Hence the family has the mission to guard, reveal and communicate love." *Familiaris Consortio* states: "The relationships between the members of the family community are inspired and guided by the law of 'free-giving.' By respecting and fostering personal dignity in each and every one as the only basis for value, this free giving takes the form of heartfelt acceptance, encounter, dialogue, disinterested availability, generous service and deep solidarity" (FC 43).

The text also states: "All members of the family, each according to his or her own gift [*munus*], have the grace and responsibility of building, day by day, the communion of persons, making the family 'a school of deeper humanity': this happens where there is care and love for the little ones, the sick, the aged; where there is mutual service every day; when there is a sharing of goods, of joys and of sorrows" (FC 21).

A key phrase for our purposes is the next line: "A fundamental opportunity for building such a communion is constituted by the education exchanged between parents and children, in which each gives and receives" and "Family communion can only be preserved and perfected through a great spirit of sacrifice. It requires, in fact, a ready and generous openness of each and all to understanding, to forbearance, to pardon, to reconciliation." These passages suggest the kinds of virtues needed for and cultivated by good family life. Successfully adapting to family life fosters love and generosity, ability to forgive, and many other related virtues. Both the parents and the children and ultimately the whole of society stand to grow in these virtues as the family attempts to be true to its nature.

The *munus* of transmitting life, of educating children, of being parents, then, yields multiple goods. Creating a family in which self-giving and all the virtues might begin to flourish is an activity that has multiple purposes. Certainly, it works toward achieving God's end of producing more individuals to share with Him eternal bliss. Having children also helps parents mature and acquire many of the virtues they need to be fully human and fully Christian. Furthermore, building families is to the good of the whole of society because generosity and love should flow from the family to the larger community, especially to the poor and needy.

What is key here for an understanding of *Humanae Vitae* is to recognize that to reject the procreative power of sexual intercourse is not simply to reject some biological power; it is to reject a God-given *munus* and all that it entails. The resistance to the procreative power of sexual intercourse that accompanies the desire to use contraception predictably involves an underestimation of the value of the family: to God, to the spouses, and to the larger society. Ultimately spouses must come to realize that to reject the *munus* of transmitting life, to limit the number of children they have for selfish reasons, is to limit the number of gifts and blessings that God gives to them; it is to limit the gifts that they return to God and their opportunities and ability to grow as Christians.

An Application of *Munus* to *Humanae Vitae*

An analogy drawn around the concept *munus* may help us better understand the teaching of *Humanae Vitae*. This analogy requires us to imagine a good and generous king of a country who has asked one of his worthy subjects to help him build his kingdom. The king needs a responsible individual to perform this task since it is important, indeed, essential, to the kingdom to keep contact with a distant borough. He chooses to honor his subject George with the *munus* (mission) of maintaining contact with one of the outlying boroughs. In order for George to perform this service, the king gives him the use of a fine horse and buggy that will enable him to travel to the distant borough. The king needs someone to spread goodwill and cheer in this community and wants George to undertake this *munus*. He makes it clear that George should never go to the borough unless he attends to the king's business when he is there. The king has another motive for providing George with the horse and buggy, for he also wishes George to prosper. The horse and buggy will enable George to attend to his own business when he travels to the distant borough. The king makes it clear that those who live in the borough, and George himself, will fare better if George uses the horse and buggy as designated, for the king knows that it is quite impossible for George and him to prosper without each other. So George achieves two ends by the use of the horse and buggy; he advances his own prosperity and that of the kingdom. The king also tells George that business is closed in the outlying borough one week of every month and during that week George may continue freely to use the horse and buggy for his own purposes. Moreover, since the horse and buggy are handsome and efficient it is pleasurable for George to employ them, but pleasure is an added benefit to the use of the horse and buggy, not its purpose. The king more or less leaves it up to George how often and when he visits the borough; he asks him to be generous but to use his own good judgment. Now, if George were to accept this *munus* and the horse and buggy that go with it but refuse to drive to the outlying borough, then he would be reneging on the *munus* that he accepted. And if he were to go to the borough but refuse to attend to the king's business while there, he would again be failing to live up to the demands of his *munus*.

There are parallels here with the *munus* of transmitting human life. God has given this *munus* to spouses because He wishes to share the goods of His kingdom with humans and He has chosen to call on spouses to share with Him the work of bringing new life into the world. This work is an honor entrusted only to those willing to embrace the responsibilities of marriage. Those who perform the responsibilities of marriage in accord with God's will benefit both themselves and the rest of society. The spouses achieve the good of strengthening their relationship through sexual intercourse, that is, the good of union, and they achieve the good of having children, that is, the good of procreation. Both goods also benefit God's kingdom for He wishes love between spouses to flourish and He desires more people with whom to share the goods of His kingdom. Thus, sexual intercourse is a part of the *munus* of transmitting human life, a *munus* that is intimately bound with other goods. Those who accept this *munus* need to respect the other goods that accompany it.

Still, in the same way that the good king allowed George to use the horse and buggy even when business was not in session in the outlying borough, God has so designed human fertility and human sexuality, that humans are sometimes fertile and sometimes not. It is permissible for spouses to enjoy marital intercourse at any time, whether they are infertile or fertile. God seems to have designed the human system this way to foster greater union and happiness between spouses. He has also asked them to be receptive to new life, generously but in accord with their best judgment, and not to fail to fulfill the *munus* that He has given them. To refuse absolutely to have children is like refusing ever to go to the outlying district. It is to renege on the *munus* that accompanies marriage. To have contraceptive sex is like driving to the outlying borough and ignoring the king's business. The contracepting couple is repudiating the *munus* of their own fertility and altering the functioning of the body. They are pursuing pleasure while emphatically rejecting the good of procreation. They may not feel that they are engaging in an act of emphatic rejection of the good of procreation, but in terms of their *munus*, that is exactly what they are doing. (It is also true that the good they achieve, pleasure, is not identical to the good of union, for that can be achieved only if the procreative good is also respected.) But the good king allowed George to use the horse and buggy when business was not in session, and that is exactly what the couple who are having sexual intercourse during the infertile period is doing. They are pursuing one good, the good of union, *when another is not available*. Again, the contracepting couple is repudiating a *munus* that they have accepted; the noncontracepting couple, on the other hand, is cooperating with the complexity of the *munus* that God has entrusted to them.

This analogy and argument allow us to see how a theological concept can "illuminate and enrich" our understanding of the Church's condemnation of contraception.

In the second portion of this chapter, we shall turn to the question of the role of conscience in a Catholic's response to *Humanae Vitae* and to the question of the infallibility of the teaching of *Humanae Vitae*.

Humanae Vitae and Conscience

When *Humanae Vitae* was issued, some Catholic theologians immediately rejected the encyclical largely on the basis of the claim that the natural law understanding of the encyclical was inadequate.[17] Yet the immediate aftermath, for the most part, was not characterized by the attempt to establish more adequate formulations of natural law. Rather, one of the chief responses to the encyclical was the development of the argument that Catholics were permitted to practice contraception if their consciences so directed them. Indeed, in 1969, one theologian, John Milhaven, announced that in a sense *Humanae Vitae* had become a dead letter: Catholics felt perfectly free to use contraception as an act of conscience.[18] As Milhaven noted, the statements of several bishops' conferences following the promulgation of *Humanae Vitae* seems to have offered support for such a response.

The statement of the French bishops portrays the reason for countenancing the use of contraception by Catholics as the result of a "conflict of duties" and states that "traditional wisdom makes provision for seeking before God which duty in the circumstances is the greater."[19] Although this statement is frequently given as an instance of justifying departure from the teaching of the encyclical on the basis of conscience, it seems rather to draw on the principle of the toleration of the lesser evil, a principle that is explicitly rejected by *Humanae Vitae* 14 as not being properly applicable to the issue of birth control.[20] Statements from other bishops' conferences, however, do seem to have a "conscience clause." The Canadian statement is perhaps the most straightforward in this regard:

> It is a fact that a certain number of Catholics, although admittedly subject to the teaching of the encyclical, find it either extremely difficult or even impossible to make their own all elements of this doctrine. . . . We must appreciate the difficulty experienced by contemporary man in understanding and appropriating some of the points of this encyclical, and we must make every effort to learn from the insights of Catholic scientists and intellectuals, who are of undoubted loyalty to Christian truth, to the church and to the authority of the Holy See. Since they are not denying any point of divine and Catholic faith nor rejecting the teaching authority of the church, these Catholics should not be considered, or consider themselves, shut off from the body of the faithful. But they should remember that their good faith will be dependent on a sincere self-examination to determine the true motives and grounds for such suspension of assent and on continued effort to understand and deepen their knowledge of the teaching of the church.[21]

Further on it states:

> Counselors may meet others who, accepting the teaching of the Holy Father, find that because of particular circumstances they are involved in what seems to them a clear conflict of duties, e.g., the reconciling of conjugal love and responsible parenthood with the education of children already born or with the health of the mother. In accord with the accepted principles of moral theology, if these persons have tried sincerely but without success to pursue a line of conduct in keeping with the given directives, they may be safely assured that whoever honestly chooses that course which seems right to him does so in good conscience.[22]

To round out the picture let us note portions of a few other statements, those by the Austrian and U.S. bishops. The Austrian bishops observe:

> Since the encyclical does not contain an infallible dogma, it is conceivable that someone feels unable to accept the judgment of the teaching authority of the Church. The answer to this is: if someone has experience in this field and has reached a divergent conviction after serious examination, free of emotion and haste, he may for the time being follow it. He does not err, if he is willing to continue his examination and otherwise affords respect and fidelity to the Church. It remains clear, however, that in such a case he has no right to create confusion among his brothers in the faith with his opinion.[23]

The U.S. bishops speak of dissent only in respect to theologians: "There exists in the Church a lawful freedom of inquiry and of thought and also general norms of licit dissent. This is particularly true in the area of legitimate theological speculation and research. When conclusions reached by such professional theological work prompt a scholar to dissent from noninfallible received teaching, the norms of licit dissent come into play." It seems fair that the next sentence be cited as well: "They [the norms of licit dissent] require of him careful respect for the consciences of those who lack his special competence or opportunity for judicious investigation."[24] This portion of the statement of the U.S. bishops, although not immediately relevant to the question of conscience, allows us to make an important distinction. What needs to be noted here is that scholarly dissent on a theoretical level by learned theologians is not at all the same as dissent on a practical level by individuals untrained in theology. Offering reasons why one thinks a teaching is faulty differs radically from living in contradiction to that teaching. Our primary concern in this section is not to determine the proper status of theological dissent but to determine whether Catholics can practice contraception in good conscience. Momentarily we shall note that the U.S. bishops had within their statement a quite developed view of conscience that does not allow much room for divergence from the Church's teaching.

The perspective of over twenty years' distance from the issuance of these statements may put them in a different light. The Austrian bishops on March 29, 1988, issued a statement that seems to repudiate their statement of 1968.[25] The recent statement emphasizes and clarifies further the acknowledgment of the 1968 document "There is freedom of conscience but no freedom from building a correct conscience." A greater stress is put on the obligation to form one's conscience in accord with what the Church teaches. The Austrian hierarchy promised further clarification of the nature, function, and formation of conscience.

The Canadian bishops seemed to have sensed the inadequacy of their statement somewhat earlier, for in 1974 they issued a statement on conscience that puts forward a view of conscience that suggests that a Catholic would have a very difficult—if not impossible—time rejecting the Church's teaching in good conscience.[26] We shall note some of the teachings of the Canadian bishops' statement on conscience shortly, but first let us review, if only in a very sketchy way, the Church's teaching.

First, it must be noted that the Church teaches that one must follow his conscience, even if this conscience is wrong.[27] Conscience and practical reason are very closely related: conscience informs an individual whether an action he is about to perform or has performed is one that is in accord with morality. If a Man is not following his conscience, he is following something (for instance, one of his passions) or someone else, and these evidently are urging him to oppose his conscience. An individual may have various passions and desires directing him to do this or that, but the conscience is an act of reason and determines whether those passions are guiding him toward what is moral or what is immoral; the conscience should also determine whether advice he is getting from another coheres with the dictates of morality; he should only follow the advice of another when this advice does not conflict with his conscience. To say that a Man should always follow his conscience is to say that he should always do what he believes to be moral and not do what he believes to be immoral. Certainly, because of ignorance, neglect, or a variety of other causes, an individual may have a conscience that is not making a good judgment about what is moral. Nonetheless, it is the conscience that says, "This is moral and that is immoral," and it should be the guide of one's action, otherwise one is acting against what one believes to be moral.

There are two other corollaries that are important to note here. Although one must follow one's conscience whether one's conscience is correct or not, this does not necessarily free one of all moral responsibility for one's action. One may be acting out of ignorance, but it may be culpable ignorance;[28] an individual may have neglected to acquire all the information necessary to make a good decision; for instance, a man may be hunting and may shoot at a moving figure that he thought to be a deer; he may be acting in good conscience; he may think he has done no wrong. But he may have killed a human being going for a walk in the woods. If the hunter failed to take due care to determine whether what he was shooting at was a deer or a human being, he may have acted in good conscience, but he is still guilty of wrongdoing. Second, even if one acts from a good conscience and is in no way culpable for wrongdoing, one's action may still be objectively evil. For instance, a woman may have an abortion without knowing that she has taken a human life. She may have consulted a doctor and even a clergyman and theologian who assured her that her action was moral. But if she has an abortion, although she may not be morally culpable, she has still performed an action that is objectively evil.[29] Thus, although one must always follow one's conscience, this does not guarantee that one is not morally responsible for what one has done or that one will never do what is objectively evil.

There is a modern distortion of the teaching that one must always follow one's conscience that is the most pernicious; some draw the false inference that if one does not feel guilty that means that one has not acted in contradiction to one's conscience. Many moderns tend to think that they are following their conscience if they feel comfortable about, or feel no guilt about, their chosen behavior. Some may steal or commit adultery and claim that they feel no guilt. It would seem that their consciences do not trouble them. But it is more likely that they have not troubled their conscience, that is, that they have never pondered whether what they are doing is moral or immoral; they have simply acted on their desires. Furthermore, some may not properly form their consciences and thus not feel guilt for what they do, but they cannot rightly be said to be acting in "good conscience."

Let us also recall that the conscience is one's guide to moral behavior; it does not *decide* the principles of moral behavior but *discovers or learns* them and then judges whether a particular action is moral or immoral.[30] One of the best and most succinct statements on conscience is to be found in *Gaudium et Spes*:

> Deep within his conscience man discovers a law which he has not laid upon himself but which he must obey. Its voice, ever calling him to love and to do what is good and to avoid evil, tells him inwardly at the right moment: do this, shun that. For man has in his heart a law inscribed by God. His dignity lies in observing this law, and by it he will be judged. His conscience is man's most secret core, and his sanctuary. There he is alone with God whose voice echoes in his depths. By conscience, in a wonderful way, that law is made known which is fulfilled in the love of God and of one's neighbor. Through loyalty to conscience Christians are joined to other men in the search for truth and for the right solution to so many moral problems which arise both in the life of individuals and from social relationships. Hence, the more a correct conscience prevails, the more do persons and groups turn aside from blind choice and try to be guided by the objective standards of moral conduct. Yet it often happens that conscience goes astray through ignorance which it is unable to avoid, without thereby losing its dignity. This cannot be said of the man who takes little trouble to find out what is true and good, or when conscience is by degrees almost blinded through the habit of committing sin. (GS 16)

Conscience, then, is not the faculty by which each man or woman tries to determine what he or she thinks moral or immoral; it is the faculty by which an individual attempts to discern what God holds to be moral or immoral.

For a Catholic, the magisterium of the Church plays a definite role in assisting him or her in determining what God holds to be moral or immoral. As the following discussion hopes to establish, if the magisterium is not forming the conscience of the Catholic, again something else (one's own reason, perhaps) or someone else is. The Catholic who rejects the teaching of the Church has, in effect (though possibly not deliberately), decided that something or someone else is a more authoritative teacher than the Church.

Although many dissenters contest it, it has been and remains the claim of the Church to be an authentic teacher on matters of morals (and faith). The Canadian bishops speak of the Catholic's relation to Church teaching in this way: "A believer has the absolute obligation of conforming his conduct first and foremost to what the Church teaches, because first and foremost for the believer is the fact that Christ, through His Spirit, is ever present in His Church—in the whole Church to be sure, but particularly with those who exercise services within the Church and for the Church, the first of which services is that of the apostles." A Catholic presumably knows and accepts the nature of the Church to which he or she belongs; this Church claims to teach for Christ and to have special guidance from the Holy Spirit in its teachings on faith and morals. This, too, is a decision of conscience; one decides that it is right to become or remain a Catholic.

Some claim that the Catholic has an obligation to follow the Church's teaching only when that teaching has been declared infallibly (the next section of this chapter will discuss the infallibility of the teaching). Those who contest this claim, as do the Canadian bishops, regularly draw on *Lumen Gentium* 25:

> Bishops who teach in communion with the Roman Pontiff are to be revered by all as witnesses of divine and Catholic truth; the faithful, for their part, are obliged to submit to their bishops' decision, made in the name of Christ, in matters of faith and morals, and to adhere to it with a ready and respectful allegiance of mind. This loyal submission of the will and intellect must be given, in a special way, to the authentic teaching authority of the Roman Pontiff, even when he does not speak *ex cathedra* in such wise, indeed, that his supreme teaching authority be acknowledged with respect, and sincere assent be given to decisions made by him, conformably with his manifest mind and intention, which is made known principally either by the character of the documents in question, or by the frequency with which a certain doctrine is proposed, or by the manner in which the doctrine is formulated.[31]

The preceding statements rest on a claim noted earlier and reiterated in these various statements: that the Church speaks for Christ. Thus, when a Catholic wrestles with a problem on which the Church speaks one way and his own thoughts or various advisers speak another, it is much as if he were to hear Christ Himself say one thing and himself and others say another. At the least, he is hearing those Christ has designated to speak for Him. Whom should he trust?

Again, as noted, one must always follow one's conscience, even if it is wrong. But should a Catholic feel free to think his conscience is correct if it departs from a Church teaching (one that adheres to the criteria of *Lumen Gentium*)? The U.S. bishops' statement that followed *Humanae Vitae* cites the famous statement of John Henry Newman in regard to what a Catholic should do when he or she disagrees with a teaching/mandate of the Church.

> I have to say again, lest I should be misunderstood, that when I speak of conscience, I mean conscience truly so called. When it has the right of opposing the supreme, though not infallible authority of the Pope, it must be something more than that miserable counterfeit which, as I have said above, now goes by the name. If in a particular case it is to be taken as a sacred and sovereign monitor, its dictate, in order to prevail against the voice of the Pope, must

follow upon serious thought, prayer, and all available means of arriving at a right judgment on the matter in question. And further, obedience to the Pope is what is called "in possession": that is the *onus probandi* (burden of proof) of establishing a case against him lies, as in all cases of exception, on the side of conscience. Unless a man is able to say to himself, as in the presence of God, that he must not, and dare not, act upon the papal injunction, he is bound to obey it and would commit a great sin in disobeying it. *Prima facie* it is his bounden duty, even from a sentiment of loyalty, to believe the Pope right and to act accordingly. . . ."[32]

What the preceding seeks to establish is that Catholics who find that they cannot agree in conscience with the Church's teaching on contraception find themselves with a second crisis of conscience on their hands: That is, what are they to make of the Church's claim to be a reliable and authoritative teacher in matters of morals when they in practice have rejected the Church as teacher? According to the Church is this a teaching that can be disobeyed in good conscience? If not, what now is their relationship to their Church?

Now let us give some caveats here. The preceding presupposes, of course, Catholics who share the traditional understanding the Church has of its role in teaching on matters of faith and morals. The reality, however, is far from the ideal. It is perhaps true to say that many if not most Catholics have not been taught what the Church claims in regard to its status as a teacher or what the proper role of conscience is. They may not realize that their decision to reject the teaching of the Church puts them in such a quandary. With the example and counsel of dissenting theologians, their subjective state may diverge considerably from the objective reality, and their culpability may in fact be slight.

The Infallibility of *Humanae Vitae*

Since the earliest moments of its promulgation, many theologians have justified dissent from *Humanae Vitae* by arguing that the document and its teaching are not infallible. Most acknowledge the teaching of the document to be authoritative and deserving of respect but not as having the claim on Catholics that an infallible teaching would have. Indeed, Monsignor Ferdinando Lambruschini, a member of the Papal Commission who sided with the majority and who presented *Humanae Vitae* to the press on its promulgation, claimed that the document did not have the "theological note of infallibility."[33] Although he was never publicly corrected on this statement, Rev. Ermenegildo Lio, reportedly one of the authors of *Humanae Vitae*, reports that Lambruschini had not been authorized to make such a statement and that the views were strictly his own. Lambruschini's statement about the "noninfallibility" of the encyclical was omitted from the report in *L'Osservatore Romano* on the press conference.[34]

Although there were multitudes of articles on the issuance of the encyclical that attempted to define the nature of the authority of the document,[35] with perhaps one or two exceptions,[36] there was no immediate attempt in the scholarly literature to challenge Lambruschini and the widespread consensus that the teaching of *Humanae Vitae* was not infallible. Lio has since taken up the challenge[37] by arguing that Pope Paul VI used language in *Humanae Vitae* meant to indicate that he was making a solemn definition of Church doctrine and that infallibility extends to such definitions. To date it seems that there have been no responses to Lio's work, a work at this time available in Italian only.

Lio was not the first to make the argument that the teaching of *Humanae Vitae* has been infallibly pronounced. On very different terms, in 1978 John C. Ford, S.J., and Germain Grisez made such an argument; they do not argue that *Humanae Vitae* was an infallible declaration; rather they argue that the condemnation of contraception was already an infallible teaching by virtue of the way it had been taught through the ordinary magisterium. Their argument has met with some vigorous criticism to which Grisez has as vigorously replied[38] Both the arguments of Grisez and Ford and those of their critics are complex and lengthy. Thus, a thorough recounting of the debate would be out of place here. A brief sketch of its nature will have to serve.

The Minority Report of the Papal Commission had included the argument that the Church could not have erred through all the centuries (not even through one century) in its condemnation of contraception, a condemnation that imposed "very heavy burdens under the grave obligation of the name of Jesus Christ." The strong implication is, that if the Church were wrong about such a matter it would have to relinquish its claim to being the authoritative interpreter of Christ's teachings. Grisez and Ford "sought to develop and complete" this argument in their study.[39] They argued that the teaching of *Humanae Vitae* meets the criteria of *Lumen Gentium* 25 for a teaching that is infallible not by virtue of being defined so in an ex cathedra fashion but by virtue of being constantly proclaimed by the universal ordinary magisterium. They articulate what they believe to be Vatican II's criteria for a teaching to be proclaimed infallibly by the universal ordinary magisterium: "First, that the bishops remain in communion with one another and with the Pope; second, that they teach authoritatively on a matter of faith or morals; third, that they agree in one judgment; and fourth, that they propose this judgment as one to be held definitively."[40] Building on the work of John Noonan that demonstrated that the Church has constantly proclaimed contraception to be evil (a nearly uncontested claim), Grisez and Ford came to the conclusion that the condemnation against contraception has infallible status:

> At least until 1962, Catholic bishops in communion with one another and with the Pope agreed in and authoritatively proposed one judgment to be held definitively on the morality of contraception: Acts of this kind are objectively, intrinsically, and gravely evil. Since this teaching has been proposed infallibly, the controversy since 1963 takes nothing away from its objectively certain truth. It is not the received Catholic teaching on contraception which needs to be rethought. It is the assumption that this teaching could be abandoned as false which needs to be rethought.[41]

Francis Sullivan, S.J., questions several claims that he believes Grisez and Ford to be making: (1) he questions the claim that throughout the centuries the faithful have accepted the Church's teaching on contraception *as a matter of faith;* (2) he objects that if their argument holds, then "If the magisterium speaks in a definitive way about something, it must necessarily be the case that what they speak about is a proper object of infallible teaching"; (3) he registers a doubt that Grisez and Ford have succeeded in showing that the teaching on contraception is a secondary object of infallibility (one that is not revealed but necessary to guard revealed truths); (4) he questions that the Church has truly taught *definitively* on contraception; (5) and he doubts that the Church has the authority to teach infallibly on "concrete norms" of natural moral law.[42]

In another extensive article, Grisez responds to each of these difficulties[43]: it would be quite otiose to cover them here. One point of central interest, though, would seem to be whether the teaching of the Church is truly rooted in norms expressed in Scripture and whether it has a necessary connection with truths that are necessary for salvation. To this point, Grisez cites a speech by John Paul, wherein he makes precisely the claims Grisez has labored to defend.

The Church teaches this norm, although it is not formally (that is, literally) expressed in Sacred Scripture, and it does this in the conviction that the interpretation of the precepts of natural law belongs to the competence of the Magisterium.

However, we can say more. Even if the moral law, formulated in this way in the Encyclical *Humanae Vitae,* is not found literally in Sacred Scripture, nonetheless, from the fact that it is contained in Tradition and—as Pope Paul VI writes—has been "very often expounded by the Magisterium" (HV, n. 12) to the faithful, it follows that this norm *is in accordance with the sum total of revealed doctrine contained in biblical sources* (cf. HV, n. 4).

4. It is a question here not only of the sum total of the moral doctrine contained in Sacred Scripture, of its essential premises and general character of its content, but of that fuller context to which we have previously dedicated numerous analyses when speaking about the "theology of the body."

Precisely against the background of this full context it becomes evident that the above-mentioned moral norm belongs not only to the natural moral law, but also to the *moral order revealed by God:* also from this point of view, it could not be different, but solely what is handed down by Tradition and the Magisterium and, in our days, the Encyclical *Humanae Vitae* as a modern document of this Magisterium.[44]

Grisez draws three points out of this passage: "The fact that the norm excluding contraception is in accord with the sum total of revelation *follows from* its being contained in tradition and its often being expounded by the magisterium; the norm belongs to the moral order *revealed by God;* and it *could* not be different." The preceding, of course, does not constitute an argument or even lay out the lines of an argument: it does, though, serve to indicate what the issues of the debate are.

Garth Hallett, S.J., is one of the few who contest that the Church has had a constant teaching against contraception. He categorizes moral expressions into those that are prescriptive (those that attempt to command or forbid behavior) and those that are descriptive (those that explain why behavior is good or bad). He argues that although the Church has consistently opposed contraception, that is, provided prescriptive teachings against it, it has not provided consistent descriptive accounts about the immorality of contraception. He claims that infallibility does not extend to prescriptive teachings.

In reply Grisez questions Hallett's acceptance of the categorization of moral expressions popular with one school of modern philosophy. Although Grisez grants (not concedes) that moral language is complex, he argues that we are not without resources to determine what the moral expressions of various periods mean. He denies that the Church is without a common criterion to determine morality. He further notes that if Hallett is correct about incoherence in the Church's teaching on contraception, the same would hold true of its teaching about any moral behavior, such as killing the innocent or loving one's enemies.

This last claim by Grisez is a challenging one. Those who uphold the Church's teaching on contraception note that the Church has taught few moral norms with as much consistency and zeal as it has the norm against contraception. Thus, they reason, if the Church is wrong about contraception, it is possible to call into question most if not all of its other moral norms. As other portions of this book [the author's *Humanae Vitae: A Generation Later*] demonstrate, since *Humanae Vitae,* most if not all of the other moral norms taught by the Church, especially those regarding sexuality, have been called into question.

One further important argument needs to be noted. Nearly all of those who assert that *Humanae Vitae* does not contain infallible teaching in fact think that that teaching is not only not infallible but wrong. But they are not troubled in the same way as their opponents for they generally believe that the Church has been wrong in its teaching many times in the past. The statement issued by Charles Curran and other dissident theologians on the issuance of *Humanae Vitae* provides a good example of this view: "The encyclical is not an infallible teaching. History shows that a number of statements or [*sic*] even greater authoritative weight have subsequently been proven inadequate or even erroneous. Past authoritative statements on religious liberty, interest-taking, the right to silence, and the ends of marriage have all been corrected at a later date."[45] What must be noted here is that there is certainly no complete agreement with the claim that teachings promulgated with the same gravity and weight as the condemnation of contraception have been "proven inadequate or even erroneous."[46] Many have contested the very examples given in the preceding statement (given with no supporting argumentation). The arguments generally take three forms: either the claim is made that the Church has not in fact changed its teaching on a given issue (arguments in this respect have been made about the Church's teaching on religious liberty);[47] or that the other teachings were wedded to certain cultural conditions that no longer exist (arguments in regard to usury generally take this line);[48] or that development of a teaching has been of a sort not to contradict or cancel an earlier teaching but to expand and illuminate it (analyses of the new emphasis on personalist values in marriage often take this form).[49]

To this day, there is much debate on what the proper response would be for a Catholic to the teaching of *Humanae Vitae*. From the moment of its promulgation it met with a very mixed response.

Notes

1. This section has been greatly assisted by the unpublished work of James Lehrberger, O.Cist.
2. In early Church condemnations of contraception, Genesis 38:1–9, the story of Onan, is often cited as a scriptural condemnation of contraception. More recent biblical scholarship identifies Onan's sin not as one of "spilling seed" but of refusing to do his duty by his brother's wife. A recent study by Charles D. Provan, *The Bible and Birth Control* (Monongahela, Pa.: Zimmer Printing, 1989), makes the case for the immorality of contraception from the Bible; Provan argues for a traditional understanding of the Onan incident.
3. Translations for Scripture are taken from *The New American Bible* (Camden, N.J.: Thomas Nelson, 1971).
4. *Humanae Vitae* cites Scripture six times, in sections 8, 18, 25 (three times), and 28; there are nine additional scriptural references in the footnotes.
5. See footnotes 31, 33, 34, 35, 36, and 37 to HV 25.
6. Much of this section is taken from my article, "The *Munus* of Transmitting Human Life: A New Approach to *Humanae Vitae*," *The Thomist* 54:3 (July 3, 1990) 385–427.
7. The translations for passages from the conciliar documents are from *Vatican II: The Conciliar and Postconciliar Documents,* ed. Austin Flannery, O.P.; hereafter the section number is given in the text.
8. See the introduction to the translation of *Humanae Vitae* in Appendix 1 [of the author's *Humanae Vitae: A Generation Later*].
9. Charlton T. Lewis and Charles Short, *A Latin Dictionary* (Oxford: Clarendon Press, 1975), lists *officium* (duty), *ministerium* (function), and *honos* (honor) as synonyms for *munus* but also notes that it is a *munus* that confers or entails *officia* ("Munus significat officium, cum dicitur quis munere fungi. Item donum quod officii causa datur" ["*munus* means 'duty' when someone is said to perform a *munus*. Also, it is a gift that is given for the sake of a duty"]). Cicero uses the phrase *munus officii,* which clearly signals a difference between the two words.
10. Austin Flannery, O.P., ed., *Vatican Council II* (Northport, N.Y.: Costello Publishing Co., 1975).
11. Walter M. Abbott, S.J., ed., *The Documents of Vatican II* (Chicago: Follett Publishing Co., 1966).

12. Roy J. Deferrari, *A Latin-English Dictionary of St. Thomas Aquinas* (Boston: St. Paul Editions, 1960) lists only "gift" as a suitable translation for *munus*.

13. The abbreviations for the texts of Vatican II are standard. The translation given here is my own.

14. Translations for *Familiaris Consortio* are from *The Role of the Christian Family in the Modern World* (Boston: St. Paul Editions, 1981).

15. Karol Wojtyla, *Sources of Renewal*, trans. P. S. Falla (San Francisco: Harper & Row, 1980) 219, originally published in Poland in 1972.

16. Ibid., 220.

17. See the statement issued by a number of Catholic theologians under the leadership of Charles Curran, in *The Birth Control Debate*, ed. Robert G. Hoyt (Kansas City, Mo.: National Catholic Reporter, 1968) 180.

18. John Giles Milhaven, "The Grounds of the Opposition to '*Humanae Vitae*,'" *Thought* 44 (1969) 343–57. Perhaps the most famous justification for the legitimacy of dissent and one of the most influential is that by Karl Rahner, S.J., "On the Encyclical 'Humanae Vitae,'" *Catholic Mind* 66 (Nov. 1968) 28–45, which also appeared in *National Catholic Reporter*, Sept. 18, 1968. For a sampling of the argumentation made in behalf of conscientious dissent, see *Conscience: Its Freedom and Limitations*, ed. William C. Bier, S.J. (New York:. Fordham University Press, 1971).

19. John Horgan, *Humanae Vitae and the Bishops* (Shannon: Irish University Press, 1972) 364.

20. See Chapter 3 [of the author's *Humanae Vitae: A Generation Later*] for a discussion of this principle.

21. Hoyt, *Birth Control Debate*, 169–70.

22. Ibid., 172.

23. Horgan, *Humanae Vitae and the Bishops*, 360.

24. The document in its entirety can be found in *The Pope Speaks* 13:4 (1969) 377–94.

25. *Verordnungsblatt der Erzdiozese Salzburg* 4 (Apr. 1988) 54–58.

26. The bishops of Manitoba in April 1989 issued a pastoral letter, "Responsible Parenthood," which expressed strong support for *Humanae Vitae*.

27. The *locus classicus* for this is Thomas Aquinas, *Summa Theologiae*, I–II, q. 19, art. 5, 6.

28. Ibid., q. 6, art. 8.

29. See the statement of the U.S. bishops, *The Pope Speaks*, 385.

30. See Carlo Caffarra, "Conscience, Truth, and Magisterium in Conjugal Morality" in *Marriage and Family* (San Francisco: Ignatius Press, 1989) 21–36.

31. Flannery, *Vatican II*, 379.

32. The U.S. bishops ("Human Life in Our Days," *The Pope Speaks* 13 [1969] 377–95) are quoting *A Letter to the Duke of Norfolk* (384). Bishop (now Cardinal) Bernardin issued a clarifying statement after the release of the bishops' statement, in which he stated, "The bishops in no way intended to imply that there is any divergence between their statement and the teaching of the Holy Father. It is true that people must form their consciences, but it is equally true that they have the responsibility to form a correct conscience." He then cited *Lumen Gentium* 25 ("Statements on the Birth Control Encyclical," *Catholic Mind* 66 [Sept. 1968] 2).

The Irish bishops have also issued a statement on conscience, and their commentary on this passage from Newman is much to the point:

The type of case Newman has in mind is where the Pope gives an injunction or precept in some matter of conduct to a member of the Church. But what he has to say applies with even greater force to the person who appeals to conscience against a declaration by the Pope on what the moral law requires in a particular matter. This is all the more true if (as happened, for example with the Encyclical *Humanae Vitae* of Paul VI, from which many claimed the right to dissent) the Pope, after long consideration, speaks formally and deliberately to settle a matter of public controversy in the Church, and in doing so confirms a doctrine traditionally held. Even a person with the necessary theological competence to judge such an issue, before claiming the right to dissent, would still have to ask himself whether his personal judgment, however reliable and well-founded he believed it to be, could possibly take precedence over such a decision of the Pope. For it is the Pope's divinely appointed task to give direction to the Church in these matters, and in so doing he is assured of the special assistance of the Spirit of Christ. (*Conscience and Morality* [Boston: St. Paul Editions, 1980] 19)

33. "Statement Accompanying Encyclical *Humanae Vitae*," *Catholic Mind* 52.

34. As reported by Brian Harrison, "Appendix III: *Humanae Vitae e Infallibilitá*," in *Religious Liberty and Contraception* (Melbourne: John XXIII Fellowship Co-op. Ltd., 1988) 175. Appendix III is a book review of Ermenegildo Lio's book, *Humanae Vitae e Infallibilitá: il Concilio, Paolo VI e Giovanni Paolo II* (Vatican City: Libreria Editrice Vaticana, 1986).

35. See, for instance, Karl Rahner, "On the Encyclical *Humanae Vitae*"; Gerard P. Kirk, S.J., "*Humanae Vitae* and the Assent Due It," *Continuum* 6 (1968) 288–94; John McHugh, "The Doctrinal Authority of the Encyclical 'Humanae Vitae,'" *Clergy Review* 54 (1969) 586–96, 680–93, 791–802; Sabbas J. Kilian, "The Question of Authority in '*Humanae Vitae*,'" and John Giles Milhaven, "The Grounds of Opposition to '*Humanae Vitae*,'" both in *Thought* 44:174 (Autumn 1969) 327–42 and 343–57; Peter Harris, "The Church and Moral Decision," *New Blackfriars* 51 (1970) 518–27; Gregory Baum, "The New Encyclical on Contraception," *Homiletic and Pastoral Review* 68 (Sept. 1968) 1001–4; Charles E. Curran and Robert E. Hunt, *Dissent In and For the Church: Theologians and Humanae Vitae* (New York: Sheed and Ward, 1969), and *The Responsibility of Dissent: The Church and Academic Freedom* (New York: Sheed and Ward, 1969); *Contraception: Authority and Dissent,* ed. Charles Curran (New York: Herder and Herder, 1969); Joseph A. Komonchak, "*Humanae Vitae* and Its Reception: Ecclesiological Reflections," *Theological Studies* 39 (1978) 221–57. All the above are by dissenters. Robert J. Dionne, who holds the teaching of *Humanae Vitae* to be true, argues that its proper theological note seems to be "*doctrina catholica*, not *de fide catholica*,": "'Humanae Vitae' Re-examined: A Response," *Homiletic and Pastoral Review* (July 1973) 57–64.

36. Joseph F. Costanzo in "Papal Magisterium and 'Humanae Vitae,'" *Thought* 44:174 (Autumn 1969) 377–412, does not argue precisely that the teaching of the document is infallible but observes:

> There is more impression than substance in pointing to the distinction between the infallibility of a solemn *ex cathedra* definition and the authentic and authoritative teaching of the Roman pontiff. The insinuating argument is that what is not formally infallible is fallible. It supposes that infallibility may not derive from another source than a solemn *ex cathedra* definition. Church documents and the "theologians" themselves have traditionally acknowledged an infallibility *ex ordinario magisterio*. This means more than mere longevity but a continuing active and constant witness of the teaching authority of the Church to the general moral principle that opposes all contraceptive practices, the novelty being only its authoritative application to specific problems as they emerged in time. Further, who could honestly question the gravity and solemnity of the historical occasion for *Humanae Vitae*? The world-wide expectation of the papal pronouncement by the faithful and non-faithful alike, the critical nature of the controversy, the largely predictable divisive consequences—all these attest to the awesome responsibility with which Pope Paul has spoken. (396–97).

He concludes: "There was no need for the formality of an *ex cathedra* definition" (397). Nicholas Halligan, O.P., "The Church as Teacher," *Thomist* 33 (1969) 675– 717, argues: "Every authentic or official teaching of pope (or local bishop) binds in conscience by virtue of its authority and not (by supposition) of its infallibility. Authority determines the obligation to give assent or obedience, infallibility only determines the kind of assent or adherence. As a matter of fact, infallibility is not of itself precluded from every non-*ex cathedra* pronouncement simply because it is in a non-*ex cathedra* mode, e.g., from the Council's teaching on episcopal collegiality; it merely cannot be verified" (705).

37. Harrison's review ("Appendix III") provides a good summary of Lio's work (*Humanae Vitae e Infallibilitá*).

38. "Contraception and the Infallibility of the Ordinary Magisterium," originally published in *Theological Studies* 39:2 (June 1978) 258–312, and reprinted in *The Teaching of Humanae Vitae: A Defense* (San Francisco: Ignatius Press, 1988). References here are to the reprint. Russell Shaw summarized this argument in "Contraception, Infallibility and the Ordinary Magisterium," *Homiletic and Pastoral Review* 78 (July 1978) 9–19. Garth Hallett, S.J., responded to the Ford-Grisez argument in "Contraception and Prescriptive Infallibility," *Theological Studies* 43 (1982) 629–50, and Francis A. Sullivan, S.J., critiqued the Ford-Grisez argument in *Magisterium: Teaching Authority in the Catholic Church* (New York: Paulist Press, 1983)

119–52. Grisez replied to Hallett in "Infallibility and Contraception: A Reply to Garth Hallett," *Theological Studies* 47 (1986) 134–45, and to Sullivan in "Infallibility and Specific Moral Norms: A Review Discussion," *Thomist* 49 (1985) 248–87. Robert J. Dionne has two lengthy footnotes commenting on the Grisez-Sullivan debate in *The Papacy and the Church* (New York: Philosophical Library, 1987) 468–69.

39. Grisez, "Infallibility and Specific Moral Norms: A Review Discussion," *Thomist*, 268.

40. Grisez and Ford, *The Teaching of Humanae Vitae: A Defense*, 145.

41. Ibid., 171.

42. Sullivan, *Magisterium*, 144.

43. Brian Harrison also replied to Sullivan in Appendix II of *Religious Liberty*.

44. Grisez, "Infallibility and Specific Moral Norms: A Review Discussion," *Thomist*, 285, citing John Paul II, "General Audience of 18 July," *L'Osservatore Romano* (Eng. ed.) (July 23, 1984) 1.

45. *Catholic Mind* 66 (Sept. 1968) 2.

46. See, for instance, Joseph Costanzo, "Academic Dissent: An Original Ecclesiology," *Thomist* 34:4 (Oct. 1970) 636–54; see particularly 648–53.

47. See, for instance, Harrison, *Religious Liberty;* William H. Marshner, "*Dignitatis Humanae* and Traditional Teaching on Church and State," *Faith & Reason* 9:3 (Fall 1983) 222–48; William G. Most, "Religious Liberty: What the Texts Demand," *Faith & Reason* 9:3 (Fall 1983) 196–209.

48. Grisez and Ford offer such an argument, *The Teaching of Humanae Vitae*, 190ff.

49. See Chapter 2 [of the author's *Humanae Vitae: A Generation Later*] and many of the sources cited therein.

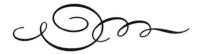

Acknowledgment of Sources

The editor and publisher thank the owners of the copyright for their permission to include the selections in this anthology.

Chapter 1. Reprinted from Eugene A. LaVerdiere, S.S.S., "The Witness of the New Testament," in *Dimensions of Human Sexuality*, ed. Dennis Doherty (Garden City, N.Y.: Doubleday and Co., 1979), 21–38. Copyright © 1979 by Dennis Doherty. Used by permission of Doubleday, a division of Random House, Inc.

Chapter 2. Reprinted from James B. Nelson, "Sexual Salvation: Grace and the Resurrection of the Body," in *Embodiment: An Approach to Sexuality and Christian Theology* (Minneapolis: Augsburg Publishing House, 1978), 70–80. Copyright © 1978 Augsburg Publishing House. Used by permission of Augsburg Fortress.

Chapter 3. Reprinted from Eric Fuchs, "Christianity and Sexuality: An Ambiguous History," in *Sexual Desire and Love: Origins and History of the Christian Ethic of Sexuality and Marriage* (Cambridge: James Clarke and Co.; New York: Seabury Publishers, 1983), 84–148. Used by permission of the publisher.

Chapter 4. Reprinted from Francis Mugavero, "Sexuality—God's Gift: A Pastoral Letter," *Catholic Mind* (May 1976): 53–59. Reprinted with permission of America Press, Inc. Copyright © 1976. All rights reserved.

Chapter 5. Reprinted from A. L. Descamps, "The New Testament Doctrine on Marriage," in *Contemporary Perspectives on Christian Marriage: Proposition and Papers from the Theological Commission*, ed. Richard Malone and John R. Connery, (Chicago: Loyola University Press, 1984) 217–72.

Chapter 6. Reprinted from Edward Schillebeeckx, O.P., "The New Testament Teaching on Marriage," in *Marriage: Human Reality and Saving Mystery* (London: Sheed and Ward, 1965), 107–40. Reprinted by permission of Sheed and Ward, an Apostolate of the Priests of the Sacred Heart.

Chapter 7. Reprinted from Theodore Mackin, "Augustine on the Nature of Marriage," in *What Is Marriage?* (New York: Paulist Press, 1982), 127–44. Copyright © 1982 by Theodore Mackin. Reprinted by permission of Paulist Press.

Chapter 8. Reprinted from Lisa Sowle Cahill, "Sex, Marriage, and Family in Christian Tradition," in *Sex, Gender and Christian Ethics* (Cambridge: Cambridge University Press, 1996), 166–216. Reprinted with the permission of Cambridge University Press.

Chapter 9. Reprinted from Carolyn Osiek, R.S.C.J., "The Family in Early Christianity: 'Family Values' Revisited," *Catholic Biblical Quarterly* 58, no. 1 (January 1996): 1–24. Reprinted with permission of *Catholic Biblical Quarterly*.

Chapter 10. Reprinted from H. J. Selderhuis, "The Theory and Practice of Marriage on the Eve of the Reformation," in *Marriage and Divorce in the Thought of Martin Bucer*, trans. John Vriend and Lyle D. Bierma (Kirksville, Mo.: Thomas Jefferson Press, Truman State University), 9–31. Copyright © 1999 Truman State University Press. Reprinted with the permission of Thomas Jefferson Press; permission conveyed through Copyright Clearance Center.

Chapter 11. Reprinted from Joseph Martos, "From Secular to Ecclesiastical Marriage," in *Doors to the Sacred: A Historical Introduction to Sacraments in the Catholic Church*, expanded edition (Liguori, Mo.: Triumph Books, 1991), 360–73. Copyright © 1991 Ligouri Publications, Ligouri, Mo.

Chapter 12. Reprinted from *Gaudium et Spes*, nn. 47–52, *Decrees of the Ecumenical Councils*, vol. 2, *Trent to Vatican II*, ed. Norman P. Tanner, S.J. (Washington, D.C.: Georgetown University Press, 1990). Reprinted with permission of Libereria Editrice Vaticana, 00120 Città del Vaticano.

Chapter 13. Reprinted from Pope John Paul II, *Familiaris Consortio*, nn. 11–72 (Vatican Polygot Press, 1981). Reprinted with permission of Libereria Editrice Vaticana, 00120 Città del Vaticano.

Chapter 14. Reprinted from Francis Schüssler Fiorenza, "Marriage," in *Systematic Theology: Roman Catholic Perspectives*, vol. 2, ed. Francis Schüssler Fiorenza and John P. Calvin (Minneapolis: Fortress Press, 1991), 307–47. Copyright © 1991 Augsburg Fortress.

Chapter 15. Reprinted from Walter Kasper, "The Sacramental Dignity of Marriage," in *Theology of Christian Marriage* (London: Burns and Oates, 1980), 25–44. Reprinted by permission of Burns and Oates.

Chapter 16. Reprinted from Karl Rahner, S.J., "Marriage as a Sacrament," in *Theological Investigations*, vol. 10, trans. David Bourke (New York: Herder and Herder, 1973), 199–221.

Chapter 17. Reprinted from Edouord Hamel, S.J., "The Indissolubility of Completed Marriage: Theological, Historical, and Pastoral Reflections," in *Contemporary Perspectives on Christian Marriage: Propositions and Papers from the Theological Commission*, ed. Richard Malone and John R. Connery (Chicago: Loyola University Press, 1984), 181–203.

Chapter 18. Reprinted from Richard A. McCormick, "Divorce, Remarriage, and the Sacraments," in *The Critical Calling: Reflections on Moral Dilemmas since Vatican II* (Washington, D.C.: Georgetown University Press, 1989), 233–53. Used by permission of the publisher.

Chapter 19. Reprinted from Kenneth R. Himes, O.F.M., and James A. Coriden, "Pastoral Care of the Divorced and Remarried," *Theological Studies* 57, no. 1 (1996): 97–123. Copyright © 1996 by *Theological Studies*. Reprinted with permission of the publisher; permission conveyed through Copyright Clearance Center.

Chapter 20. Reprinted from John T. Noonan, "Contraception: The Doctrine and the Context," in *Contraception: A History of Its Treatment by the Catholic Theologians and Canonists*, enlarged edition (Cambridge: Belknap Press of Harvard University Press, 1986), 477–533. Copyright © 1965, 1986 by the President and Fellows of Harvard College. Reprinted by permission of the publishers.

Chapter 21. Reprinted from Pope Paul VI, *Humanae Vitae* (Vatican Polygot Press, 1930). Reprinted with permission of Libereria Editrice Vaticana, 00120 Città del Vaticano.

Chapter 22. Reprinted from Richard A. McCormick, "*Humanae Vitae* 25 Years Later," *America*, 17 July 1993, 6–12. Copyright © 1993 by America Press, Inc. All rights reserved. Used with permission.

Chapter 23. Reprinted from Janet E. Smith, "Some Theological Considerations on *Humanae Vitae*," in *Humanae Vitae: A Generation Later* (Washington, D.C.: Catholic University of America Press, 1991), 129–60. Reprinted by permission of the publisher.